HYPERTENSION IN THE ELDERLY

CLINICAL HYPERTENSION
AND VASCULAR DISEASES

WILLIAM B. WHITE, MD
SERIES EDITOR

HYPERTENSION IN THE ELDERLY

Edited by

L. MICHAEL PRISANT, MD

Medical College of Georgia, Augusta, GA

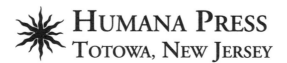

HUMANA PRESS
TOTOWA, NEW JERSEY

© 2005 Humana Press Inc.
999 Riverview Drive, Suite 208
Totowa, New Jersey 07512

humanapress.com

For additional copies, pricing for bulk purchases, and/or information about other Humana titles, contact
Humana at the above address or at any of the following numbers: Tel.: 973-256-1699; Fax: 973-256-8341;
E-mail: orders@humanapr.com; or visit our Website: www.humanapress.com

Production Editor: Robin B. Weisberg
Cover design by Patricia F. Cleary

This publication is printed on acid-free paper. ∞
ANSI Z39.48-1984 (American National Standards Institute) Permanence of Paper for Printed Library Materials.

Printed in the United States of America. 10 9 8 7 6 5 4 3 2 1
eISBN: 1-59259-911-7

Library of Congress Cataloging-in-Publication Data
Hypertension in the elderly / edited by Michael L. Prisant.
    p. ; cm. -- (Clinical hypertension and vascular diseases)
Includes bibliographical references and index.
ISBN 1-58829-197-9 (alk. paper)
1. Hypertension in old age.
[DNLM: 1. Hypertension--drug therapy--Aged. 2. Hypertension--etiology--Aged.
3. Antihypertensive Agents--therapeutic use--Aged. 4. Clinical Trials--Aged.
WG 340 H99517 2005] I. Prisant, Michael L. II. Series.
RC685.H8H7872 2005
618.97'6132--dc22

                                                                                    2004019019

DEDICATION

With love to my wife,
Rose Corinth Trincher, MD

ACKNOWLEDGMENT

Without my mentor, Dr. Albert A. Carr, there would be no book, research, publications, teaching skills, or cognitive patient care. I was fortunate to have him as my friend and teacher.

In Memoriam

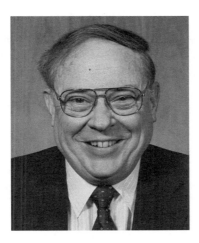

In memory of Dr. Ray W. Gifford, 1923–2004

Dr. Gifford was the former chairman of the Department of Hypertension and Renal Disease at The Cleveland Clinic and a renowned clinician, pioneering researcher, leader of medical professional societies, and internationally recognized expert on the nature and treatment of hypertension, nephrology, and cardiovascular disease. As a researcher, Dr. Gifford investigated the causes and treatments of hypertension. As chairman and a member of the Joint National Committee on Detection, Evaluation and Treatment of Hypertension, he coordinated and produced standards for medical professionals across America in the diagnosis and treatment of hypertension and related disorders.

While Dr. Gifford was chairman of Hypertension and Renal Disease, he linked the Clinic's strong research programs in the humoral, hemodynamic, and neurologic aspects of hypertension, with clinical programs that focused on treatment options and their benefits, as well as patient and physician education. The author of more than 460 scientific papers, and the textbook *Pheochromocytoma* (with William M. Manger, MD), Dr. Gifford performed long-term studies of patients with hypertension, evaluated medications and surgical treatments for hypertension, contributed to knowledge of arteriosclerosis and aneurysms, Raynaud's disease, renal artery disease, renal transplantation, the effect of hypertension on the extremities, and the effects of dietary sodium, among many other subjects.

Dr. Gifford enjoyed great rapport with his patients and was beloved by a large and loyal practice. Although he attempted to retire from the Clinic in 1993, strong demand from his patients brought him back to active practice until 1999. His influence on the discipline of hypertension will be felt for many years. He will missed by his family and colleagues.

SERIES EDITOR'S INTRODUCTION

The importance of treating hypertension in the elderly has been greatly appreciated by physicians and scientists since the results of the Medical Research Council studies of the 1970s and the isolated systolic hypertension trials SHEP and Syst-Eur that followed in the 1980s and 1990s. Despite this appreciation of the severity of the complications of this common disorder during advancing age, treatment rates to control blood pressure in elderly patients with hypertension have been quite low. Dr. Prisant's volume on *Hypertension in the Elderly* is therefore a most clinically relevant contribution in the area of management of hypertension in older people. This book brings together the basic pathophysiological, epidemiological, diagnostic, and therapeutic advances in the evaluation of high blood pressure in this population.

The editor, Dr. Prisant, has astutely organized this volume into sections that cover age-related changes in the cardiovascular system including the development of reductions in arterial compliance, overviews of the epidemiology of hypertension in the older patient, clinical evaluation that covers a variety of topics such as blood pressure measurement and hypertensive complications characteristic of the older patient, and nonpharmacological and pharmacological approaches to the treatment of hypertension in the elderly.

Substantial coverage has been appropriately given to the impact of pharmacological treatments based on clinical trials in the elderly in Chapters 15 through 20. There are also a few chapters devoted to special patient populations that highlight problems of particular concern in older patients, including cerebrovascular disease, diabetes mellitus, heart failure, and chronic arthritis. These sections contribute to the novelty of this book because they are grounded in clinical investigations that have led to enhanced understanding of the management of hypertension during advancing age. The complications of hypertension in older patients are complex, clinically challenging, and have led to much improved therapies targeted towards disease regression or prevention, as outlined in Chapters 12–14, and 22.

The chapters in *Hypertension in the Elderly* have been written by a number of well-known, expert authors who have provided comprehensive, scientifically sound, and clinically appropriate information. As series editor of *Clinical Hypertension and Vascular Diseases*, I am pleased by the publication of this timely, well-organized book and know that *Hypertension in the Elderly* will become a highly utilized textbook for all specialists in cardiovascular and geriatric medicine as well as all physicians who take care of older adults.

William B. White, MD
Professor of Medicine and Chief
Division of Hypertension and Clinical Pharmacology
Pat and Jim Calhoun Cardiology Center
University of Connecticut School of Medicine
Farmington, CT

PREFACE

Hypertension in the Elderly attempts to focus attention on the group of hypertensive patients with the largest body of outcomes trial data, but the poorest blood pressure control. Research data continue to recognize the importance of hypertension for contributing to both the morbidity and mortality of older patients. The outcomes trials document the benefits of blood pressure treatment in reducing the rate of myocardial infarction, heart failure, and stroke.

The organization of *Hypertension in the Elderly* is separated into basic concepts, epidemiology and trials, evaluation and management, pharmacologic treatment, special populations, and adherence. The contributors have provided detailed current information that is useful for the management of patients. Several chapters are state-of-the-art reviews that integrate a large body of information.

The four chapters in Part I impart to the reader an important overview. The late Dr. Gifford and I underscore the importance and the challenge of treating elderly hypertensive patients. As emphasized, most elderly hypertensives in the United States and in the world are not getting the maximum benefit from antihypertensive medications. Drs. Webb and Inscho describe the physiology of the age-related changes of the cardio-renal system, and Dr. Izzo applies that information to give insight into the mechanisms of hypertension in the elderly. Age-related changes in vascular stiffness are a central factor of hypertension and target organ damage. Finally, Dr. Sica describes the pharmacological and pharmaco-dynamic changes in older patients that influence how drugs are handled. There is merit in the clinical maxim of drug therapy in the elderly "to start low and go slow."

Part II covers the epidemiology and trials of older patients. It is appropriate that Drs. Kannel and Wilson should remind us of the Framingham Heart Study experience. The Framingham Heart Study has always maintained the importance of systolic blood pressure as a risk factor for cardiovascular disease, a finding that has been rediscovered over the last 10 yr. Dr. Harrell and I methodically review the lifestyle trials in older patients. Except for TONE, most of these trials are small; thus, more work needs to be done. These data document that nonpharmacologic therapy can decrease the need for drug therapy. Finally, I review the hypertension outcomes trials that were conducted in older persons. Except for ALLHAT, I have included only trials that were conducted on elderly hypertensive patients. It is my opinion that the double-blind trials provide the best data for decision making.

Part III is an ambitious section covering blood pressure measurement, clinical evaluation, secondary hypertension, and target organ damage. Drs. Arias-Vera and White correctly point out that blood pressure determination is one of the most important parts of the clinical evaluation of an older patient. Therefore, the physician must make every effort to measure blood pressure accurately. Dr. Jackson and I provide a practical approach for evaluating the elderly hypertensive patient. Dr. Isales reports that most endocrine causes of secondary hypertension in elderly are rare, except for thyroid disease; however, he provides a useful clinical approach for evaluation. Drs. Vongpatanasin and Victor provide a thoughtful approach to both renovascular hypertension and hypertensive renal disease. Drs. Landolfo, Thornton, Robinson, and I reviewed the heart failure trials in elderly patients and have concluded that our knowledge base is limited. Indeed, about 50% of elderly patients with heart failure have a preserved ejection fraction, for which there are scanty outcomes trials. Dr. Houghton emphasizes a comprehensive approach to risk factors in hypertensive patients with and without ischemic heart disease. Finally, Dr. Nichols examines the relationship of hypertension and various cerebrovascular events. His discussion of dementia and hypertension highlights the complexity of the relationship.

Part IV covers pharmacological therapy. The role of individual drug classes, including diuretics and β-blockers (Dr. Cushman), angiotensin-converting enzyme inhibitors (Dr. Sica), angiotensin receptor blockers (my assignment), calcium antagonists (Drs. White and Thavarajah), and α_1-blockers (Dr. Pool) are described, as is how they should be used to treat the elderly hypertensive. Dr. Mulloy and I reviewed the sparse individual trials of combination drug therapy in the elderly hypertensive patients and concluded that combination drug therapy achieves a higher control rate.

Part V focuses on special populations, including African-Americans, patients with diabetes, and patients with arthritis. Drs. Johnson and Saunders support a more culturally sensitive approach to treating older African-Americans. Various drug classes are evaluated. The use of the treatment algorithm of the International Society for Hypertension on Blacks is highlighted. Dr. Sowers and I cover the elderly diabetic hypertensive. This group will enlarge and require multiple drugs to achieve blood pressure, glucose, lipid, and antiplatelet control. Drs. Thavarajah and White address a topic that plagues thoughtful physicians and hypertensionologists—arthritis pain control vs blood pressure control. Clearly, we need antiarthritics that do not impair blood pressure control when acetaminophen and salicylate fail. Chronic requirements for these anti-inflammatory agents may necessitate a change in the class of anti-hypertensive agent or an up titration of current antihypertensive agents to prevent clinically significant untoward effects.

Part VI addresses adherence. Drs. Egan and Okonofua speak to the clinician's role in improving therapeutic adherence and blood pressure control in older hypertensive patients. The behavioral science of this topic is a neglected area in the training of most health care providers.

I am grateful to the individual authors who have contributed their expertise and time to *Hypertension in the Elderly* with their outstanding manuscripts. I would also like to acknowledge others who have influenced the content of this book in various ways: Drs. George Bakris, Henry Black, Bill Elliott, Bill Frishman, Tom Giles, Marvin Moser, Suzanne Oparil, Donald Vidt, Michael Weber, and many others. However, without my mentor Dr. Albert A. Carr, there would be no book. Humana Press was kind enough to provide the opportunity to work on this book as one of series in the field of hypertension.

I offer my first book, *Hypertension in the Elderly*, to the reader with some trepidation. As with any new undertaking, the feedback of the readers will improve further editions. Thus, I ask readers to forward to me your comments for any additions, omissions, or errors.

L. Michael Prisant, MD

CONTENTS

PART III: EVALUATION AND MANAGEMENT

PART IV: PHARMACOLOGICAL MANAGEMENT

CONTRIBUTORS

JOSE RAMIRO ARIAS-VERA, MD • *Rhode Island Department of Corrections, Warwick, RI*

WILLIAM C. CUSHMAN, MD • *Department of Preventive Medicine and Medicine, University of Tennessee College of Medicine and Preventive Medicine Section, Veterans Affairs Medical Center, Memphis, TN*

BRENT M. EGAN, MD • *Department of Medicine and Pharmacology, Medical University of South Carolina, Charleston, SC*

RAY W. GIFFORD, JR., MD • *Department of Nephrology and Hypertension, Cleveland Clinic Foundation, Cleveland, OH*

DEAN U. HARRELL, MD • *Senior Health Center, Department of Medicine, Medical College of Georgia, Augusta, GA*

JAN LAWS HOUGHTON, MD • *Division of Cardiology, Albany Medical College, Albany, NY*

EDWARD W. INSCHO, PhD • *Department of Physiology, Medical College of Georgia, Augusta, GA*

CARLOS M. ISALES, MD, FACP • *Department of Medicine, Institute of Molecular Medicine and Genetics, Medical College of Georgia, Augusta, GA*

JOSEPH L. IZZO, JR., MD • *Division of Clinical Pharmacology, School of Medicine and Biomedical Sciences, State University of New York at Buffalo, Buffalo, NY*

THOMAS W. JACKSON, MD • *Senior Health Center, Department of Medicine, Medical College of Georgia, Augusta, GA*

WALLACE R. JOHNSON, JR., MD • *Section of Hypertension, University of Maryland School of Medicine, Baltimore, MD*

WILLIAM B. KANNEL, MD, MPH • *Department of Medicine and Public Health, Boston University School of Medicine; Framingham Heart Study, Framingham, MA*

CAROLYN LANDOLFO, MD, FACC • *Section of Cardiology, Department of Medicine, Medical College of Georgia, Augusta, GA*

LAURA LYNGBY MULLOY, DO, FACP • *Section of Nephrology, Hypertension, and Transplantation, Department of Medicine, Medical College of Georgia, Augusta, GA*

FENWICK T. NICHOLS III, MD, FACP • *Department of Neurology, Medical College of Georgia, Augusta, GA*

ENI C. OKONOFUA, MD • *Department of Medicine, Medical University of South Carolina, Charleston, SC*

JAMES L. POOL, MD • *Departments of Medicine and Pharmacology, Baylor College of Medicine, Houston, TX*

L. MICHAEL PRISANT, MD, FACC, FACP, FAHA • *Hypertension and Clinical Pharmacology, Department of Medicine, Medical College of Georgia, Augusta, GA*

VINCENT J. B. ROBINSON, MBBS, FACC • *Section of Cardiology, Department of Medicine, Medical College of Georgia, Augusta, GA*

ELIJAH SAUNDERS, MD • *Section of Hypertension, University of Maryland School of Medicine, Baltimore, MD*

DOMENIC A. SICA, MD • *Section of Clinical Pharmacology and Hypertension, Division of Nephrology, Medical College of Virginia of Virginia Commonwealth University, Richmond, VA*

JAMES R. SOWERS, MD, FACE, FACP, FAHA • *Department of Internal Medicine, University of Missouri Health Care, Columbia, MO*

SUMESKA THAVARAJAH, MD • *Department of Nephrology, John Hopkins School of Medicine. Baltimore, MD*

JOHN THORNTON, MD, FACC • *Section of Cardiology, Department of Medicine, Medical College of Georgia, Augusta, GA*

RONALD G. VICTOR, MD • *Hypertension Division, University of Texas Southwestern Medical Center, Dallas, TX*

WANPEN VONGPATANASIN, MD • *Divisions of Hypertension and Cardiology, University of Texas Southwestern Medical Center, Dallas, TX*

R. CLINTON WEBB, PhD • *Department of Physiology, Medical College of Georgia, Augusta, GA*

PETER W. F. WILSON, MD • *Department of Endocrinology, Diabetes, and Medical Genetics, General Clinical Research Center, Medical University of South Carolina, Charleston, SC*

WILLIAM B. WHITE, MD • *Section of Hypertension and Clinical Pharmacology, University of Connecticut School of Medicine, Farmington, CT*

1

The Importance of Hypertension in the Geriatric Population

Ray W. Gifford, Jr., MD and L. Michael Prisant, MD, FACC, FACP

THE PROBLEM

A 50% increase in the 1995 US population size by the year 2050 has been projected *(1)*. Although 12.5% of the population was 65 years or older in 1990, it is estimated the percentage will increase to 20% by 2050 (Fig. 1). The number of elderly will increase from 39 million in 2010 to 69 million by 2030 *(1)*. The projected population growth of older patients will certainly increase the prevalence of hypertension in the elderly, which accounts for two-thirds of the elderly population *(2)*. The prevalence of hypertension has increased since 1988 (Fig. 2) *(3)*.

It is unfortunate, but true, that elderly people have a disproportionate share of hypertension in this country (Fig. 3) and in the other industrialized countries of the world *(4)*. The increase in systolic blood pressure (SBP) with aging is so conspicuous and consistent that it is sometimes mistaken as a normal phenomenon and is not treated (Fig. 4).

In medical school, we were taught that isolated systolic hypertension should not be treated. A normal SBP was 100 mmHg plus the person's

From: *Clinical Hypertension and Vascular Diseases: Hypertension in the Elderly*
Edited by: L. M. Prisant © Humana Press Inc., Totowa, NJ

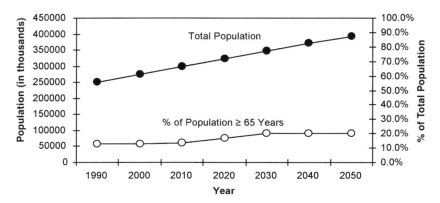

Fig. 1. Population projections in the United States. (Data derived from ref. *1*.)

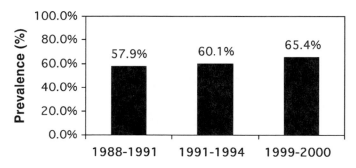

Fig. 2. Prevalence of hypertension for persons 60 years or older in the United States, 1988–2000. The change of 7.5% from 1988 to 2000 was highly significant (*p* = 0.002). (Data derived from ref. *3*.)

age. Prevailing opinion at that time held that diastolic blood pressure (DBP) was the culprit causing the organ damage frequently associated with high blood pressure. Now, it is widely recognized that SBP is more important than DBP in determining cardiovascular and renal complications of hypertension. In contrast to young patients, 80% of elderly patients have isolated systolic hypertension *(5)*.

After analyzing data from the National Health and Nutrition Examination Survey, Hyman and Pavlik *(6)* concluded that most cases of uncontrolled hypertension in the United States consisted of mild isolated systolic hypertension in older adults, most of whom have access to health care and relatively frequent contact with physicians (Fig. 5). In an accompanying editorial, Chobanian stated that "despite very effective antihypertensive therapies and data from clinical trials demonstrating that lowering

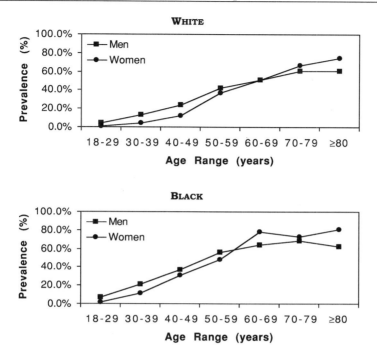

Fig. 3. Prevalence of hypertension in the United States by age, gender, and race. (Data from ref. *4*.)

blood pressure reduces cardiovascular and renal complications, more than one-fourth of the estimated 42 million people with hypertension in the United States remain unaware that they have the disorder, and approximately three-fourths of those with known hypertension have blood pressure that exceeds recommended levels" *(7)*.

THE TRIALS

It has been more than 12 years since Applegate *(8)* advised physicians that drug treatment of isolated systolic hypertension or predominant systolic hypertension reduced cardiovascular morbidity; this advice was based on the results of the Systolic Hypertension in the Elderly Program trial *(9)* and the Medical Research Council's Trial on Hypertension in the Elderly *(10)*. Because many physicians apparently have been reluctant to treat isolated systolic hypertension in elderly patients (Fig. 5), the Coordinating Committee of the National High Blood Pressure Education Program issued a clinical advisory statement, "Importance of Sys-

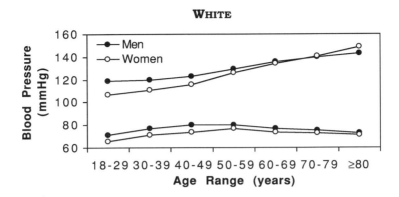

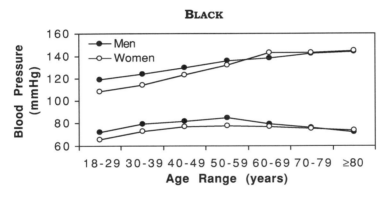

Fig. 4. Mean systolic and diastolic blood pressure by age, race, and gender in the United States. (Data from ref. *4*.)

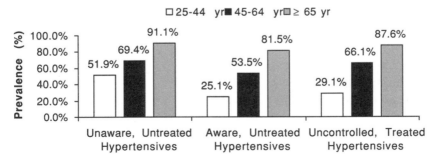

Fig. 5. Prevalence of uncontrolled isolated systolic hypertension according to age. Isolated systolic hypertension is defined as diastolic blood pressure less than 90 mmHg and systolic blood pressure 140 mmHg or greater. (Data derived from ref. *6*.)

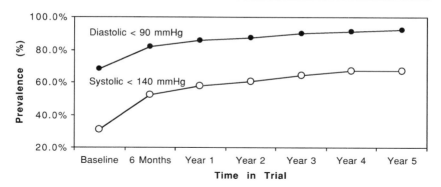

Fig. 6. Blood pressure control in the Antihypertensive and Lipid-Lowering Treatment to Prevent Heart Attack Trial (ALLHAT). Systolic and diastolic blood pressure were controlled, respectively, in 67 and 92% of participants. (Data derived from ref. *17.*)

tolic Blood Pressure in Older Americans" *(11)*. This report emphasized the importance of controlling systolic as well as diastolic hypertension, especially in elderly patients.

Evidence from controlled clinical trials showed reduced cardiovascular and renal events in elderly patients treated to recommended goal SBP and DBP *(9,10,12–15)*. The recently published results of the Antihypertensive Lipid-Lowering Heart Attack Trial may change physicians' attitudes about treating hypertension in the elderly *(15)*. There were 42,448 participants, of which 80.9% were 60 years or older and 35.3% were 70 years or older *(16)*. The study was conducted by physicians in their own offices with their own hypertensive patients. After an average of 4.9 years, blood pressure was reduced from an average of 146/84 to 134/75 mmHg, and more than 60% achieved goal blood pressure of less than 140/90 mmHg (Fig. 6) *(17)*, which is decidedly better than 27.4% reported recently (Fig. 7) *(3)*.

THE GOALS

If these community physicians can get blood pressure to goal in more than 60% of elderly hypertensive patients, why can't the rest of us? The answer is that it often requires two or more medications to control hypertension in elderly patients *(18)*, one of the important messages of the most recent Joint National Committee's report *(19)*.

Unfortunately, hypertension tends to beget hypertension. High normal SBP (i.e., 130–140 mmHg) pounding at the aorta with each heartbeat, year after year, damages elastic tissue in the aorta and its large

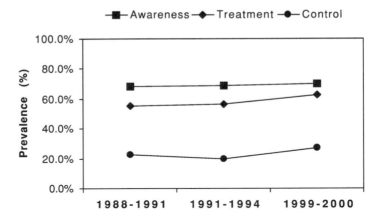

Fig. 7. Awareness, treatment, and control among persons 60 years or older in the United States, 1988–2000. Although there was no improvement in awareness of hypertension from 1988 to 2000, there has been a 7.6% improvement in treatment ($p = 0.006$) and a 4.9% improvement in control of all hypertensives ($p = 0.02$). (Data derived from ref. *3.*)

branches, reducing aortic and arterial compliance. Hence, SBP tends to rise with age in the United States and other acculturated societies. Regrettably, most elderly hypertensives in this country and in the world are not getting the maximum benefit from antihypertensive medications.

ACKNOWLEDGMENT

Sandra Bronoff provided helpful comments for the revision of this chapter.

REFERENCES

1. Day JC. Population Projections of the United States by Age, Sex, Race, and Hispanic Origin: 1995 to 2050. Washington, DC: US Government Printing Office; 1996. US Bureau of Census, Current Population Reports P25-1130.
2. The sixth report of the Joint National Committee on prevention, detection, evaluation, and treatment of high blood pressure. *Arch Intern Med* 1997;157:2413–2446.
3. Hajjar I, Kotchen TA. Trends in prevalence, awareness, treatment, and control of hypertension in the United States, 1988–2000. *JAMA* 2003;290:199–206.
4. Burt VL, Whelton P, Roccella EJ, et al. Prevalence of hypertension in the US adult population. Results from the Third National Health and Nutrition Examination Survey, 1988–1991. *Hypertension* 1995;25:305–313.
5. Franklin SS, Jacobs MJ, Wong ND, L'Italien GJ, Lapuerta P. Predominance of isolated systolic hypertension among middle-aged and elderly US hypertensives: analysis based on National Health and Nutrition Examination Survey (NHANES) III. *Hypertension* 2001;37:869–874.

6. Hyman DJ, Pavlik VN. Characteristics of patients with uncontrolled hypertension in the United States. *N Engl J Med* 2001;345:479–486.
7. Chobanian AV. Control of hypertension—an important national priority. *N Engl J Med* 2001;345:534–535.
8. Applegate WB. The relative importance of focusing on elevations of systolic vs diastolic blood pressure. A definitive answer at last. *Arch Intern Med* 1992;152: 1969–1971.
9. Prevention of stroke by antihypertensive drug treatment in older persons with isolated systolic hypertension. Final results of the Systolic Hypertension in the Elderly Program (SHEP). SHEP Cooperative Research Group. *JAMA* 1991;265:3255–3264.
10. Medical Research Council trial of treatment of hypertension in older adults: principal results. MRC Working Party. *BMJ* 1992;304:405–412.
11. Izzo JL Jr, Levy D, Black HR. Clinical Advisory Statement. Importance of systolic blood pressure in older Americans. *Hypertension* 2000;35:1021–1024.
12. Mulrow CD, Cornell JA, Herrera CR, Kadri A, Farnett L, Aguilar C. Hypertension in the elderly. Implications and generalizability of randomized trials. *JAMA* 1994;272:1932–1938.
13. Liu L, Wang JG, Gong L, Liu G, Staessen JA. Comparison of active treatment and placebo in older Chinese patients with isolated systolic hypertension. Systolic Hypertension in China (Syst-China) Collaborative Group. *J Hypertens* 1998;16(12 Pt 1):1823–1829.
14. Staessen JA, Fagard R, Thijs L, et al. Randomised double-blind comparison of placebo and active treatment for older patients with isolated systolic hypertension. The Systolic Hypertension in Europe (Syst-Eur) Trial Investigators. *Lancet* 1997;350:757–764.
15. Major outcomes in high-risk hypertensive patients randomized to angiotensin-converting enzyme inhibitor or calcium channel blocker vs diuretic: the Antihypertensive and Lipid-Lowering Treatment to Prevent Heart Attack Trial (ALLHAT). *JAMA* 2002;288:2981–2997.
16. Grimm RH Jr, Margolis KL, Papademetriou VV, et al. Baseline characteristics of participants in the Antihypertensive and Lipid Lowering Treatment to Prevent Heart Attack Trial (ALLHAT). *Hypertension* 2001;37:19–27.
17. Cushman WC, Ford CE, Cutler JA, et al. Success and predictors of blood pressure control in diverse North American settings: the Antihypertensive and Lipid-Lowering treatment to prevent Heart Attack Trial (ALLHAT). *J Clin Hypertens (Greenwich)* 2002;4:393–404.
18. Prisant LM, Moser M. Hypertension in the elderly: can we improve results of therapy? *Arch Intern Med* 2000;160:283–289.
19. Chobanian AV, Bakris GL, Black HR, et al. The Seventh Report of the Joint National Committee on Prevention, Detection, Evaluation, and Treatment of High Blood Pressure: the JNC 7 report. *JAMA* 2003;289:2560–2572.

2

Age-Related Changes in the Cardiovascular System

R. Clinton Webb, PhD and Edward W. Inscho, PhD

INTRODUCTION

According to the US Census Bureau, the proportion of people in the United States over the age of 65 years is increasing. Current estimates indicate that approximately 30 to 35 million people are 65 years of age or older. In the year 2030, it is estimated that there will be approximately 55 to 60 million people in this age category. This aspect of our population has an important impact on the understanding of cardiovascular disease (CVD) because it is known that advancing age confers the major risk. The incidence and prevalence of CVD increases dramatically with advancing age in both men and women.

Aging is a complicated event, and most individuals consider the process a loss in general function that impairs ability. Epidemiological studies have demonstrated that the process of aging is the major risk factor

From: *Clinical Hypertension and Vascular Diseases: Hypertension in the Elderly*
Edited by: L. M. Prisant © Humana Press Inc., Totowa, NJ

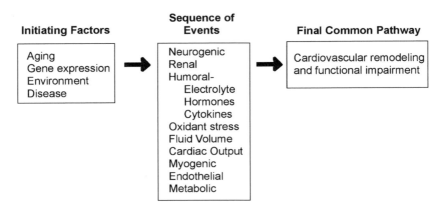

Fig. 1. Mechanisms of cardiovascular changes in aging. Aging is an independent risk factor for cardiovascular disease. The effects of aging are diverse and can be identified at the molecular, cellular, tissue, organ, and system levels as contributing to the altered function of the intact organism. The effects of aging act with other variables (initiating factors), such as gene expression, environment, and disease, to alter various organ systems. With respect to cardiovascular remodeling and impaired function in older individuals (final common pathway), it is known that the changes are modulated by other systems in the body (sequence of events).

for cardiovascular impairment (Fig. 1). The reason for this dominance is that aging occurs while an individual is responding to various stressors by changing patterns of gene expression (genetic traits) on a background of environmental factors and disease states.

The effects of aging are diverse and can be identified at the molecular, cellular, tissue, organ, and system levels as contributing to the altered function of the intact organism. With respect to the cardiovascular system (Fig. 1), it is known that the changes that occur with age are modulated by other systems in the body. For example, functional changes in the autonomic nervous system during aging affect the overall function of the cardiovascular system owing to the fact that the latter is controlled in large part by the former. Another example is that changes in the endocrine system can have an important impact on cardiovascular function. Testosterone levels decrease with age, and it is known that this hormone alters the distribution of contractile proteins in the heart. It should also be recognized that age-related changes in the cardiovascular system differ in male and female subjects.

This brief review summarizes several aspects of cardiovascular aging. The goal is to separate those changes in the heart and vasculature associated with aging in healthy individuals from those associated with disease

processes. Clearly, it is nearly impossible to dissociate all the components of aging from those that are characteristic of disease processes.
Aging of the cardiovascular system is the platform from which CVDs are
launched. Thus, the reader is directed to other reviews of these topics for
a more complete treatment of the subject (*see* refs. *1–16*). Other chapters
within this volume also address adaptive and pathological changes in the
cardiovascular system brought on by disease.

AGE-RELATED CHANGES IN VASCULAR FUNCTION

Increased Wall Thickening and Arterial Stiffening

Extensive evidence has demonstrated that wall thickening and dilation are the major structural changes that occur in the large elastic arteries during aging (Fig. 2; *see* refs. *1, 4, 7,* and *14* for review). The wall
thickening involves both the tunica intima and the tunica media. As a
consequence of this remodeling, there is a reduction in arterial compliance with an increase in vessel stiffness. Increased pulse wave velocity
reflects this vascular stiffening because it is determined by the intrinsic
stress/strain relationship of the vascular wall and by the mean arterial
pressure.

Factors that contribute to the increased wall thickening and stiffening
in aging include increased collagen, reduced elastin, and calcification.
The amount of extracellular matrix increases and becomes particularly
rich in glucosaminoglycans. These changes should not be considered
"atherosclerotic" even though the factors are associated with this disease
process (*17*). Age-dependent thickening of the arteries occurs in the
absence of atherosclerosis and with aging in nonhuman primates and
rodents. Thus, aging of the arteries is likely an adaptive mechanism to
maintain conditions of blood flow and wall tension.

When the large arteries become stiffer, there is an increase in systolic
arterial pressure, a decrease in diastolic pressure, and a widening of the
pulse pressure (*see* ref. *1* for review). This pattern of changes in the
vasculature with respect to indices of blood pressure is much different
from that seen in hypertension, for which there is an increase in total
peripheral resistance. An increase in total peripheral resistance tends to
increase both systolic and arterial pressure to a similar degree.

Endothelial Dysfunction

A portion of the stiffening of large arteries during the aging process
can be attributed to a reduction in endothelial function, which normally
opposes contraction of the underlying vascular smooth muscle (*5,18–
23*). The principle finding is that with aging there is a reduction in the

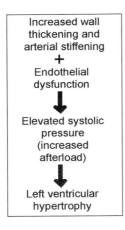 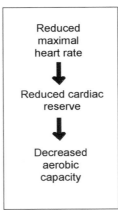 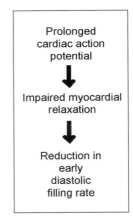

Fig. 2. Age-related changes in the cardiovascular system. The major age-related changes in the cardiovascular system are (a) arterial stiffening; (b) endothelial dysfunction, which promotes vasoconstriction; (c) elevated systolic blood pressure and increased pulse pressure; (d) increased left ventricular wall thickness; (e) reduced early diastolic filling of the ventricles; (f) impaired cardiac reserve; (g) alterations in heart rate rhythm; (h) prolonged cardiac action potential; and (i) a decline in renal function that contributes to improper maintenance of extracellular fluid volume and composition. These age-associated changes in cardiovascular function contribute to morbidity and mortality brought about by various disease states (i.e., hypertension, atherosclerosis, heart failure, etc.).

amount of nitric oxide (NO) produced by the endothelial cells. NO is produced from L-arginine by endothelial nitric oxide synthase (eNOS). This enzyme is constitutively active and regulated by the intracellular concentration of calcium (Ca^{2+}). eNOS is inhibited competitively by analogs of L-arginine such as $N\omega$-nitro-L-arginine. Asymmetric dimethylarginine, an endogenous inhibitor of eNOS, is increased in older individuals and may therefore serve as an additional mechanism to lower NO production by the endothelium *(19)*.

In addition to a reduction in the production of NO by the endothelial cells, it has been demonstrated that the bioavailability of NO is reduced with aging *(5)*. This reduction is thought to be mainly the result of an increase in oxidative stress during aging. Presumably, superoxide anion quenches endothelium-derived NO through a chemical reaction to form peroxynitrite *(5,15,22)*. Thus, vasoconstriction is promoted because the dilator activity of NO is removed. However, this is not the only mechanism by which superoxide acts because it is known to cause contraction of vascular smooth muscle in the absence of the endothelium or in the presence of inhibitors of nitric oxide synthase.

Once produced, endothelium-derived NO diffuses to the smooth muscle cells. NO binds to smooth muscle cell-soluble guanylate cyclase, leading to an increase in cyclic guanosine 3'5' monophosphate (cGMP) and the subsequent activation of cGMP-dependent protein kinase. NO/cGMP/cGMP-dependent protein kinase signaling has been proposed to decrease intracellular Ca^{2+} concentration via the inhibition of L-type Ca^{2+} channels and the activation of sarcoplasmic reticulum $Ca^{2+}G$ adenosine triphosphatases (ATPases), as well as induce cellular hyperpolarization through the activation of membrane K^+ channels. NO has other actions, such as activation of ribosyl transferases and nitration of proteins, which could also contribute to inhibitory effects and vasodilation. Reductions in many of the components of these NO-dependent cell-signaling pathways have been observed in the vasculature of aging animals and humans.

The barrier function of the endothelium also changes during the aging process *(5)*. Compared to vessels of young animals, the permeability of the endothelium is increased in older animals.

AGE-RELATED CHANGES IN CARDIAC FUNCTION

Heart Rate and Cardiac Output

Resting heart rate does not change dramatically with age (*see* ref. *2* for review). In the supine position at rest, heart rate in older men does not differ from that in younger men. In changing from the supine to the sitting position, heart rate increases; the magnitude of this change is somewhat less in older men.

During exercise, the maximal heart rate attainable is lower in older individuals than in younger individuals. This inability to raise the heart rate to high levels during exercise is reflected in lower cardiac output reserve in older subjects and contributes to declining aerobic capacity in advancing age. Other factors that contribute to the reduction in aerobic capacity in older individuals include the following: (a) an increase in body fat, (b) a reduction in muscle mass, and (c) impaired oxygen extraction.

It should also be noted that a considerable portion of the diminished hemodynamic response during vigorous exercise is related to the inability of the sympathetic nervous system to provide adequate modulation of cardiac output. As noted by Lakatta and Sollott *(4)*, the reduced β-adrenergic modulation of cardiac function is one of the best-characterized changes that occur in the cardiovascular system during aging, and it has been characterized at the molecular, cellular, organ, and system levels with integration into the intact organism.

The variability in heart rate (beat-to-beat fluctuation) declines during aging (*see* refs. *2* and *14* for review). This alteration in heart rhythm is a reflection of dysregulation of the autonomic nervous system commonly found in older individuals. Based on the accumulated evidence, it is widely believed that the dramatic change in cardiac function attributable to altered heart rhythm places the aging population at increased risk of morbidity and mortality.

Left Ventricular Wall Function

The stiffening of arteries during aging affects cardiac structure and function (*see* refs. *2* and *14* for review). As noted in the section "Increased Wall Thickening and Arterial Stiffening," systolic blood pressure increases with age. This increase in afterload contributes to a moderate increase in left ventricular mass observed in many individuals between the third and ninth decades of life. A large portion of this hypertrophy is caused by an enlargement of cardiac myocytes because of the addition of sarcomeres. There is a decrease in myocyte number in the aging myocardium, but the mechanism for this myocyte loss is unclear *(24)*.

Left ventricular filling during the early phase of diastole slows after the age of 20 years, and by the 80 years of age, the rate is approximately 50% of its peak value observed in early life (*see* refs. *2* and *14* for review). Accumulation of fibrous material in the left ventricle and slowing in Ca^{2+} activation from the preceding systole are possible mechanisms contributing to this reduced early diastolic filling rate. Regardless, adequate filling of the left ventricle occurs in late diastole because of an increase in atrial contraction. Thus, the atria are often hypertrophied in older individuals because of this augmented atrial contraction. Left ventricular systolic function is preserved during aging.

Myocardial Contraction

Contraction of the cardiac myocyte is initiated by an action potential that causes an increase in intracellular Ca^{2+} concentration to activate interaction between contractile proteins. The activator Ca^{2+} comes from several sources, including a transmembrane flux of the cation and a release from storage sites inside the cell (sarcoplasmic reticulum). During relaxation of the cardiac myocyte, the intracellular concentration of Ca^{2+} is reduced by pumping it back into the sarcoplasmic reticulum and by extrusion from the cell (sodium–calcium exchange, plasma membrane Ca^{2+} ATPase).

Excitation–contraction coupling in the cardiac myocyte changes during aging *(2,25–28)*. The action potential becomes prolonged, and the cytosolic Ca^{2+} transient after excitation is increased, leading to prolonged contraction. The prolonged action potential is caused by slower inactivation of L-type Ca^{2+} current and reduction in outwardly directed potassium currents (26,27). The prolonged Ca^{2+} transient is caused partly by a reduction in uptake of the cation by the sarcoplasmic reticulum (2). There is also an increase in the transcripts for the sodium–calcium exchanger, which serves to extrude calcium from the cell. These age-associated changes in Ca^{2+} movements impair myocardial relaxation and contribute to the aforementioned reduction in early diastolic filling rate characterizing the aging heart.

KIDNEY FUNCTION AND THE CONTROL OF EXTRACELLULAR FLUID VOLUME IN AGING

Normal aging is accompanied by alterations in many aspects of renal morphology and function in both humans and animals (29–32). Whereas the prevalence of declining renal function in aging is recognized, the mechanisms responsible for the decline remain obscure and highly controversial. Renal mass decreases by 20 to 25% between the ages of 30 and 80 years (30). Glomerular filtration rate declines by approximately 10% each decade after 30 years of age and is accompanied by an increase in renal vascular resistance and a decrease in glomerular number. The decline in glomerular filtration rate and glomerular number stimulates a compensatory increase in the size of the remaining glomeruli (30,31, 33,34). Age-related sclerosis of the remaining glomeruli, thickening of basement membrane, accumulation of extracellular matrix, expansion of the glomerular mesangium, and alteration of tubular epithelial transporters are also commonly reported (35). These factors contribute to an overall decline in glomerular filtration rate and impairment of tubular reabsorptive function that compromises the ability of the kidneys to maintain proper extracellular fluid volume and composition. This progressive loss of renal functional reserve develops over decades and may be unnoticed until the subject is faced with significant cardiovascular or extracellular fluid challenge (31). The addition of other cardiovascular risk factors, such as salt sensitivity, hypertension, and diabetes, accelerates the loss of functioning nephrons and increases the susceptibility of elderly individuals to end-stage renal injury (36).

Regulation of glomerular perfusion, glomerular capillary pressure, medullary blood flow, and renal hemodynamics all occur through adjustments in renal microvascular resistance (37). Resistance changes are controlled by intrinsic mechanisms such as autoregulation and locally released autocrine and paracrine factors as well as through extrinsic mechanisms, which include sympathetic nerves or circulating vasoactive agents *(37)*. In normal kidneys, locally produced NO, adenosine, prostaglandins, endothelin, angiotensin II, and myriad tubular and endothelial factors combine to modulate intrarenal vascular function. Studies have shown that the influence of these regulatory systems on renal vascular function is reduced in aged subjects, possibly exposing glomeruli to inappropriately high blood pressures and promoting glomerular and vascular inflammation and sclerosis *(38,39)*. Thus, age-related impairment of renal vascular control can account for some of the reduction in glomerular number and glomerular filtration rate known to define the senescent kidney.

Kidney-related volume and electrolyte disturbances also represent a significant clinical challenge in elderly individuals *(30,31,40)*. The genesis of such disturbances remains poorly understood, but includes both renal tubular and neurological mechanisms. Renal tubular function is reduced in elderly subjects, leading to a reduced ability to excrete a sodium or an acid load and a compromised ability to maintain potassium balance. As the excretory capacity of the kidney declines, the ability of the kidney to eliminate drug metabolites also declines. Accordingly, therapeutic regimens need to be adjusted to account for reduced renal clearance to prevent drug toxicity or overdose *(35)*.

Paradoxically, the aged kidney also exhibits reduced urinary-concentrating ability, leading to polyuria and reduced ability to conserve filtered sodium *(30,31,40)*. This is coupled with a reduced thirst sensation, leading to overall volume contraction and susceptibility to hyponatremia, hyperkalemia, and acidosis. Thus, cardiovascular management of elderly individuals can be complicated by conditions of volume and electrolyte overload or volume and electrolyte deficit. Diagnosis and treatment of such conditions certainly require consideration of both renal and cardiovascular issues to correct clinical and physiological abnormalities safely in elderly patients.

ETIOLOGY OF AGING
IN THE CARDIOVASCULAR SYSTEM

The mechanistic explanation for aging of the cardiovascular system is an area of intense study. Most investigators believe that aging is the result of cumulative damage brought on by a variety of insults. Oxidative stress, nonenzymatic glycation, and changes in gene expression influence aging of the cardiovascular system *(2,5,41,42)*. Thus, it is often stated that aging of the cardiovascular system resembles the morphological and biochemical changes seen in inflammation. This is reasonable because the two processes share many common features, such as alterations in reactive oxygen species and cytokine expression.

Many of the changes in the aging cardiovascular system are not fixed. Indeed, endurance training has a beneficial effect on maximum oxygen consumption, diastolic filling, myocardial relaxation, and vascular stiffening *(43–45)*.

SUMMARY

This brief review provides an overview of the major age-related changes in the cardiovascular system. These changes include the following:

- arterial stiffening
- endothelial dysfunction promoting vasoconstriction
- elevated systolic blood pressure and increased pulse pressure
- increased left ventricular wall thickness
- reduced early diastolic filling
- impaired cardiac reserve
- alterations in heart rate rhythm
- prolonged cardiac action potential
- a decline in renal function that contributes to improper maintenance of extracellular fluid volume and composition.

These age-associated changes in cardiovascular function precede clinical disease (hypertension, stroke, atherosclerosis, etc.).

ACKNOWLEDGMENT

This work was supported by grants from the National Institutes of Health (HL-18575, HL-71138 and DK-44628).

REFERENCES

1. Lakatta EG, Levy D. Arterial and cardiac imaging: major shareholders in cardiovascular disease enterprises. Part I: Aging arteries: A "set up" for vascular disease. *Circulation* 2003;107:139–146.
2. Lakatta EG, Levy D. Arterial and cardiac imaging: major shareholders in cardiovascular disease enterprises. Part II: The aging heart in health: links to heart disease. *Circulation* 2003;107:346–354.
3. Lakatta EG. Arterial and cardiac imaging: major shareholders in cardiovascular disease enterprises. Part III: cellular and molecular clues to heart and arterial aging. *Circulation* 2003;107:490–497.
4. Lakatta EG, Sollott SJ. Perspectives on mammalian cardiovascular aging: humans to molecules. Comp Biochem Physiol A Mol Integr Physiol 2002;132:699–721.
5. Yu BP, Chung HY. Oxidative stress and vascular aging. *Diabetes Res Clin Pract* 2001;54(suppl 2):S73–S80.
6. Isoyama S. Age-related changes before and after imposition of hemodynamic stress in the mammalian heart. *Life Sci* 1996;58:1601–1614.
7. Ferrari AU. Modifications of the cardiovascular system with aging. *Am J Geriatr Cardiol* 2002;11:30–33.

8. Pugh KG, Wei JY. Clinical implications of physiological changes in the aging heart. *Drugs Aging* 2001;18:263–276.
9. Lakatta EG. Cardiovascular aging research: the next horizons. *J Am Geriatr Soc* 1999;47:613–625.
10. Franklin SS, Gustin W 4th, Wong ND, et al. Hemodynamic patterns of age-related changes in blood pressure. The Framingham Heart Study. *Circulation* 1997;96: 308–315.
11. Aviv A. Salt consumption, reactive oxygen species and cardiovascular aging: a hypothetical link. *J Hypertens* 2002;20:555–559.
12. Kass DA. Age-related changes in ventricular-arterial coupling: pathophysiologic implications. *Heart Fail Rev* 2002;7:51–62.
13. Schutzer WE, Mader SL. Age-related changes in vascular adrenergic signaling: clinical and mechanistic implications. *Ageing Res Rev* 2003;2:169–90.
14. Lakatta EG. Cardiovascular regulatory mechanisms in advanced age. *Physiol Rev* 1993;73:413–467.
15. Matz RL, Schott C, Stoclet JC, Andriantsitohaina R. Age-related endothelial dysfunction with respect to nitric oxide, endothelium-derived hyperpolarizing factor and cyclooxygenase products. *Physiol Res* 2000;49:11–18.
16. Lundberg MS, Crow MT. Age-related changes in the signaling and function of vascular smooth muscle cells. *Exp Gerontol* 1999;34:549–557.
17. Homma S, Hirose N, Ishida H, Ishii T, Araki G. Carotid plaque and intima-medica thickness assesses by b-mode ultrasonography in subjects ranging from young adults to centenarians. *Stroke* 2001;32:830–835.
18. Asai K, Kudej RK, Shen YT, et al. Peripheral vascular endothelial dysfunction and apoptosis in old monkeys. *Arterioscler Thromb Vasc Biol* 2000;20:1493–1499.
19. Challah M, Nadaud S, Philippe M, et al. Circulating and cellular markers of endothelial dysfunction with aging in rats. *Am J Physiol* 1997;273 (4Pt 2):H1941–H1948.
20. Cernadas MR, Sanchez de Miguel L, Garcia-Duran M, et al. Expression of constitutive and inducible nitric oxide synthases in the vascular wall of young and aging rats. *Circ Res* 1998;83:279–286.
21. Celermajer DS, Sorensen KE, Spiegelhalter DJ, Georgakopoulos D, Robinson J, Deanfield JE. Aging is associated with endothelial dysfunction in healthy men years before the age-related decline in women. *J Am Coll Cardiol* 1994;24:471–476.
22. van der Loo B, Labugger R, Skepper JN, et al. Enhanced peroxynitrite formation is associated with vascular aging. *J Exp Med* 2000;192:1731–1744.
23. Chen J Brodsky SV, Goligorsky DM, Hampel DJ, Li H, Gross SS, Goligorsky MS. Glycated collagen I induces premature senescence-like phenotypic changes in endothelial cells. *Circ Res* 2002;90:1290–1298.
24. Anversa P, Palackal T, Sonnenblick EH, Olivetti G, Meggs LG, Capasso JM. Myocyte cell loss and myocyte cellular hyperplasia in the hypertrophied aging rat heart. *Circ Res* 1990;67:871–885.
25. Orchard CH, Lakatta EG. Intracellular calcium transients and developed tensions in rat heart muscle. A mechanism for the negative interval-strength relationship. *J Gen Physiol* 1985;86:637–651.
26. Josephson IR, Guia A, Stern MD, Lakatta EG. Alterations in properties of L-type Ca channels in aging rat heart. *J Mol Cell Cardiol* 2002;34:297–308.
27. Walker KE, Lakatta EG, Houser SR. Age associated changes in membrane currents in rat ventricular myocytes. *Cardiovasc Res* 1993;27:1968–1977.
28. Janczewski AM, Spurgeon HA, Lakatta EG. Action potential prolongation in cardiac myocytes of old rats is an adaptation to sustain youthful intracellular Ca2+ regulation. *J Mol Cell Cardiol* 2002;34:641–648.

29. Baylis C, Corman B. The aging kidney: insights from experimental studies. *J Am Soc Nephrol* 1998;9:699–709.
30. Beck LH. Changes in renal function with aging. *Clin Geriatr Med* 1998;14:199–209.
31. Beck LH. The aging kidney: defending the delicate balance of fluid and electrolytes. *Geriatrics* 2000;55:26–32.
32. Herrera AH, Davidson RA. Renovascular disease in older adults. *Clin Geriatr Med* 1998;14:237–254.
33. Fliser D, Ritz E. Relationship between hypertension and renal function and its therapeutic implications in the elderly. *Gerontology* 1998;44:123–131.
34. Hill GS, Heudes D, Bariety J. Morphometric study of arterioles and glomeruli in the aging kidney suggests focal loss of autoregulation. *Kidney Int* 2003;63:1027–1036.
35. Muhlberg W, Platt D. Age-dependent changes of the kidneys: pharmacological implications. *Gerontology* 1999;45:243–253.
36. Ruilope LM. Prevalence of renal disease in elderly hypertensive patients with cardiovascular problems. *Coron Artery Dis* 1997;4:483–488.
37. Navar LG, Inscho EW, Majid SA, Imig JD, Harrison-Bernard LM, Mitchell KD. Paracrine regulation of the renal microcirculation. *Physiol Rev* 1996;76:425–536.
38. Ungar A, Castellani S, Di Serio C, et al. Changes in renal autacoids and hemodynamics associated with aging and isolated systolic hypertension. *Prostaglandins Other Lipid Mediat* 2000;62:117–133.
39. Drew B, Leeuwenburgh C. Aging and the role of reactive nitrogen species. *Ann NY Acad Sci* 2002;959:66–81.
40. Stout NR, Kenny RA, Baylis PH. A review of water balance in ageing in health and disease. *Gerontology* 1999;45:61–66.
41. Lucas D, Szweda LI. Cardiac reperfusion injury: aging, lipid peroxidation and mitochondrial dysfunction. *Proc Natl Acad Sci USA* 1998;95:510–514.
42. Barja G. Endogenous oxidative stress: relationship to aging, longevity and caloric restriction. *Ageing Res Rev* 2002;1:397–411.
43. Brenner DA, Apstein CS, Saupe KW. Exercise training attenuates age-associated diastolic dysfunction in rats. *Circulation* 2001;104:221–226.
44. Vaitkevicius PV, Fleg JL, Engel JH, et al. Effects of age and aerobic capacity on arterial stiffness in healthy adults. *Circulation* 1993;88:1456–1462.
45. Tanaka H, DeSousza CA, Seals DR. Absence of age-related increase in central arterial stiffness in physically active women. *Arterioscler Thromb Vasc Biol* 1998;18:127–132.

3

Aging, Arterial Stiffness, and Systolic Hypertension

Joseph L. Izzo, Jr., MD

CONTENTS

INTRODUCTION
POPULATION STUDIES
PATHOPHYSIOLOGY
NONINVASIVE MEASUREMENT OF ARTERIAL STIFFNESS
REFERENCES

INTRODUCTION

Within the past few years, the paradigm in hypertension has shifted from an emphasis on diastolic blood pressure (DBP) to one that emphasizes the importance of systolic blood pressure (SBP), especially in individuals over age 50 years *(1–4)*. The rationale for this shift is based on a large body of observational and clinical trial data demonstrating that SBP is a better risk predictor, and that SBP control markedly reduces cardiovascular morbidity and mortality. At the same time, there has been relatively little information available to practitioners about the many new concepts that underlie this new approach to cardiovascular pathophysiology. Most important is the notion that age-related changes in vascular stiffness are at the center of future efforts to provide important new diagnostic and therapeutic advances in hypertension care.

From: *Clinical Hypertension and Vascular Diseases: Hypertension in the Elderly*
Edited by: L. M. Prisant © Humana Press Inc., Totowa, NJ

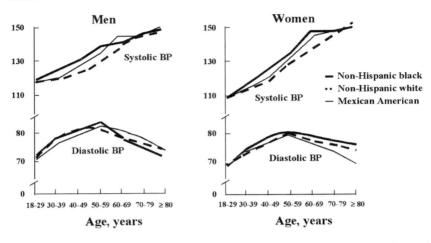

Fig. 1. Mean systolic and diastolic blood pressures (BPs) by age and race/ethnicity for men and women, US population ≥18 years old. (From ref. 5.)

POPULATION STUDIES

Age, Blood Pressure, and Cardiovascular Risk

Cross-sectional population studies showed that SBP increases throughout life, whereas DBP increases until about age 50 years and then declines in men and women and in all racial groups *(5)* (Fig. 1). Of interest, the relationship of age and SBP is only found in complex industrialized societies; primitive peoples and cloistered groups such as nuns or institutionalized people do not experience this effect. By age 60 years, about two-thirds of those with hypertension have isolated systolic hypertension (ISH); by age 75 years, almost all hypertensives have systolic hypertension, and about three-fourths of hypertensives have ISH *(3)*.

It is now widely recognized that the risk of cardiovascular diseases (CVDs) in individuals beyond 50 years of age is best predicted by SBP *(1-4,6)*. In fact, some studies in individuals 50 to 79 years of age suggested that the risk of coronary artery disease is *inversely* related to DBP at any given level of SBP. Wide pulse pressure (PP; PP = SBP – DBP) has been found to be an independent predictor of CVD risk in people over 60 years of age, even after adjusting for previous clinical CVD, age, gender, and other cardinal risk factors *(7)*. PP is a stronger predictor of CVD risk in those with dyslipidemia, left ventricular hypertrophy (LVH), albuminuria, chronic kidney disease, or prior cardiovascular events (myocardial infarction, ventricular dysfunction, or heart failure) *(8–10)*.

Yet, there are important limitations to using PP as a reliable risk indicator. In middle-aged, healthy populations or older individuals with both systolic and diastolic hypertension, any blood pressure (BP) component (systolic, diastolic, or mean arterial pressure [MAP]) may be equal or superior to PP as a risk predictor *(6)*.

Impact on Classification of Hypertension

There are important implications of aging effects on the value of SBP and DBP as diagnostic indices in hypertension. After age 50 years, SBP becomes more reliable in the classification of hypertension and in risk stratification, as was shown in the Framingham Heart Study *(11)*. By convention, when both SBP and DBP are considered, the higher value determines the correct stage of hypertension. For example, using the current classification system, a person with a BP of 162/90 mmHg would be classified as having stage 2 hypertension because the 162 mmHg exceeds the threshold for stage 2 hypertension (>160 mmHg) and thus "upstages" the diastolic value (which would by itself be considered stage 1). When used as the sole classifier of the stage of hypertension, SBP is accurate more than 90% of the time, whereas the diastolic value accurately predicts the stage of hypertension only about 60% *(11)*.

Benefits of SBP Control

The best study conducted in systolic hypertension is the Systolic Hypertension in the Elderly Program, a 4-year intervention that included 4694 individuals over age 60 with pretreatment SBP over 160 and DBP under 90 mmHg. Compared to placebo, individuals treated with chlorthalidone (with or without β-blocker) achieved favorable benefits in the primary end point of stroke (–36%), as well as reductions in heart failure events (–54%), myocardial infarctions (–27%), and overall CVD events (–32%) *(12)*. Using a similar design and sample size, the Systolic Hypertension in Europe trial compared a regimen based on nitrendipine (a dihydropyridine calcium antagonist) to a placebo-based regimen and found a significant benefit on stroke (–41%) as well as overall CVD events (–31%) *(13)*. A meta-analysis of eight placebo-controlled trials in 15,693 elderly patients followed for 4 years found that active antihypertensive treatment reduced coronary events (23%), strokes (30%), cardiovascular deaths (18%), and total deaths (13%), with the benefit particularly high in those older than 70 years of age *(14)*. Most experts now feel that the choice of initial agent is less important than the level of BP reduction achieved *(4,15)*.

PATHOPHYSIOLOGY

Why is there such a great benefit of treating systolic hypertension? The answer becomes clearer after a review of basic cardiovascular pathophysiology. Although it is currently fashionable to describe hypertension as a complex metabolic syndrome that involves insulin resistance and other derangements; in the main, hypertension remains a hemodynamic syndrome with properties that change with age.

Steady-State Hemodynamics

Basic teaching of the hemodynamics of hypertension has historically ignored the intrinsic pulsatility of the circulation. Typically, a steady-state flow model has been used to approximate circulatory hemodynamics, and MAP has been used as a surrogate for systemic vascular resistance (SVR) and the integrated pressure burden on the vasculature. MAP is analogous to voltage in the electrical steady-state model (Ohm's law), where Voltage = Current × Resistance. Thus, MAP = Total flow (Cardiac output) × SVR. In this simplified model, MAP is more closely related to DBP than SBP. Parallel increases in SBP and DBP up to age 50 years are primarily the result of age-related increases in SVR, but it is common to find systolic hypertension associated with increased cardiac stroke volume in younger hypertensives *(16)*.

Pulsatility and Blood Flow

To understand the pathophysiological relevance of systolic hypertension, it is necessary to review the physiology of circulatory pulsatility. In conjunction with cardiac contraction, the arterial system serves two basic interrelated functions: conveyance of a sufficient quantity of blood to various tissues (the conduit function) and damping of pulsatile flow to provide a smoother flow profile in the microcirculation. The pulsatile or dynamic component of blood pressure is the summation of three major factors: cardiac contractility (stroke volume), aortic impedance (central arterial stiffness), and late systolic pressure augmentation caused by pulse wave reflection from the distal circulation (Fig. 2).

Central Arterial Stiffness

Large central arteries, predominantly the thoracic aorta and its proximal branches, fulfill the damping function by expanding during systole, storing some but not all of each stroke volume, and utilizing elastic recoil to propel the residual of each stroke volume to the periphery during diastole. The resulting damping of pulsatility in normal young arteries creates a relatively narrow PP (Fig. 3). When central arteries are stiffer,

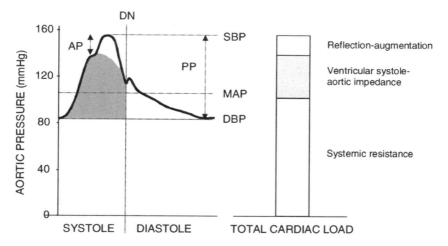

Fig. 2. Components of blood pressure (BP) and cardiac load. Various parameters are needed to describe pulsatile phenomena. DN, dicrotic notch, the division between systole and diastole. Left-hand panel demonstrates a typical aortic pulse contour in an individual with hypertension. Pulse pressure (PP) represents the maximal difference between systolic BP (SBP) and diastolic BP (DBP); mean arterial pressure (MAP) = DBP + 1/3 PP. Major components of PP include (a) cardiac stroke volume, (b) aortic impedance to early systolic outflow, and (c) late systolic augmentation pressure (AP) caused by arterial stiffening and premature return of reflected waves. Total cardiac load, the integral of the systolic pulse contour, depends mainly on the interactions of three factors proportionally represented by the bar graph at the right: DBP, coupled effects of ventricular contraction and aortic impedance, and AP.

two related events occur: (a) SBP increases because more blood is delivered to the periphery during systole, and (b) DBP decreases because there is less residual stroke volume to be delivered to the periphery during diastole. Thus, central arterial stiffness causes PP to increase, a phenomenon that is independent of any change in MAP.

The cellular basis of age-related arterial stiffening is only partly understood. The elastic behavior of arteries depends primarily on the composition and arrangement of collagen, elastin, and vascular smooth muscle cells in the tunica media of the arterial wall. An elastin matrix attached to vascular smooth muscle cells acts to damp changes in intraluminal pressure and tension. There is a functional dependency of arterial wall tension and stiffness on the distending pressure; increased BP stretches the load-bearing elastic lamellae, making the arteries functionally stiffer. Over a lifetime, other structural changes occur, including loss of elastin and increased collagen deposition. This degenerative process is some-

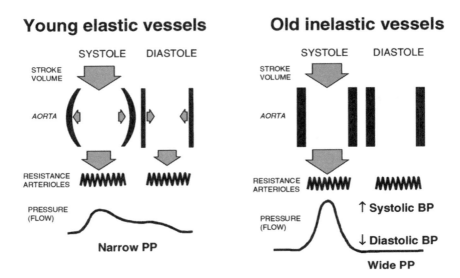

Fig. 3. Effect of central arterial stiffness on pulse pressure (PP). Age-related increases in central arterial stiffness convert a smooth peripheral pressure wave with a narrow PP to a more pulsatile peripheral pressure wave with increased PP. Changes in PP are independent of changes in stroke volume or systemic vascular resistance. The central problem is the loss of aortic elasticity; systolic pressure is increased and diastolic blood pressure (BP) is decreased because of the loss of elastic recoil of the aorta. (Adapted from ref. *26*.)

times called *arteriosclerosis* to differentiate it from *atherosclerosis*, the occlusive result of endovascular inflammatory disease caused by lipid oxidation and plaque formation. Hypertension, diabetes, and chronic renal failure accelerate the aging of central elastic arteries and cause premature arterial stiffening.

Reflection, Augmentation, and Amplification

A fundamental property of stiff arteries is that they conduct pulse waves faster than more elastic vessels. Arterial stiffness thus can be approximated by measuring pulse wave velocity (PWV). Another fundamental property of pulse wave transmission is that pulse waves can be reflected within arterial walls, leading to both forward and backward transmission of pulse waves *(17)* (Fig. 4). Reflected waves have their origins at points of "impedance mismatch," where the flow and pressure waves are not perfectly matched, especially from branch points, constrictions, or areas of turbulence.

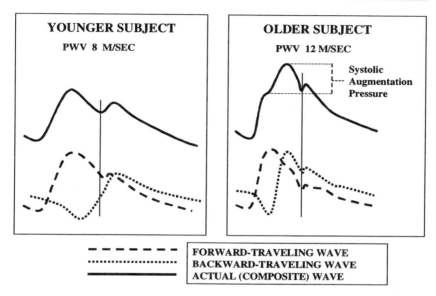

Fig. 4. Components of arterial pulse waves in older and younger subjects. Because of the property of wave reflection, any pulse wave can be decomposed into a forward-traveling and backward-traveling wave. The velocity of travel of these pulse waves (PWV) is directly proportional to the stiffness of the arterial wall. In older people, increased PWV causes early return of the principal reflected wave, which summates with the incident wave to augment late systolic pressure. Vertical line is the dicrotic notch that separates systole from diastole. (Modified from ref. *17*.)

Wave reflection can have important effects on cardiac function and structure. In young people with elastic arteries, the primary reflected wave returns to the aortic root during early diastole, where it serves to augment coronary artery filling. In older people with stiffer arteries, the high PWV causes the primary reflected wave to return to the aortic root before the end of systole, where it summates with the forward-traveling pulse wave and augments late SBP (Fig. 4).

Another interesting and poorly understood property of the arterial tree is PP amplification *(18)* (Fig. 5). In normal young individuals with highly elastic arterial walls, PP at distal arterial sites is greater than that measured centrally. This contrasts with MAP, which is relatively constant throughout the arterial tree. PP amplification is the result of the progressive increase in impedance that occurs in the distal circulation and the corresponding differences in the summation of incident and reflected waves along the arterial tree. In normal young people, it is not uncom-

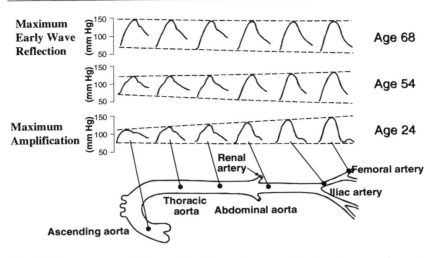

Fig. 5. Pulse pressure (PP) amplification and wave reflection. In normal young individuals, PP is amplified as the wave travels downstream because of a progressive increase in impedance, and mean arterial pressure remains constant. With age and increased central pressure augmentation, the difference between central and peripheral PP decreases. Thus, peripheral PP is not always equivalent to central PP. (From ref. *27.*)

mon to observe a brachial PP that is 20 to 30 mmHg higher than that at the aortic root. With aging, however, the greater magnitude of the reflected waves and the increased PWV contribute to a progressive diminution of the apparent central–peripheral PP differential (Fig. 5). The importance of this effect is that brachial SBP (or PP) is not always a reliable surrogate for central SBP *(19).*

The Integrated Hemodynamic Model

Age-related increases in SBP and widening of PP usually signify that arterial stiffness has become the dominant hemodynamic lesion. There remains a role for excessive vasoconstriction in the syndrome of hypertension, however, because systemic vasoconstriction and increased SVR contribute to both systolic and diastolic hypertension (Fig. 6). Overall, increased SBP can be the result of increases in stroke volume, arterial stiffness, or SVR, whereas DBP is *decreased* when central arterial stiffness increases. DBP thus varies directly with SVR and inversely with central arterial stiffness.

The ability of increased SVR to cause increases in either SBP or DBP (depending on the degree of central arterial stiffness) causes otherwise unexpected differences in the therapeutic responses of SBP and DBP to

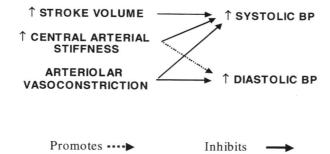

Fig. 6. Integrated hemodynamic model of hypertension. Factors promoting increased systolic blood pressure (BP) are increased cardiac contractility (stroke volume), increased central arterial stiffness, and increased arteriolar constriction (systemic vascular resistance). Peripheral arteriolar constriction directly increases diastolic BP and mean arterial pressure, whereas central artery stiffness lowers diastolic BP.

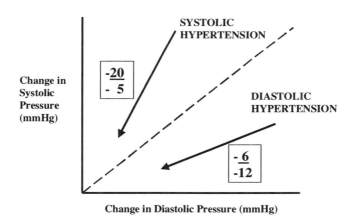

Fig. 7. Effect of arterial stiffness on BP responses to vasodilation. The net effect of an arteriolar dilator drug on systolic and diastolic BP can be very different depending on the stiffness of an individual's central arteries. For the same degree of vasodilation, an individual with stiff arteries and isolated systolic hypertension (ISH) will respond with a marked reduction in systolic BP (-20/-5 mmHg = -10 mmHg MAP), whereas an individual with isolated diastolic hypertension will experience a predominant effect on diastolic BP (–6/–12 mmHg = –10 mmHg MAP). (Modified from ref. 20.)

vasodilators *(20)*. In ISH, a vasodilator causes a disproportionate drop in SBP; the same vasodilator in a person with diastolic hypertension decreases DBP. If both SBP and DBP are elevated, both will be decreased by the vasodilator therapy (Fig. 7).

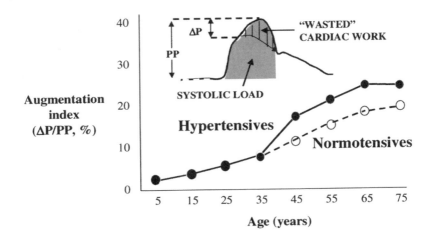

Fig. 8. Effect of age and central pressure augmentation on cardiac load. Increased arterial stiffness causes increased pulse wave velocity and promotes late systolic pressure augmentation. Augmentation index increases with age, but this effect is accelerated by the presence of hypertension. Increased late systolic pressure contributes to the overall cardiac load and can be considered "wasted" cardiac work. Increased cardiac load contributes directly to left ventricular hypertrophy.

Pathological Implications

Systolic hypertension and increased PP are strong surrogate markers for CVD morbidity and mortality. Increased pulsatile load is the major factor in increased left ventricular systolic wall stress and LVH, both of which impair left ventricular relaxation and contribute to diastolic dysfunction. Increased ventricular mass increases coronary blood flow requirements and decreases coronary flow reserve. Late systolic pressure augmentation further increases ventricular load; in elderly persons with ISH, late systolic pressure can be increased by as much as 20 to 40 mmHg as a result of wave reflection. In general, central systolic augmentation is age dependent and contributes to "wasted cardiac output" and LVH (Fig. 8). Simultaneously, as PP widens, decreases in DBP further compromise coronary filling. At the same time, greater shear stress on the central arteries accentuates aortic, carotid, and coronary atherosclerosis and probably contributes to rupture of unstable atherosclerotic plaques. The distal vasculature is also affected because increased pulsatile stress promotes endothelial dysfunction, thus affecting the balance in the forces controlling arteriolar constriction and dilation and favoring arteriolar smooth muscle hypertrophy and arteriolar remodeling.

NONINVASIVE MEASUREMENT OF ARTERIAL STIFFNESS

As discussed in this review, information related to the assessment of SBP, PP, and central arterial stiffness is fundamentally different from that related to DBP or MAP. Thus, the elastic properties of the arteries and the impact of arterial stiffness on pulse wave transmission and reflection are of increasing interest to researchers and clinicians. Because brachial PP is only loosely related to central PP and wide PP in general is a late indicator of CVD risk, many investigators are searching for more sensitive measures of earlier changes in arterial wall properties.

Changes in central artery stiffness can be quantitated using research methods that measure PWV, aortic impedance, and analysis of arterial waveform morphology. Increased PWV has been correlated with increased CVD mortality *(21)*, and aortic impedance can be affected differently by different antihypertensive agents *(22)*. In the future, it may be possible to use these indicators of central artery stiffness to allow targeted primary prevention of CVD or improved therapeutic monitoring of antihypertensive drugs or new compounds that directly reduce arterial stiffness. At present, all techniques that assess arterial stiffness should be considered primarily research tools not ready for immediate clinical application *(23–25)*.

REFERENCES

1. Kannel WB, Gordon T, Schwartz MJ. Systolic vs diastolic blood pressure and risk of coronary heart disease. *Am J Cardiol* 1971;27:335–345.
2. Izzo JL Jr, Levy D, Black HR. Clinical advisory statement: importance of systolic blood pressure in older Americans. *Hypertension* 2000;35:1021–1024.
3. Franklin SS, Jacobs MJ, Wong ND, L'Italien GJ, Lapuerta P. Predominance of isolated systolic hypertension among middle-aged and elderly US hypertensives: analysis based on National Health and Nutrition Examination Survey (NHANES) III. *Hypertension* 2001;37:869–874.
4. Chobanian AV, Bakris GL, Black HR, et al. Seventh report of the Joint National Committee on the Prevention, Detection, Evaluation, and Treatment of High Blood Pressure—JNC VII Express. *JAMA* 2003;289:2560–2572.
5. Burt VL, Whelton P, Roccella EJ, et al. Prevalence of hypertension in the US adult population: results from the Third National Health and Nutrition Examination Survey, 1988–1991. *Hypertension* 1995;25:305–313.
6. Lewington S, Clarke R, Qizilbash N, Peto R, Collins R. Age-specific relevance of usual blood pressure to vascular mortality: a meta-analysis of individual data for one million adults in 61 prospective studies. *Lancet* 2002;360:1903–1913.
7. Franklin SS, Khan SA, Wong ND, Larson MG, Levy D. Is pulse pressure more important than systolic blood pressure in predicting coronary heart disease events. *Circulation* 1999;100:354–360.
8. Mitchell GF, Moye LA, Braunwald E, et al. Sphygmomanometrically determined pulse pressure is a powerful independent predictor of recurrent events after myocar-

dial infarction in patients with impaired left ventricular function. *Circulation* 1997;96:4254–4260.

9. Blacher J, London GM, Safar ME, Mourad JJ. Influence of age and end-stage renal disease on the stiffness of carotid wall material in hypertension. *J Hypertens* 1999;17:237–244.

10. Asmar R, Rudnichi A, Blacher J, London GM, Safar ME. Pulse pressure and aortic pulse wave are markers of cardiovascular risk in hypertensive populations. *Am J Hypertension* 2001;14:91–97.

11. Lloyd-Jones DM. Impact of systolic vs diastolic blood pressure level of JNC-VI blood pressure stage classification. *Hypertension* 1999;34:381–385.

12. SHEP Cooperative Research Group. Prevention of stroke by antihypertensive drug treatment in older patients with isolated systolic hypertension. *JAMA* 1991;265: 3255–3264.

13. Staessen JA, Fagard R, Thijs L, et al. Randomised double-blind comparison of placebo and active treatment for older patients with isolated systolic hypertension. The Systolic Hypertension in Europe (Syst-Eur) Trial Investigators. *Lancet* 1997;350:757–764.

14. Staessen JA, Wang JG, Thijs L, Fagard R. Overview of the outcome trials in older patients with isolated systolic hypertension. *J Hum Hypertens* 1999;13:859–863.

15. Fagard RH, Staessen JA, Thijs L, et al. Response to antihypertensive therapy in older patients with sustained and nonsustained systolic hypertension. Systolic Hypertension in Europe (Syst-Eur) Trial Investigators. *Circulation* 2000;102:1139–1144.

16. Julius S, Krause L, Schork NJ, et al. Hyperkinetic borderline hypertension in Tecumseh, Michigan. *J Hypertens* 1991;9:77–84.

17. Asmar R. Arterial pulse waves. In: Asmar R, ed. Arterial stiffness and pulse wave velocity: clinical applications. Amsterdam: Elsevier; 1999:17–23.

18. Nichols WW, O'Rourke MF. McDonald's blood flow in arteries: theoretical, experimental and clinical principles. 4th ed. London: Arnold; 1998:220–222.

19. Wilkinson IB, Franklin SS, Hall IR, Tyrrell S, Cockcroft JR. Pressure amplification explains why pulse pressure is unrelated to risk in young subjects. *Hypertension* 2001;38:1461–1466.

20. Koch-Weser J. Correlation of pathophysiology and pharmacology in primary hypertension. *Am J Cardiol* 1973;32:499–499.

21. Blacher J, Asmar R, Djane S, London GM, Safar ME. Aortic pulse wave velocity as a marker of cardiovascular risk in hypertensive patients. *Hypertension* 1999;33:1111–1117.

22. Mitchell GF, Izzo JL Jr, Lacourciere Y, et al. Omapatrilat reduces pulse pressure and proximal aortic stiffness in patients with systolic hypertension: results of the conduit hemodynamics of omapatrilat international research study. *Circulation* 2002;105: 2955–2961.

23. Izzo JL Jr, Shykoff BE. Arterial stiffness: clinical relevance, measurement, and treatment. *Rev Cardiovasc Med* 2001;2:29–34, 37–40.

24. Izzo JL Jr, Manning TS, Shykoff BE. Office blood pressures, arterial compliance characteristics, and estimated cardiac load. *Hypertension* 2001;38:1467–1470.

25. Manning TS, Shykoff BE, Izzo JL Jr. Validity and reliability of diastolic pulse contour analysis (windkessel model) in humans. *Hypertension* 2002;39:963–968.

26. Williams TF, Foerster JE, Proctor JK, Hahn A, Izzo AJ, Elliott GA. A new double-layered launderable bed sheet for patients with urinary incontinence. *J Am Geriatr Soc* 1981;29:520–527.

27. Nichols WW, et al. Arterial vasodilation. Philadelphia; 1993:32.

28. Fleg/Kelly. Hypertension primer.

4

Pharmacological and Pharmacodynamic Alterations in the Elderly
Application to Cardiovascular Therapies

Domenic A. Sica, MD

CONTENTS

INTRODUCTION

Except for drugs eliminated predominantly by renal excretion, it is not possible to generalize on the type, magnitude, or importance of age-related differences in pharmacokinetics. Conflicting data in the literature for various drugs may be attributed to small numbers of subjects studied, differences in selection criteria for subjects, and variation in protocol design. Apparent age-related differences in drug disposition are multifactorial and influenced by environmental, genetic, physiological, and pathological factors.

This chapter addresses relevant pharmacokinetic and, if available, pharmacodynamic considerations in the elderly, with an emphasis on the interplay of cardiovascular medications in these processes. In this chapter,

From: *Clinical Hypertension and Vascular Diseases: Hypertension in the Elderly*
Edited by: L. M. Prisant © Humana Press Inc., Totowa, NJ

the term *cardiovascular medications* encompasses all antihypertensives. Cardiovascular compounds other than antihypertensives are described in an agent- or class-specific manner.

Aging, characterized by periods of growth, development, and senescence, is a source of interindividual variability in drug response and is one of several factors that influence the optimization of therapy. This is more so in the very aged, a patient group often in most critical need of safe and effective medication administration. However, any agewise stratification into elderly or very elderly categories is quite arbitrary. Life is a continuous process, with the distinction between one time period and the next often quite arbitrary.

It is also clear that chronological age does not necessarily dictate functional age; thus, population-based pharmacokinetic suppositions do not always reflect how an individual patient will change with age. In this regard, the process of aging may begin as early as the fourth decade and can proceed at different rates from person to person. In addition, with age many individuals can develop any of several systemic illnesses that can compound age-related changes in physiology and lead to serious therapeutic challenges.

EPIDEMIOLOGY

Demographic trends at least partly dictate the relevance of age-related pharmacological changes. In this regard, the world's population is aging at an unprecedented rate. Since 1900, there has been an 11-fold increase in the number of Americans above the age of 65 years (12.6% of the population), whereas the number of those younger than 65 years has only tripled. By 2030, one in five of all Americans will be older than 65 years *(1)*.

The elderly are more susceptible to drug effects; adverse drug reactions are at least two to three times more frequent in geriatric patients than in adults younger than 30 years *(2)*. Unwanted adverse drug effects are responsible for many hospital admissions in elderly patients. In one series, one in six elderly patients admitted to a general ward experienced adverse drug reactions; severe reactions occurred in 24%, with orthostatic hypotension a common cause of admission *(3)*.

PHARMACOKINETICS IN THE ELDERLY

Drug Absorption

Drug absorption is not dramatically altered with age despite the age-related change in several variables that influence drug absorption. With aging, gastric pH tends to increase, although the change can be quite variable from patient to patient. In this regard, calcium channel blockers (CCBs) have been suggested to increase the frequency of gastroesophageal reflux but do not *per se* increase acid production *(4)*. When present, an increase in gastric pH can alter the lipid solubility or dissolution characteristics of some drugs, thereby reducing absorption. This is seldom clinically relevant. Gastric emptying also slows with aging. The age-related change in gastric emptying has a poorly quantified effect on the pharmacokinetics and/or pharmacodynamics of cardiovascular medications; however, when age-related changes are combined with those attributable to disease states, such as diabetes, drug delivery to more distal intestinal absorptive sites may be delayed to a sufficient degree to influence the onset of drug effect. In this regard, prior observations have suggested that clonidine has a prokinetic effect; however, when formally studied, clonidine did not increase the rate of gastric emptying *(5)*.

Intestinal motility/gut blood flow is reduced in the elderly, which can further impact drug absorption. Certain therapies, such as verapamil, can substantially reduce intestinal motility and exaggerate this *de novo* process in the elderly *(6)*. However, this motility effect with verapamil predominates in the colon, where little drug absorption typically occurs and therefore is unlikely to influence overall drug absorption. The converse, increased intestinal motility, does not commonly occur with cardiovascular medications.

Cardiovascular medications can also have an impact on drug absorption by reducing blood pressure (BP) in the setting of already-compromised gut blood flow. Several cardiovascular medications have been considered regarding their ability to increase regional intestinal blood flow, with inconclusive findings. These studies have generally been carried out under acute conditions and cannot be generalized to the usual circumstances of cardiovascular medication administration in the elderly *(7,8)*.

Transdermal Absorption

The barrier function characteristics of human skin change dramatically with increasing age *(9)*. Any pharmacological penetrant has three potential pathways to the underlying viable tissue: through hair follicles with associated sebaceous glands, via sweat ducts, or across continuous stratum corneum between these appendages. The intact stratum corneum provides the main barrier; its "brick-and-mortar" structure is analogous to a wall. Most molecules penetrate through skin via this intercellular microroute *(10)*.

Two cardiovascular medications can be given via the transdermal route: nitroglycerin and clonidine. The transdermal absorption of each of these compounds has not been specifically studied in the elderly. However, despite the absence of such information, no reports exist to suggest altered clinical outcomes when these drugs are given by the transdermal route in the elderly.

Body Weight

Body weight compartmentalization changes with aging, with a variable overall effect on total body weight. Body fat increases at the expense of a loss in lean body mass (muscle) *(11)*. A weight adjustment in dosing is only considered if the weight of an individual differs by more than 30% from the average 70-kg adult weight. This is most pertinent to the emaciated or petite individual, for whom standard medication doses may lead to high plasma concentrations and potential excess pharmacological effect.

Drug Distribution

The aging process is accompanied by changes in body composition that can influence drug volume of distribution. With aging, lean body mass diminishes, and adipose tissue increases. In addition, total body water, both in absolute terms and as a percentage of body weight, declines by 10 to 15% coincident to aging; thus, drugs restricted to a space approximating total body water, such as ethanol, have a smaller volume in which to distribute and will reach a higher blood level relative to dose in elderly patients *(12)*. Conversely, highly lipid-soluble drugs such as diazepam have relatively more adipose tissue in which to distribute and therefore have larger volumes of distribution in elderly patients *(13)*. However, in very elderly individuals, who lose body weight and become frail, the proportion of fat can decrease. In such individuals, the result can be an increase in the plasma concentration of lipophilic drugs *(14)*. In the elderly, drug volume of distribution has been poorly studied as it may apply to the pattern of response to antihypertensives *(15)*. If a relationship exists between volume of distribution and the BP-reducing effect of an antihypertensive medication, it is more likely a function of drug half-life because drug half-life varies directly with the volume of distribution.

Protein Binding

Although protein binding is a major determinant of drug action, it is only one of several such factors. Highly protein-bound drugs are impacted most by alterations in binding. The extent of protein binding is a function of drug and protein concentrations, the affinity constant for the drug–protein interaction, and the number of protein-binding sites per class of binding site *(16)*. Age-related changes in protein binding appear not to influence antihypertensive drug effect *(17–19)*. Albumin levels are often decreased in the elderly, whereas α_1-acid glycoprotein levels are not altered by age *per se*. Alterations in plasma protein binding found in the elderly are generally not attributed to age, but rather to physiological and pathophysiological changes/disease states and drug–drug interactions *(20)* that occur more frequently in the elderly. Age-related physiological changes, such as decreased renal, hepatic, and cardiac function, generally produce more clinically significant alterations in drug disposition than plasma protein binding.

Drug Metabolism

PHYSIOLOGICAL CHANGES INFLUENCING HEPATIC METABOLISM

Aging is accompanied by marked changes in the physiology of many organs, as well as in the functions of their constituent cells. These nonpathological alterations in structure or function may affect normal physiological processes in the elderly as relates to drug disposition. On the basis of a variety of clinical evaluation tools, most liver function tests in humans appear to be well preserved in the absence of underlying disease. However, liver parenchymal volume declines in an absolute (and relative to body weight) fashion; in addition, regional blood flow to the liver via the portal system falls off with age in humans and no doubt contributes to the diminished clearance of drugs that exhibit significant first-pass pharmacokinetic profiles *(21)*. In this regard, age is associated with a reduction in the presystemic metabolism of propranolol and labetalol, drugs that both have high extraction ratios. Accordingly, the bioavailability of these drugs increases with age *(22,23)*.

As mentioned, the liver plays a major role in drug clearance, and aging has been reported to diminish intrinsic metabolic function. The absolute cytochrome P450 (CYP) content of the human liver has been variably reported to be either unchanged *(24)* or diminished *(25)*. In vivo drug metabolism *per se* is variably modified in the course of aging. Phase I reactions that involve oxidation by the microsomal CYP-dependent mono-oxygenase systems more times than not are slowed *(26,27)*. Alternatively, there is little to no change in phase II conjugative processes with aging *(25)*. The most consistent characteristic of hepatic metabolic function in the elderly is the large interindividual variability, a feature that easily obscures age-related differences. In addition, a range of factors, including diet, concurrent illness, smoking, and alcohol, can confound interpretation of age-related changes in CYP activity on an age basis alone.

Among the antihypertensive drug classes in common use, CCBs most often exhibit age-related slowing of metabolism. CCB pharmacokinetics have a wide interindividual variability, particularly in the elderly, which clouds the possible detection of pure age-related metabolic differences. Observed pharmacokinetic changes for CCBs with aging include increased maximum plasma concentrations C_{max}, area under the curve, and absolute bioavailability $(28–33)$. These alterations are of a sufficient magnitude to influence both the starting and maximum dose of several CCBs in the elderly (34). In addition, this age relationship with CCB metabolism is the more probable explanation for many of the altered pharmacokinetic patterns for CCBs in renal failure because most patients with renal failure are older than the general population (35).

RENAL EXCRETION

With age, renal cortical mass, renal blood flow, and glomerular filtration rate (GFR) decline significantly, particularly if hypertension has been present for any period of time (36). With aging, renal plasma flow typically declines to a greater degree than GFR, resulting in a rise in the filtration fraction (37). After age 30, creatinine clearance decreases an average of 8 mL per minute per 1.73 m^2 per decade in about 65% of persons, but remains unchanged in the remainder. This last observation is clinically important in that it suggests that loss of renal function with aging is not an immutable process (37).

Importantly, with aging serum creatinine levels can often remain within so-called normal limits because the elderly match declining renal function with a consistent and parallel loss of muscle mass (the source of serum creatinine). This lends itself to the perception of "normal" renal function when in fact significant renal disease may exist. A decrease in tubular processing and endocrinological functions tracks with changes in glomerular function in the elderly. The most important of these tubular changes involves sodium and water handling: urinary-concentrating ability declines, and the capacity to attain sodium balance in the face of a reduction in dietary sodium intake is timewise very sluggish.

These pathophysiological changes decrease the capacity for renal elimination of drugs. This is particularly important for compounds cleared by filtration and tubular secretion, as is the case for many of the angiotensin-converting enzyme (ACE) inhibitors (38). The clinical implications of decreased renal clearance of any compound depends on the contribution that renal elimination makes to total body clearance of a drug and thereafter on the drug's therapeutic index (ratio of the maximum tolerated dose to the minimum effective dose). The latter is somewhat difficult to predict reliably in the hypertensive patient because the relationship between drug levels and response can be unstructured. Accumulation of active metabolites (e.g., *N*-acetylprocainamide, morphine-6-glucuronide) increases the risk of toxicity in the elderly because of age-related decreases in renal clearance. There are few active metabolites of antihypertensive medications other than ACE inhibitors that are renally cleared, so this consideration has limited application.

Because renal function is dynamic, maintenance doses of drugs should be adjusted if a patient becomes acutely ill or dehydrated or has recently recovered from dehydration. Also, because renal function may continue to decline with age, the dose of drugs given long term should be reviewed periodically. Concomitant medications can be a problem for many elderly patients. In particular, the more frequent need for long-term nonsteroidal anti-inflammatory drug therapy in many elderly patients presents a particular challenge *(39)*. These compounds attenuate the antihypertensive effects of many compounds, diminish the renal capacity to excrete sodium and potassium loads effectively, and reversibly (for the most part) diminish renal function if even the slightest degree of volume contraction occurs *(40)*. The ready availability as over-the-counter compounds increases use and thereby risk with this drug class.

MEASUREMENT OF RENAL FUNCTION

The timewise measurement of GFR provides a quantitative assessment of filtration capacity and has become a popular way to track stability or rate of decline in renal function with age. Measurement of true GFR is complicated; therefore, as a substitute for direct *in situ* measurement, GFR is indirectly estimated with serum creatinine values. Normal serum creatinine concentrations for a typical population range from 0.5–1.3 mg/dL (40–110 μmol/L) in males to 0.5–1.1 mg/dL (40–100 μmol/L) in females. Elevated serum creatinine measurements, when indexed for muscle mass, are indicative of renal insufficiency and are easier to interpret. However, interpretation of a normal serum creatinine value requires some skill because renal failure can still be present with normal values.

Creatinine is a product of creatine metabolism in muscle, and its daily production correlates closely with muscle mass. Thus, the greater the muscle mass, the more creatinine generated and the higher the "normal serum creatinine." For example, in a well-muscled older male, a serum creatinine value of 1.2 mg/dL can be considered normal, although such a value may be viewed as grossly abnormal in an individual with less muscle mass. An individual with a small muscle mass, such as an elderly female, with normal renal function should have a serum creatinine value close to 0.6 mg/dL or less. If a serum creatinine value of 1.2 mg/dL is present, although this value falls in the normal "population" range, it represents a significant deviation from this individual's expected normal value. Because creatinine clearance is reciprocally related to serum creatinine concentrations, in this patient the doubling of serum creatinine would correspond to an approximate halving of renal function.

Because of the inherent limitations to serum creatinine values and the problems with obtaining accurate timed creatinine clearance determinations, estimated creatinine clearance values using the Cockcroft-Gault or similar formulas are used to guide drug dosing *(41)*. The Cockcroft-Gault formula uses the serum creatinine concentration, age, and weight to calculate creatinine clearance:

$$Cl_{creat} \text{ (mL/min)} = \frac{(140\text{-age [yr]}) \times (\text{body weight [kg]})}{(72) \times (\text{serum creatinine [mg/dL]})}$$

For women, the calculated values are multiplied by 0.85, although this arbitrarily presumes all women have less muscle mass (or source of creatinine) than do males *(41)*. This is an incorrect presumption and is often the source of a systematic error in estimating renal function with this formula. Also, use of urine-free formulas (such as the Cockcroft-Gault formula) for estimation of renal function fails to detect early renal function change, particularly in the elderly.

PHARMACODYNAMICS IN THE ELDERLY

The basis for altered drug response in the elderly can be pharmacokinetic as discussed in a previous section, or pharmacodynamic. In many instances, the elderly experience a highly individualized combination of both, which makes the treatment of hypertension in the elderly as much an art as a science. There is a series of age-related changes in physiology that in combination with age-related pharmacokinetic alterations creates very specific pharmacodynamic tendencies in the elderly.

First, there are alterations in body composition such that total body water decreases; therein resides an important consideration for diuretic therapy in the elderly, particularly in light of poorly responsive thirst-sensing mechanisms in the elderly. Second, there are noteworthy changes in a variety of neurohumoral systems, the most important of which include a decline in activity of the renin–angiotensin–aldosterone system and an age-associated rise in circulating catecholamines, which suggests a reduction in responsiveness to sympathetic stimulation. Third, structural alterations are accompanied by baseline and adaptive change in hemodynamic responses. Left ventricular hypertrophy, diastolic dysfunction, and a loss of elasticity in the central and peripheral circulation occur. Resting heart rate remains unchanged or declines slightly in old age. In addition, baroreceptor reflex sensitivity and responsiveness decreases with age, which makes elderly patients more prone to exaggerated orthostatic drops in BP. Finally, receptor function changes with a decrease in β-receptor-mediated systemic and vascular responses *(42)*.

The following discussion does not specifically address the efficacy of various drug classes in the treatment of the elderly hypertensive; rather, it offers selective comments on each drug class as relates to pharmacodynamics, efficacy, and safety.

Diuretics

Diuretic use in the elderly generally occurs for two reasons. First, thiazide-type diuretics are administered for their ability to reduce BP; second, loop diuretics are given for volume control in disease states, such as congestive heart failure. The BP-lowering response to thiazide-type diuretics seems not to be modified by the aging process *(43)*, and if diuretics are dose adjusted, this is prompted by the onset of a negative fluid balance state. Adaptation to loss of volume is poor in the elderly, enough so that volume contraction can occur without careful thought about the dose amount and frequency of diuretic administration *(44)*. Moreover, with aging there is a decline in the thirst-sensing mechanism, which can further increase the risk of sustaining a volume-contracted state *(45)*. In a positive sense, this abnormality in thirst drive can be viewed as a counterbalancing factor preventing diuretic-related hyponatremia, a not-uncommon finding in elderly females *(46)*.

Regarding diuretics used for volume control, loop diuretic action derives from the amount of diuretic delivered to its thick ascending limb site of action. Such tubular delivery first requires entry into the luminal compartment, which can be characteristically altered because of the underlying loss of tubular secretion capacity with aging, with the elderly delivering on average one-half the amount of diuretic into the urine as do younger patients *(47)*. However, when the response to furosemide is indexed as a function of the amount of furosemide in the urine, it is clear that the elderly follow the same relationship as do young patients with normal renal function. Thus, for the elderly to achieve the same diuretic response as a younger individual, twice the diuretic dose generally needs to be given. This is contrary to the usual recommendation for drug dosing in the elderly. The usual admonition is to reduce doses in the elderly. Diuretics represent a special and unique exception simply because their mechanism of action depends on a urinary site of effect.

ACE Inhibitors

ACE inhibitors exhibit predictable pharmacokinetic alterations in the elderly, particularly because their total body clearance is so heavily dependent on renal function and renal function declines in parallel with the aging process *(48)*. There is some class heterogeneity in this regard because the ACE inhibitors fosinopril and trandolapril are both moderately hepatically cleared and do not accumulate in patients with renal dysfunction whatever the etiology *(49)*.

The BP-lowering effect of ACE inhibitors is not mechanistically influenced by age *per se (50)*. However, this statement needs some qualification. Plasma renin activity and blood/urine aldosterone level decline with age, both at baseline and in response to position or volume changes *(51)*. This neurohumoral quiescence has fueled speculation that low renin forms of hypertension, such as observed in the elderly, may be less responsive to drugs like ACE inhibitors, which primarily reduce activity in the renin–angiotensin–aldosterone axis.

Although this may be the case, two separate processes will influence the final BP response to an ACE inhibitor in the elderly. First, age slows the renal clearance of these compounds and therefore significantly increases systemic exposure (at the same dose given to a younger subject) *(51)*. Second, the systolic BP value in the older hypertensive is typically higher than that found in young hypertensives, a characteristic that guides BP lower once treatment is initiated. Hemodynamic side effects observed with ACE inhibitors, such as first-dose hypotension and functional renal insufficiency, can be expected to occur more commonly in the elderly *(52)*. A lengthier discussion of ACE inhibitor-related hemodynamic side effects is available in Chapter 16.

Angiotensin-Receptor Blockers

There are currently seven angiotensin-receptor blockers available in the United States. The systemic handling of these compounds is such that there is typically a more balanced renal and hepatic mode of elimination than is the case with ACE inhibitors *(53)*; accordingly, dosage adjustment of these compounds is not warranted on the basis of the potential for systemic accumulation in the renally compromised elderly patient. Rather, dosage adjustment in the elderly should occur on the basis of achieving and maintaining the desired hemodynamic response. This approach is similar to the one employed for ACE inhibitor administration in the elderly.

α-Blockers

The peripheral α-blockers, prazosin, terazosin, and doxazosin, undergo extensive hepatic metabolism, and their pharmacokinetics are not altered by the presence of renal insufficiency. Peripheral α-blocker use will occasionally be accompanied by orthostatic hypotension, and these drugs should be given cautiously in patients so prone, such as the elderly *(54)*.

Use of α-adrenergic antagonists in the treatment of hypertension has been limited by their tendency to increase plasma volume; this pseudoresistance may be more evident at higher doses *(55)*. The peripheral α-blocker doxazosin has been associated with an excess of new-onset congestive heart failure, which may relate partly to its tendency to induce salt and water retention *(56)*.

β-*Blockers*

The BP-lowering effect of β-blockers is somewhat unpredictable in the elderly patient unless combined with a diuretic *(57)*, unlike the effects in the postmyocardial infarction circumstance, for which mortality and recurrent events are clearly favorably impacted *(58)*. The irregular response to β-blockers in the elderly likely relates to the hemodynamic mismatch caused by β-blockade. Many elderly patients exhibit a hemodynamic profile characterized by a low normal cardiac output and increased peripheral vascular resistance. Most β-blockers lower BP by additional reduction in cardiac output in association with an increase (or no change) in peripheral vascular resistance *(59)*.

The β-blockers differ pharmacologically on the basis of lipid solubility, cardioselectivity, and intrinsic sympathomimetic activity. In clinical practice, these differences may not affect antihypertensive efficacy or the side effect profile in a major away. The β-blocker pharmacodynamics do not substantially differ on the basis of age *(60)*.

The selection of a β-blocker for an elderly patient should also occur with some knowledge of the elimination characteristics of the drug as well as whether the compound has active metabolites *(61)*. β-Blockers such as acebutolol, atenolol, betaxolol, nadolol, and sotalol undergo significant degrees of renal clearance and are liable to accumulation in the elderly with compromised renal function *(51,60)*.

β-Blocker accumulation in a patient with chronic renal failure does not generally improve BP control because β-blockers have a flat dose–response curve; alternatively, β-blocker accumulation can be associated with more frequent side effects, such as fatigue and central nervous system effects. If such side effects occur, two options exist: to continue the offending β-blocker with empiric dose reduction or to convert to a hepatically cleared β-blocker and reassess both the response and side effects. The latter is generally the preferable approach.

Calcium Channel Blockers

CCBs are commonly used drugs in the elderly patient; this relates to the predictability of their BP-lowering response and their utility as antianginal agents. Dihydropyridine CCBs are not remarkably different in their ability to reduce BP in the elderly patient in comparison to nondihydropyridine CCBs, such as verapamil and diltiazem. Although it has been suggested that elderly hypertensives are more responsive to CCBs, this may not be an independent age-related effect. Responsiveness to CCBs during long-term treatment appears to be correlated directly with the starting BP and response to the initial dosage (62). Conduction system effects with verapamil do not have an obvious age difference (63).

The volume of distribution, protein binding, and plasma half-life of CCBs are fairly variable subject to subject among the elderly. However, these drugs do have a tendency to reach higher blood concentrations in the elderly compared to young individuals (64–66). Although CCB pharmacokinetics have a wide interindividual variability in the elderly, they typically have a delayed clearance and reach higher plasma concentrations. Consideration should be given to initiating therapy in the elderly at low doses with these compounds, particularly with dihydropyridine CCBs (63). The heart rate response to potent vasodilators, such as dihydropyridine CCBs, may be lacking; as a result, the drop in BP with these compounds can be significant, particularly with short-acting forms of these drugs. Nifedipine immediate-release dosage form use in elderly hypertensives has been associated with a nearly fourfold increased risk for all-cause mortality when compared to β-blockers, ACE inhibitors, or other classes of CCBs (67). The basis for this mortality difference is likely related to the manner in which BP was reduced.

CCB-related side effects have to be considered when these drugs are used in the elderly patient. Many elderly patients tend to be constipated, and this can be aggravated by verapamil. Also, CCBs can produce peripheral edema on a vasodilatory basis. This form of edema is more common in the elderly. Age is a determinant of edema in that interstitial tissue typically serves a barrier role to hydrostatically driven edema formation, and the counterbalancing nature (to prevent edema) of such tissue diminishes with age (68).

CONCLUSION

The aging process is characterized by numerous pathophysiological changes, with many of these alterations having the potential to modify drug handling or effect. In the individual patient, such changes are not easily determined other than for the measurement of renal function. The status of renal function can be fairly accurately approximated by an understanding of the relationship among muscle mass, serum creatinine, and level of renal function. To the extent that renal failure in the elderly decreases excretion of renally cleared compounds and such drug accumulation exaggerates the desired hemodynamic effect, then dose adjustment should occur; otherwise, dosing of cardiovascular medications for the elderly is fairly empiric and is driven by the need to reach specific goal BP values while minimizing concentration-dependent side effects.

REFERENCES

1. Demographics of aging in the United States. *Arch Dermatol* 2002;138:1427–1428.
2. Nolan L, O'Malley K. Prescribing in the elderly: I. Sensitivity of the elderly to adverse drug reactions. *J Am Geriatric Soc* 1988;36:142–149.
3. Mannesse CK, Derkx FH, de Ridder MA, et al. Contribution of adverse drug reactions to hospital admission of older patients. *Age Ageing* 2000;29:35–39.
4. Wu JH, Chang CS, Chen GH, et al. Felodipine does not increase the reflux episodes in patients with gastroesophageal reflux disease. *Hepatogastroenterology* 2000;47: 1328–1331.
5. Huilgol V, Evans J, Hellman RS, Soergel KH. Acute effect of clonidine on gastric emptying in patients with diabetic gastropathy and controls. *Aliment Pharmacol Ther* 2002;16:945–950.
6. Krevsky B, Maurer AH, Niewiarowski T, Cohen S. Effect of verapamil on human intestinal transit. *Dig Dis Sci* 1992;37:919–924.
7. Parviainen I, Rantala A, Ruokonen E, Tenhunen J, Takala J. Angiotensin converting enzyme inhibition has no effect on blood pressure and splanchnic perfusion after cardiac surgery. *J Crit Care* 1998;13:73–80.
8. Kincaid EH, Miller PR, Meredith JW, Chang MC. Enalaprilat improves gut perfusion in critically injured patients. *Shock* 1998;9:79–83.
9. Roskos KV, Maibach HI. Percutaneous absorption and age. Implications for therapy. *Drugs Aging* 1992;2:432–449.
10. Barry BW. Novel mechanisms and devices to enable successful transdermal drug delivery. *Eur J Pharm Sci* 2001;14:101–114.
11. Forbes G, Reina J. Adult lean body mass declines with age: some longitudinal observations. *Metabolism* 1970;19:653–663.
12. Vestal RE, McGuire EA, Tobin JD, et al. Aging and ethanol metabolism. *Clin Pharmacol Ther* 1977;21:343–354.
13. Ochs HR, Greenblatt DJ, Divoll M, et al. Diazepam kinetics in relation to age and sex. *Pharmacology* 1981;23:24–30.
14. Norris AH, Lundy T, Shock NW. Trends in selected indices of body composition in men between the ages of 30 and 80 years. *Ann NY Acad Sci* 1963;110:623–639.
15. Cheymol G, Poirier JM, Carrupt PA, et al. Pharmacokinetics of β-adrenoceptor blockers in obese and normal volunteers. *Br J Clin Pharmacol* 1997;43:563–570.
16. Grandison MK, Boudinot FD. Age-related changes in protein binding of drugs: implications for therapy. *Clin Pharmacokinet* 2000;38:271–290.
17. Sugioka N, Koyama H, Kawakubo M, et al. Age-dependent alteration of the serum-unbound fraction of nicardipine, a calcium-channel blocker, in man. *J Pharm Pharmacol* 1996;48:1327–1331.
18. Gilmore DA, Gal J, Gerber JG, Nies AS. Age and gender influence the stereoselective pharmacokinetics of propranolol. *J Pharmacol Exp Ther* 1992;261:1181–1186.
19. Andros E, Detmar-Hanna D, Suteparuk S, et al. The effect of aging on the pharmacokinetics and pharmacodynamics of prazosin. *Eur J Clin Pharmacol* 1996;50:41–46.
20. Wallace S, Whiting B, Runcie J. Factors affecting drug binding in plasma of elderly patients. *Br J Clin Pharmacol* 1976;3:327–330.
21. Wynne HA, Cope LH, Mutch E, et al. The effect of age on liver volume and apparent blood flow in healthy males. *Hepatology* 1989;9:297–301

22. Castleden CM, George CF. The effect of ageing on the hepatic clearance of propranolol. *Br J Clin Pharmacol* 1979:7:49–54.
23. Kelly JG, McGarry K, O'Malley K, O'Brien ET. Bioavailability of labetalol increases with age. *Br J Clin Pharmacol* 1982;14:304–305.
24. O'Mahony MS, Woodhouse KW. Age, environmental factors and drug metabolism. Pharmacol Ther 1994;61:279–287.
25. Sotamieni EA, Arranto AJ, Pelkonen O, et al. Age and cytochrome P450-linked drug metabolism in humans: an analysis of 2267 subjects with equal histopathological conditions. *Clin Pharmacol Ther* 1997;61:331–339.
26. Schmucker DL. Liver function and phase I drug metabolism in the elderly: a paradox. *Drugs Aging* 2001;18:837–851.
27. Schmucker DL. Aging and drug disposition: an update. *Pharmacol Rev* 1985;37: 133–148.
28. Muck W, Breuel HP, Kuhlmann J. The influence of age on the pharmacokinetics of nimodipine. *Int J Clin Pharmacol Ther* 1996;34:293–298.
29. Kelly JG, O'Malley K. Clinical pharmacokinetics of calcium antagonists. *Clin Pharmacokinet* 1992;22:416–433.
30. Robertson DRC, Walker DG, Renwick AG, George CF. Age-related changes in the pharmacokinetics and pharmacodynamics of nifedipine. *Br J Clin Pharmacol* 1988;25:297–305.
31. Meredith PA, Elliott HL, Ahmed JH, Reid JL. Age and the antihypertensive efficacy of verapamil: an integrated pharmacokinetic-pharmacodynamic approach. *J Hypertens* 1987;5(suppl 5):S219–S221.
32. Elliott HL, Meredith PA, Reid JL, Faulkner JK. A comparison of the disposition of single oral doses of amlodipine in young and elderly subjects. *J Cardiovasc Pharmacol* 1988;12 (suppl 7):S64–S66.
33. Edgar B, Lundborg P, Regardh CG. Clinical pharmacokinetics of felodipine: a summary. *Drugs* 1987;34(suppl 3):16–27.
34. Abernethy DR, Schwartz JB. Calcium-antagonist drugs. *N Engl J Med* 1999;341: 1447–1457.
35. Ellis PA, Cairns HS. Renal impairment in elderly patients with hypertension and diabetes. *Q J Med* 2001;94:261–265.
36. Lindeman RD, Tobin J, Shock NW. Longitudinal studies on the rate of decline of renal function with age. *J Am Geriatr Soc* 1985;33:278–285.
37. Landahl S, Aurell M, Jagenburg R. Glomerular filtration rate at the age of 70 and 75. *J Clin Exp Gerontol* 1982;3:29–45.
38. Sica DA. Kinetics of angiotensin converting enzyme inhibitors in renal failure. *J Cardiovasc Pharmacol* 1992;20(suppl 10):S13–S20.
39. Baum C, Kennedy D, Forbes M. Utilization of nonsteroidal anti-inflammatory drugs. *Arthritis Rheum* 1985;28:686–692.
40. Unworth J, Sturman S, Lunec J, et al. Renal impairment associated with nonsteroidal anti-inflammatory drugs. *Ann Rheum Dis* 1987;46:233–236.
41. Cockcroft DW, Gault MH. Prediction of creatinine clearance from serum creatinine. *Nephron* 1976;16:31–41.
42. Hammerlein A, Derendorf H, Lowenthal DT. Pharmacokinetic and pharmacodynamic changes in the elderly. Clinical implications. *Clin Pharmacokinet* 1998;35: 49–64.
43. Prevention of stroke by antihypertensive drug treatment in older persons with isolated systolic hypertension. Final results of the Systolic Hypertension in the Elderly Program (SHEP). SHEP Cooperative Research Group. *JAMA* 1991;265:3255–3264.
44. Epstein M, Hollenberg NK. Age as a determinant of renal sodium conservation in normal man. *J Lab Clin Med* 1976;87:411–417.

45. Phillips PA, Phil D, Rolls BJ, et al. Reduced thirst after water deprivation in healthy elderly men. *N Engl J Med* 1984;311:753–759.
46. Sharabi Y, Illan R, Kamari Y, et al. Diuretic induced hyponatremia in elderly hypertensive women. *J Hum Hypertens* 2002;16:631–635.
47. Kerremans AL, Tan Y, van Baars H, et al. Furosemide kinetics and dynamics in aged patients. *Clin Pharmacol Ther* 1983;34:181–189.
48. Tomlinson B. Optimal dosage of ACE inhibitors in older patients. *Drugs Aging* 1996;9:262–273.
49. Brown NJ, Vaughn DE. Angiotensin-converting enzyme inhibitors. *Circulation* 1998;97:1411–1420.
50. Weidmann P, De Myttenaere-Bursztein S, Maxwell M, et al. Effects of aging on plasma renin and aldosterone in normal man. *Kidney Int* 1975;8:325–333.
51. Williams BR, Kim J. Cardiovascular drug therapy in the elderly: theoretical and practical considerations. *Drugs Aging* 2003;20:445–463.
52. Schoolwerth A, Sica DA, Ballermann BJ, Wilcox CS. Renal considerations in angiotensin converting enzyme inhibitor therapy. A statement for healthcare professionals from the Council on the Kidney in Cardiovascular Disease and the Council for High Blood Pressure Research of the American Heart Association. *Circulation* 2001;104:1985–1991.
53. Sica DA. Renal handling of angiotensin receptor blockers: clinical relevance. *Curr Hypertens Rep* 2003:5:337–339.
54. Cleophas TJ, Marum R. Age-related decline in autonomic control of blood pressure. *Drugs Aging* 2003;20:313–319.
55. Bryson CL, Psaty BM. A review of the adverse effects of peripheral α-1 antagonists in hypertension therapy. *Curr Control Trials Cardiovasc Med.* 2002;3:7–13.
56. Sica DA. Doxazosin and congestive heart failure. *Congest Heart Fail* 2002;8:178–184.
57. Messerli FH, Grossman E, Goldbourt U. Are β-blockers efficacious as first-line therapy for hypertension in the elderly? A systematic review. *JAMA* 1998;279:1903–1907.
58. Di Bari M, Marchionni N, Pahor M. β-Blockers after acute myocardial infarction in elderly patients with diabetes mellitus: time to reassess. *Drugs Aging* 2003;20:13–22.
59. Man in't Veld AJ, Van Den Meiracker AH, Schalekamp MA. Do β-blockers really increase peripheral vascular resistance? *Am J Hypertens* 1988;1:91–96.
60. Sowinski K, Forrest A, Wilton J, et al. Effect of aging on atenolol pharmacokinetics and pharmacodynamics. *J Clin Pharmacol* 1995;35:807–814.
61. McCullough PA, Sandberg KR, Borzak S, et al. Benefits of aspirin and β-blockade after myocardial infarction in patients with chronic kidney disease. *Am Heart J* 2002;144:226–232.
62. Donnelly R, Elliott H. Factors influencing the response to calcium antagonists in elderly patients with hypertension and ischaemic heart disease. *Exp Gerontol* 1990;25:375–381.
63. Elliott H. Calcium antagonists in the treatment of hypertension and angina pectoris in the elderly. *J Cardiovasc Pharmacol* 1989;13(suppl 4):S12–S16.
64. Abernethy DR, Montamat SC. Acute and chronic studies of diltiazem in elderly vs young hypertensive patients. *Am J Cardiol* 1987;60:116I–120I.
65. Schwartz JB, Troconiz IF, Verotta D, et al. Aging effects on stereoselective pharmacokinetics and pharmacodynamics of verapamil. *J Pharmacol Exp Ther* 1993;265:690–698.
66. Robertson D, Waller A, Renwick C, et al. Age-related changes in the pharmacokinetics and pharmacodynamics of nifedipine. *Br J Clin Pharmacol* 1099;25:297–305.
67. Pahor M, Guralnik JM, Corti MC, et al. Long-term survival and use of antihypertensive medications in older persons. *J Am Geriatr Soc* 1995;43:1191–1197.

68. Fogari R, Malamani GD, Zoppi A, et al. Comparative effect of lercanidipine and nifedipine gastrointestinal therapeutic system on ankle volume and subcutaneous interstitial pressure in hypertensive patients: a double-blind, randomized, parallel-group study. *Curr Ther Res* 2000;61:850–862.

II EPIDEMIOLOGY AND TRIALS

5 Epidemiology of Hypertension in the Older Patient

William B. Kannel, MD, MPH and Peter W. F. Wilson, MD

CONTENTS

INTRODUCTION
HYPERTENSION PREVALENCE AND INCIDENCE
CARDIOVASCULAR IMPACT
COMPONENTS OF BLOOD PRESSURE
RISK STRATIFICATION
SPECIAL SUBGROUPS
PREVENTIVE IMPLICATIONS
SUMMARY AND CONCLUSIONS
REFERENCES

INTRODUCTION

Disease, disability, and death from cardiovascular disease (CVD) represent major problems in the elderly. As the elderly population continues to grow and constitute a larger proportion of the general population, the magnitude of the problem is expected to increase and to place a heavy burden on existing medical care resources. Heart disease and stroke continue to be the first and third leading causes of death in the United States, respectively. CVD becomes the leading cause of death by age 40 years, whereas in women this is delayed until age 70 years, accounting for the predominance of women in the elderly population (1).

From: *Clinical Hypertension and Vascular Diseases: Hypertension in the Elderly*
Edited by: L. M. Prisant © Humana Press Inc., Totowa, NJ

Table 1
Increment in Incidence of Atherosclerotic Cardiovascular Disease Events
by Age and Gender, 44-Year Follow-Up Framingham Study[a]

| | Age-adjusted average annual incidence per 1000 | | | | | | | | | |
| | All CVD | | CHD | | Stroke | | CHF | | PAD | |
Age, years	Men	Women	Men	Women	Men	Women	Men	Women	Men	Women
35–64	17	9	12	5	2	2	2	1	3	2
65–94	44	30	27	16	13	11	12	9	8	5
Risk ratio										
>65/<65	2.6	3.3	2.3	3.2	6.5	5.5	6.0	9.0	2.7	2.5

[a]Includes 20-year follow-up of Framingham Offspring cohort.
CHD, coronary heart disease; CHF, congestive heart failure; CVD, cardiovascular disease; PAD, peripheral artery disease.

The incidence of atherosclerotic CVD triples from age 35–64 to age 65–94 years (Table 1). The increments are greatest for heart failure and stroke, but coronary disease is the most common and lethal hazard, equaling in incidence all the other atherosclerotic CVD outcomes combined. The absolute risk for CVD is lower in women than men, but the risk ratio imposed by age is just as great for women as for men, and there is a steep increase in CVD incidence with advancing age. This increase is largely attributable to a greater burden of the major risk factors, longer exposure to them, and a diminished ability to cope with them in advanced age. The proportion of coronary events manifesting as myocardial infarction (MI) increases with age, and one in three of these heart attacks goes unrecognized (2).

Framingham Study data indicated that most elderly persons do not die at the time of their first CVD event, but live on, often with debilitating illness and poor quality of life. Over the age of 65 years, three-fourths who have a heart attack survive with disability (3). Most risk factors increase with age and more so in women than men. The risk factors that predispose to CVD in the elderly are the same as those that operate in the middle aged (4). These need to be measured and treated to protect the elderly from their high rate of CVD. However, there is unjustified pessimism about the efficacy of preventive measures for the elderly. Some doubt that it is possible to mitigate the effect of prolonged exposure to CVD risk factors beginning late in life or to do so without inducing intolerable side effects.

HYPERTENSION PREVALENCE AND INCIDENCE

The blood pressure (BP) of adults in Western society increases with age. Systolic pressure continues to rise after the diastolic peaks and then declines, resulting in a widening pulse pressure (PP) and isolated systolic hypertension in older persons. This variety of hypertension, resulting from the disproportionate rise in systolic blood pressure (SBP) induced by diminished arterial compliance, comprises 60% of the hypertension in the elderly.

National data in the United States indicates a rise in the prevalence of hypertension (140/90 mmHg) from 4% under age 30 years to 65% over age 80 years *(5)*. Each year, about 2 million people add to the pool of hypertensive people needing treatment. In the Framingham Study cohort, 25 to 50% of normotensive persons developed stage 2 or greater hypertension during 26 years of surveillance *(6)*. Those with normal pressures developed hypertension at only half the rate of those with high-normal pressure *(7)*. Persons with a high-normal diastolic pressure are three times more likely to progress to hypertension than those with optimum diastolic blood pressure (DBP).

Recent Framingham Study data indicated a stepwise increase in hypertension incidence going from optimum ($\leq$120/80) to normal (120/ 80–129/84) to high normal (130/85–139/89). Of the elderly with a high-normal BP, 50% developed hypertension, a rate 5.5 times that of persons with optimum BP (Table 2). Older persons were more likely to progress to hypertension within 4 years than younger ones, with similar rates in men and women *(8)*.

Multivariable analysis indicates that baseline body mass index and weight gain are important determinants of future hypertension, and that systolic rather than diastolic baseline BP is the major determinant of progression. The Framingham Study suggested that persons with normal or high-normal BP return for follow-up BP checkups at 5-year intervals *(9)*. In the Framingham Study, 87% of elderly men and women with untreated high BP had mild-to-moderate hypertension. The effects of high-normal BP and mild-to-moderate BP elevations both on the development of more severe forms of hypertension and on damage to target organs are not fully appreciated.

CARDIOVASCULAR IMPACT

Because of its high prevalence and sustained impact in advanced age, hypertension is a dominant contributor to CVD in the elderly. Data from the Framingham Study indicated that in men about 30% of atherosclerotic CVD in the population, including those on treatment, is attributable

Table 2
4-Year Hypertension Incidence Rate by Baseline Blood Pressure Category,
Subjects Aged 65–94 Years, Framingham Study

Baseline Blood pressure category	4-year rate, %	Odds ratio
Optimum (<120/80 mmHg)	16.0 (12.0–20.9)	Referent
Normal (120–129/80–84 mmHg)	25.5 (20.4–31.4)	2.0 (1.4–2.7)
High normal (130–139/85–89 mmHg)	49.5 (42.6–56.4)	5.5 (4.0–7.4)

Adjusted for gender, age, body mass index, and baseline systolic and diastolic blood pressure. (From ref. 8.)

to all grades of "hypertension" (Table 3). As much as 15%, or half this contribution, is attributable to BPs of 140–179/90–109 mmHg. In women, almost one-fifth of the 26% contribution comes from this level of elevated BP. It is noteworthy that about one-third of the CVD in men and 65% of that in women is arising from persons in the population on treatment, reflecting inadequate BP control. For an individual, the absolute risk and odds ratio of developing CVD increase sharply with the degree of hypertension. On a population basis, most CVD occurs in persons with moderate hypertension.

Hypertension is a powerful predisposing condition for the development of all the major clinical manifestations of atherosclerotic CVD that commonly afflicts the elderly, including coronary disease, stroke, peripheral artery disease (PAD), and heart failure (Table 4). The hypertensive CVD risk ratios are greatest for stroke and heart failure, but coronary disease is the most common and lethal hazard. The decrease in CVD risk ratio for hypertension that occurs with advancing age is offset by the doubled CVD incidence in the elderly compared to the middle aged. The CVD mortality rate of elderly hypertensive persons is triple that of normotensive persons of the same age. Hypertension ranks high among the major established correctable risk factors for CVD in the elderly, outranking cholesterol and cigarette smoking and rivaling diabetes in absolute and relative risk. Unrecognized MIs, which are particularly common in the elderly, occur more frequently in those who are hypertensive. About 35% of all MIs in hypertensive men and 49% in hypertensive women go unrecognized (10).

Left ventricular hypertrophy (LVH) is most often a consequence of long-standing or severe hypertension in the elderly. It is no longer accepted that LVH is an incidental compensatory feature of hypertension that helps the heart cope with an increased pressure load. LVH

Table 3
Hypertensive Population Attributable Cardiovascular Disease Risk
by JNC V Blood Pressure Status, Framingham Study Subjects Aged 65–94 Years

Hypertensive	Exposed, %		Odds ratio		Attributable risk, %	
Status (mmHg)	Men	Women	Men	Women	Men	Women
Normal (130/85)	23	19	Referent	Referent	—	—
High normal (130–139/85–89)	17	13	1.2	1.1	2.1	0.6
Stage 1 (140–159/90–99)	24	21	1.5	1.3	7.9	4.8
Stage 2 (160–179/100–109)	9	10	2.1	1.2	7.1	1.3
Stage 3 (180–210/110–120)	3	4	2.6	1.9	3.1	2.8
Stage 4 (<210/120)	2	1	4.3	—	1.0	0.02
On high blood pressure treatment	22	32	1.7	1.7	10.4	17.0

Adapted from ref. 36.

Table 4
Relation of Hypertension to Specified Cardiovascular Disease Outcomes
in the Elderly, Framingham Study Subjects Aged 65–94 Years,
36-Year Follow-up

	Biennial Age Adjusted			
	Rate per 1000		Risk ratio[a]	
Cardiovascular disease outcome	Men	Women	Men	Women
Coronary disease	72.6	44.2	1.6	1.9
Stroke	36.0	38.8	1.9	2.3
Peripheral artery disease	16.5	9.6	1.6	2.0
Heart failure	33.0	23.5	1.9	1.9

[a]Compared to normal blood pressure.
Note. All estimates statistically significant, $p < 0.0001$, except for peripheral artery disease, $p < 0.03$.

discerned by chest film, echocardiogram, or electrocardiogram (ECG) is an ominous harbinger of CVD morbidity and mortality in the elderly. The risk of CVD events such as heart failure, MI, and stroke increase an additional two- to threefold after hypertension induces LVH (Table 5).

A population-based study of persons with essential hypertension added to the data quantifying the influence of LVH as a powerful independent predictor of CVD morbidity (11). For each 39-g increase in left ventricular mass per square meter of body surface area, there is a 40%

Table 5

Risk of Cardiovascular Events in Hypertensive Subjects
(Blood Pressure >160/95 mmHg) by Electrocardiographic Left Ventricular
Hypertrophy Status, 32-Year Follow-Up Framingham Study

| | Age-adjusted biennial rate per 1000 | | | |
| | Age 35–64 years | | Age 65–94 years | |
ECG LVH	Men	Women	Men	Women
None	58	31	128	67
Voltage only	52	41	162	114
Voltage plus S-T & T	198*	125*	335*	205*

*$p < 0.01$. Cardiovascular events: coronary heart disease, stroke, and peripheral artery disease.

ECG, electrocardiographic; LVH, left ventricular hypertrophy.

increase in CVD events. LVH is a prominent feature of hypertensive heart failure in the elderly. About 20% of heart failure cases have ECG LVH, and 60 to 70% exhibit it on the more sensitive echocardiogram. Adjusted for age and other risk factors, it increases hypertensive heart failure risk an additional two- to threefold *(12)*.

Altered diastolic filling and detrimental structural remodeling occur in isolated systolic hypertension. The increased pulsatile load imposed by isolated systolic hypertension plays a major role in LVH and, eventually, heart failure. Cardiac hypertrophy is predictable from high PP and elevated SBP accompanied by low DBP *(13,14)*. There is also evidence that LVH is associated with the development of hypertension, suggesting common factors promote both outcomes. Altered regulation of renin–angiotensin and catecholamines has been proposed as such an antecedent *(15–17)*.

BP, not categorically defined hypertension, promotes CVD. CVD risk increases incrementally with the BP at all ages, including the elderly. No clear boundary delineates normal from pathological BP. The continuous and graded relationship between CVD and BP extends into what is regarded as high-normal and even normal BP.

CVD risk predictions are traditionally based on current BP. The Framingham Study assessed the incremental impact of long-term antecedent BP on the risk for ischemic stroke *(18)*. Antecedent BP contributed significantly to the future risk of such strokes even after adjusting for current BP level at age 70 years. This investigation indicated that midlife BP continues to affect future stroke risk over long periods.

COMPONENTS OF BLOOD PRESSURE

For most of the 20th century, medical research and clinical practice were preoccupied with the diastolic component of BP as the chief hazard of hypertension *(19)*. The focus has finally shifted to the systolic and PP as of paramount importance. DBP rises with peripheral arterial resistance and falls as the central arterial circulation stiffens and the relative contributions of these opposing forces determine the PP.

When assessed in the Framingham Study, increments in PP at most systolic pressures were associated with greater risk of coronary disease than increments in systolic pressure at given PPs *(20)*. Despite the high correlation of PP with SBP, the PP appears to predominate as a predictor of coronary disease, especially in the elderly. Increased pulsatile load plays a major role in large artery atherosclerosis, vascular remodeling of small resistance arteries, LVH, and eventually heart failure.

PP and systolic pressure have great relevance in the elderly because the importance of diastolic pressure wanes and that of SBP increases as a predictor of coronary disease. A Framingham Study investigation of the impact of components of BP indicated that with increasing age there is a shift from diastolic to systolic and then to PP as the dominant predictor of coronary disease *(21)*. Most, but not all, investigations of the influence components of BP on CVD agree with the Framingham Study findings on the importance of PP in the elderly *(22–24)*. Nevertheless, it is clear that CVD morbidity and mortality increase with the PP (Table 6).

The classification of geriatric hypertension overemphasizes peripheral vascular resistance and underestimates the influence of large artery stiffness. It is a mistake to rely on the DBP to evaluate the need for treatment in persons with elevated SBP. Recent analysis of Framingham Study data was undertaken to determine the relative roles of SBP and DBP in determining Sixth Report of the Joint National Committee on the Prevention, Detection, Evaluation, and Treatment of High Blood Pressure (JNC 6) BP stage and eligibility for treatment. Examination of the effect of disparate SBP and DBP on staging and eligibility for treatment showed that SBP is more accurate in classifying persons as hypertensive, high-normal, or normal *(25)*. SBP alone correctly classified 95% of persons aged 60 years or older.

RISK STRATIFICATION

Hypertension per se may induce encephalopathy, renal insufficiency, and acute heart failure; its promotion of accelerated atherogenesis is more complex, involving lipid atherogenesis, thrombogenesis, insulin resistance, and endothelial dysfunction. Evaluation of the hypertensive

Table 6
Cardiovascular Morbidity and Mortality by Pulse Pressure (PP),
Rate per 1000 Person-Years, Tertile of PP

Event	PP 1 (n − 735)	PP 2 (n = 726)	PP 3 (n = 746)	Risk ratio: PP3/PP1
Myocardial infarction	3.5	2.9	7.5	2.8 (1.1–4.2)
Stroke	1.2	2.3	2.9	2.5 (0.8–7.7)
Cardiovascular disease	5.2	6.6	13.6	2.6 (1.6–4.4)
Cardiovascular disease deaths	1.7	4.3	7.5	4.3 (1.9–9.6)

PP 1 < 46 mmHg; PP 2 = 47–62 mmHg; PP 3 > 63 mmHg. (From ref. 37.)

hazard for development of atherosclerotic CVD requires consideration of other metabolically linked risk factors. Despite the 1.5- to 2.0-fold increased risk associated with moderate (stages 1 and 2) hypertension, the absolute hazard is modest, making it necessary to treat many such persons to prevent one case of CVD.

Efficient selection for aggressive treatment with medication requires multivariable global risk assessment of the urgency for treatment. Also, the goal of therapy should be to improve the global risk profile as well as the BP. Targeted therapy based on a composite risk profile improves the cost–benefit ratio of antihypertensive therapy.

Hypertension occurs in isolation in only 20% of patients. Clusters of three or more additional risk factors occur at four times the rate expected by chance (26). Insulin resistance, induced by visceral adiposity and weight gain, promotes this cluster of associated risk factors. Hypertension in the elderly is often a consequence of loss of arterial compliance and an insulin-resistance syndrome characterized by abdominal obesity, hypertension, glucose intolerance, and dyslipidemia (27).

Risk of CVD in older persons with hypertension varies widely, depending on the associated burden of other risk factors. Substantial risk in hypertensive elderly with mild-to-moderate hypertension is concentrated in those with coexistent dyslipidemia, diabetes, and left ventricular hypertrophy. For stroke, the most feared hazard of hypertension in the elderly, risk varies over a wide range and reaches substantial proportions when accompanied by diabetes, LVH, atrial fibrillation, and coronary disease or heart failure (Fig. 1).

Hypertensive elderly commonly have target organ damage such as LVH, impaired renal function, silent MI, strokes, transient ischemic attacks, retinopathy, or PAD. At least 60% of older men and 50% of elderly women with hypertension in the Framingham Study had one or more of these conditions.

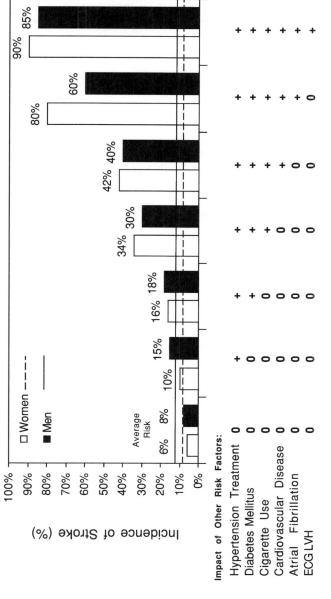

Fig. 1. Probability of a stroke (%) during 10 years in men and women aged 70 years, systolic blood pressure 160 mmHg. (Modified from ref. 38.)

Instruments for the global assessment of multivariable risk of coronary disease, stroke, PAD, and heart failure have been produced using Framingham Study data *(28)*. This makes it convenient to estimate the global risk of hypertensive elderly patients using ordinary office procedures and standard laboratory tests.

SPECIAL SUBGROUPS

Diabetics

Type 2 diabetes is one of the most common chronic diseases in the United States that increased in older persons from 8.9% in 1976–1980 (Second National Health and Nutrition Examination Survey [NHANES II]) to 12.3% in (NHANES III) in 1988–1994. Hypertension is twice as common in diabetics as it is in persons the same age without diabetes, and both are associated with an increased risk of atherosclerotic CVD and chronic renal failure. In patients with diabetes, as much as 75% of CVD, including renal impairment, is attributable to accompanying hypertension. The presence of diabetes further enhances the hypertensive propensity to develop LVH.

End-Stage Renal Disease

Hypertension directly promotes development of end-stage renal disease, and it accelerates decline in renal function from other kidney disease *(29)*. Early subclinical renal dysfunction in hypertensive persons is readily detected by testing for microalbuminuria, an abnormality that is reported in 10 to 25% of hypertensive persons *(30)*. Proteinuria is also an indicator of increased CVD risk in persons with hypertension. Elderly hypertensive persons with diabetes or renal dysfunction are at exceptionally high risk for CVD, warranting aggressive antihypertensive therapy.

PREVENTIVE IMPLICATIONS

Although the onset and progression of atherosclerotic CVD and renal disease are related to chronic hypertension, the pathophysiology is complex and requires assessment of coexisting atherogenic risk factors. Global risk assessment to estimate the multivariable risk is required to target candidates efficiently for aggressive antihypertensive therapy. The most recent update of the JNC guidelines (JNC 7) emphasizes that elevated BP is only one of many risk factors predisposing hypertensive persons to CVD. They argue that the goal of therapy is not only to reduce the BP, but also to primarily lower the risk of cardiovascular events *(31)*.

The JNC 7 guidelines in concert with epidemiological data emphasize the need to be aware of the hazards of even high-normal elevations of BP (designated prehyper-tensive) and the dangers of isolated systolic hypertension in the elderly.

The report also recommends focusing more attention on the absolute risk. It further specifies that some patients need their BPs reduced to below 140/90 mmHg, particularly if they have heart failure, diabetes, or renal insufficiency. It recommends that thiazide should be used either alone or in combination with drugs from other classes for most patients with uncomplicated hypertension. The report signifies certain high-risk conditions as compelling indications for the use of other antihypertensive drugs, such as angiotensin-converting enzyme inhibitors, angiotensin-receptor blockers, β-blockers, and calcium channel blockers. These considerations are particularly relevant for elderly hypertensive patients. They point out that most patients will require two or more medications to achieve the recommended goal of 140/90 mmHg or less than 130/80 mmHg for those with diabetes or renal disease.

Fear of reducing the BP in the elderly was shown to be ill founded by major trials investigating the efficacy of antihypertensive therapy for isolated systolic hypertension *(32,33)*. Hypertension therapy is safe, well tolerated, and efficacious for CVD without any penalty of overall mortality. Worldwide statistics indicate the need for more aggressive BP control because studies found that, in clinical practice, not enough effort is made to reach recommended target BP goals. Despite the epidemiological and trial evidence indicating the importance of systolic hypertension, surveys showed that DBP and not SBP guides most treatment decisions, particularly in older patients *(34,35)*. The elderly deserve greater effort because clinical data indicate that equivalent BP reduction provides greater benefit in the elderly. Vigorous BP control is merited, particularly for diabetic and proteinuric hypertensive patients, for whom tight control of BP has been particularly efficacious.

Data suggested that more attention needs to be given to SBP, and PP may have to be controlled in the older hypertensive person. Information now available makes choices of therapy and indications for treatment more complex. The variety of antihypertensive agents for monotherapy and combination therapy has increased, and there is controversy about first-choice agents and whether treatment should be tailored to each patient's CVD risk profile. Pharmacotherapy now includes recommendations for low-dose combination therapy, and there is concern about the cost of lifelong therapy, with the more expensive agents shown to be particularly beneficial.

SUMMARY AND CONCLUSIONS

In the elderly, the predominant variety of hypertension, resulting from a disproportionate rise in systolic compared to diastolic pressure with advancing age, is isolated systolic hypertension. This is too often regarded as an incidental feature of advancing age. There is no justification for the emphasis on the diastolic component of the BP in evaluation and treatment of hypertension in the elderly. The rise in BP with advancing age is no longer considered inevitable, necessary, or normal. The focus on DBP was based on unfounded concepts reinforced by clinical trials that arbitrarily based selection for inclusion and treatment goals on the diastolic pressure. Population-based epidemiological data and even data from clinical trials using diastolic pressure entry criteria and goals for therapy consistently show a greater impact of systolic than diastolic pressure in the elderly.

Of particular importance in older persons is the recognition and treatment of isolated systolic hypertension and widened PP. Reliance on the DBP to determine the urgency for treatment in older persons with elevated BP is imprudent. Elevated SBP exerts a continuous graded influence on CVD occurrence, so that the concept of normal BP in the elderly has changed from that which is usual to that which confers the greatest freedom from CVD. Most CVD events in elderly hypertensive persons occur in those with only modest elevations of BP, making it important to select high-risk candidates for aggressive treatment by global risk assessment.

Hypertension in the elderly seldom occurs in isolation from other risk factors or associated target organ damage. Hypertension is best regarded as one component of a CVD multivariable risk profile comprised of metabolically linked risk factors because the hazard varies widely, contingent on the associated burden of risk factors. Epidemiological and trial data indicate that more aggressive therapy is needed for high-risk elderly hypertensive persons who have diabetes, left ventricular hypertrophy, or evidence of renal involvement.

Despite the demonstration of the efficacy of treating systolic hypertension in the elderly, poor BP control is overwhelmingly caused by lack of reduction of the SBP. The benefit of treating isolated systolic hypertension, and by inference PP, is established, but it is not clear whether the benefit derives more from the reduction of the SBP or narrowing of the widened PP.

ACKNOWLEDGMENT

Framingham Study research is supported by the National Institutes of Health/National Heart, Lung, and Blood Institute (N01-HC-25195) and the Visiting Scientist Program, which is supported by Servier Amerique.

REFERENCES

1. National Institutes of Health and National Heart, Lung, and Blood Institute. Chartbook on Cardiovascular, Lung and Blood Disease. Washington, DC: US Dept of Health and Human Services, Public Health Services.
2. Kannel WB, Abbott RD. Incidence and prognosis of unrecognized myocardial infarctions: An update from the Framingham Study. *N Engl J Med* 1984;34:1144–1147.
3. Kannel WB, Wolf PA, Garrison RJ. The Framingham Study, Section 34: Some Risk Factors Related to the Incidence of Cardiovascular Disease and Death Using Pooled Repeated Biennial Measurements; Framingham Heart Study, 30-year Follow-up. Bethesda, MD: National Heart, Lung, and Blood Institute; 1987. NIH Publication 87-2703.
4. Kannel WB, D'Agostino RB. The importance of cardiovascular risk factors in the elderly. *Am J Geriatr Cardiol* 1995;2:10–23.
5. Centers for Disease Control and Prevention. National Center for Health Statistics Third National Health and Nutrition Examination Survey. 1988–1991.
6. Dannenberg AL, Garrison RJ, Kannel WB. Incidence of hypertension in the Framingham Study. *Am J Public Health* 1988;78:676–679.
7. Leitschuh M, Cupples LA, Kannel WB, et al. High-normal blood pressure progression to hypertension in the Framingham Heart Study. *Hypertension* 1991;17:22–27.
8. Vasan RS, Larson MG, Leip EC, Kannel WB, Levy D. Assessment of frequency of progression to hypertension in non-hypertensive participants in the Framingham Heart Study: a cohort study. *Lancet* 2001;358:1682–1686.
9. Wood D, DeBacker G, Faergeman O, Graham I, Mancia G, Pyorala K. Prevention of coronary heart disease in clinical practice: summary of recommendations of the second joint task force of European and other societies on coronary prevention. *J Hypertens* 1998;16:1407–1414.
10. Kannel WB, Dannenberg AL, Abbott RD. Unrecognized myocardial infarction and hypertension: the Framingham Study. *Am Heart J* 1985;109:581–585.
11. Verdecchia P, Carini G, Circo A, et al. Left ventricular mass and cardiovascular morbidity in essential hypertension. The MAVI Study. *J Am Coll Cardiol* 2001;38:1829–1835.
12. Kannel WB. Vital epidemiologic clues in heart failure. *J Clin Epidemiol* 2000;53:229–235.
13. Pannier B, Brunel P, Aroussey WE, et al. Pulse pressure and echocardiographic findings in essential hypertension. *J Hypertens* 1989;7:127–132.
14. Garden JM, Gottdiener JS, Wong ND, et al. Left ventricular mass in the elderly. The Cardiovascular Health Study. *Hypertension* 1997;29:1095–1103.
15. Post W, Larson MG, Levy D. Impact of left ventricular structure on the incidence of hypertension. The Framingham Heart Study. *Circulation* 1994;90:179–185.

16. Davidman M, Opsahl J. Mechanisms of elevated blood pressure in human essential hypertension. Med Clin North Am 1984;68:301–320.

17. Hachamovich R, Sonnenblick EH, Strom JA, Frishman WH. Left ventricular hypertrophy in hypertension, and the effects of antihypertensive drug therapy. Curr Probl Cardiol 1988;13:375–421.

18. Seshardri S, Wolf PA, Beiser A, et al. Elevated mid-life blood pressure increases stroke risk in elderly persons. The Framingham Study. Arch Intern Med 2001;161: 2343–2350.

19. Rutan G, McDonald RH, Kuller LH. A historical perspective of systolic vs diastolic blood pressure from an epidemiological and clinical trial viewpoint. J Clin Epidemiol 1989;42:663–673.

20. Franklin SS, Kahn SA, Wong ND, Larson MG, Levy D. Is pulse pressure useful for predicting coronary disease? The Framingham Heart Study. Circulation 1999;100: 253–360.

21. Franklin SS, Larson MG, Kahn SA, et al.. Does the relation of blood pressure to coronary heart disease change with aging? Circulation 2001;103:1245–1249.

22. Madhaven S, Ooi WL, Cohen H, Alderman MH. Relation of pulse pressure and blood pressure reduction to the incidence of myocardial infarction. Hypertension 1994;23:395–401.

23. Chae CU, Pfeffer MA, Glynn RJ, Mitchell GF, Taylor JO, Hennekens CH. Increased pulse pressure and risk of heart failure in the elderly. JAMA 1999;281:634–639.

24. Psaty BM, Furberg CD, Kuller LH, et al. Association between blood pressure level and the risk of myocardial infarction, stroke and total mortality. The Cardiovascular Health Study. Arch Intern Med 2001;161:1183–1192.

25. Lloyd-Jones DM, Evans JC, Larson MG, O'Donnel CJ, Levy D. Differential impact of systolic and diastolic blood pressure on JNC-VI staging. Hypertension 1999;34:381–385.

26. Kannel WB, Wilson PWF, Silbershatz H. D'Agostino RB. Epidemiology of risk factor clustering in elevated blood pressure. In: Gotto AM, Lenfant C, Paoletti R, Eds. Multiple Risk Factors in Cardiovascular Disease. Dordrecht, The Netherlands: Kluwer Academic Publishers and Fondazione Giovanni Lorenzini; 1998:325–333.

27. Reaven GM. Insulin resistance, hyperinsulinemia, and hypertriglyceridemia in the etiology clinical course of hypertension. Am J Med 1991;90:7S–12S.

28. Anderson KM, Odell PM, Wilson PWF, Kannel WB. Cardiovascular disease risk profiles. Am Heart J 1990;121:293–298.

29. Moore MA, Epstein M, Agoda L, Dwarkin LD. Current strategies for management of hypertensive renal disease. Arch Intern Med 1999;159:23–28.

30. Mimran A. Microalbuminuria in essential hypertension. Clin Exp Hypertens 1997;19:23–28.

31. The Seventh Report of the Joint National Committee on Prevention, Detection, Evaluation and Treatment of High Blood Pressure JNC 7. JAMA 2003;289:2560–2572.

32. SHEP Cooperative Research Group. Prevention of stroke by antihypertensive drug treatment in older persons with isolated systolic hypertension. JAMA 1991;265: 3255–3264.

33. Staessen JA, Fagard R, Thijs L, et al. Randomized double blind comparison of placebo and active treatment for older patients with isolated systolic hypertension. Lancet 1997;350:757–764.

34. Berlowitz DR, Ash AS, Hickey EC, et al. Inadequate management of blood pressure in a hypertensive population. N Engl J Med 1998;339:1957–1963.

35. Coppola WG, Whincup PH, Walker M, Ebrahim S. Identification and management of stroke risk in older people: a national survey of current practice in primary care. J Hum Hypertens 1997;11:185–191.
36. Kannel WB. Prospects for prevention of cardiovascular disease in the elderly. Prev Cardiol 1998;1;32–39.
37. Madhavan S, Ooi WL, Cohen H, Alderman MH. Relation of pulse pressure and blood pressure reduction to the incidence of myocardial infarction. Hypertension 1994;23:395–401.
38. Wolf PA, D'Agostino RB, Belanger AJ, Kannel WB. Probability of stroke: a risk profile from the Framingham study. Stroke 1991;22:312–318.

6 Nonpharmacological Trials in the Older Hypertensive Patient

L. Michael Prisant, MD, FACC, FACP and Dean U. Harrell, MD

INTRODUCTION

Lifestyle modification (Table 1) is recommended for adults with prehypertension (120–139/80–89 mmHg) for the primary prevention of hypertension (1). However, lifestyle changes are also adjunctive to antihypertensive drug therapy (2,3). The National High Blood Pressure Education Program Working Group included reduced alcohol intake, tobacco abstinence, reduction of saturated fat, and adequate dietary intake of potassium, calcium, and magnesium as nonpharmacological modalities in the elderly (4).

From: *Clinical Hypertension and Vascular Diseases: Hypertension in the Elderly*
Edited by: L. M. Prisant © Humana Press Inc., Totowa, NJ

Table 1
Lifestyle Modification for the Prevention and Treatment of Hypertension

Intervention	Goal	Systolic blood pressure change
Aerobic activity	30 minutes per day	4 to 9 mmHg
Alcohol consumption	30 mL (men)[a] 15 mL (women)[a]	2 to 4 mmHg
Dietary Approaches to Stop Hypertension diet	Increase fruits, low-fat dairy foods, and vegetables; reduce total and saturated fats	8 to 14 mmHg
Sodium restriction	<100 mmol per day[b]	2 to 8 mmHg
Weight reduction	18.5–24.9 kg/m^2	5 to 20 mmHg per10 kg

[a]30 mL (1 oz) ethanol is 24 oz beer, 10 oz wine, and 2 oz 100-proof whiskey.
[b]100 mmol sodium = 2.4 g sodium or 6 g NaCl.

These guidelines are often repeated, but are there data for managing older patients with nondrug therapy? Will older patients implement this approach to treatment, and will nonpharmacological therapy be effective? Surprisingly, there are not many nonpharmacological trials that have been conducted in the elderly (5–7).

EARLY STUDIES

Recognizing the lack of data, Applegate and colleagues conducted a randomized, controlled trial (RCTs) to reduce blood pressure (BP) in older patients with mild hypertension (8). Men and women aged 60 to 85 years were screened. The requirements for enrollment included a diastolic blood pressure (DBP) from 85 to 100 mmHg, a weight 115% or more of ideal body weight, a Folstein (Mini-Mental Status Exam) score of 22 or more, suitable vision, and ample physical health. Antihypertensive medications were discontinued. The 47 subjects received nondrug therapy (n = 21) or no treatment (n = 26). Treatment assignment was blinded to the personnel measuring BP. The intervention group, through individual and group counseling, was instructed to restrict daily sodium intake to 1400 mg, reduce weight 4.5 kg, reduce caloric intake (1200 calories per day for women and 1500 calories per day for men), and increase physical activity by walking 30 minutes 4 days a week.

Subjects were evaluated monthly for 6 months after randomization. BP and weight were measured at each visit. Urine sodium was collected over 24 hours at baseline and at 2, 3, and 6 months. As shown in Fig. 1,

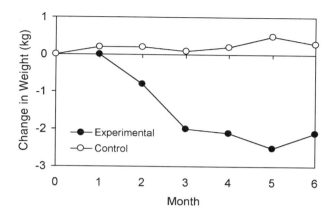

Fig. 1. Randomized trial of older hypertensives: weight outcomes. The experimental group lost 2.1 kg more than the control group ($p = 0.0009$). (Data from ref. *8*.)

weight increased in the control group and decreased in the experimental group by 2.1 kg ($p = 0.0009$). There was no significant difference in the change in sodium excretion between treatment groups, although each group declined. There was a significant reduction in systolic blood pressure (SBP; $p = 0.02$) and DBP ($p = 0.003$) in the lifestyle intervention group (Fig. 2). Participation in the counseling sessions ranged from 71 to 86%. This study supported the potential for a large trial.

SODIUM RESTRICTION

The Rotterdam Study, a population-based study to assess diseases of aging, assessed 1006 men and women older than 55 years without hypertension or treatment with antihypertensive drugs *(9)*. An overnight urine collection was performed and analyzed for sodium and potassium. An independent inverse relationship was observed between urine potassium and SBP and DBP. After adjustment for urinary potassium excretion, urine sodium was positively correlated with SBP. The Intersalt trial and a meta-analysis suggested that sodium restriction might reduce BP in the elderly *(10,11)*.

In a randomized, placebo-controlled, double-blind study, seven elderly men in an independent-living health care facility received either 43 or 175 mmol sodium per day for 4 weeks and then received the alternative intervention *(12)*. Their average age was 85 years, and the entry BP was 140–180/80–95 mmHg. Single-blind, low-sodium periods of 4 weeks preceded and followed the 8-week double-blind crossover phase

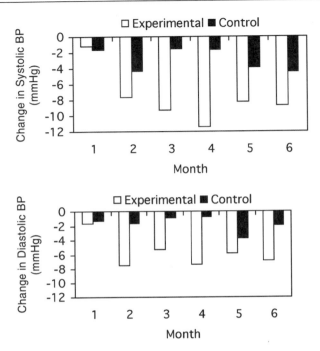

Fig. 2. Randomized trial of older hypertensives: change in blood pressure. The experimental group had a greater reduction in blood pressure of –4.2/–4.9 mmHg more than the control group ($p = 0.02$ for systolic and $p = 0.003$ for diastolic). (Data from ref. 8.)

of the study. There was a decrease in BP on the low-sodium diet (–11.0/ –8.9 mmHg). Only the change in DBP was significant ($p < 0.01$).

A double-blind, randomized, placebo-controlled, crossover trial was conducted in 17 white hypertensive subjects (13). Antihypertensive medications were discontinued for 4 weeks. All subjects met with a dietitian to achieve a daily sodium intake of 80 to 100 mmol over the 14 weeks of investigation. After a 4-week placebo run-in period, subjects received 80 mmol sodium chloride or placebo for 5 weeks and subsequently were crossed over to the alternative strategy. After each of the treatment periods, 24-hour ambulatory BP was performed. Supine clinic SBP was 8 mmHg higher in the high-sodium group ($p < 0.05$). However, there was no difference in the mean 24-hour ambulatory ($n = 16$) SBP or DBP for low- vs high-sodium treatment groups despite increased urinary sodium excretion and lower peripheral renin activity and plasma aldosterone in the high-sodium group.

An additional analysis separated subjects into salt-sensitive ($n = 6$) and salt-resistant groups ($n = 16$) based on a mean 24-hour ambulatory SBP decline of 5 mmHg or greater while on the low-sodium diet *(14)*. During the sodium-restricted period, renin was lower among the salt-sensitive group compared to the salt-resistant group (0.8 vs 1.9 ng/mL per hour, $p = 0.05$). However, there was no difference in lipid parameters and calcium, phosphorus, parathyroid hormone, glucose, creatinine, and urine albumin levels. Also, orthostatic changes were not more common among salt-sensitive subjects.

Using a double-blind, randomized, crossover design, 47 untreated older persons were given 120 mmol sodium or placebo for 4 weeks after a lead-in period on their usual diet for 4 weeks and a low-sodium diet for 2 weeks *(15)*. The average decline in supine BP on placebo was –8.2/ –3.9 mmHg for 18 normotensive patients and –6.6/–2.7 mmHg for 29 hypertensive patients. Although the change in supine BP was significant for both groups, this was not the case for standing BP.

The limited data from these studies and others suggest a benefit of sodium restriction and a hazard of an increase in BP with excess sodium chloride intake *(16)*.

POTASSIUM SUPPLEMENTATION

Potassium supplementation reduces cerebral hemorrhage in stroke-prone rats *(17)*. Thus, there has been an interest in potassium supplementation in humans. Twenty-one elderly subjects were taken off their routine antihypertensive medications for 2 weeks and then admitted to a clinical research unit for 8 days *(18)*. Subjects received an isocaloric diet with 22 mmol sodium, 70 mmol potassium, and 500 mg calcium. Treatment consisted of 40 mmol of microencapsulated potassium chloride dosed three times daily for 4 days or placebo. Then, each patient received the alternative for an additional 4 days. The mean change in BP in the placebo group was +0.7/–0.1 mmHg vs –8.6/–4.0 mmHg in the potassium supplementation group ($p < 0.02$ for both SBP and DBP). Both urinary potassium and sodium excretion increased during treatment with potassium; however, glomerular filtration rate, atrial natriuretic peptide, renin, urine thromboxane B_2, and urine 6-keto-prostaglandin were unchanged.

In another double-blind, randomized, placebo-controlled, crossover trial, 18 hypertensive elderly patients were studied after a 4-week placebo run-in period following withdrawal of all medications *(19)*. Flavored potassium chloride (20 mmol three times daily) or flavored placebo for 4 weeks was given, and then subjects were crossed over to the alternative treatment. Ambulatory BP was performed at the end of each treatment period. Compared to the placebo period, the clinic BP during potassium supplementation was significantly decreased (−10/−6 mmHg). However, only SBP was significantly decreased by 24-hour ambulatory BP during potassium treatment (−6/−2 mmHg). Urinary potassium but not urinary sodium excretion increased. In an unblinded extension of the study, eight subjects were given 48 mmol potassium chloride for 4 months *(20)*. The reduction in 24-hour ambulatory SBP was maintained.

In a randomized, double-blind trial, 100 untreated hypertensive men and women between the ages of 55 and 75 years received mineral salt or common salt for 24 weeks *(21)*. The mineral salt consisted of 17% magnesium salt, 41% KCl, 41% NaCl, and 1% trace minerals. Both salts were given for cooking and incorporated into provided foods. The mean decline in BP was −8.7/−3.6 mmHg, favoring the mineral salt group. Also, urinary sodium excretion decreased, and urinary potassium increased. The mineral salt was well tolerated.

Twenty elderly hypertensive patients in a nursing home had ambulatory BP performed before and after the introduction of low-sodium, high-potassium salt, consisting of 57% NaCl, 28% KCl, 12% MgSO$_4$, and 2% L-lysine HCl *(22)*. This special mineral salt was substituted for table and cooking salt for 6 months. Of the 20 subjects, 45% had a reduction in their daytime and nighttime BPs.

Although these trials showed a modest benefit, there may be other reasons to maintain a normal potassium level in elderly patients. Among diuretic users, a potassium level less than 4.1 mEq/L was associated with an increased risk of atherothrombotic and embolic strokes in the Cardiovascular Health Study, a prospective, multicenter study of 5888 men and women 65 years of age or older *(23)*. This supports the *post hoc* observation from the Systolic Hypertension in the Elderly Population study that a potassium level less than 3.5 mEq/L among participants receiving active treatment was associated with a higher rate of coronary heart disease and stroke events *(24)*.

CALCIUM SUPPLEMENTATION

Utilizing data from the first National Health and Nutrition Examination Survey (1971–1975), several variables were associated with high BP in older adults *(25)*. These included body mass index (BMI), alcohol consumption, and dietary calcium and phosphorus. There have been several trials to assess the role of supplemental calcium in elderly patients *(26–29)*.

An early uncontrolled study stopped all antihypertensive medications for eight elderly subjects for 1 month *(26)*. Then, the subjects were hospitalized for 10 weeks. The daily dietary intake consisted of 120 mEq sodium and 40 mEq potassium. The first 2 weeks, a placebo was given; for the last 8 weeks, 22.4 g per day of calcium gluconate was given, divided among three daily meals. The mean change in BP was a significant reduction (−24/−15 mmHg) as measured by an automatic sphygmomanometer.

Another study was conducted of nine hospitalized elderly patients *(27)*. Subjects were given a diet for 4 weeks that included 500 mg calcium, 2 g sodium, and 3 g potassium. Using a crossover design, subjects were treated with 1 g elemental calcium in the form of oyster shell electrolyte for 8 weeks with a washout period of 4 weeks. Ambulatory BP measurements for 24 hours were performed every 4 weeks. The mean change in blood was −13.6/−5 mmHg in the calcium period and −1.5/+1.0 mmHg in the control period ($p < 0.005$ for SBP and $p < 0.05$ for DBP). Ionized calcium increased, and parathyroid hormone levels declined. Both urinary sodium and calcium excretion increased.

A single-blind study enrolled 125 hypertensive subjects between 50 and 80 years of age (mean age 62.4 years) after a baseline observation period of 4 weeks. Then, subjects received placebo for 4 weeks followed by 12 weeks of 1 g calcium carbonate *(28)*. Compared to placebo, calcium supplementation did not lower supine or standing BP. Of the 103 subjects who completed the 12-week period of calcium treatment, 42 (41%) had 5 mmHg or greater decrease in either SBP or DBP. These subjects were treated for an additional 36 weeks with calcium. After the 48th week of treatment, their BP measurements were similar to those of the placebo period.

In an ambulatory setting, 148 women 70 years or older with serum 25-OHD$_3$ below 50 nmol/L were recruited for an 8-week, double-blind trial of 600 mg of elemental calcium with or without 400 IU vitamin D$_3$ *(29)*. Approximately 50% of subjects were hypertensive. The mean change in BP was −5.7/−6.9 mmHg in the calcium-only group compared to −13.1/−7.2 mmHg in the vitamin D$_3$-calcium group ($p = 0.02$ for SBP and $p = 0.10$ for DBP).

VITAMIN C

There has also been interest in using vitamin C for vascular protection of the elderly. A 20-year follow-up study of 730 British men and women found that mortality from stroke occurred more commonly with the lowest vitamin C intake or plasma ascorbic acid concentration *(30)*. In a study of 541 British elderly subjects not taking antihypertensive medications, there was an inverse relationship between plasma ascorbate levels and heart rate, SBP, and DBP *(31)*.

In a randomized, double-blind trial, 27 treated but uncontrolled hypertensive patients received 200 mg vitamin C dosed twice daily or matching placebo for 4 weeks and then received the alternative treatment for an additional 4 weeks *(32)*. The average fall in BP was –3/–0.4 mmHg. The change in DBP was not significant, and the change in SBP was not interpretable because of a treatment period interaction.

After a 2-week run-in period, 48 untreated hypertensive subjects received 250 mg vitamin C ($n = 22$) dosed twice daily or placebo ($n = 26$) for 6 weeks *(33)*. The change in BP in the vitamin C group was –10.3/–5.9 vs –7.7/–4.7 mmHg. The change from baseline was not significant between the groups.

Another study examined the effect of 250 mg vitamin C twice daily or placebo in a double-blind, crossover study *(34)*. Each treatment phase lasted 3 months. Ambulatory and clinic BPs were measured at baseline and at the end of each treatment period. Although plasma ascorbate levels increased from 49 mmol/L to 85 mmol/L, vitamin C did not lower clinic BP. However, daytime ambulatory SBP was lowered by 3.7 mmHg among the 17 hypertensive subjects, but not among the 23 normotensive subjects. There was no decline in DBP.

One randomized, double-blind trial followed 31 treated hypertensive patients (mean age 62 years and 80% elderly) for 8 months *(35)*. After a 4-week placebo period, they received 500 mg, 1000 mg, or 2000 mg vitamin C taken every 12 hours as two capsules. The mean decline in BP from the placebo period was –4.5/–2.8 mmHg ($p < 0.05$ for both systolic and diastolic). However, the maximal BP decrease was seen at 1 month (–6.1/–3.8 mmHg), which declined to –1.0/–1.7 mmHg by 6 months. There was no dose-dependent change in BP.

These trials in aggregate suggest a small benefit on SBP.

EXERCISE

Exercise is generally recommended by national guidelines to reduce weight and lower BP *(1,2,4)*. A meta-analysis of RCTs that assessed the effect of aerobic exercise on BP reported a change in BP of –4.9/–3.7 mmHg in 15 studies of hypertensive subjects and –4.0/–2.3 mmHg in 27 studies of normotensive subjects *(36)*.

There are numerous benefits of exercise for older patients in absence of hypertension *(37–40)*. One study conducted an RCT of 4 months among subjects 60 years or older *(41)*. This study assigned 247 subjects to 40 minutes of supervised exercise three times a week or a control group for 16 weeks. The target heart rate was about 70% of the peak heart rate. The mean reduction in BP was –5.6/–2.7 mmHg.

Another RCT study of 62 elderly subjects (50% with SBP 140 or greater) compared moderate aerobic exercise and T'ai Chi (Yang style) over 12 weeks *(42)*. There was no difference in the change in BP from baseline comparing the moderate aerobic exercise (–8.4/–3.2 mmHg) and the T'ai Chi (–7.0/–2.4 mmHg, p = 0.54) groups. A study randomized 39 older Japanese persons to exercise 2 to 3 days per week or lectures for 25 weeks *(43)*. Using home BP measurements, the exercise group had a significantly lower BP (–7.7/–4.2 mmHg) than the control group.

Finally, among 24 elderly hypertensives undergoing 45 minutes of low-intensity exercise, BP decreased and persisted 22 hours postexercise as assessed by ambulatory BP monitoring *(44)*. More studies are needed to evaluate this intervention.

MISCELLANEOUS INTERVENTIONS

The recommendation to reduce alcohol intake is based on the increase in BP observed in epidemiological studies *(45)*. Heavy alcohol use has been viewed as a risk factor for hemorrhagic and nonhemorrhagic strokes *(46)*, but this has not been observed in all studies *(47)*. Although the estimated benefit of alcohol reduction on BP reduction is –3.3/–2.0 mmHg, there are no RCTs among elderly subjects *(48)*.

It is hypothesized that ω-3 fatty acids stimulate vasodilating prostaglandins and lower BP. Two meta-analyses of RCTs observed a significant decline of BP in hypertensive subjects (–3.4/–2.0 mmHg and –5.5/–3.5 mmHg) *(49,50)*. One 4-week, double-blind study in 106 normotensive elderly subjects reported that fish oil (–8.1/–2.8 mmHg) and sunflower oil (–6.4/–2.4 mmHg) lowered BP significantly on a 70 mmol/day sodium-restricted diet, but not during normal sodium intake *(51)*.

Coffee consumption was found in one meta-analysis to increase BP +2.4/+1.2 mmHg compared with control *(52)*. One study randomized 22 normotensive and 26 hypertensive subjects to a caffeine-free diet or 300 mg per day of caffeine for 2 weeks after a 2-week caffeine-free diet *(53)*. The mean age of the study population was 72 years (range 54 to 89 years), and all were nonsmokers. A 24-hour ambulatory BP measurement was performed at the end of each 2-week period. BP was increased significantly in the hypertensive subjects receiving caffeine (+4.8/+3.0 mmHg) but not in the normotensive group.

A meta-analysis of randomized clinical trials of magnesium supplementation observed only a nonsignificant decline in BP (–0.6/–0.8 mmHg) *(54)*. However, higher doses reduced SBP (–4.3 mmHg, $p <$ 0.001). These 20 studies did not provide information on the effects of magnesium supplementation in elderly hypertensives.

TRIAL OF NONPHARMACOLOGICAL INTERVENTION IN ELDERLY

The Trial of Nonpharmacologic Intervention in Elderly (TONE) was designed to determine whether sodium restriction, weight loss, or both could maintain BP goals after withdrawal of antihypertensive drug therapy *(55)*. The four-center trial assessed each treatment variable in hypertensive subjects between the ages of 60 and 80 years. Treated patients taking one antihypertensive drug (or a combination drug with a diuretic) with a mean BP less than 145/85 mmHg after three visits were eligible. If the subject was on two drugs and one drug could be stopped and the BP criteria met, the subject was also eligible. Patients with angina, insulin-requiring diabetes mellitus, heart failure, and recent myocardial infarction or stroke were excluded from participation.

Obesity was defined as a BMI of 27.8 kg/m^2 or more for men and 27.3 kg/m^2 or more for women. The control groups included overweight subjects not assigned to weight reduction or sodium restriction and nonobese subjects not assigned to the sodium-restriction group. The interventions were designed to achieve a 24-hour urine sodium of 80 mEq (1800 mg) or less and/or a weight loss of 4.5 kg (10 lb) or more after randomization. Individual (4 sessions) and group counseling (12 sessions) were used to attain the goals of treatment during an initial 4-month intensive phase followed by a 4-month extended (biweekly group and individual sessions) and maintenance phases (monthly group or individual sessions). Usual care participants met for monthly sessions for issues unrelated to the interventions. The staff responsible for data collection wase blinded to the treatment assignment, BP, and drug withdrawal status.

The trial end points included an average BP of at least 150/90 mmHg on three visits, 170/100 mmHg or above on two visits, or at least 190/110 mmHg on one visit. Additional trial end points included (a) symptoms requiring resumption of antihypertensive drugs; (b) personal physician resumption of drug therapy; and (c) cardiovascular complications (angina, myocardial infarction, congestive heart failure, hypertensive encephalopathy, or stroke) or coronary revascularization after randomization.

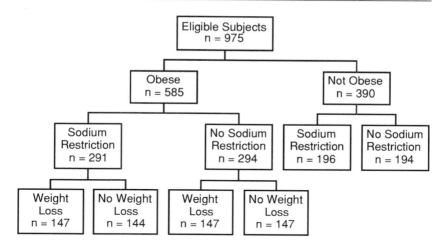

Fig. 3. Trial of Nonpharmacologic Interventions in Elderly (TONE): treatment group allocation. (Derived from ref. *57.*)

Initially, 8787 potential subjects were contacted for screening *(56)*. There were 975 participants randomized to one of six treatments determined by BMI *(57)*. The trial assignments are displayed in Fig. 3. Antihypertensive medication was stopped on average 90 ± 14 days after the assigned intervention. Patients were seen weekly during drug withdrawal and biweekly for 6 weeks after medication cessation. Six months after randomization, follow-up visits occurred every 3 months. During follow-up visits, the following were assessed: BP, weight, girth, 24-hour urine, interval history including current medications, psychological and physical activity questionnaires, and 24-hour diet recall. BP was measured three times at each visit *(58,59)*. Mean follow-up was 27.6 months (range 15.6 to 35.9 months).

The average age of the study population was 66.5 years, with 78% of subjects between 60 and 69 years. Of the cohort, 48% were female. There were 24% black participants. The duration of antihypertensive therapy was about 12 years. Fewer than 7% smoked, and 32% or more had one or more alcoholic drinks daily. Entry medications are displayed in Fig. 4. As seen, diuretics and calcium channel blockers were the most commonly prescribed antihypertensive drugs. Attendance rate at follow-up visits was outstanding.

Figure 5 shows the mean reduction in sodium at 9, 18, and 30 months for participants salt restricted or not salt restricted. The net achieved sodium reduction was significant ($p < 0.001$) at each collection period.

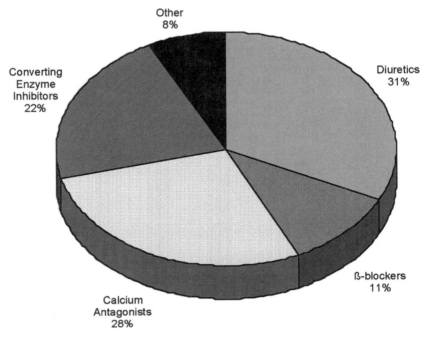

Fig. 4. Medications of TONE Participants at baseline. (Derived from ref. 57.)

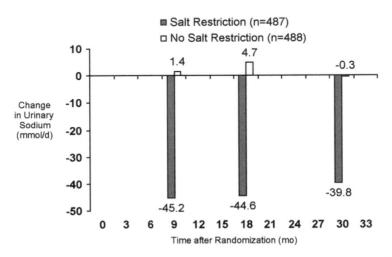

Fig. 5. Trial of Nonpharmacologic Interventions in Elderly (TONE): sodium restriction—change in urinary sodium. The net achieved sodium reduction was significant ($p < 0.001$) at each collection period. (Derived from ref. 57.)

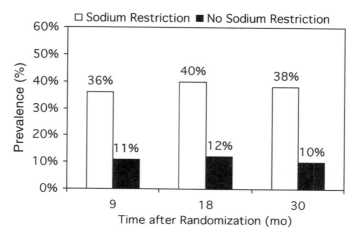

Fig. 6. Trial of Nonpharmacologic Interventions in Elderly (TONE): prevalence of urinary sodium of 80 mmol/day or less according to treatment assignment. (Derived from ref. *57*.)

The mean reduction in sodium excretion was 28.7 mmol lower in obese subjects in the sodium-restriction group than in the combined intervention group. Figure 6 shows the prevalence of urine sodium reduction of no more than 80 mmol per day.

The average weight change over time is shown in Fig. 7. The net reduction in weight varied from 3.6 to 3.9 kg. Figure 8 shows the prevalence of weight reduction of no less than 4.5 kg. However, there were differences in the extent of weight reduction among the 421 white and 164 black study participants *(60)*. Comparing the net change in weight from the weight loss-only group minus the usual care group, blacks lost an average of 2.7 kg compared to 5.9 kg among white subjects at 6 months ($p = 0.0002$). Additional weight loss occurred later for black participants compared with weight gain for white participants. The net change at the end of the study was −2.0 kg for blacks and −4.9 kg for whites ($p = 0.007$). Comparing the net change in weight from combined weight and sodium group minus the sodium-only group, there was no significant difference in blacks (−2.1 kg) and whites (−2.8 kg, $p = 0.51$) at 6 months. Approximately 41% of blacks and 66% of whites achieved the 4.5 kg weight loss goal.

One of the four centers examined the effect of weight reduction on bone mineral density (BMD) of the total body, lumbar spine, and femoral neck using dual-energy X-ray absorptiometry *(61)*. Sixty-seven women underwent an examination at baseline, 6 months, and 12 months.

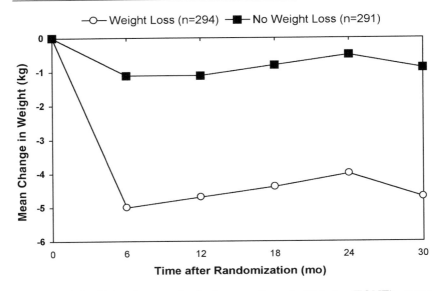

Fig. 7. Trial of Nonpharmacologic Interventions in Elderly (TONE): mean change in body weight. The net reduction of weight among the weight loss participants was 3.6 kg or greater ($p < 0.001$). (Derived from ref. 57.)

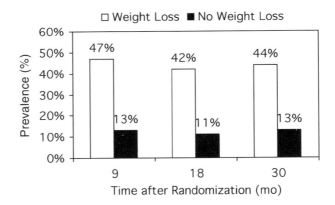

Fig. 8. Trial of Nonpharmacologic Interventions in Elderly (TONE): prevalence of achieved weight loss of 4.5 kg or more. (Derived from ref. 57.)

Weight loss was associated with modest decrease in BMD of the total body, but not the lumbar spine or the femoral neck. The change in BMD was associated with an increase in osteocalcin.

Most trial end points (74%) resulted from elevated BP measurements; 5.6% were cardiac or other clinical events (62). The non-BP-related end

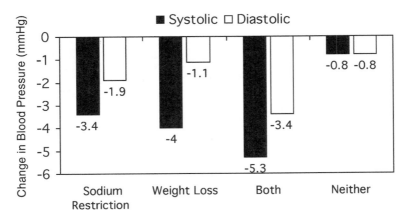

Fig. 9. Trial of Nonpharmacologic Interventions in Elderly (TONE): change in blood pressure by treatment. The change in systolic and diastolic blood pressure from baseline was significant ($p < 0.001$) for each intervention compared to no intervention. (Derived from ref. *57.*)

points occurred most frequently in women, those subjects with a cardiac disease history, and the subjects who did not reduce their sodium intake. The rate of cardiovascular events was 5.5, 5.5, and 6.8 per 100 person-years in nonoverweight subjects ($p = 0.84$) and 7.2, 5.2, and 5.6 per 100 person-years in obese subjects ($p = 0.08$) for the time periods of randomization to the onset of drug withdrawal, during or after drug withdrawal, and after resumption of antihypertensive drugs, respectively *(63)*. The remaining 20.5% were the result of either patient or their physician not tapering medication or resuming antihypertensive drugs. After 30 months, 38% of the sodium-restriction group ($n = 487$) compared with 24% of the group with no salt restriction ($n = 488$) were free of trial end points ($p < 0.001$) *(57)*. For the weight-loss ($n = 291$) and no weight-loss ($n = 294$) groups, 39 and 26% were free of trial end points ($p = 0.001$). Among obese participants, the combined intervention (44%) was less likely to achieve trial end points compared to the no-intervention group (16%) at 30 months ($p < 0.001$). Combined treatment modalities were not more effective than either sodium restriction (34%, $p < 0.001$) or weight loss (37%, $p = 0.002$) alone. The change in BP from baseline to the last visit is shown in Fig. 9. There were no adverse cardiovascular events associated with the treatment interventions vs usual care.

The sodium excretion rate was more reduced in men than in women (53 vs 27%, respectively, $p < 0.001$); however, there was no difference between overweight vs nonobese subjects, 60- to 69-year age group vs the 70- to 80-year age group, and black vs non-black subjects *(64)*. All

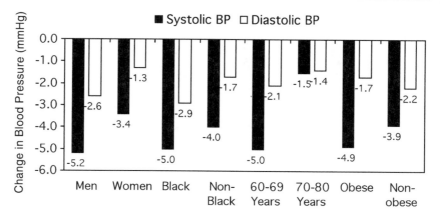

Fig. 10. Trial of Nonpharmacologic Interventions in Elderly (TONE): subset analysis of restricted sodium group. The change in blood pressure in sodium-restricted group is corrected from the usual care group. The change in systolic blood pressure was significant ($p < 0.05$) for each group except for subjects 70 to 80 years old. The change in diastolic blood pressure was significant ($p < 0.05$) for each group except women, obese individuals, and subjects 70 to 80 years old. (Data from ref. *64.*)

subgroups (Fig. 10) experienced a significant placebo-corrected decline in SBP, except the 70- to 80-year age group. For women, overweight subjects, and the 70- to 80-year age group, there was no significant drop in DBP. After 30 months, 43% of the cohort in the reduced-sodium group compared to 27% in the usual care group ($p < 0.001$) had their BP controlled without medication. The greater the reduction in urinary sodium excretion, the lower the risk of reaching a trial end point ($p = 0.002$).

Predictors of long-term withdrawal from antihypertensive drugs included assignment to an active intervention *(62)*. Having a lower baseline SBP, treatment with one antihypertensive drug, and treatment for a shorter duration of time were also significant predictors of successful drug withdrawal.

The long-term effect of individual and group counseling after discontinuation of the study was assessed by one of the four participating centers (Fig. 11) *(65,66)*. There were 108 study participants available for the urinary sodium excretion and weight measurements 6 to 13 months after the completion of TONE for extended follow-up. Although there was 1.1 kg weight gain in the weight-loss group ($n = 53$) during follow-up, the net loss compared to baseline in the weight-loss group was –3.9 kg compared to the –2.2 kg in no weight-loss group ($n = 55$; $p = 0.07$) *(65)*. Alternatively, sodium excretion was reduced from baseline to 52

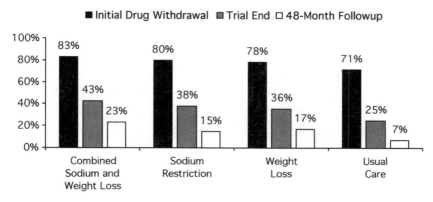

Fig. 11. Follow-up from one Trial of Nonpharmacologic Interventions in Elderly (TONE) center: persistence of normotension. (Data from refs. *64* and *66*.)

mmol per day in the sodium-restriction group ($n = 44$) compared to 13 mmol/day in the no sodium-restriction group ($n = 55$; $p = 0.008$). Thus, sodium restriction persists in effectiveness, unlike weight reduction. On completion of TONE, 43% of the combined sodium-restriction and weight-loss group was off medication compared to 25% of the usual care group ($p = 0.011$ by χ^2) *(66)*. Follow-up was obtained for 222 of the 244 randomized subjects an average of 48.4 months after study termination. The combined intervention group was associated with superior BP control compared to usual care ($p = 0.012$).

SUMMARY

In aggregate, these data document that nonpharmacological therapy can decrease the need for drug therapy. Many of the trials were not blinded, well-controlled, or adequately powered. TONE proved that sodium restriction and weight loss are effective in elderly patients. Sodium restriction is more likely to be continued over longer periods of time than weight reduction. More data are needed for other nonpharmacological interventions in the elderly. However, it is likely that an approach to comprehensive lifestyle modification would be beneficial *(67,68)*.

REFERENCES

1. Whelton PK, He J, Appel LJ, et al. Primary prevention of hypertension: clinical and public health advisory from the National High Blood Pressure Education Program. *JAMA* 2002;288:1882–1888.

 2. Chobanian AV, Bakris GL, Black HR, et al. The Seventh Report of the Joint National Committee on Prevention, Detection, Evaluation, and Treatment of High Blood Pressure: the JNC 7 report. *JAMA* 2003;289:2560–2572.
 3. Chobanian AV, Bakris GL, Black HR, et al. Seventh Report of the Joint National Committee on Prevention, Detection, Evaluation, and Treatment of High Blood Pressure. *Hypertension* 2003;42:1206–1252.
 4. National High Blood Pressure Education Program Working Group Report on Hypertension in the Elderly. National High Blood Pressure Education Program Working Group. *Hypertension* 1994;23:275–285.
 5. Black HR. Nonpharmacologic therapy for hypertension in the elderly. *Geriatrics* 1989;44(suppl B):20–29.
 6. Prisant LM. Nutritional treatment of blood pressure: nonpharmacologic therapy. In: Berdanier CD, ed. *CRC Handbook of Nutrition and Food.* Boca Raton, FL: CRC Press; 2002:961–998.
 7. Prisant LM. Nutritional treatment of blood pressure: major nonpharmacologic trials of prevention or treatment of hypertension. In: Berdanier CD, ed. *CRC Handbook of Nutrition and Food.* Boca Raton, FL: CRC Press; 2002:999–1010.
 8. Applegate WB, Miller ST, Elam JT, et al. Nonpharmacologic intervention to reduce blood pressure in older patients with mild hypertension. *Arch Intern Med* 1992;152:1162–1166.
 9. Geleijnse JM, Witteman JC, Hofman A, Grobbee DE. Electrolytes are associated with blood pressure at old age: the Rotterdam Study. *J Hum Hypertens* 1997;11:421–423.
10. Stamler J, Rose G, Elliott P, et al. Findings of the International Cooperative INTERSALT Study. *Hypertension* 1991;17(suppl):I9–I15.
11. Law MR, Frost CD, Wald NJ. By how much does dietary salt reduction lower blood pressure? III—Analysis of data from trials of salt reduction. *BMJ* 1991;302:819–824.
12. Palmer RM, Osterweil D, Loon-Lustig G, Stern N. The effect of dietary salt ingestion on blood pressure of old-old subjects. A double-blind, placebo-controlled, crossover trial. *J Am Geriatr Soc* 1989;37:931–936.
13. Fotherby MD, Potter JF. Effects of moderate sodium restriction on clinic and 24-hour ambulatory blood pressure in elderly hypertensive subjects. *J Hypertens* 1993;11:657–663.
14. Fotherby MD, Potter JF. Metabolic and orthostatic blood pressure responses to a low-sodium diet in elderly hypertensives. *J Hum Hypertens* 1997;11:361–366.
15. Cappuccio FP, Markandu ND, Carney C, Sagnella GA, MacGregor GA. Double-blind randomised trial of modest salt restriction in older people. *Lancet* 1997;350: 850–854.
16. Alam S, Johnson AG. A meta-analysis of randomised controlled trials (RCT) among healthy normotensive and essential hypertensive elderly patients to determine the effect of high salt (NaCl) diet of blood pressure. *J Hum Hypertens* 1999;13:367–374.
17. Tobian L, Lange J, Ulm K, Wold L, Iwai J. Potassium reduces cerebral hemorrhage and death rate in hypertensive rats, even when blood pressure is not lowered. *Hypertension* 1985;7(3 pt 2):I110–I114.
18. Smith SR, Klotman PE, Svetkey LP. Potassium chloride lowers blood pressure and causes natriuresis in older patients with hypertension. *J Am Soc Nephrol* 1992;2: 1302–1309.
19. Fotherby MD, Potter JF. Potassium supplementation reduces clinic and ambulatory blood pressure in elderly hypertensive patients. *J Hypertens* 1992;10:1403–1408.
20. Fotherby MD, Potter JF. Long-term potassium supplementation lowers blood pressure in elderly hypertensive subjects. *Int J Clin Pract* 1997;51:219–222.

21. Geleijnse JM, Witteman JC, Bak AA, den Breeijen JH, Grobbee DE. Reduction in blood pressure with a low sodium, high potassium, high magnesium salt in older subjects with mild to moderate hypertension. *BMJ* 1994;309:436–440.

22. Katz A, Rosenthal T, Maoz C, Peleg E, Zeidenstein R, Levi Y. Effect of a mineral salt diet on 24-hour blood pressure monitoring in elderly hypertensive patients. *J Hum Hypertens* 1999;13:777–780.

23. Green DM, Ropper AH, Kronmal RA, Psaty BM, Burke GL. Serum potassium level and dietary potassium intake as risk factors for stroke. *Neurology* 2002;59:314–320.

24. Franse LV, Pahor M, Di Bari M, Somes GW, Cushman WC, Applegate WB. Hypokalemia associated with diuretic use and cardiovascular events in the Systolic Hypertension in the Elderly Program. *Hypertension* 2000;35:1025–1030.

25. Harlan WR, Hull AL, Schmouder RL, Landis JR, Larkin FA, Thompson FE. High blood pressure in older Americans. The First National Health and Nutrition Examination Survey. *Hypertension* 1984;6(6 pt 1):802–809.

26. Tabuchi Y, Ogihara T, Hashizume K, Saito H, Kumahara Y. Hypotensive effect of long-term oral calcium supplementation in elderly patients with essential hypertension. *J Clin Hypertens* 1986;2:254–262.

27. Takagi Y, Fukase M, Takata S, Fujimi T, Fujita T. Calcium treatment of essential hypertension in elderly patients evaluated by 24 hour monitoring. *Am J Hypertens* 1991;4(10 pt 1):836–839.

28. Morris CD, McCarron DA. Effect of calcium supplementation in an older population with mildly increased blood pressure. *Am J Hypertens* 1992;5(4 pt 1):230–237.

29. Pfeifer M, Begerow B, Minne HW, Nachtigall D, Hansen C. Effects of a short-term vitamin D(3) and calcium supplementation on blood pressure and parathyroid hormone levels in elderly women. *J Clin Endocrinol Metab* 2001;86:1633–1637.

30. Gale CR, Martyn CN, Winter PD, Cooper C. Vitamin C and risk of death from stroke and coronary heart disease in cohort of elderly people. *BMJ* 1995;310:1563–1566.

31. Bates CJ, Walmsley CM, Prentice A, Finch S. Does vitamin C reduce blood pressure? Results of a large study of people aged 65 or older. *J Hypertens* 1998;16:925–932.

32. Lovat LB, Lu Y, Palmer AJ, Edwards R, Fletcher AE, Bulpitt CJ. Double-blind trial of vitamin C in elderly hypertensives. *J Hum Hypertens* 1993;7:403–405.

33. Ghosh SK, Ekpo EB, Shah IU, Girling AJ, Jenkins C, Sinclair AJ. A double-blind, placebo-controlled parallel trial of vitamin C treatment in elderly patients with hypertension. *Gerontology* 1994;40:268–272.

34. Fotherby MD, Williams JC, Forster LA, Craner P, Ferns GA. Effect of vitamin C on ambulatory blood pressure and plasma lipids in older persons. *J Hypertens* 2000;18:411–415.

35. Hajjar IM, George V, Sasse EA, Kochar MS. A randomized, double-blind, controlled trial of vitamin C in the management of hypertension and lipids. *Am J Ther* 2002;9:289–293.

36. Whelton SP, Chin A, Xin X, He J. Effect of aerobic exercise on blood pressure: a meta-analysis of randomized, controlled trials. *Ann Intern Med* 2002;136:493–503.

37. Katzel LI, Bleecker ER, Colman EG, Rogus EM, Sorkin JD, Goldberg AP. Effects of weight loss vs aerobic exercise training on risk factors for coronary disease in healthy, obese, middle-aged and older men. A randomized controlled trial. *JAMA* 1995;274:1915–1921.

38. King AC, Haskell WL, Taylor CB, Kraemer HC, DeBusk RF. Group- vs home-based exercise training in healthy older men and women. A community-based clinical trial. *JAMA* 1991;266:1535–1542.

39. Hamdorf PA, Withers RT, Penhall RK, Haslam MV. Physical training effects on the fitness and habitual activity patterns of elderly women. *Arch Phys Med Rehabil* 1992;73:603–608.
40. Okumiya K, Matsubayashi K, Wada T, Kimura S, Doi Y, Ozawa T. Effects of exercise on neurobehavioral function in community-dwelling older people more than 75 years of age. *J Am Geriatr Soc* 1996;44:569–572.
41. Posner JD, Gorman KM, Windsor-Landsberg L, et al. Low to moderate intensity endurance training in healthy older adults: physiological responses after four months. *J Am Geriatr Soc* 1992;40:1–7.
42. Young DR, Appel LJ, Jee S, Miller ER 3rd. The effects of aerobic exercise and T'ai Chi on blood pressure in older people: results of a randomized trial. *J Am Geriatr Soc* 1999;47:277–284.
43. Ohkubo T, Hozawa A, Nagatomi R, et al. Effects of exercise training on home blood pressure values in older adults: a randomized controlled trial. *J Hypertens* 2001;19:1045–1052.
44. Brandao Rondon MU, Alves MJ, Braga AM, et al. Postexercise blood pressure reduction in elderly hypertensive patients. *J Am Coll Cardiol* 2002;39:676–682.
45. Klatsky AL, Friedman GD, Armstrong MA. The relationships between alcoholic beverage use and other traits to blood pressure: a new Kaiser Permanente study. *Circulation* 1986;73:628–636.
46. Gill JS, Shipley MJ, Tsementzis SA, et al. Alcohol consumption—a risk factor for hemorrhagic and non-hemorrhagic stroke. *Am J Med* 1991;90:489–497.
47. Berger K, Ajani UA, Kase CS, et al. Light-to-moderate alcohol consumption and risk of stroke among US male physicians. *N Engl J Med* 1999;341:1557–1564.
48. Xin X, He J, Frontini MG, Ogden LG, Motsamai OI, Whelton PK. Effects of alcohol reduction on blood pressure: a meta-analysis of randomized controlled trials. *Hypertension* 2001;38:1112–1117.
49. Appel LJ, Miller ER 3rd, Seidler AJ, Whelton PK. Does supplementation of diet with "fish oil" reduce blood pressure? A meta-analysis of controlled clinical trials. *Arch Intern Med* 1993;153:1429–1438.
50. Morris MC, Sacks F, Rosner B. Does fish oil lower blood pressure? A meta-analysis of controlled trials. *Circulation* 1993;88:523–533.
51. Cobiac L, Nestel PJ, Wing LM, Howe PR. A low-sodium diet supplemented with fish oil lowers blood pressure in the elderly. *J Hypertens* 1992;10:87–92.
52. Jee SH, He J, Whelton PK, Suh I, Klag MJ. The effect of chronic coffee drinking on blood pressure: a meta-analysis of controlled clinical trials. *Hypertension* 1999;33:647–652.
53. Rakic V, Burke V, Beilin LJ. Effects of coffee on ambulatory blood pressure in older men and women: a randomized controlled trial. *Hypertension* 1999;33:869–873.
54. Jee SH, Miller ER 3rd, Guallar E, Singh VK, Appel LJ, Klag MJ. The effect of magnesium supplementation on blood pressure: a meta-analysis of randomized clinical trials. *Am J Hypertens* 2002;15:691–696.
55. Appel LJ, Espeland M, Whelton PK, et al. Trial of Nonpharmacologic Intervention in the Elderly (TONE). Design and rationale of a blood pressure control trial. *Ann Epidemiol* 1995;5:119–129.
56. Whelton PK, Babnson J, Appel LJ, et al. Recruitment in the Trial of Nonpharmacologic Intervention in the Elderly (TONE). *J Am Geriatr Soc* 1997;45:185–193.
57. Whelton PK, Appel LJ, Espeland MA, et al. Sodium reduction and weight loss in the treatment of hypertension in older persons: a randomized controlled trial of nonpharmacologic interventions in the elderly (TONE). TONE Collaborative Research Group. *JAMA* 1998;279:839–846.

58. Espeland MA, Kumanyika S, Kostis JB, et al. Antihypertensive medication use among recruits for the Trial of Nonpharmacologic Interventions in the Elderly (TONE). *J Am Geriatr Soc* 1996;44:1183–1189.
59. Anderson RT, Hogan P, Appel L, Rosen R, Shumaker SA. Baseline correlates with quality of life among men and women with medication-controlled hypertension. The Trial of Nonpharmacologic Interventions in the Elderly (TONE). *J Am Geriatr Soc* 1997;45:1080–1085.
60. Kumanyika SK, Espeland MA, Bahnson JL, et al. Ethnic comparison of weight loss in the Trial of Nonpharmacologic Interventions in the Elderly. *Obes Res* 2002;10:96–106.
61. Chao D, Espeland MA, Farmer D, et al. Effect of voluntary weight loss on bone mineral density in older overweight women. *J Am Geriatr Soc* 2000;48:753–759.
62. Espeland MA, Whelton PK, Kostis JB, et al. Predictors and mediators of successful long-term withdrawal from antihypertensive medications. TONE Cooperative Research Group. Trial of Nonpharmacologic Interventions in the Elderly. *Arch Fam Med* 1999;8:228–236.
63. Kostis JB, Espeland MA, Appel L, Johnson KC, Pierce J, Wofford JL. Does withdrawal of antihypertensive medication increase the risk of cardiovascular events? Trial of Nonpharmacologic Interventions in the Elderly (TONE) Cooperative Research Group. *Am J Cardiol* 1998;82:1501–1508.
64. Appel LJ, Espeland MA, Easter L, Wilson AC, Folmar S, Lacy CR. Effects of reduced sodium intake on hypertension control in older individuals: results from the Trial of Nonpharmacologic Interventions in the Elderly (TONE). *Arch Intern Med* 2001;161:685–693.
65. Kostis JB, Wilson AC, Shindler DM, Cosgrove NM, Lacy CR. Non-drug therapy for hypertension: do effects on weight and sodium intake persist after discontinuation of intervention? *Am J Med* 2000;109:734–736.
66. Kostis JB, Wilson AC, Shindler DM, Cosgrove NM, Lacy CR. Persistence of normotension after discontinuation of lifestyle intervention in the trial of TONE. Trial of Nonpharmacologic Interventions in the Elderly. *Am J Hypertens* 2002;15:732–734.
67. Svetkey LP, Harsha DW, Vollmer WM, et al. Premier: a clinical trial of comprehensive lifestyle modification for blood pressure control: rationale, design and baseline characteristics. *Ann Epidemiol* 2003;13:462–471.
68. Appel LJ, Champagne CM, Harsha DW, et al. Effects of comprehensive lifestyle modification on blood pressure control: main results of the PREMIER clinical trial. JAMA 2003;289:2083–2093.

7 Clinical Trials of Hypertension in the Older Patient

L. Michael Prisant, MD, FACC, FACP

CONTENTS

INTRODUCTION
THE TRIALS
ANALYSIS
REFERENCES

INTRODUCTION

Outcomes trials have established the benefit of treating hypertension in the older patient but not the very elderly *(1,2)*. These trials are reviewed because they represent the cornerstone of care of these patients. Subset analyses of early studies suggested a potential benefit for reducing blood pressure (BP) in older patients *(3–8)*.

In this chapter, only prospective trials are considered (Table 1). The strongest proof is derived from prospective, randomized, double-blind trials. Single-blind trials (e.g., Medical Research Council in Old Patients) provide weaker data for assessing optimal patient therapy. The prospective, randomized, open-label, blinded end point (PROBE) design offers some improvement over prospective, single-blind trials (e.g., Second Australian National Blood Pressure Trial) *(9)*. Although PROBE trials are less expensive to implement, the design has a major disadvantage of investigator bias.

From: *Clinical Hypertension and Vascular Diseases: Hypertension in the Elderly*
Edited by: L. M. Prisant © Humana Press Inc., Totowa, NJ

Table 1
Prospective Hypertension Outcomes Trials in the Elderly: Baseline Characteristics

Trial	Year	Design	n	Follow-up, yr	Entry age, yr	Entry SBP, mmHg	Entry DBP, mmHg	Mean age, yr	Women, %	Target SBP, mmHg	Target DBP, mmHg
ANBP2	2003	PROBE	6083	4.1	65–84	≥160	≥90	71.9	51	<160 and <140, if tolerated	<90 and <80, if tolerated
CASTEL	1994	Random allocation	655	7	≥65	≥160	≥95	73.7	64.7	NS	NS
EWPHE	1985	Double blind	840	4.7	≥60	160–239	90–119	72	69.8	NA	<90
HEP	1986	Random allocation	884	4.4	60–79	≥170	≥105	68.8	69.1	<170	<105
HYVET Pilot	2003	PROBE	1283	1.1	≥80	160–219 and st SBP ≥ 140	95–119	83.8	62.9	<150	<80
MRC-Older	1992	Single blind	4396	5.8	65–74	160–209	≤114	70.3	58.2	If ≥180, then ≤160; if <180, then ≤150	NA
NCS-EH	1999	Double blind	414	3.9–4.5	≥60	160–220	<115	69.8	33.1	?	?
SCOPE	2003	Double blind	4969	3.7	70–89	160–179	90–99	76.4	64.5	<160	<90
SHELL	2003	PROBE	1882	2.7	≥60	≥160	≤95	72.4	61.3	≤160 and >20	NA
SHEP	1991	Double blind	4736	4.5	≥60	160–219	<90	71.6	56.8	If >180, then <160; if 160–180, then −20	NA
STONE	1996	Alternate allocation, single blind	1632	3	60–79	≥160	>95	66.4	53.1	140–159	<90

STOP-Hypertension	1991	Double blind	1627	2.1	70–84	180–230 and DBP≥90	105–120	75.7	63	<160	<90
STOP-Hypertension 2	1999	PROBE	6614	5	70–84	≥180	≥105	76	66.8	<160	<95
Syst-China	1998	Alternate allocation Single blind	2394	3	≥60	160–219	<95	66.5	35.6	<150 and ≥20	NA
Syst-Eur	1997	Double blind	4695	2	>60	160–219 and st SBP ≥140	<95	70.3	66.8	<150 and ≥20	NA

See text for definitions of trial abbreviations. DBP, diastolic blood pressure; NA, not applicable; NS, not stated; SBP, systolic blood pressure; St SBP, standing blood pressure.

THE TRIALS

European Working Party on High Blood Pressure in the Elderly

The European Working Party on High Blood Pressure in the Elderly (EWPHE) was the first randomized, double-blind, placebo-controlled trial to study patients older than 60 years *(10,11)*. This trial was conducted when there was uncertainty about lowering BP in elderly patients *(3–5,12–14)*. It was designed to detect a reduction in fatal and nonfatal strokes. The entry BP was a sitting diastolic blood pressure (DBP) of 90–119 mmHg and a systolic blood pressure (SBP) of 160–239 mmHg. Patients were allocated to active drugs or matching placebo. Initial treatment was a once-daily dose capsule of 25 mg hydrochlorothiazide and 50 mg of triamterene, which could be doubled after 2 weeks to achieve a BP goal of less than 160/90 mmHg. If the BP target was not achieved, methyldopa could be titrated from 250 to 2000 mg daily after 4 weeks.

The mean age of the 840 patients was 72 years. Average follow-up exceeded 4.6 years. BP was reduced from 183/101 to 148/85 mmHg in the active treatment group and 182/101 to 167/90 mmHg in the placebo group. More than 35% of subjects stopped treatment prematurely. There was no significant reduction of stroke mortality ($-43\%, p = 0.15$) or overall mortality ($-26\%, p = 0.08$), but there was a significant reduction of fatal MI (MI; $-60\%, p = 0.043$) and nonfatal heart failure ($-63\%, p = 0.01$).

Hypertension in the Elderly in Primary Care Trial

In the Hypertension in the Elderly in Primary Care (HEP) trial, Coope and Warrender conducted a prospective, random allocation study in 884 general practice patients aged 60–79 years *(15)*. The entry BP was an SBP of 170–280 mmHg and a DBP of 105–120 mmHg. Active treatment started with 100 mg of atenolol once daily and progressively added 5 mg of bendrofluazide once daily, 500 mg of methyldopa at bedtime, and 20 mg of nifedipine sustained release twice daily to achieve the treatment goal of less than 170/105 mmHg. The control group did not receive a placebo. The mean reduction of BP in the treatment group was $-18/-11$ mmHg. After a follow-up period of 4.4 years, the rate of fatal strokes in the treatment group was reduced by 70% (2.2 vs 7.3 per 1000 patient-years, $p < 0.025$), but cardiovascular and total mortality did not decrease.

Systolic Hypertension in the Elderly Program

The Systolic Hypertension in the Elderly Program (SHEP) was designed as a randomized, double-blind, placebo-controlled study to assess the benefit of reducing BP in 4736 patients 60 years or older with isolated systolic hypertension *(16)*. Isolated systolic hypertension was defined as an SBP greater than 160 mmHg and a DBP less than 90 mmHg based on four measurements at two visits. The primary objective was a reduction in fatal and nonfatal strokes. Patients with a SBP between 160 and 219 mmHg were enrolled. Active drugs or matching placebos were titrated (a) to reduce SBP greater than 180 mmHg to below 160 mmHg and (b) to reduce SBP by 20 mmHg for those patients with SBP below 180 mmHg. Active treatment was initiated with 12.5–25 mg of chlorthalidone dosed once daily. Supplemental therapy included 25–50 mg of atenolol dosed once daily or 0.05–0.1 mg of reserpine dosed once daily if atenolol was contraindicated.

The mean age of subjects was 71.6 years, and the baseline BP was 170/77 mmHg. In the active treatment group, 46% of subjects received diuretic monotherapy, and 9% received no medication. Overall BP was lowered by –26/–9 mmHg. In the placebo group, 44% of subjects received antihypertensive drugs by year 5. Drug therapy was well tolerated *(17)*. After a mean follow-up of 4.5 years, active treatment reduced fatal and nonfatal strokes (Fig. 1) by 36% (5.5 vs 9.2 per 100 persons, $p = 0.0003$). Nonfatal MI and fatal and nonfatal heart failure were significantly lowered by 33 and 49%, respectively *(18)*. There were 81 cases of dementia, yielding a rate of 1.6% in the active treatment group and 1.9% in the placebo group ($p > 0.05$). The 13% total mortality reduction was not significant.

There were 583 patients (12.3%) with non-insulin-dependent diabetes in SHEP *(19)*. After adjustment in baseline differences, the diabetic subjects had a significant reduction in the composite of nonfatal MI and fatal coronary heart disease events (54%) and major coronary heart disease events (56%). There was no reduction in all-cause mortality and total strokes. In contrast, the nondiabetic persons had a significant reduction in nonfatal and fatal strokes (38%).

Swedish Trial in Old Patients With Hypertension

Previous outcomes trials established the benefit of reducing BP in patients less than 70 years. Thus, the Swedish Trial in Old Patients With Hypertension (STOP-Hypertension) study enrolled 1627 patients aged 70–84 years with (a) an SBP between 180 and 230 mmHg and a DBP of 90 mmHg or higher or (b) a DBP of 105–120 mmHg *(20)*. The trial excluded older patients with an SBP greater than 230 mmHg and/or DBP greater than 120 mmHg. Isolated systolic hypertension, defined as 180 or higher systolic and below 90 mmHg diastolic pressure, was also an exclusion.

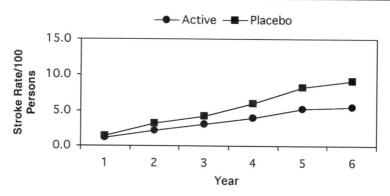

Fig. 1. Systolic Hypertension in the Elderly Program: cumulative stroke rate by year. After a mean follow-up of 4.5 years, active treatment reduced fatal and nonfatal strokes by 36% (5.5 vs 9.2 per 100 persons, p = 0.0003). (Data from ref. *16*.)

STOP-Hypertension was conducted as a double-blind, multicenter, randomized study to compare antihypertensive treatment to placebo. Initial drug therapy consisted of a once-daily diuretic (25 mg of hydrochlorothiazide and 2.5 mg of amiloride), a β-blocker (50 mg of atenolol, 100 mg of controlled-release metoprolol, or 5 mg of pindolol), or a matching placebo after a 1- to 6-month washout period. Both active treatment drugs could be combined if BP exceeded 160/95 mmHg after 2 months. For the placebo group, open-label antihypertensive therapy could be added if the BP exceeded 230/120 mmHg. The primary outcome was MI, stroke, and other cardiovascular death.

Baseline BP was 195/102 mmHg. The average follow-up period was 25 months. Fewer than one-third of the active treatment patients received monotherapy. The β-blocker monotherapy was less effective than diuretic monotherapy for lowering SBP but not DBP *(21)*. At 12 months, the placebo-corrected changes in BP were greatest when the β-blocker was combined with a diuretic. BP was reduced to 186/96 in the placebo group and 167/87 mmHg in the active treatment group. The composite of the primary end points was reduced by 40% (p = 0.0031). As shown in Fig. 2, treatment reduced total mortality 43% (p = 0.0079) and strokes 47% (p = 0.0081). The rate of all MIs was not reduced over the short duration of follow-up. There are no data in this trial to suggest either a benefit or risk of β-blocker treatment in terms of mortality *(22)*.

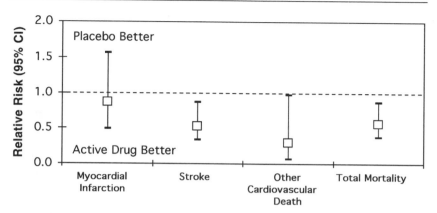

Fig. 2. Swedish Trial of Older Patients With Hypertension. Active treatment reduced total mortality 43% ($p = 0.0079$) and strokes 47% ($p = 0.0081$). (Data from ref. *55*.)

Medical Research Council Trial in Older Adults

The Medical Research Council (MRC) trial was a randomized, placebo-controlled, single-blind trial ($n = 4396$) designed to compare a diuretic, β-blocker, and placebo for reducing strokes, coronary artery disease, and total mortality *(23)*. Patients aged 65–74 years were randomized if their DBP was less than 115 mmHg and the SBP was 160–209 mmHg after an 8-week period off antihypertensive drugs. They received 50–100 mg of atenolol, 25 mg of hydrochlorothiazide with 2.5 mg of amiloride, or matching placebo dosed once daily. If the target SBP of less than 150–160 mmHg was not achieved, the alternative active drug could be added and further supplemented by 20 mg nifedipine dosed once daily. Subjects were followed 5.8 years.

The benefits of treatment in the MRC trial were confined to diuretic-assigned patients. There was no difference in the total stroke rate between active treatments ($p = 0.33$); however, the rate of fatal strokes was the same for the β-blocker and placebo groups (Fig. 3). The rate of coronary events was lower in the diuretic group than in the β-blocker group ($p = 0.006$). The cardiovascular death rate was higher in the β-blocker group than in the diuretic group ($p = 0.03$). Active treatment did not lower all-cause mortality.

For multiple reasons, the MRC trial is difficult to interpret *(24–27)*. The single-blind study design may have influenced the results *(22)*. At 5 years, 52% of patients receiving β-blockers and 38% receiving diuretics required additional drugs. There was a higher rate of patients treated

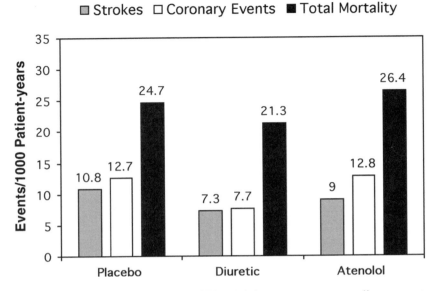

Fig. 3. Medical Research Trial in Older Adults: outcomes according to treatment. The rate of coronary events was lower in the diuretic group than the β-blocker group ($p = 0.006$). The rate of fatal strokes was the same for the β-blocker and placebo groups. The cardiovascular death rate was higher in the β-blocker group than in the diuretic group ($p = 0.03$). (Data from ref. *23*.)

with atenolol (63%) that stopped medication or were lost to follow-up compared to those treated with a diuretic (48%) or placebo (53%). Among smokers, BP control was poorer in patients assigned to β-blocker treatment, and overall cardiovascular events were worse (Fig. 4). These differences are explained by the acceleration of the metabolism of β-blockers by smoking. Overall, 25% of subjects were lost to follow-up. The choice of a hydrophilic β-blocker may have also influenced outcome *(24)*.

Cardiovascular Study in the Elderly

The Cardiovascular Study in the Elderly (CASTEL) was a prospective, single-blind study conducted in northern Italy to evaluate the prevalence of hypertension, the cardiovascular risk, and the effectiveness of drug therapy to reduce mortality in subjects 65 years or older *(28,29)*. The study population consisted of 1404 normotensives and 655 hypertensives. The hypertensives received no intervention ($n = 304$) or drug therapy ($n = 351$), which included 0.15 mg of clonidine per day ($n = 61$), 20 mg of nifedipine per day ($n = 146$), or the fixed combina-

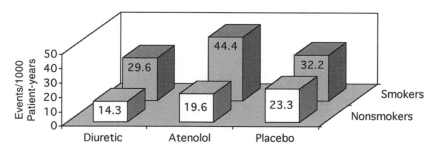

Fig. 4. Medical Research Trial in Older Adults: all cardiovascular events in smokers and nonsmokers. Among smokers, blood pressure control was poorer in patients assigned to β-blocker treatment, and overall cardiovascular events were worse. (Data from ref. *23*.)

tion of 100 mg of atenolol and 25 mg of chlorthalidone (*n* = 144). After 7 years, the overall mortality was 36.9% in the no intervention group, 22.5% in the drug-therapy group, and 24.2% in the normotensive group (*p* = 0.0001). The cardiovascular mortality was 23.7% in the no intervention group, 12.2% in the drug-therapy group, and 11.9% in the normotensive group (*p* = 0.0001). The fixed-dose combination reduced mortality the most.

The Shanghai Trial of Nifedipine in the Elderly

The Shanghai Trial of Nifedipine in the Elderly (STONE) was a single-blind trial that used alternate treatment allocation *(30)*. After a 4-week placebo period, 1632 Chinese patients aged 60–79 years received 10–30 mg of nifedipine twice daily or matching placebo. Captopril, dihydrochlorothiazide, or both could be added to either treatment arm if the BP exceeded 160/90 mmHg. Average follow-up was 30 months. The average decline in BP was –22/–12 mmHg for nifedipine and –12/–8 mmHg for placebo (*p* ≤ 0.0001 for both SBP and DBP). There were more strokes, arrhythmias, and noncardiovascular events in the placebo group, but there was no difference in cardiovascular or overall mortality.

Systolic Hypertension in Europe Trial

The Systolic Hypertension in Europe (Syst-Eur) was planned as a randomized, double-blind, placebo-controlled study to test whether reducing SBP in patients 60 years or older with isolated systolic hypertension would reduce fatal and nonfatal strokes *(31)*. Patients were eligible for randomization if their sitting SBP was 160–219 mmHg, standing SBP was 140 mmHg or higher, and sitting DBP was less than 95 mmHg after

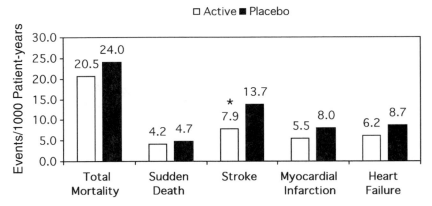

Fig. 5. Systolic Hypertension in Europe Trial. Active therapy reduced all strokes by 42%. *p = 0.003. (Data from ref. *31*.)

a 3-month run-in period. The 4695 patients received active drug or matching placebo to reduce sitting SBP by 20 mmHg to less than 150 mmHg. Active treatment for titration consisted of 10–40 mg of nitrendipine, 5–20 mg of enalapril, and 12.5–25 mg of hydrochlorothiazide.

The mean age was 70 years, and baseline BP was 174/85 mmHg. Median follow-up was 24 months. The average reduction in BP in the placebo group was –13/–2 mmHg, and in the active treatment group was –23/–7 mmHg. Many patients in the placebo group were treated with antihypertensive therapy. The target BP was achieved in 43.5% of subjects assigned to drug therapy compared to 21.4% assigned to placebo. As shown in Fig. 5, active therapy reduced all strokes by 42% ($p = 0.003$). There was no significant reduction in total mortality. MI, heart failure, and sudden death were not significantly reduced individually; however, when combined as a composite cardiac end point, the reduction was 26% ($p = 0.03$).

There were 492 diabetic (10.5%) patients in the Syst-Eur trial *(32)*. Although the placebo-corrected decline of BP in diabetic and nondiabetic persons was similar (8.6/3.9 vs 10.3/4.5 mmHg, $p = 0.4$), there were significant differences in outcomes. The diabetic patients had a significant reduction in overall mortality (55%), cardiovascular mortality (76%), stroke (73%), and cardiac events (63%) after adjustment in baseline variables. Nondiabetic subjects had only a significant reduction in strokes (38%).

The relationship of cognitive impairment, dementia, and hypertension is controversial *(34)*. This was based on 32 cases, 21 in the placebo group and 11 in the active treatment group (7.7 vs 3.8 cases per 1000 patient-years). In an open-label, active treatment extension involving 2902 patients, the rate of dementia, based on 64 cases, was reduced by 55%, from 7.4 to 3.3 cases per 1000 patient-years ($p < 0.001$) *(35)*.

Systolic Hypertension in China

The Systolic Hypertension in China (Syst-China) study used alternate allocation rather than randomization to assess 2394 Chinese hypertensive patients aged 60 years or older with isolated systolic hypertension *(36)*. After a single-blind, placebo run-in phase, patients were enrolled if their SBP was 160–219 mmHg and the DBP was less than 95 mmHg. Nitrendipine (10–40 mg alone or in combination with 12.5–50 mg of captopril), 12.5–50 mg of hydrochlorothiazide, or a combination of both was given to reduce sitting SBP by 20 mmHg or greater and to less than 150 mmHg. The control group received a matching placebo. The average entry BP was 171/86 mmHg. The median follow-up was 3 years. With treatment, the BP declined –11/–2 mmHg in the placebo group and –20/–5 mmHg in the nitrendipine group. Total mortality (17.4 vs 28.4 events per 1000 patient-years, $p = 0.003$) and stroke mortality (2.9 vs 6.9 events per 1000 patient-years, $p = 0.03$) were significantly lower in the active treatment group. Fatal and nonfatal strokes were reduced by 38% ($p = 0.01$). There was no reduction in MI, heart failure, or sudden death.

Swedish Trial in Old Patients With Hypertension-2

The purpose of the STOP-Hypertension-2 study was to examine conventional antihypertensive treatment with newer drugs (angiotensin-converting enzyme [ACE] inhibitors or calcium channel blockers) on cardiovascular events in older patients *(37)*. Using a PROBE design, 6614 patients 70–84 years old were randomly assigned to active treatment if their SBP was 180 mmHg or higher, DBP was 105 mmHg or higher, or both. Unlike the STOP-Hypertension study, patients with isolated systolic hypertension were included in the STOP-Hypertension-2 study. Conventional treatment consisted of once-daily 50 mg of atenolol, 100 mg of controlled-release metoprolol, 5 mg of pindolol, or the combination of 25 mg of hydrochlorothiazide and 2.5 mg of amiloride, which could be combined with the β-blocker monotherapy if the target BP of 160/95 mmHg was not achieved. The ACE inhibitors 10 mg of enalapril or 10 mg of lisinopril dosed once daily were supplemented with 12.5–25 mg of hydrochlorothiazide to achieve treatment goals. The calcium antagonists 2.5 mg of felodipine or 2.5 mg of isradipine dosed once daily were augmented with any of the above β-blockers to achieve the target BP.

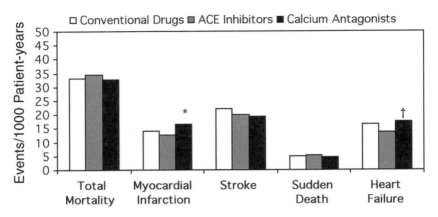

Fig. 6. Outcomes in the Swedish Trial of Older Patients With Hypertension-2. Compared to the angiotensin-converting enzyme (ACE)inhibitor group, there were more fatal and nonfatal myocardial infarctions and a higher frequency of heart failure among patients treated with calcium antagonists. *p = 0.018 vs ACE inhibitor. †p = 0.025 vs ACE inhibitor. (Data from ref. *37.*)

Baseline BP was 194/98 mmHg. After 24 months, there was no difference in the reduction of BP among the three treatment groups. Combination therapy was used in 46% of subjects. There was no difference among the three groups for the primary end point of cardiovascular death after 60.3 months (Fig. 6). However, compared to the ACE inhibitor group, there were more fatal and nonfatal MIs and a higher frequency of heart failure among patients treated with calcium antagonists (Fig. 6). The primary end point did not differ significantly among the 719 diabetic elderly patients *(38)*.

National Intervention Cooperative Study in Elderly Hypertensives

The National Intervention Cooperative Study in Elderly Hypertensives (NICS-EH) compared trichlormethiazide dosed once daily and sustained-release nicardipine hydrochloride dosed twice daily in preventing cardiovascular events in hypertensive patients 60 years or older in Japan*(39,40)*. NICS-EH was a randomized, double-blind, comparison trial *(39)*. After a 4-week placebo period, either 20–40 mg of sustained-release nicardipine or 2–4 mg of trichlormethiazide daily were given to 414 patients with a SBP 160–220 mmHg and a DBP less than 115 mmHg. Medication was administered using the double-dummy technique. Median follow-up differed between treatments, 4.6 years in the nicardipine group and 3.9 years in the diuretic group. However, BP

Table 2
Second Australian National Blood Pressure Study Treatment Algorithm

ACE inhibitor group
    Step 1   ACE inhibitor (enalapril recommended)
    Step 2 β-blocker, α_1-blocker, or calcium antagonist
    Step 3   Drug from class not used in step 2 or diuretic
    Step 4   Drug from class not used in step 2 or 3
Diuretic Group
    Step 1   Thiazide-type diuretic (low dose)
    Step 2 β-blocker, α_1-blocker, or calcium antagonist
    Step 3   Drug from class not used in step 2
    Step 4   Drug from class not used in step 2 or 3

control was similar. There was no difference in the rate of cardiovascular end points in the calcium antagonist and diuretic groups.

Second Australian National Blood Pressure Study

The Second Australian National Blood Pressure Study (ANBP2) trial was designed to compare a diuretic-based and an ACE inhibitor-based regimen in the reduction of all cardiovascular events or total mortality*(41)*. Utilizing a PROBE design, 6083 subjects 65–84 years of age were enrolled and followed for a median of 4.1 years. Entry BP was an SBP of 160 mmHg or higher and/or a DBP of 90 mmHg or higher after the individual was off all antihypertensive medication for at least 1 week. The therapeutic goal was to reduce (a) SBP by 20 mmHg to less than 160 mmHg and below 140 mmHg, if tolerated, and (b) DBP by 10 mmHg to less than 90 mmHg and below 80 mmHg, if tolerated. The treatment protocol required that an ACE inhibitor or diuretic be used as initial therapy (Table 2) *(42)*. Interestingly, the protocol allowed a diuretic to be added to the ACE inhibitor group.

The mean age at randomization was 72 years, and the average BP was 168/91 mmHg. At the end of the study, 58% of subjects in the ACE inhibitor group and 62% in the diuretic group were still receiving their assigned therapy; 65% of the ACE inhibitor-treated and 67% of the diuretic-treated participants took monotherapy. The average reduction in BP was 26/12 mmHg at year 5. There was no difference in total mortality between treatments (Fig. 7). There were fewer first cardiovascular events in the ACE inhibitor group compared with the diuretic group (33.7 vs 37.1 per 1000 patient-years, $p = 0.07$), which was because of a lower MI rate (4.7 vs 6.7 per 1000 patient-years, $p = 0.04$). However,

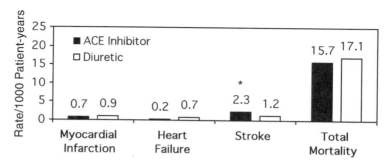

Fig. 7. The Second Australian National Blood Pressure Study: fatal first events and total mortality. There were more first fatal strokes in the angiotensin-converting enzyme inhibitor group compared with the diuretic group. *$p = 0.04$. (Data from ref. *41*.)

there were more first fatal strokes (Fig. 7) in the ACE inhibitor group compared with the diuretic group (2.3 vs 1.2 per 1000 patient-years, $p = 0.04$).

The Study on Cognition and Prognosis in the Elderly

The purpose of the Study on Cognition and Prognosis in the Elderly (SCOPE) was to assess whether the angiotensin-receptor blocker (ARB) candesartan would reduce the first major cardiovascular event (nonfatal stroke, nonfatal MI, and cardiovascular death), cognitive decline, and dementia in 4964 patients aged 70–89 years *(43)*. This double-blind, randomized, parallel group study enrolled patients with a SBP of 160–179 mmHg and/or a DBP of 90–99 mmHg. SCOPE originally was designed to compare candesartan vs placebo, but the protocol was changed to allow open-label active drugs in both groups based on a change in the World Health Organization-International Society of Hypertension guidelines for therapy.

After an open run-in period of 1–3 months, 8–16 mg of candesartan dosed once daily or placebo was given. The initial treatment goal was to lower the SBP below 160 mmHg, decrease the SBP by 10 mmHg from the baseline, and decrease the DBP 85 mmHg or less. If the BP was 160/90 mmHg or higher, then 12.5 mg of hydrochlorothiazide once daily could be added. Except for ACE inhibitors or ARBs, other drug classes could be supplemented to achieve the target BP.

The baseline BP was 166/90 mmHg. After 44.6 months, the adjusted mean difference in BP was −3.2/−1.6 mmHg lower in the candesartan group ($p < 0.001$ for both SBP and DBP). Only 25% of the candesartan-

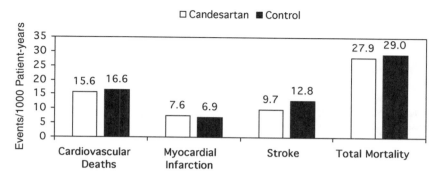

Fig. 8. Study on Cognition and Prognosis in the Elderly. There was no significant reduction in the composite of major cardiovascular events or total mortality with candesartan. (Data from ref. *43*.)

treated patients and 16% of the placebo group received their assigned treatment. Add-on antihypertensive drugs were received by 49% of the candesartan group and 66% of the placebo group.

There was no significant reduction in the composite of major cardiovascular events or total mortality with candesartan (Fig. 8). There was a lower rate of nonfatal strokes in the candesartan group (7.4 vs 10.3 events/1000 patient-years, $p = 0.04$) but not fatal stroke. There was no difference in cognitive function as assessed by the Mini Mental State Examination or the rate of dementia.

Systolic Hypertension in the Elderly: Lacidipine Long-Term Study

The Systolic Hypertension in the Elderly: Lacidipine Long-Term (SHELL) study was planned to compare lacidipine and chlorthalidone on cardiovascular outcome in patients 60 years or older with isolated systolic hypertension, defined as a SBP 160 mmHg or higher and a DBP 95 mmHg or less *(44,45)*. The primary outcome was a composite of cardiovascular and cerebrovascular events. SHELL used a PROBE design; however, 12 sites followed a double-blind design for the first year. Patients ($n = 1882$) were randomly assigned to the administration of 12.5 mg of chlorthalidone or 4 mg of lacidipine dosed once daily after a 2-week washout period. If there was not a 20-mg or greater reduction in SBP and SBP exceeded 160 mmHg after 4 weeks, chlorthalidone was increased to 25 mg or lacidipine to 6 mg daily. If BP control was not achieved after 1 month, then the dose of the assigned drug was reduced to the starting dose, and 10 mg fosinopril once daily was added. The planned sample size of 4800 patients was not achieved.

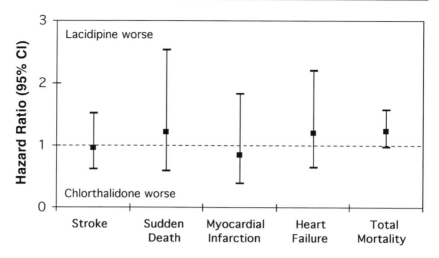

Fig. 9. Systolic Hypertension in the Elderly: Lacidipine Long-Term (SHELL) study. There was no significant difference for individual cardiovascular events. (Data from ref. *44*.)

Baseline BP was 178/87 mmHg. After 32 months, BP was reduced to 142/79 mmHg in chlorthalidone-treated patients and 143/79 mmHg in the lacidipine-treated patients. Low-dose monotherapy was taken by 72% of lacidipine-treated and 47% of diuretic-treated patients. The overall incidence of the primary end points was 9.3%, with no difference according to treatment. As shown in Fig. 9, there was no significant difference for individual cardiovascular events. Total mortality, a secondary end point, was comparable.

Hypertension in the Very Elderly Trial Pilot

The Hypertension in the Very Elderly Trial (HYVET) Pilot trial was a multicenter, PROBE design study in which hypertensive patients over the age of 80 years were randomly assigned to determine if treatment would reduce fatal and nonfatal strokes *(46–49)*. After 2 months of observation, subjects were enrolled with a sitting SBP of 160–219 mmHg and DBP of 95–109 mmHg, based on four readings, and a standing BP greater than 140 mmHg, based on two readings. Patients received no treatment (*n* = 426) or treatment with 2.5–5 mg of a bendrofluazide dosed once daily (*n* = 426) or 2.5–5 mg of lisinopril dosed once daily (*n* = 431). Titration of drug doses and the addition of 120–240 mg of slow-release diltiazem dosed once daily were allowed to achieve a seated

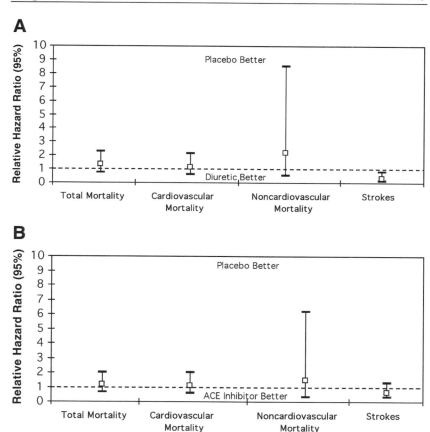

Fig. 10. Hypertension in the Very Elderly Trial (HYVET) pilot. Treatment with a diuretic significantly reduced the risk of fatal and nonfatal strokes by 69% ($p = 0.01$). This benefit was not seen with the angiotensin-converting enzyme inhibitor. (Data from ref. *49.*)

BP of less than 150/80 mmHg. Patients were followed for a mean duration of 13 months. The average change in the sitting and standing BP, respectively, was −30/−16 and −26/−15 mmHg for the diuretic group, −30/−16 and −27/−16 mmHg for the ACE inhibitor group, and −7/−5 and −3/−4 mmHg for the placebo group.

Antihypertensive treatment (Fig. 10) with a diuretic significantly reduced the risk of fatal and nonfatal strokes by 69% ($p = 0.01$). The number of events was too small to compare treatments. There was an insignificant increase in total mortality with hypertensive treatment: 7.0, 6.3, and 5.2% for the diuretic, ACE inhibitor, and placebo groups, respectively. The results were consistent with the previously published meta-analysis *(2)*. The main double-blind HYVET trial is actively enrolling subjects.

Antihypertensive and Lipid-Lowering
Treatment to Prevent Heart Attack Trial

The Antihypertensive and Lipid-Lowering Treatment to Prevent Heart Attack Trial (ALLHAT) has not been mentioned because it was not entirely a trial of the elderly. Enrollment included hypertensive patients 55 years or older with one other cardiovascular risk factor. There were 42,448 participants, of whom 80.9% were 60 years or older and 35.3% were 70 years and older *(50)*. Mean age was 67 years. Thus, ALLHAT should not be ignored compared with the 43,104 patients listed in Table 1, which included only 17,281 patients in double-blind trials.

The purpose of ALLHAT was to determine whether new antihypertensives, calcium antagonists, ACE inhibitors, and α_1-blockers reduced fatal and nonfatal heart attacks compared with a diuretic *(51–53)*. The trial was conducted as a randomized, double-blind trial. The goal was to titrate the BP to less than 140/90 mmHg. Initial drug therapy (Table 3) was blinded, but the drug choice for step 2 was left to the physician. The effectiveness of the treatment protocol is displayed in Fig. 11 *(54)*. Among the elderly patients 70 years and older, 26.2% were controlled to less than 140/90 mmHg on enrollment. After 5 years, the control rate increased to 64.4%, which required three or more drugs among 27% of the patients.

After a mean follow-up of 3.2 years, the α_1-blocker (doxazosin) arm was terminated because of more cardiovascular events compared to the diuretic arm *(51,53)*. There were 12,382 patients 60 years and older assigned to chlorthalidone and 7341 assigned to doxazosin. BP control was better in the diuretic than α_1-blocker arm after 4 years. Although there was no difference in total mortality or the primary end point of fatal and nonfatal MI, there was a significantly higher rate of stroke events, heart failure, angina, and coronary revascularization in the doxazosin group. Among participants 65 years or older, the rate of heart failure was 89% higher, and combined cardiovascular disease was 23% higher among doxazosin-treated patients *(53)*.

After a mean follow-up of 4.9 years, the results of the comparison of the ACE inhibitor and calcium antagonist arms were compared to the diuretic arm *(52)*. There were 8784, 5204, and 5185 subjects 65 years and older in the chlorthalidone, amlodipine, and lisinopril groups, respectively. Chlorthalidone was more effective for SBP control than ei-

Table 3
Antihypertensive and Lipid-Lowering Treatment to Prevent Heart Attack Trial
(ALLHAT) Initial Treatment and Titration Protocol

Step 1 drug	Initial dose, mg	Dose 1, mg	Dose 2, mg	Dose 3, mg
Chlorthalidone	12.5	12.5	12.5	25
Amlodipine	2.5	2.5	5	10
Lisinopril	10	10	20	40
Doxazosin	1	2	4	8

Step 2 drug choice	Dose 1, mg	Dose 2, mg	Dose 3, mg
Reserpine	0.05 qd or 0.1 qod	0.1 qd	0.2 qd
Oral clonidine	0.1 bid	0.2 bid	0.3 bid
Atenolol	25 qd	50 qd	100 qd

Step 3 drug			
Hydralazine	25 bid	50 bid	100 bid

qd, every day; qod, every other day; bid, twice a day.

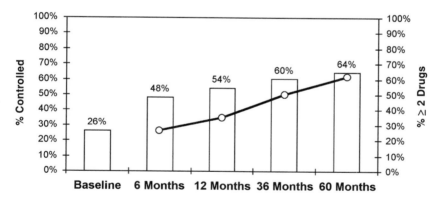

Fig. 11. Antihypertensive and Lipid-Lowering Treatment to Prevent Heart
Attack Trial (ALLHAT): rate of blood pressure control (<140/90 mmHg) among
patients 70 years and older. The bars show the percentage of subjects controlled.
The line shows the percentage of subjects requiring two or more drugs after
enrollment. (Data from ref. *49*.)

ther amlodipine or lisinopril over the 5 years of the study. As shown in
Figs. 12 and 13, there was no difference in the primary end point or all-
cause mortality, but there was a higher risk of heart failure: 33% for
amlodipine-treated patients and 20% for lisinopril-treated patients.

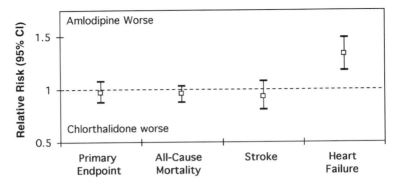

Fig. 12. Antihypertensive and Lipid-Lowering Treatment to Prevent Heart Attack Trial (ALLHAT): outcomes comparing amlodipine and chlorthalidone in patients 65 years and older. There was no difference in the primary end point or all-cause mortality, but there was a 33% higher risk of heart failure for amlodipine-treated patients compared to those treated with chlorthalidone. (Data from ref. *52*.)

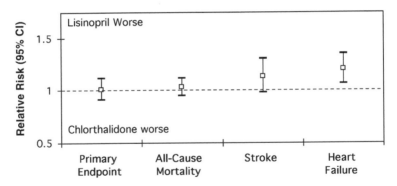

Fig. 13. Antihypertensive and Lipid-Lowering Treatment to Prevent Heart Attack Trial (ALLHAT): outcomes comparing lisinopril and chlorthalidone in patients 65 years and older. There was no difference in the primary end point or all-cause mortality, but there was a 20% higher risk of heart failure for amlodipine-treated patients compared to those treated with chlorthalidone. (Data from ref. *52*.)

ANALYSIS

The completed trials in the elderly have been summarized. There are difficulties in interpreting the data from single-blind and PROBE design trials, especially in the presence of solid, well-designed, double-blind trials to guide decisions. Thus, the information from EWPHE, NICS-EH, SCOPE, SHEP, STOP-Hypertension, Syst-Eur, and ALLHAT should guide thinking depending on the outcome that is examined. The double-blind, placebo-controlled trials are shown in Table 4. The inclu-

Table 4
Double-Blind, Placebo-Controlled Outcome Trials in the Elderly: Percentage Change

Trial	Total mortality	Cardiovascular mortality	Stroke mortality	Fatal myocardial infarctions	Heart failure	All myocardial infarctions	Fatal and nonfatal stroke	All cardiovascular events
EWPHE	-26	-38*	-43	-47*	-63*	NS	-46	-34*
SCOPE	-4	-6	-7	-5	NS	+10	-24	-11
SHEP	-13	-20	-29	-43	-54*	-27*	-36*	-32*
STOP-Hypertension	-43*	NS	-73*	-25	-51*	-13	-47*	-40*
Syst-Eur	-14	-27	-27	-56	-29	-30	-42*	-31*

See text for trial abbreviation definitions. NS, not stated.
*Significant reduction.

sion of SCOPE in this table is controversial because the protocol changed during the trial. As displayed, only one trial reported a reduction in total mortality as a secondary end point. All trials except SCOPE reduced total fatal and nonfatal cardiovascular events. Only EWPHE and SCOPE did not observe a reduction in fatal and nonfatal strokes. Heart failure was not decreased with the calcium antagonist nitrendipine but was decreased with the diuretic-based therapy used in EWPHE, SHEP, and STOP-Hypertension.

ALLHAT provided the strongest data for the comparison of initial antihypertensive therapy. The results of the PROBE trials ANBP2 and STOP-Hypertension-2 were not inconsistent with ALLHAT. It should be recalled that none of these studies was a monotherapy trial. Multiple drugs will be required to achieve BP goals necessary to avoid premature disability and death.

REFERENCES

1. Mulrow CD, Cornell JA, Herrera CR, Kadri A, Farnett L, Aguilar C. Hypertension in the elderly. Implications and generalizability of randomized trials. *JAMA* 1994;272:1932–1938.
2. Gueyffier F, Bulpitt C, Boissel JP, et al. Antihypertensive drugs in very old people: a subgroup meta-analysis of randomised controlled trials. INDANA Group. *Lancet* 1999;353:793–796.
3. Effects of treatment on morbidity in hypertension. 3. Influence of age, diastolic pressure, and prior cardiovascular disease; further analysis of side effects. *Circulation* 1972;45:991–1004.
4. Five-year findings of the hypertension detection and follow-up program. II. Mortality by race-sex and age. Hypertension Detection and Follow-up Program Cooperative Group. *JAMA* 1979;242:2572–2577.
5. Treatment of mild hypertension in the elderly. A study initiated and administered by the National Heart Foundation of Australia. *Med J Aust* 1981;2:398–402.
6. Birkenhäger WH, de Leeuw PW, Amery A, Staessen J. Treatment of hypertension in the elderly. *Cardiovasc Drugs Ther* 1988;2:275–279.
7. Smith WM. The case for treating hypertension in the elderly. *Am J Hypertens* 1988;1(3 pt 3):173S–178S.
8. Beard K, Bulpitt C, Mascie-Taylor H, O'Malley K, Sever P, Webb S. Management of elderly patients with sustained hypertension. *BMJ* 1992;304:412–416.
9. Hansson L, Hedner T, Dahlöf B. Prospective randomized open blinded end-point (PROBE) study. A novel design for intervention trials. Prospective Randomized Open Blinded End-Point. *Blood Press* 1992;1:113–119.
10. Amery A, Birkenhäger W, Brixko P, et al. Mortality and morbidity results from the European Working Party on High Blood Pressure in the Elderly trial. *Lancet* 1985;1:1349–1354.
11. Prisant LM, Carr AA. Overview of the findings of the European Party on High Blood Pressure in the Elderly. *Geriatr Med Today* 1990;9:35–38.
12. Carter AB. Hypotensive therapy in stroke survivors. *Lancet* 1970;1:485–489.
13. Effect of antihypertensive treatment on stroke recurrence. Hypertension-Stroke Cooperative Study Group. *JAMA* 1974;229:409–418.

14. Sprackling ME, Mitchell JR, Short AH, Watt G. Blood pressure reduction in elderly: a randomised controlled trial of methyldopa. *Br Med J (Clin Res Ed)* 1981;283:1151–1153.
15. Coope J, Warrender TS. Randomised trial of treatment of hypertension in elderly patients in primary care. *Br Med J (Clin Res Ed)* 1986;293:1145–1151.
16. Prevention of stroke by antihypertensive drug treatment in older persons with isolated systolic hypertension. Final results of the Systolic Hypertension in the Elderly Program (SHEP). SHEP Cooperative Research Group. *JAMA* 1991;265:3255–3264.
17. Applegate WB, Pressel S, Wittes J, et al. Impact of the treatment of isolated systolic hypertension on behavioral variables. Results from the systolic hypertension in the elderly program. *Arch Intern Med* 1994;154:2154–2160.
18. Kostis JB, Davis BR, Cutler J, et al. Prevention of heart failure by antihypertensive drug treatment in older persons with isolated systolic hypertension. SHEP Cooperative Research Group. *JAMA* 1997;278:212–216.
19. Curb JD, Pressel SL, Cutler JA, et al. Effect of diuretic-based antihypertensive treatment on cardiovascular disease risk in older diabetic patients with isolated systolic hypertension. Systolic Hypertension in the Elderly Program Cooperative Research Group. *JAMA* 1996;276:1886–1892.
20. Dahlof B, Lindholm LH, Hansson L, Schersten B, Ekbom T, Wester PO. Morbidity and mortality in the Swedish Trial in Old Patients with Hypertension (STOP-Hypertension). *Lancet* 1991;338:1281–1285.
21. Ekbom T, Dahlöf B, Hansson L, Lindholm LH, Scherstén B, Wester PO. Antihypertensive efficacy and side effects of three beta-blockers and a diuretic in elderly hypertensives: a report from the STOP-Hypertension study. *J Hypertens* 1992;10:1525–1530.
22. Prisant LM. Should beta blockers be used in the treatment of hypertension in the elderly? *J Clin Hypertens (Greenwich)* 2002;4:286–294.
23. Medical Research Council trial of treatment of hypertension in older adults: principal results. MRC Working Party. *BMJ* 1992;304:405–412.
24. Kendall MJ. Treatment of hypertension in older adults. *BMJ* 1992;304:639.
25. Mitchell AB. MRC trial of treating hypertension in older adults. *BMJ* 1992;304:1631.
26. Swedberg K. MRC trial of treating hypertension in older adults. *BMJ* 1992;304:1630–1631.
27. Tuomilehto J. MRC trial of treating hypertension in older adults. *BMJ* 1992;304:1631.
28. Casiglia E, Spolaore P, Mormino P, et al. The CASTEL project (Cardiovascular Study in the Elderly) : protocol, study design, and preliminary results of the initial survey. *Cardiologia* 1991;36:569–576.
29. Casiglia E, Spolaore P, Mazza A, et al. Effect of two different therapeutic approaches on total and cardiovascular mortality in a Cardiovascular Study in the Elderly (CASTEL). *Jpn Heart J* 1994;35:589–600.
30. Gong L, Zhang W, Zhu Y, et al. Shanghai trial of nifedipine in the elderly (STONE). *J Hypertens* 1996;14:1237–1245.
31. Staessen JA, Fagard R, Thijs L, et al. Randomised double-blind comparison of placebo and active treatment for older patients with isolated systolic hypertension. The Systolic Hypertension in Europe (Syst-Eur) Trial Investigators. *Lancet* 1997;350:757–764.
32. Tuomilehto J, Rastenyte D, Birkenhäger WH, et al. Effects of calcium-channel blockade in older patients with diabetes and systolic hypertension. Systolic Hypertension in Europe Trial Investigators. *N Engl J Med* 1999;340:677–684.

33. Birkenhager WH, Forette F, Seux ML, Wang JG, Staessen JA. Blood pressure, cognitive functions, and prevention of dementias in older patients with hypertension. *Arch Intern Med* 2001;161:152–156.

34. Forette F, Seux ML, Staessen JA, et al. Prevention of dementia in randomised double-blind placebo-controlled Systolic Hypertension in Europe (Syst-Eur) trial. *Lancet* 1998;352:1347–1351.

35. Forette F, Seux ML, Staessen JA, et al. The prevention of dementia with antihypertensive treatment: new evidence from the Systolic Hypertension in Europe (Syst-Eur) study. *Arch Intern Med* 2002;162:2046–2052.

36. Liu L, Wang JG, Gong L, Liu G, Staessen JA. Comparison of active treatment and placebo in older Chinese patients with isolated systolic hypertension. Systolic Hypertension in China (Syst-China) Collaborative Group. *J Hypertens* 1998;16(12 pt 1) :1823–1829.

37. Hansson L, Lindholm LH, Ekbom T, et al. Randomised trial of old and new antihypertensive drugs in elderly patients: cardiovascular mortality and morbidity the Swedish Trial in Old Patients with Hypertension-2 study. *Lancet* 1999;354:1751–1756.

38. Lindholm LH, Hansson L, Ekbom T, et al. Comparison of antihypertensive treatments in preventing cardiovascular events in elderly diabetic patients: results from the Swedish Trial in Old Patients with Hypertension-2. STOP Hypertension-2 Study Group. *J Hypertens* 2000;18:1671–1675.

39. Kuramoto K. Treatment of elderly hypertensives in Japan: National Intervention Cooperative Study in Elderly Hypertensives. The National Intervention Cooperative Study Group. *J Hypertens Suppl* 1994;12:S35–S40.

40. Randomized double-blind comparison of a calcium antagonist and a diuretic in elderly hypertensives. National Intervention Cooperative Study in Elderly Hypertensives Study Group. *Hypertension* 1999;34:1129–1133.

41. Wing LM, Reid CM, Ryan P, et al. A comparison of outcomes with angiotensin-converting—enzyme inhibitors and diuretics for hypertension in the elderly. *N Engl J Med* 2003;348:583–592.

42. Australian comparative outcome trial of angiotensin-converting enzyme inhibitor- and diuretic-based treatment of hypertension in the elderly (ANBP2) : objectives and protocol. Management Committee on behalf of the High Blood Pressure Research Council of Australia. *Clin Exp Pharmacol Physiol* 1997;24:188–192.

43. Lithell H, Hansson L, Skoog I, et al. The Study on Cognition and Prognosis in the Elderly (SCOPE) : principal results of a randomized double-blind intervention trial. *J Hypertens* 2003;21:875–886.

44. Malacco E, Mancia G, Rappelli A, Menotti A, Zuccaro MS, Coppini A. Treatment of isolated systolic hypertension: the SHELL study results. *Blood Press* 2003;12: 160–167.

45. Malacco E, Gnemmi AE, Romagnoli A, Coppini A. Systolic hypertension in the elderly: long-term lacidipine treatment. Objective, protocol, and organization. SHELL Study Group. *J Cardiovasc Pharmacol* 1994;23(suppl 5) :S62–S66.

46. Bulpitt CJ, Fletcher AE, Amery A, et al. The Hypertension in the Very Elderly Trial (HYVET). *J Hum Hypertens* 1994;8:631–632.

47. Bulpitt CJ, Fletcher AE, Amery A, et al. The Hypertension in the Very Elderly Trial (HYVET). Rationale, methodology and comparison with previous trials. *Drugs Aging* 1994;5:171–183.

48. Bulpitt C, Fletcher A, Beckett N, et al. Hypertension in the Very Elderly Trial (HYVET) : protocol for the main trial. *Drugs Aging* 2001;18:151–164.

49. Bulpitt CJ, Beckett NS, Cooke J, et al. Results of the pilot study for the Hypertension in the Very Elderly Trial. *J Hypertens* 2003;21:2409–2417.
50. Grimm RH Jr, Margolis KL, Papademetriou VV, et al. Baseline Characteristics of Participants in the Antihypertensive and Lipid Lowering Treatment to Prevent Heart Attack Trial (ALLHAT). *Hypertension* 2001;37:19–27.
51. Major cardiovascular events in hypertensive patients randomized to doxazosin vs chlorthalidone: the antihypertensive and lipid-lowering treatment to prevent heart attack trial (ALLHAT). ALLHAT Collaborative Research Group. *JAMA* 2000;283: 1967–1975.
52. Major outcomes in high-risk hypertensive patients randomized to angiotensin-converting enzyme inhibitor or calcium channel blocker vs diuretic: the Antihypertensive and Lipid-Lowering Treatment to Prevent Heart Attack Trial (ALLHAT). *JAMA* 2002;288:2981–2997.
53. Diuretic vs α-blocker as first-step antihypertensive therapy: final results from the Antihypertensive and Lipid-Lowering Treatment to Prevent Heart Attack Trial (ALLHAT). *Hypertension* 2003;42:239–246.
54. Cushman WC, Ford CE, Cutler JA, et al. Success and predictors of blood pressure control in diverse North American settings: the antihypertensive and lipid-lowering treatment to prevent heart attack trial (ALLHAT). *J Clin Hypertens (Greenwich)* 2002;4:393–404.
55. Dahlöf B, Lindholm LH, Hansson L, Scherstén B, Ekbom T, Wester PO. Morbidity and mortality in the Swedish Trial in Old Patients with Hypertension (STOP-Hypertension). *Lancet* 1991;338:1281–1285.

III

EVALUATION AND MANAGEMENT

8 Blood Pressure Measurement in Older Patients With Hypertension

Jose Ramiro Arias-Vera, MD
and William B. White, MD

INTRODUCTION

Accurate measurement of blood pressure (BP) in older patients is vitally important for prognosis and intervention; however, obtaining reliable measurement data in this population is not always an easy task. The office BP in older patients is often difficult to measure for a variety of reasons. For example, in older patients accurate BP measurement is challenging because alterations in cardiovascular physiology with the aging process produce an increase in BP variability. Furthermore, certain structural changes in the blood vessel can add to the imprecision of many types of BP determination.

The objective of this chapter is to detail some of the specific age-related factors that play an important role in BP measurement and to review the benefits and pitfalls of self-BP (home) and ambulatory BP monitoring (ABPM) in the elderly.

From: *Clinical Hypertension and Vascular Diseases: Hypertension in the Elderly*
Edited by: L. M. Prisant © Humana Press Inc., Totowa, NJ

OFFICE BLOOD PRESSURE

Most large outcome trials in hypertension utilized data obtained with the BP measured under standardized conditions at office visits and using the auscultatory method and a mercury column sphygmomanometer. Thus, many physicians feel strongly that to apply these studies of prognosis and interventions, similar standard conditions and methods of BP determination should be used in clinical practice. However, there are inherent inaccuracies of office BP measurements that cause misdiagnoses and lead toward treatment that may not always be appropriate. Defective equipment, poor measurement technique, and observer bias all may contribute as sources of error in measurement.

In an effort to minimize the potential error for BP measurement in practice, a number of guidelines have been published over the years that have focused on standardizing the technique. One of the most widely accepted of the guidelines has been by the American Heart Association (AHA) in 1993 (1). However, many studies showed that the majority of physicians and ancillary medical personnel in fact do not measure BP correctly as recommended by these guidelines. The potential medical, economic, and even legal implications of incorrect BP measurement are substantial. The AHA guidelines in the elderly are not different from those for other age groups. Thus, next we focus on certain age-specific conditions that need special attention when measuring BP in the elderly at the office. These include the issues of the auscultatory gap, orthostatic hypotension, pseudohypertension, and white-coat hypertension (WCH).

The Auscultatory Gap

A lengthy disappearance of the Korotkoff sounds between the systolic blood pressure (SBP) and diastolic blood pressure (DBP) is referred to as the *auscultatory gap*. The auscultatory gap has a diagnostic significance because, if it is not recognized, it becomes a source of error in BP measurement; in addition, some data suggest it may be a marker of cardiovascular morbidity (2).

When the auscultatory gap is analyzed by wideband external pulse recording added to clinical auscultation, three types of gaps are identified (3): G1, G2, and G3. G1 and G2 are related to the intermittent variation in BP produced by the respiratory cycle. G1 is the intermittent disappearance of the Korotkoff sounds when the cuff pressure is just below the SBP and is produced by the phasic decrease in SBP during inspiration. G2 is the intermittent disappearance of the Korotkoff sounds when the cuff pressure is just above DBP produced by the phasic increase in BP during expiration.

G3 is the classically described auscultatory gap for which the disappearance of audible sounds between SBP and DBP is independent of respiratory variations. Missing the auscultatory gap will produce an underestimation of SBP and occasionally an overestimation of the DBP. To avoid the incorrect assessment of the SBP level, estimation of SBP by palpation must be performed before auscultation. To avoid the overestimation of the DBP, auscultation should be continued for at least 10 mmHg after the first disappearance of the Korotkoff sounds.

The physiological etiology of the auscultatory gap is not fully understood, but it appears to be related to the physical properties of the arterial wall (3). There is a study that suggested that the G3 auscultatory gap may be associated with increased arterial stiffness and carotid atherosclerosis independent of age or BP level (2). Although this study did not find age to be an independent predictor of the gap, increased arterial stiffness is more common in the elderly. Increased arterial stiffness and atherosclerosis are independent risk factors for cardiovascular morbidity; thus, the presence of a G3 gap might be a surrogate marker for these conditions and may have an indirect correlation with increased cardiovascular morbidity.

Orthostatic Blood Pressure Changes

The maintenance of BP on standing is the result of complex physiological mechanisms that require intact function of the autonomic and cardiovascular systems. The BP response to postural changes in healthy individuals is characterized by a transient initial decrease in pressure during the first 15 seconds after standing followed by progressive increases in BP over 30 seconds that ultimately reach a value that is higher than the initial supine pressure (4). Orthostatic hypotension is typically defined as a fall of 20 mmHg or more in SBP or 10 mmHg or more in DBP after 3 minutes of standing (5). However, this definition has limited clinical significance because many patients can experience symptoms of cerebral hypoperfusion with smaller decreases in the SBP, when they might be at risk for falls and syncope. Furthermore, there may be fairly marked intraindividual variability in the absolute change in orthostatic pressure at different times of the day (6,7) and on different days of the week (8).

Orthostatic hypotension becomes more common with increasing age (9–11). With aging, there are decreases in baroreflex responsiveness and reductions in the cardiovascular response to sympathetic stimuli as well. However, these alterations in physiology do not fully explain the level and frequency of orthostatic hypotension that occurs in older people.

Many pathological conditions common in the elderly affect the autonomic system and produce more severe orthostatic hypotension, such as Parkinson's disease, multiple system atrophy, or peripheral neuropathies. In fact, the orthostasis may occur before overt neurological symptoms develop.

Therefore, evaluation of postural BP changes should form a part of the initial evaluation of elderly patients, and a significant drop in BP after 1 or more minutes of standing should be considered abnormal. Even if the orthostatic reduction in BP is initially asymptomatic, it is important to identify those individuals with varying degrees of postural hypotension because they are susceptible to significant BP falls induced by changes in clinical status or in response to vasoactive medications (12–14).

A particularly challenging group of patients are those who develop both hypotension on standing and supine hypertension. In fact, there is a direct correlation between the level of the supine BP and the degree of BP decrease on standing (8,15). Thus, in these hypertensive patients, carefully lowering the supine or seated BP may decrease the degree of orthostatic hypotension (7). The group of patients who have significant autonomic failure caused by conditions such as Parkinson's disease and multiple system atrophy not only has supine hypertension and standing hypotension, but also can manifest severe abnormalities in BP regulation and may have a highly variable circadian BP (16,17). Beyond the more obvious clinical consequences of the hypotensive episodes, there are even data suggesting that orthostatic hypotension in the elderly may be a predictor of all-cause mortality (18,19).

Pseudohypertension

A significant overestimation of BP when measured noninvasively by the cuff as compared to directly measured (intra-arterial) BP has been termed *pseudohypertension*. Pseudohypertension is generally thought to be secondary to increased arterial wall stiffness; thus, the external pressure needed to occlude the artery is increased independent of internal arterial pressure. In extreme cases, when the artery is highly calcified, the vessel may become noncompressible by an external cuff. Most investigators have defined pseudohypertension using an absolute cuff pressure of no less than 10 mmHg systolic and/or diastolic pressure above the directly measured pressure. However, given the lack of evidence of the clinical significance of directly measured BP, any value used to define pseudohypertension is relatively arbitrary.

The prevalence of pseudohypertension in the elderly is highly variable among different studies, ranging between as low as 1.7% and as high as 70% (20). Despite the methodological differences among these studies, the major factor accounting for the different results has been the selection of individuals studied. Thus, in the group of elderly subjects in whom pseudohypertension was suspected, the incidence of confirmed pseudohypertension was the highest. On the other hand, on groups of randomly selected older individuals, pseudohypertension was relatively rare. Pseudohypertension is also more common in patients with accelerated atherosclerosis, such as those with end-stage renal failure *(21)*.

It is often quite difficult to identify those patients with pseudo-hypertension. The condition should be suspected clinically in older hypertensive patients who lack a correlation between hypertension-related end target organ damage and the level of BP or when a patient with elevated arm BP experiences signs and symptoms of hypotension induced by antihypertensive medications.

The Osler's sign has been recommended as a means to screen potential patients for pseudohypertension *(1)*. This sign is basically a finding associated with large arterial sclerosis and is positive when either the brachial or radial artery is still palpable after the BP cuff has been inflated above systolic pressure. Although an initial study conducted in selected patients with suspected pseudohypertension found significant correlation between a positive Osler's sign and pseudohypertension *(22)*, other studies in randomly selected individuals showed that this correlation is usually not significant *(23,24)*. Thus, for general screening, the Osler's sign lacks reliability and has poor predictive value for pseudohypertension.

White-Coat Effect and White-Coat Hypertension

With the increased use of out-of-office BP measurements in the elderly, it has become evident that a large proportion of patients have an office BP that is higher than the measured BP value outside the medical environment. The prevalence of WCH is approximately 15–30% *(25,26)*. This condition should be suspected clinically when the office BP is high and when there is a lack of hypertension-related end target organ damage or when patients develop side effects from antihypertensive therapy typically associated with excessive reduction in BP.

WHITE-COAT EFFECT

The phenomenon of transient BP elevations when the individual is in a medical environment is called the *white-coat effect*. The exact prevalence of individuals who develop the white-coat effect is not known, but it seems to increase with increasing age *(27)*. The white-coat effect is a qualitative definition independent of absolute values, and it may be present as assessed by office readings in both normotensive and hypertensive individuals. Use of home self-measured BP (SMBP) is an acceptable means to start the evaluation for a white-coat effect but as described below should be confirmed with 24-hour ambulatory BP recordings.

REVERSE WHITE-COAT EFFECT

The phenomenon in which the office BP is lower than the ambulatory BP is called *reverse white-coat effect* or, more recently, *masked hypertension (28)*. Although far less studied than WCH, Wing et al. *(29)* reported that 21% of older patients studied had lower office than ambulatory systolic pressures.

WHITE-COAT HYPERTENSION

WCH is defined when an untreated patient has a persistent office BP greater than 140/90 mmHg with an average daytime ambulatory BP below 135/85 mmHg *(30)*. Most recent studies suggest that WCH is more common in the elderly individual than in middle-aged patients. ABPM in conjunction with carefully measured office BPs is the only means to accurately diagnose a patient as having WCH. Self- or home BP measurements might suggest this condition but are not considered definitive.

OUT-OF-OFFICE BLOOD PRESSURE MEASUREMENTS

Monitoring of BP outside the medical care environment has become an important part of clinical hypertension assessment and management. There are two main forms of out-of-office BP monitoring: (a) self- or home monitoring, usually performed by the patient with a portable automatic or semiautomatic device or aneroid manometer plus stethoscope and (b) ABPM, which uses automatic devices for repeated determinations during an extended time period, typically 24 hours. Both techniques have been shown to substantially enhance the clinician's understanding of BP behavior and aid in diagnosis and therapeutic decision making.

Self-Measured Blood Pressure

The self-measurement of BP at home is a useful tool and adds to office BP in the evaluation and management of the hypertensive patient. However, knowledge in this area is yet evolving. At this time, there is no absolute consensus about distribution of values of home BP in the general population, comparison of SMBP and office BP, standardization of devices and technique for SMBP, and the diagnostic or prognostic value of out-of-office BPs. Therefore, decisions for management of the hypertensive patient should not be done based solely on out-of-office BP determinations. In this section, we describe this method and the current evidence about its value and indications focused in the elderly.

DEVICES FOR SELF-MEASURED BLOOD PRESSURE

Several types of BP monitors are available for use at home, including aneroid manometers, semiautomatic electronic sphygmomanometers, and mercury column sphygmomanometers. Aneroid manometers with a stethoscope are relatively simple to use and generally are the most economical type of self-monitoring units available. However, all the concerns about technique and biased readings with auscultatory BP measurement are even greater when patients perform the readings. For these reasons, they are usually not recommended. They are even less suitable in older patients lacking manual dexterity or when hearing loss is an issue.

Automatic electronic devices are the most convenient and during the past few years have clearly become the devices of choice for home or SMBP. Most electronic devices are of the oscillometric type and can be applied to the brachial or radial artery. Finger devices use the plethysmographic technique and are the least accurate, so are not recommended for self-measurements. A number of the oscillometric brachial or radial devices have demonstrated accuracy under standard measuring conditions. However, wrist devices become inaccurate when the wrist is not maintained at heart level or is in extreme flexion or extension. Given this potential error in measuring technique, they are better used only when a brachial device is not a suitable option, such as in very obese patients. Therefore, automatic brachial oscillometric devices are the first choice for self-measured BP.

A number of these devices are commercially available; however, only a few have been independently validated. The responsibility in certifying that the device used is accurate currently falls on the physician in charge. The Association for the Advancement of Medical Instrumentation and the British Hypertension Society have rigorous protocols for validation *(31,32)*. One special consideration in older patients is the fact that many oscillometric devices are less accurate in the elderly, probably because of increased arterial stiffness. Therefore, devices for use in the elderly need to have demonstrated accuracy in this age group. Added to this initial validation, a clinical comparison against a mercury column sphygmomanometer should be performed on a regular basis by the physician. It is also important to certify that the patient uses a cuff size correct for his or her arm circumference. The recommended bladder width should be 40% of the arm circumference, as recommended by the AHA (Table 1).

Table 1
Acceptable Bladder Dimensions (cm) for Arms of Different Size in Adults

Cuff	Bladder width	Bladder length	Arm circumference range at midpoint
Small adult	10	24	22–26
Adult	13	30	27–34
Large adult	16	38	35–44
Adult thigh	20	42	45–52

Adapted from the American Heart Association (1).

TECHNIQUE AND MEASUREMENTS

There is no consensus about the number and time of self-BP measurements. Some experts recommend that, for the initial evaluation of a patient, BP should be taken three consecutive times in the morning and three in the evening for 3 days a week for 2 weeks (33) and to have measurements performed both during the work period and during off-work days. Patients are usually fairly accurate when transcribing their own pressures, but underreporting or missed reporting of the readings is not that uncommon. Devices with memory capability that store multiple readings for future evaluation overcome this problem. Some devices are also able to transmit data telephonically to a receiving central unit, but they are not commonly used because of cost issues.

NORMAL VALUES FOR SELF-BLOOD PRESSURE

What represents normality for home BP is still a matter of debate. There is consensus, however, about the fact that home BP should be lower than office BP in normotensive and hypertensive subjects. The American Hypertension Society recommends the value of 135/85 mmHg as the upper limit of normal for home BP (34). This is in agreement with studies showing that this value is roughly equivalent to an office BP of 140/90 mmHg (35).

INDICATIONS FOR SELF-MONITORING OF THE BLOOD PRESSURE

Although the theoretical advantages of self-monitoring are obvious, there is not yet sufficient prospective data to make a definitive conclusion about SMBP and end target organ damage, prediction of cardiovascular risk, or association with clinical outcomes. The available data suggest, however, that self-monitored BP does correlate better with echocardiographically determined left ventricular mass than clinic pressures in patients with mild hypertension (36,37), and that it is a better predictor of cardiovascular risk than office BP in older patients (38).

Table 2
Usefulness of Self- or Home Blood Pressure Monitoring

- Distinguishes sustained hypertension from white-coat effect suggesting white-coat hypertension
- Assesses response to antihypertensive therapy
- Improves patient adherence to treatment
- Potentially reduces management costs

The self-monitored BP has the potential for reducing the bias and error in assessing the "true" pressure in a patient (which may be quite large if a small number of readings in the doctor's office are used) (Table 2). In some studies, the self-monitored pressure has been shown to be similar to the attenuated BP seen with repeated measurements over time (i.e., weeks and months) in the clinic *(39,40)*. Moreover, SMBP seems to correlate with mean daytime pressures as measured by ABPM better than office BP. Once antihypertensive therapy has been initiated, self-monitoring of the BP is an excellent way to evaluate the effectiveness of the therapy and avoid multiple doctor or nurse visits. Furthermore, the relationship between time of dosing of antihypertensive therapy and BP levels may be easier to assess with self-monitoring patients. As a final attribute, adherence to therapy and BP control have been shown to improve when patients (even previously noncompliant ones) self-monitor their BP.

One important limitation of SMBP is that readings are usually taken under rested and relaxed conditions, so they might not accurately reflect BP in other situations. This is apparent when home readings are normal, yet ABPM demonstrates high values. Another limitation is that BP cannot be measured during sleep and, as discussed regarding relationship with disease, nocturnal BP alterations seem to be independently related to cardiovascular and cerebrovascular outcomes.

Ambulatory Blood Pressure Monitoring

The use of ABPM with devices able to record readings for 24 hours has had significant value in the evaluation of the hypertensive patient. It is an accurate and unbiased method of measuring BP while the subject is engaged in his or her regular daily activities. It also gives information about BP while the subject is sleeping, a factor of significant importance in cardiovascular morbidity that can only be measured by ABPM.

Before discussing the clinical utility of ambulatory BP recordings, one must develop a frame of reference for the values derived from the ambulatory BP recordings. Usually, physicians set the recorders to measure 50–100 BPs in 24 hours. There is a reproducible diurnal/nocturnal pattern to BP during a 24-hour period of measurement in about 80% of patients. Typically, the pressure is highest while awake (especially during work) and lowest during sleep. The data are expressed as 24-hour mean BP and often as the values during wakefulness and sleep. BP during sleep is quite low compared to the office or clinic pressure, and BP during wakefulness is similar to the values obtained in the office. These differences must be kept in mind when trying to interpret ambulatory BP recordings. Most consensus groups have used a 24-hour BP greater than 135/85 mmHg as clearly abnormal based on several new outcome studies comparing ambulatory vs clinic BP in patients with hypertension.

RELATIONSHIP BETWEEN THE AMBULATORY BLOOD PRESSURE AND HYPERTENSIVE DISEASE

One of the most important findings regarding the ambulatory BP has been its relationship to hypertension-related target organ disease. The majority of cross-sectional studies published to date have shown the ambulatory BP is superior to office BP in predicting target organ involvement. The most striking evidence has come from assessment of the relations among office BP, ambulatory BP, and indexes of left ventricular hypertrophy (41–44). Large studies have demonstrated that ABPM is a better predictor of cardiovascular morbidity than conventional office BP (45,46). More recent data have also demonstrated that ambulatory BP is superior to office pressure in predicting hypertensive cerebrovascular disease (47). Most of these studies demonstrated that a loss of nocturnal decline in BP (so-called nondippers) conveys excessive risk for stroke and myocardial infarction.

Vascular dementia is also of major importance in the elderly. Although less clear, nocturnal hypertension or hypotension seem to play a role in the development of lacunar infarcts and deep white matter lesions. Most studies have shown that a nondipping status correlates with lacunar infarcts and white matter lesions (48–53), whereas others suggested that extreme dipping (>20% decline in nocturnal BP) might also be implicated in the development of lacunar infarcts (54). A nondipping pattern was an independent predictor for lacunar infarcts, diffuse white matter lesions, and vascular dementia (55).

One other area of interest in ABPM is the analysis of BP variability by conventional intermittent or by beat-to-beat BP measurements. Studies suggested that increased BP variability is an independent risk factor for cardiovascular morbidity (56,57). Older patients and those with severe hypertension might be among those with excessive BP variability.

Table 3
Clinical Diagnoses or Problems for Which Noninvasive
Ambulatory Blood Pressure Monitoring May Be Useful

- Office or white-coat hypertension
- Borderline hypertension with or without target organ involvement
- Evaluation of patients refractory to antihypertensive therapy
- Episodic hypertension
- Hypotensive symptoms associated with antihypertensive medications
- Autonomic dysfunction/nocturnal hypertension

Adapted from ref. *58*.

CLINICAL USEFULNESS OF AMBULATORY BLOOD PRESSURE

Several subsets of hypertensive diagnoses have been elucidated as a result of ABPM (Table 3). Clinical problems seen more often by practicing physicians that are appropriate for ABPM include the assessment of possible WCH, which can be only diagnosed with ABPM; borderline hypertension (with and without evidence for target organ damage); and refractory hypertension in patients on complex antihypertensive regimens. ABPM is the only available method for diagnosis of nocturnal hypertension. Less often, ABPM can be used in the evaluation of patients with hypotensive symptoms while on antihypertensive drugs or caused by autonomic dysfunction and in those with suspected episodic hypertension. Patients might benefit clinically when the ambulatory BP is known in addition to the measurements made in the medical care environment.

WCH and Borderline Hypertension. As described in this chapter, WCH can only be diagnosed by ABPM when the office BP is persistently over 140/90 and the average daytime BP is less than 135/85 mmHg. This condition is suspected when office readings are high (usually, but not necessarily, in the high-normal range) and there is lack of evidence of hypertension-related end target organ damage. In these patients, home self-measured BP readings should be tried first. If SMBP is normal, ABPM is needed to confirm WCH; however, if it is high, WCH is ruled out. As discussed here, the subgroup of patients with WCH seems to have a lower cardiovascular risk than those with persistent hypertension. However, given that their risk compared to normotensives is less clear, these patients should be closely followed. Furthermore, any patient with WCH can later develop persistent hypertension.

Reverse White-Coat Effect. Patients in any range of BP by the office readings can be found to have higher values by ABPM. This condition is also known as reverse white-coat effect. A recent study in older individuals with hypertension reported an incidence of 21% of reverse white-coat effect. Thus, it is likely that many patients with normal or high-normal readings at the office could be found to have hypertension by ABPM or what could be called white coat normotension. This phenomenon highlights the importance of the clinical evaluation for assessing hypertension-related end target organ damage and, if present, considering use of ABPM to diagnose hypertension when other methods show normality.

Refractory Hypertension. There is evidence that, in both middle-aged and older patients with hypertension, changes in ambulatory BP are better correlated than office BP to regression of left ventricular hypertrophy. Therefore, ABPM is a good method to evaluate the patient with refractory hypertension and to assess therapy. ABPM might also identify those with pseudorefractory hypertension caused by the white-coat effect vs those with real refractory hypertension. Moreover, in those patients with genuine refractory hypertension, ABPM can help to tailor therapy by identifying the specific time or times during the 24-hour period in which BP is not controlled.

Hypotension. As described in a separate section, orthostatic hypotension is more common in the elderly. Typically, evaluation of positional BP changes in the office is sufficient to make this diagnosis. However, it has also been shown that orthostatic hypotension is poorly reproducible when checked at different office visits or times of the day. Moreover, symptomatic hypotension may be induced by medications during their peak effect and not necessarily be discovered during an office visit. Patients with autonomic dysfunction of any etiology might have severe orthostatic hypotension associated with significant supine hypertension. Therefore, ABPM is useful for further evaluation of all these scenarios.

Nocturnal Hypertension. As discussed in the section on the relationship of ambulatory blood pressure and hypertensive disease, nocturnal hypertension and extreme nocturnal hypotension seem to be related to lacunar infarcts, ischemia of the periventricular white matter and dementia *(48–55)*. Nocturnal hypertension is also an independent risk factor for cardiovascular morbidity. ABPM is the only method that has the capability to evaluate BP during sleep.

CONCLUSION

Blood pressure determination is one of the most important parts in the clinical evaluation of an older patient. Therefore, the physician must make every effort to measure the BP accurately. Given that clinic or office BP is a highly variable parameter in the elderly, clinicians are slowly but progressively moving away from decision making based solely on isolated readings at the office. The combined evaluation of office and self-measurements as well as use of 24-hour readings in selected cases often prove invaluable in the management of older patients with hypertension. As more information is accumulated about the diagnostic utility, prognostic significance, and added benefits in disease modification and management with the use of out-of-office BP measurements, the indications for SMBP and ABPM will be better defined. The elderly, for whom hypertension is so common and hypertension-related complications are so frequently manifested, will be the population that will benefit the most from better assessment and management of BP-related pathology.

REFERENCES

1. Perloff D, Grim C, Flack J, et al. Human blood pressure determination by sphygmomanometry. *Circulation* 1993;88:2460–2470.
2. Cavallini MC, Roman MJ, Blank SG, Pini R, Pickering TG, Devereux RB. Association of the auscultatory gap with vascular disease in hypertensive patients. *Ann Intern Med* 1996;124:877–883.
3. Blank SG, West JE, Muller FB, Pecker MS, Laragh JH, Pickering TG. Characterization of auscultatory gaps with wideband external pulse recording. *Hypertension* 1991;17:225–233.
4. Sprangers RL, Wesseling KH, Imholz AL, Imholz BP, Wieling W. Initial blood pressure fall on stand up and exercise explained by changes in total peripheral resistance. *J Appl Physiol* 1991;70:523–530.
5. Consensus statement on the definition of orthostatic hypotension, pure autonomic failure, and multiple system atrophy. *Neurology* 1996;46:1470.
6. Puisieux F, Boumbar Y, Bulckaen H, Bonnin E, Houssin F, Dewailly P. Intra-individual variability in orthostatic blood pressure changes among older adults: the influence of meals. *J Am Geriatr Soc* 1999;47:1332–1336.
7. Auseon A, Ooi WL, Hossain M, Lipsitz LA. Blood pressure behavior in the nursing home: implications for diagnosis and treatment of hypertension. *J Am Geriatr Soc* 1999;47:285–290.
8. Lipsitz LA, Storch HA, Minaker KL, Rowe JW. Intra-individual variability in postural blood pressure in the elderly. *Clin Sci* 1985;69:337–341.
9. Alli C, Avanzini F, Bettelli G, et al. Prevalence and variability of orthostatic hypotension in the elderly. Results of the "Italian Study on Blood Pressure in the Elderly (SPAA)." The "Gruppo di Studio Sulla Pressione Arteriosa nell'Anziano." *Eur Heart J* 1992;13:178–182.
10. Tilvis RS, Hakala SM, Valvanne J, Erkinjuntti T. Postural hypotension and dizziness in a general aged population: a 4-year follow-up of the Helsinki Aging Study. *J Am Geriatr Soc* 1996;44:809–814.
11. Weiss A, Grossman E, Beloosesky Y, Grinblat J. Orthostatic hypotension in acute geriatric ward: is it a consistent finding? *Arch Intern Med* 2002;162:2369–2374.
12. Mets TF. Drug-induced orthostatic hypotension in older patients. *Drugs Aging* 1995;6:219–228.

13. Lipsitz LA, Connelly CM, Kelley-Gagnon M, Kiely DK, Abernethy D, Waksmonski C. Cardiovascular adaptation to orthostatic stress during vasodilator therapy. *Clin Pharmacol Ther* 1996;60:461–471.

14. Mukai S, Lipsitz LA. Orthostatic hypotension. *Clin Geriatr Med* 2002;18:253–68.

15. James MA, Potter JF. Orthostatic blood pressure changes and arterial baroreflex sensitivity in elderly subjects. *Age Ageing* 1999;28:522.

16. Plaschke M, Trenkwalder P, Dahlheim H, Lechner C, Trenkwalder C. Twenty-four-hour blood pressure profile and blood pressure responses to head-up tilt tests in Parkinson's disease and multiple system atrophy. *J Hypertens* 1998;16:1433–1441.

17. Frongillo D, Stocchi F, Buccolini P, et al. Ambulatory blood pressure monitoring and cardiovascular function tests in multiple system atrophy. *Fundam Clin Pharmacol* 1995;9:187–196.

18. Masaki KH, Schatz IJ, Burchfiel CM, et al. Orthostatic hypotension predicts mortality in elderly men: the Honolulu Heart Program. *Circulation* 1998;98:2290–2295.

19. Raiha I, Luutonen S, Piha J, Seppanen A, Toikka T, Sourander L. Prevalence, predisposing factors, and prognostic importance of postural hypotension. *Arch Intern Med* 1995;155:930–935.

20. Zweifler AJ, Shahab ST. Pseudohypertension: a new assessment. *J Hypertens* 1993;11:1–6.

21. Jacobs LJ, Manten H, Myerburg RJ, Sheps DS. Pseudohypertension due to diffuse vascular calcification in chronic renal failure. *Ann Intern Med* 1979;90:353–354.

22. Messerli FH, Ventura HO, Amodeo C. Osler's maneuver and pseudohypertension. *N Engl J Med* 1985;312:1548–1551.

23. Kuwajima I, Hoh E, Suzuki Y, Matsushita S, Kuramoto K. Pseudohypertension in the elderly. *J Hypertens* 1990;8:429–432.

24. Belmin J, Visintin JM, Salvatore R, Sebban C, Moulias R. Osler's maneuver: absence of usefulness for the detection of pseudohypertension in an elderly population. *Am J Med* 1995;98:42–49.

25. Pickering TG, James GD, Boddie C, et al. How common is white coat hypertension? JAMA 1988;259:225–228.

26. Staessen JA, O'Brien ET, Amery AK, et al. Ambulatory blood pressure in normotensive and hypertensive subjects: results from an international database. *J Hypertens* 1994;12(suppl 7):S1–S12.

27. Rasmussen SL, Torp-Pedersen C, Borch-Johnsen K, Ibsen H. Normal values for ambulatory blood pressure and differences between casual blood pressure and ambulatory blood pressure: results from a Danish population survey. *J Hypertens* 1998;16:1415–1424.

28. Pickering TG, Davidson K, Gerin W, Schwartz JE. Masked hypertension. *Hypertension* 2002;40:795–796.

29. Wing LM, Brown MA, Beilin LJ, Ryan P, Reid CM. ANBP2 Management Committee and Investigators. Second Australian National Blood Pressure Study. "Reverse white-coat hypertension" in older hypertensives. *J Hypertens* 2002;20:639–644.

30. Verdecchia P, Staessen JA, White WB, Imai Y, O'Brien ET. Properly defining white coat hypertension. *Eur Heart J* 2002;23:106–109.

31. O'Brien E, Petrie J, Littler WA, et al. The British Hypertension Society Protocol for the evaluation of blood pressure measuring devices. *J Hypertens* 1993;11(suppl 2):S43–S63.

32. Association for the Advancement of Medical Instrumentation. American National Standard. Electronic or Automated Sphygmomanometers. Arlington, VA: AAMI; 1993.

33. Pickering T. Self monitoring of blood pressure. In: White WB, ed. *Blood Pressure Monitoring in Cardiovascular Medicine and Therapeutics*. Totowa, NJ: Humana Press; 2001:3–28.
34. Pickering T. Recommendations for the use of home (self) and ambulatory blood pressure monitoring. American Society of Hypertension Ad Hoc Panel. *Am J Hypertens* 1996;9:1–11.
35. Weisser B, Grune S, Burger R, et al. The Dubendorf Study: a population-based investigation on normal values of blood pressure self-measurement. *J Hum Hypertens* 1994;8:227–231.
36. Mule G, Caimi G, Cottone S, et al. Value of home blood pressures as predictor of target organ damage in mild arterial hypertension. *J Cardiovasc Risk* 2002;9:123–129.
37. Kleinert HD, Harshfield GA, Pickering TG, et al. What is the value of home blood pressure measurement in patients with mild hypertension? *Hypertension* 1984;6: 574–578.
38. Ohkubo T, Imai Y, Tsuji I, et al. Home blood pressure measurement has a stronger predictive power for mortality than does screening blood pressure measurement: a population-based observation in Ohasama, Japan. *J Hypertens* 1998;16:971–975.
39. James GD, Pickering TG, Yee LS, Harshfield GA, Riva S, Laragh JH. The reproducibility of average ambulatory, home, and clinic pressures. *Hypertension* 1988;11:545–549.
40. Jyothinagaram SG, Rae L, Campbell A, Padfield PL. Stability of home blood pressure over time. *J Hum Hypertens* 1990;4:269–271.
41. Prisant LM, Carr AA. Ambulatory blood pressure monitoring and echocardiographic left ventricular wall thickness and mass. *Am J Hypertens* 1990;3:81–89.
42. Verdecchia P, Schillaci G, Guerrieri M, et al. Circadian blood pressure changes and left ventricular hypertrophy in essential hypertension. *Circulation* 1990;81:528–536.
43. Cox J, Amery A, Clement D, et al. Relationship between blood pressure measured in the clinic and by ambulatory monitoring and left ventricular size as measured by electrocardiogram in elderly patients with isolated systolic hypertension. *J Hypertens* 1993;11:269–276.
44. Thijs L, O'Brien ET, Staessen JA. Systolic Hypertension in Europe (Syst-Eur) Trial Investigators. Ambulatory and conventional pulse pressures and mean pressures as determinants of the Sokolow-Lyon ECG voltage index in older patients with systolic hypertension. *Blood Press Monit* 2001;6:197–202.
45. Verdecchia P, Schillaci G, Borgioni C, Ciucci A, Pede S, Porcellati C. Ambulatory pulse pressure. A potent predictor of total cardiovascular risk in hypertension. *Hypertension* 1998;32:983–988.
46. Staessen JA, Thijs L, Fagard R, et al. Predicting cardiovascular risk using conventional and ambulatory blood pressure in older patients with systolic hypertension. *JAMA* 1999;282:539–546.
47. Ohkubo T, Hozawa A, Nagai K, et al. Prediction of stroke by ambulatory blood pressure monitoring versus screening blood pressure measurements in a general population: the Ohasama study. *J Hypertens* 2000;18:847–854.
48. Tomonaga M, Yamanouchi H, Tohgi H, Kameyama M. Clinicopathological study of progressive subcortical encephalopathy (Binswanger type) in the elderly. *J Am Geriatr Soc* 1982;30:961–965.
49. Tohgi H, Chiba K, Kimura M. Twenty-four-hour variation of blood pressure in vascular dementia of Binswanger type. *Stroke* 1991;7:477–483.
50. Yamamoto Y, Akiguchi I, Oiwa K, Satoi H, Kimura J. Diminished nocturnal blood pressure decline and lesion site in cerebrovascular disease. *Stroke* 1995;26:829–833.

51. Goldstein IB, Bartzokis G, Hance DB, Shapiro D. Relationship between blood pressure and subcortical lesions in healthy elderly people. *Stroke* 1998;29:765–772.

52. Kukla C, Sander D, Schwarze J, Wittich I, Klingelhofer J. Changes of circadian blood pressure patterns are associated with the occurrence of lacunar infarction. *Arch Neurol* 1998;55:683–688.

53. Sander D, Winbeck, Klingelhofer J, Conrad B. Extent of cerebral white matter lesions is related to changes of circadian blood pressure rhythmicity. *Arch Neurol* 2000;57:1302–1307.

54. Kario K, Matsuo T, Kobayashi H, Imiya M, Mastuo M, Shimada K. Nocturnal fall of blood pressure and silent cerebrovascular damage in elderly hypertensive patients: advanced silent cerebrovascular damage in extreme dippers. *Hypertension* 1996;27:130–135.

55. Yamamoto Y, Akiguchi I, Oiwa K, Hayashi M, Kasai T, Ozasa K. Twenty-four-hour blood pressure and MRI as predictive factors for different outcomes in patients with lacunar infarct [erratum appears in Stroke 2002;33:883]. *Stroke* 2002;33:297–305.

56. Frattola A, Parati G, Cuspidi C, Albini F, Mancia G. Prognostic value of 24-hour blood pressure variability. *J Hypertens* 1993;11:1133–1137.

57. Sega R, Corrao G, Bombelli M, et al. Blood pressure variability and organ damage in a general population: results from the PAMELA study (Pressioni Arteriose Monitorate E Loro Associazioni). *Hypertension* 2002;39:710–714.

58. National High BP Education Program Working Group report on ambulatory blood pressure monitoring. *Arch Intern Med* 1990;150:2270–2280.

9

Clinical Evaluation of the Elderly Hypertensive

L. Michael Prisant, MD, FACC, FACP and Thomas W. Jackson, MD

CONTENTS

MEASUREMENT OF BLOOD PRESSURE AND CONFIRMATION

When confronted with an elevation in blood pressure (BP) in an elderly patient, additional measurements are necessary because of increased variability in older persons possibly caused by impaired baroreceptor sensitivity (Fig. 1) *(1)*. In addition to lability of BP, there should be consideration given to the presence of an auscultatory gap *(2)*, orthostatic hypotension *(3)*, and pseudohypertension *(4)*.

Orthostatic hypertension increases with aging and hypertension and is associated with impairment of baroceptor sensitivity *(5)*. Among elderly persons with isolated systolic hypertension, a systolic decline of 20 mmHg or greater was observed in 17.3% of subjects at 1 or 3 minutes after standing (Fig. 2) *(3)*. After a high-carbohydrate meal, supine BP

From: *Clinical Hypertension and Vascular Diseases: Hypertension in the Elderly*
Edited by: L. M. Prisant © Humana Press Inc., Totowa, NJ

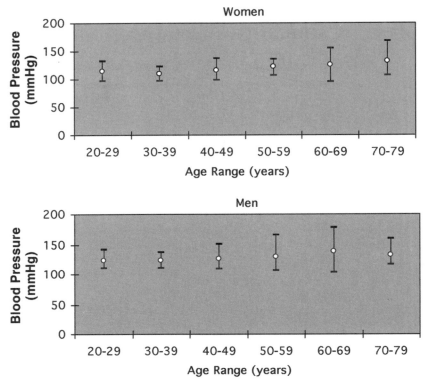

Fig. 1. Variability of blood pressure. Both the upper panel (women) and lower panel (men) show the increasing blood pressure with increasing standard deviation with aging. (Data from ref. *1*.)

declines, and heart rate increases without an increase in plasma norepinephrine levels *(6)*. Standing postmeal ingestion magnifies the BP decline *(7)*. In addition to the risk of falls and fractures, the risk of vascular death is increased *(8)*.

The quality of BP measurement is of prime importance for the initial diagnosis and the adjustment of medication *(9)*. For the diagnosis of systemic hypertension, the initial set of sitting BP measurements should occur after 5 minutes of rest and the abstinence of both caffeine and tobacco for 30 minutes. BP should be measured in nontalking patients seated with their back supported and their legs uncrossed. Also, the arm should be bared and supported at heart level. The use of a mercury sphygmomanometer remains the gold standard for routine determination of BP *(10)*.

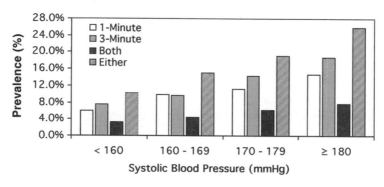

Fig. 2. Prevalence of standing systolic blood pressure decline of 20 mmHg or greater. The prevalence of a decline in systolic blood pressure at 1 and 3 minutes increase with higher levels of systolic blood pressure. (Data from ref. *3*.)

Palpation of the radial artery for the initial cuff inflation will help determine the level of systolic BP. This will avoid unnecessary cuff pressure that might cause pain and the potential underestimation of systolic blood pressure (SBP) that could occur in the presence of an auscultatory gap. Not recognizing an auscultatory gap can result in an underestimation of SBP or an overestimation of diastolic blood pressure (DBP). An auscultatory gap is associated with older age, female gender, increased arterial stiffness, and carotid atherosclerotic plaque *(11)*.

If the pulseless radial or brachial artery is palpable after ipsilateral occlusion by the cuff, then the patient is described as "Osler positive," which was a sign of pseudohypertension caused by atherosclerosis *(12,13)*. Pseudohypertension is an elevation in cuff measurement with a normal intra-arterial measurement; thus, the implication of an Osler-positive patient is that the patient is receiving inappropriate treatment *(13)*. However, despite a higher cuff pressure of +15.8/+16.4 mmHg in Osler-positive vs −3.0/+5.3 mmHg in Osler-negative patients, most subjects in this study had SBP measurements greater than 140 mmHg.

Another study of geriatric patients identified a prevalence of 11% of Osler-positive patients of 205 screened *(14)*. When Osler-positive and -negative patients were compared with intra-arterial measurements, there was no significant difference in BP. Furthermore, Osler's maneuver did not predict the presence or absence of pseudohypertension *(14)*.

The failure to use a large cuff in an obese patient is another cause of pseudohypertension.

Auscultation should be performed with the bell of the stethoscope lightly applied over the brachial artery because Korotkoff sounds are low pitched *(9)*. BP measurements are recorded to the nearest 2 mmHg. A good procedure is to perform three measurements and take the average of the last two measurements as the value for that visit. Three visits with a total of six measurements are required to diagnose systemic hypertension *(15)*.

Before the initiation of drug therapy, there should be a determination whether postural changes are present. Patients with symptoms of lightheadedness or dizziness; patients taking certain medications, including antipsychotic medications, antiparkinsonian drugs, α_1-blockers, diuretics, and nitrates; and patients with Parkinson's disease and diabetes mellitus with autonomic insufficiency need their BP and heart rate measured in the supine position and standing after 1 and 3 minutes. Measurement of BP in the contralateral arm, which is lower, suggests subclavian stenosis.

EVALUATION CONSIDERATIONS

The assessment of older patients is more complex than for younger patients. A lifetime history is likely to require more time. The reported details may not be as accurate, even if dementia is not present. In addition, altered vision and hearing can present difficulties for the examiner. Believing a symptom is caused by aging, the patient if asked directly may not acknowledge the symptom. Also, the manifestations of a disease may differ in older patients. An assessment of mental status to screen for dementia on initial examination can provide a baseline and provide important information regarding the ability of a patient to follow a medical regimen. The history of older patients should be verified with a family member. Discrepancies in the history often point to dementia. Failure to verify the history can impede the accuracy of diagnosis.

HISTORY

The purpose of the history is to determine potential symptoms associated with or suggesting causes of hypertension, evaluate the presence of target organ damage, determine other cardiovascular risk factors, assess concomitant diseases that might interfere with the treatment of hypertension, seek clues suggestive of secondary hypertension, catalogue all medications used (including over-the-counter medications and herbal remedies), assess resources, assess mental status, and determine general ability to implement the activities of daily living *(4,15–17)*.

Specific questions may provide important diagnostic clues *(16)*. The duration and ease of hypertension control are important. For instance, a long history of hypertension that has been well controlled and is now

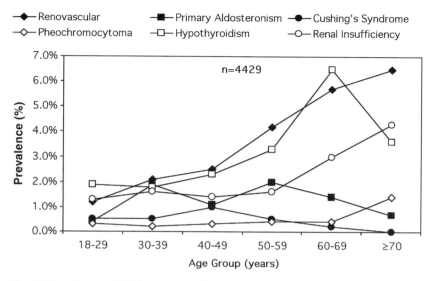

Fig. 3. Prevalence of different secondary causes of hypertension in patients 18 years or older. There was an increased prevalence of renovascular hypertension, renal insufficiency, and hypothyroidism with increasing age. (Data from ref. *18*.)

uncontrolled suggests superimposed secondary hypertension, an interfering substance (e.g., nonsteroidal anti-inflammatory drugs [NSAIDs], ethanol), or noncompliance (possibly because of finances or dementia). Essential hypertension accounts for most cases of hypertension in the elderly *(18)*. The three most common secondary causes of hypertension are chronic renal insufficiency, hypothyroidism, and renovascular hypertension (Fig. 3). The abrupt onset of severe hypertension associated with declining renal function and recurrent pulmonary edema suggests renovascular hypertension *(19–21)*.

Generally, hypertension is asymptomatic. Symptoms caused by secondary hypertension include (a) headaches, pallor, and diaphoresis (pheochromocytoma); (b) weight loss, tremor, anxiety, tachycardia, fatigue, weakness (hyperthyroidism); (c) confusion, anorexia, weakness, myalgias, constipation, depression (hypothyroidism); (d) urinary frequency, nocturia, hematuria, fatigue (renal parenchymal disease); and (e) muscle cramps, muscle weakness, nocturia, hypokalemia (primary aldosteronism).

Symptoms secondary to diabetes and hypertensive target organ damage, ischemic heart disease, heart failure, cerebrovascular disease, aortic and peripheral vascular disease, renal failure, and retinal disease must be determined to choose the most appropriate initial antihypertensive drug.

Vascular symptoms of exertional fatigue, dyspnea, orthopnea, edema, angina, palpitations, claudication, transient ischemic attacks, and syncope need to be evaluated in terms of daily activities. Heart failure, either systolic or diastolic, and atrial fibrillation are common in the elderly (*see* Chapter 12). Some patients experience postprandial hypotension associated with either dizziness or fatigue.

Patients should be asked about side effects of medications previously taken as well as allergies. It is wise to have the patient bring all medications to the clinic, including over-the-counter medications and herbal remedies. NSAIDs precipitate heart failure and interfere with the treatment of hypertension. Venlafaxine raises BP also. Quantitation of alcohol ingestion is important because excessive consumption increases BP. Long-standing tobacco use, vascular events (including myocardial infarction, strokes, and claudication), and renal insufficiency increase the likelihood of renovascular hypertension.

PHYSICAL EXAMINATION

The physical examination is conducted in a methodical fashion *(16)*. Routine vital signs of BP, heart rate, and weight are recorded at each visit. A funduscopic examination is performed as a part of the initial examination or at visits associated with very high BP measurements. The presence of retinal flame-shaped hemorrhages, retinal infarcts ("cotton wool" spots), and papilledema provides important information regarding the urgency of therapy and a clue to secondary hypertension. The neck is examined for jugular venous distention, the rate of rise of the carotid upstroke, the presence of carotid bruits, and thyromegaly. Auscultation of the lungs is targeted for the presence of wheezes and rales.

Inspection of the chest may localize the point of maximum impulse of the heart. Cardiac enlargement is suggested by its displacement past the midclavicular line. An enlarged and sustained apical impulse suggests left ventricular hypertrophy (LVH). A palpable S_4 is occasionally present. An irregularly irregular rhythm suggests atrial fibrillation or frequent atrial or ventricular ectopy. A tambour S_2 suggests aortic root dilatation. Systolic ejection murmurs are not uncommon with hypertension; however, an increased SBP, a wide pulse pressure, and a diastolic decrescendo murmur over the aortic area in the seated position support the diagnosis of aortic insufficiency. An S_3 gallop associated with dyspnea, rales, and tachycardia supports the diagnosis of heart failure.

The abdominal examination should include liver size, assessment for enlarged kidneys (polycystic kidney disease), enlarged aorta, ascites, and the presence of bruits to suggest the presence of atherosclerosis. In asymptomatic patients, the sensitivity of physical examination as assessed by ultrasonography is a function of the diameter of the aneurysm: 29% for 3.0–3.9 cm, 50% for 4.0–4.9 cm, and 76% for 5 cm or greater *(22)*. The positive predictive value is only 43%. However, if the waist circumference exceeds 40 inches, then the sensitivity is significantly reduced. Interobserver agreement between two examinations is 77% *(23)*. A high pitch epigastric systolic–diastolic bruit of long duration that lateralizes suggest renal artery stenosis *(24)*. However, 4.9% of normal individuals above age 55 years will have a bruit. The absence of a bruit does not exclude a diagnosis of renovascular hypertension. Periumbilical bruits are frequently associated with abdominal aortic aneurysms *(24)*.

Femoral pulsations and bruits and pedal pulses should be determined. The presence of peripheral edema may be caused by medications (NSAIDs, dihydropyridine calcium antagonist, or minoxidil), heart failure, decreased albumin, chronic renal insufficiency, or venous insufficiency. A careful neurological examination should define preexistent neurological deficits, including previous strokes, Parkinson's disease, and dementia.

LABORATORY ASSESSMENT

A fasting complex metabolic profile, lipid profile, complete blood count, urinalysis with microscopic examination, and electrocardiogram are reasonable for an initial evaluation. Unprovoked hypokalemia suggests primary aldosteronism, but hypokalemia is also observed with Cushing's syndrome and diuretic use. Hyperkalemia is associated with renal failure, potassium-sparing diuretics, angiotensin-converting enzyme (ACE) inhibitors, angiotensin receptor blockers (ARBs), type IV renal tubular acidosis, salt substitutes, and oral potassium supplements. A confirmed fasting glucose greater than 125 mg/dL is consistent with diabetes mellitus *(25)*, but hyperglycemia is also seen with Cushing's syndrome, acromegaly, and pheochromocytoma. Hypercalcemia may be caused by thiazide diuretics or hyperparathyroidism. Hyperuricemia is an early sign of renal disease, but is also associated with gout, diuretic use, chronic renal failure, polycythemia, hyperparathyroidism, hypothyroidism, and polycystic kidney disease. Elevated cholesterol may be caused by a secondary lipid disorder, such as hypothyroidism, nephrotic syndrome, or hypercortisolism. A creatinine greater than 1.3 mg/dL should be viewed as abnormal because older patients have less muscle mass. In addition to primary renal disease, renovascular disease, acromegaly, ACE inhibitors, ARBs, NSAIDs, and over-diuresis may also elevate the serum creatinine.

The electrocardiogram is an economical adjunct to assess target organ damage in hypertensive patients *(26,27)*. The rate, rhythm, PR and QT intervals, diagnostic Q waves, and voltage criteria of LVH provide information that can influence treatment. Although sick sinus syndrome may be present, sinus bradycardia should also suggest hypothyroidism and would preclude the use of α_2-stimulants, β-blockers, and nondihydropyridine calcium channel blockers. Alternatively, sinus tachycardia could be caused by heart failure, hyperthyroidism, pheochromocytoma, or overdiuresis. Atrial fibrillation may be caused by underlying ischemic heart disease, hypertension, or thyroid disease. A prolonged PR interval raises concern about prescribing either verapamil or diltiazem. A short QT interval may be caused by the hypercalcemia associated with hyperparathyroidism.

The gender-specific Cornell voltage criteria (for men, $R_{aVL} + S_{V3} > 35$ mm; for women, $R_{aVL} + S_{V3} > 25$ mm) have the best overall accuracy *(28)*. One of the earliest electrocardiographic findings of hypertensive heart disease is the duration of the negative phase of the P wave in chest lead $V_1 > 0.04$ seconds, a manifestation of left atrial enlargement or abnormality. There is no other classic cardiovascular risk factor more potent and dismal than LVH with "strain pattern" *(29)*. The strain pattern is characterized by ST depression ≥ 1 mm in lead I, aVL, and $V_4–V_6$. The direction of the T wave is in the opposite direction of the upright QRS complex.

INTEGRATION OF INFORMATION

Integrating information from the history, physical examination, and laboratory exam suggests additional evaluations to be performed *(15)*. These include measurement of creatinine clearance, 24-hour urinary protein excretion, plasma renin activity, thyroid-stimulating hormone, glycosylated hemoglobin, and ambulatory BP and an echocardiogram *(15)*. However, these tests do not need to be ordered routinely.

REFERENCES

1. Wiinberg N, Hoegholm A, Christensen HR, et al. Twenty-four-hour ambulatory blood pressure in 352 normal Danish subjects, related to age and gender. *Am J Hypertens* 1995;8(10 pt 1):978–986.
2. Askey JM. The auscultatory gap in sphygmomanometry. *Ann Intern Med* 1974;80:94–97.
3. Applegate WB, Davis BR, Black HR, Smith WM, Miller ST, Burlando AJ. Prevalence of postural hypotension at baseline in the Systolic Hypertension in the Elderly Program (SHEP) cohort. *J Am Geriatr Soc* 1991;39:1057–1064.
4. Franklin SS. Geriatric hypertension. *Med Clin North Am* 1983;67:395–417.

5. Ooi WL, Barrett S, Hossain M, Kelley-Gagnon M, Lipsitz LA. Patterns of orthostatic blood pressure change and their clinical correlates in a frail, elderly population. *JAMA* 1997;277:1299–1304.

6. Haigh RA, Harper GD, Burton R, Macdonald IA, Potter JF. Possible impairment of the sympathetic nervous system response to postprandial hypotension in elderly hypertensive patients. *J Hum Hypertens* 1991;5:83–99.

7. Maurer MS, Karmally W, Rivadeneira H, Parides MK, Bloomfield DM. Upright posture and postprandial hypotension in elderly persons. *Ann Intern Med* 2000;133:533–536.

8. Luukinen H, Koski K, Laippala P, Kivela SL. Prognosis of diastolic and systolic orthostatic hypotension in older persons. *Arch Intern Med* 1999;159:273–280.

9. Perloff D, Grim C, Flack J, et al. Human blood pressure determination by sphygmomanometry. *Circulation* 1993;88(5 pt 1):2460–2470.

10. Jones DW, Frohlich ED, Grim CM, Grim CE, Taubert KA. Mercury sphygmomanometers should not be abandoned: an advisory statement from the Council for High Blood Pressure Research, American Heart Association. *Hypertension* 2001;37:185–186.

11. Cavallini MC, Roman MJ, Blank SG, Pini R, Pickering TG, Devereux RB. Association of the auscultatory gap with vascular disease in hypertensive patients. *Ann Intern Med* 1996;124:877–883.

12. Messerli FH, Ventura HO, Amodeo C. Osler's maneuver and pseudohypertension. *N Engl J Med* 1985;312:1548–1551.

13. Messerli FH. Osler's maneuver, pseudohypertension, and true hypertension in the elderly. *Am J Med* 1986;80:906–910.

14. Belmin J, Visintin JM, Salvatore R, Sebban C, Moulias R. Osler's maneuver: absence of usefulness for the detection of pseudohypertension in an elderly population. *Am J Med* 1995;98:42–49.

15. Chobanian AV, Bakris GL, Black HR, et al. The Seventh Report of the Joint National Committee on Prevention, Detection, Evaluation, and Treatment of High Blood Pressure: the JNC 7 report. *JAMA* 2003;289:2560–2572.

16. Prisant LM, Carr AA. Initial evaluation of the hypertensive patient. *Postgrad Med* 1988;84:197–202, 215–217.

17. Prisant LM, Carr AA. Over-the-counter drugs that may increase blood pressure. *Postgrad Med* 1989;86:205–208.

18. Anderson GH Jr, Blakeman N, Streeten DH. The effect of age on prevalence of secondary forms of hypertension in 4429 consecutively referred patients. *J Hypertens* 1994;12:609–615.

19. Pickering TG, Herman L, Devereux RB, et al. Recurrent pulmonary oedema in hypertension due to bilateral renal artery stenosis: treatment by angioplasty or surgical revascularisation. *Lancet* 1988;2:551–552.

20. Olin JW, Vidt DG, Gifford RW Jr, Novick AC. Renovascular disease in the elderly: an analysis of 50 patients. *J Am Coll Cardiol* 1985;5:1232–1238.

21. Novick AC, Ziegelbaum M, Vidt DG, Gifford RW Jr, Pohl MA, Goormastic M. Trends in surgical revascularization for renal artery disease. Ten years' experience. *JAMA* 1987;257:498–501.

22. Lederle FA, Simel DL. The rational clinical examination. Does this patient have abdominal aortic aneurysm? *JAMA* 1999;281:77–82.

23. Fink HA, Lederle FA, Roth CS, Bowles CA, Nelson DB, Haas MA. The accuracy of physical examination to detect abdominal aortic aneurysm. *Arch Intern Med* 2000;160:833–836.

24. Turnbull JM. Is listening for abdominal bruits useful in the evaluation of hypertension? *JAMA* 1995;274:1299–1301.
25. Diagnosis and classification of diabetes mellitus. *Diabetes Care* 2004;27(suppl 1):S5–S10.
26. Prisant LM, Carr AA. Beyond diagnosis of left ventricular hypertrophy in patients with essential hypertension. *Am J Hypertens* 1992;5(12 pt 1):927–929.
27. Prisant LM. Hypertension images: electrocardiographic left ventricular hypertrophy. *J Clin Hypertens (Greenwich)* 2001;3:389–391, 398.
28. Casale PN, Devereux RB, Alonso DR, Campo E, Kligfield P. Improved sex-specific criteria of left ventricular hypertrophy for clinical and computer interpretation of electrocardiograms: validation with autopsy findings. *Circulation* 1987;75:565–572.
29. Kannel WB. Left ventricular hypertrophy as a risk factor: the Framingham experience. *J Hypertens Suppl* 1991;9:S3–S8; discussion S8–S9.

10 Hypertension in the Elderly
Endocrine Causes of Secondary Hypertension

Carlos M. Isales, MD, FACP

INTRODUCTION

According to the Third National Health and Nutrition Examination Survey (1988–1994), 20.4% of the US population had an elevated blood pressure (BP >140/90 mmHg), and 14.2% of the US population had a frankly elevated BP (≥ 160/95 mmHg) (*1*). Hypertension prevalence was higher in African Americans than in Caucasians and in males than in females, and the prevalence increased with increasing age. Interestingly, the rate of rise of the BP correlated with the initial BP, with faster rates of rise seen in those patients with an elevated initial BP (*2*).

Although essential hypertension remains by far the most common form of hypertension, those with secondary hypertension can represent between 10% and 20% of the hypertensive population. Renovascular causes are the most commonly identifiable in this group.

From: *Clinical Hypertension and Vascular Diseases: Hypertension in the Elderly*
Edited by: L. M. Prisant © Humana Press Inc., Totowa, NJ

Comparison between studies is hampered by differences in grouping according to age (by decade or arbitrary groups) and definition of hypertension (particularly in the older studies). Danielson and Dammstrom *(3)* examined 1000 consecutive patients between 20 and 70 years of age in the Hypertension Unit of their hospital in Sweden. They defined hypertension as greater than 160/95 mmHg (for patients under 40 years of age), 170/105 mmHg (for patients between 40 and 60 years of age), and 180/110 mmHg. Of these individuals, they identified 47 patients with secondary causes (34 patients with renal and 13 patients with endocrine causes of hypertension). Interestingly, of the 13 patients identified as having an endocrine cause of hypertension, 8 were felt to be hypertensive secondary to use of oral contraceptives, there was 1 patient with acromegaly, 1 with primary hyperaldosteronism, 1 with Cushing's syndrome, and 2 with pheochromocytoma.

In a study by Anderson et al. *(4)*, 4429 patients were evaluated at the State University of New York Syracuse for secondary causes of hypertension and how the prevalence of these diseases varied with age. The evaluation included a basal metabolic panel, thyroid function tests, stimulated plasma renin activity (PRA), BP response to an angiotensin II (Ang II) receptor antagonist (saralasin), plasma catecholamines and cortisol, and measurement of aldosterone after saline infusion. If any of these screening tests were abnormal, more comprehensive testing was done. Interestingly, these investigators found that the incidence of secondary hypertension increased with age (*see* Fig. 1), bringing into question the old maxim of only evaluating younger patients for secondary causes of hypertension. Overall, 10.2% of patients had an identifiable cause for their hypertension (*see* Fig. 2A,B) of which the most common causes were renal, including renovascular hypertension (3.1%) and an elevated serum creatinine (>2 mg/dL in 1.8% of patients), and endocrine causes, including primary hypothyroidism (3%), primary aldosteronism (1.4%), Cushing's syndrome (0.5%), and pheochromocytoma (0.3%) *(4)*.

Multiple endocrine conditions can result in an elevation in BP. The prevalence of many endocrine problems, such as type 2 diabetes mellitus and primary hyperparathyroidism, increases with age, as does hypertension. So, sometimes causality is not clear-cut. In other cases, even when there is clear causality between an endocrine condition and hypertension, the mechanism responsible for development of the elevation in BP is not known. In addition, the prevalence of some conditions varies depending on how elderly is defined (Fig. 1). This review is limited to the more common endocrine conditions and does not discuss all endocrine conditions that result in hypertension. For example, elevations in growth hormone (acromegaly) result in hypertension, but the incidence

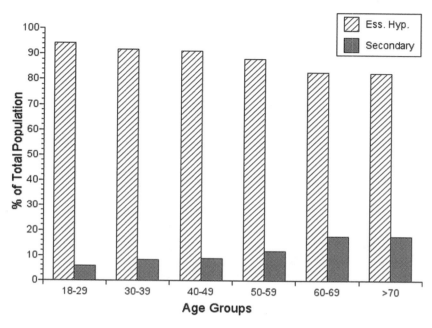

Fig. 1. There were 4429 patients evaluated; of these, 451 were determined to have secondary causes of hypertension. As seen, the prevalence of secondary hypertension increased from 5.6% of the study population between 18 and 29 years of age to 17.4% of the study population 70 years or older. (Modified from ref. *4*.)

of acromegaly does not increase with age. As seen in Fig. 1, the most common endocrine causes of secondary hypertension are abnormal thyroid hormone levels, primary aldosteronism, Cushing's syndrome, and pheochromocytoma. Appropriate treatment of these four conditions can lead to complete or partial reversal of the elevated BP. These four conditions are discussed in more detail.

ABNORMAL THYROID HORMONE LEVELS

Thyroid hormone has widespread effects in the body, affecting multiple organ systems. Thyroid hormone influences calorigenesis, modulates cellular growth, modulates carbohydrate and lipid metabolism, and has cardiovascular effects (*5*). Thyroid hormone (thyroxine, T_4) action requires conversion to a more active form, tri-iodothyronine (T_3), and binding to nuclear receptors in the cells. Nuclear binding of thyroid hormone leads to ribonucleic acid (RNA) transcription and protein synthesis. Thyroid hormone also activates cellular sodium-potassium adenosine triphosphatase (ATPase).

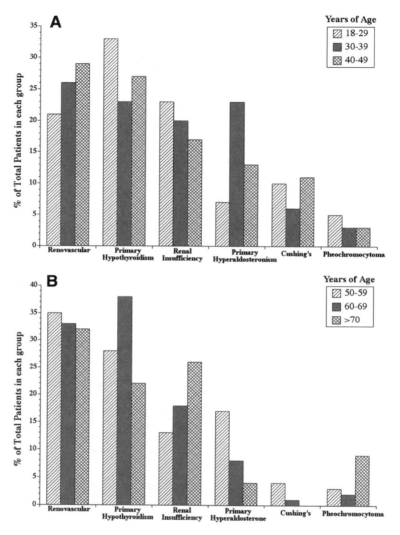

Fig. 2. If patients from this study are arbitrarily divided into two groups: less than 50 years of age and greater than 50, hypothyroidism is the major endocrine cause of secondary hypertension in both groups (27% of those under 50 and 31% of those over 50 years of age. Primary hyperaldosteronism has a similar prevalence between those under 50 (15%) and those over 50 years of age (12%), however, there are relatively fewer patients with bilateral hyperplasia as the cause of hyperaldosteronism in those patients over 60 years of age. The prevalence of Cushing's is 9% in those under 50 and 2% of those over 50 years of age. The prevalence of pheochromocytoma is similar in both groups, 3%. If the cutoff age is extended to those below vs those older than 60 years of age then hypothyroidism is the only endocrine condition that increases with increasing age (27% vs 35%). (Modified from refs. *4* and *25*.)

Pathogenesis of the Hypertension

The cardiovascular effects of thyroid hormone are multiple. It is clear that either an increase or a decrease in thyroid hormone has an impact on BP, although the mechanisms are different. Patients with hypothyroidism have, predominantly, an elevation in diastolic BP related to an increase in total peripheral resistance (TPR) and a decrease in cardiac output *(6)*. The increase in TPR in hypothyroidism is multifactorial. The increase in TPR in hypothyroidism appears to be at least partly related to an increase in sympathetic nervous tone and a relative increase in α-adrenergic tone *(6)*.

Coloumbe et al. *(7,8)* reported that patients with hypothyroidism have higher plasma norepinephrine levels than control patients, consistent with the proposed increase in sympathetic tone. In addition, as mentioned here thyroid hormone influences calorigenesis. Thus, a decrease in calorigenesis, as would be seen in hypothyroidism, leads to an increase in TPR as a mechanism for heat conservation, and the increase in calorigenesis observed in hyperthyroidism leads to a decrease in TPR as a means of dissipating some of the increased heat production. T_3 may also have direct nongenomic effects on vascular smooth muscle, which result in smooth muscle contraction *(9)* and increase TPR.

Potential indirect effects of thyroid hormone on BP, mediated by thyroid hormone-induced increases in vasoactive hormone synthesis and/or secretion, have also been studied. Thyroid hormone does not seem to exert its cardiovascular actions either through endothelin-1 (a potent vasoconstrictor released from endothelial cells) or adrenomedullin (a natriuretic and vasodilator peptide released from endothelial cells) *(9)*. However, numerous studies have shown an effect of thyroid hormone on natriuretic peptides. Atrial natriuretic peptide (ANP) is synthesized in the cardiac atria, but brain natriuretic peptide (BNP) is synthesized in the cardiac ventricles. Both ANP and BNP are potent natriuretic and vasorelaxant peptides, and their use as potential diagnostic or therapeutic agents in congestive heart failure is an area of active investigation *(10–12)*. They are normally released from the heart in response to atrial or ventricular stretch *(10)*.

In a study by Gardner et al. *(13)* in thyroidectomized rats, administration of thyroid hormone increased ANP levels about twofold. In addition, cardiac ANP messenger RNA (mRNA) was also increased, demonstrating that thyroid hormone affected both ANP synthesis and release.

The serum levels of ANP of hypothyroid patients increases when they are treated with thyroid hormone *(9,14)*. A study by Bernstein et al. *(15)* addressed whether the increase in ANP levels seen in patients with hypothyroidism on treatment with thyroid hormone was a direct effect of thyroid hormone on the cardiac myocyte or whether this was an indirect effect of thyroid hormone through an increase in heart rate and cardiac function. These investigators examined 11 hypothyroid patients with normal cardiac function at baseline and started them on thyroid hormone replacement. After 10 days of treatment, no change in ANP levels was observed. However, after 2 months of treatment with thyroid hormone, they observed an increase in the levels of proatrial natriuretic factor (1-98 amino acids), suggesting that the thyroid hormone effect was a direct one on the cardiac myocytes rather than an indirect effect through changes in vascular hemodynamics. Thus, a decrease in ANP levels in hypothyroid patients may play an important role in the fluid retention and diastolic hypertension seen in these patients *(16)*.

A study by Kohno et al. *(17)* examined BNP levels in hyperthyroid patients and BNP levels in hypo- and hyperthyroid rats. These investigators found that BNP levels were higher in both the hyperthyroid patient and animal, and the hypothyroid rat had lower BNP levels.

Patients with hyperthyroidism have predominantly systolic hypertension related to a decrease in the TPR and increase in cardiac output; they have a widened pulse pressure *(2)*. The increased cardiac output is secondary to an increase in both heart rate and stroke volume and probably contributes to the pathogenesis of systolic hypertension in the patients with hyperthyroidism *(6)*. The increased heart rates seen in patients with hyperthyroidism has been felt to be mediated by thyroid hormone effects on β_1-receptors in the heart because administration of β-blockers to patients with hyperthyroidism is clinically beneficial. Thus, the effects of thyroid hormone on β-adrenergic receptors have been studied extensively. Multiple studies have found an increase in β-adrenergic receptor expression in response to an increase in thyroid hormone levels *(5)*.

However, a study by Ojamaa et al. *(18)* examined the effects of thyroid hormone on adenylate cyclase isoform expression in cardiac rat ventricles. These investigators found that mRNA levels of adenylate cyclase isoforms V and VI were increased in hypothyroid animals compared to control euthyroid animals. In contrast, although the levels of these adenylate cyclase isoforms in hyperthyroid animals were the same as controls, the activation of these isoforms in the hyperthyroid animals was significantly reduced (35%) compared to control animals, demonstrating that, although hyperthyroidism leads to an increase in the number of β-adrenergic receptors, there is a compensatory decrease in the ability of these receptors to activate cyclic adenosine 5'-monophosphate in response to catecholamines. Thus, despite extensive investigations into thyroid hormone effects on heart rate, the mechanism is still poorly understood.

A study by Everett et al. *(19)* using cardiac ventricles of hypo- and hyperthyroid rabbits found that hypothyroid animals only expressed the heavy chain of β-myosin. Thyroid hormone increased mRNA expression of the heavy chain of α-myosin and decreased expression of the heavy chain of β-myosin. This change in myosin isoform expression leads to an increase in the activity of the calcium-ATPase activity and more forceful cardiac contraction, which contributes to the increased cardiac output seen in patients with hyperthyroidism.

Prevalence

Up to 7% of the adult population in the United States may have subclinical hypothyroidism (defined as an elevated thyroid-stimulating hormone [TSH] value with a normal T_4 value) *(20)*. It is estimated that it currently affects 10 million people in the United States *(21)*. The prevalence of subclinical hypothyroidism is highest in women over the age of 60 years (approximately 20%) but gradually increases in men with increasing age, reaching a prevalence of 16% in men over the age of 74 years. Most of these patients (75%) have only mild hypothyroidism, with TSH values between 5 and 10 μU/mL *(22)*. The Anderson et al. study *(4)* found that 6.5% of the hypertensive patients between 60 and 69 years of age (and 38% of the secondary hypertension subgroup) and 3.6% of the patients older than 70 years (and 22% of the secondary hypertension subgroup) were hypothyroid (defined as a TSH value greater than 7 μU/mL).

This makes hypothyroidism the most common endocrine condition associated with arterial hypertension. It is also the only endocrine diagnosis in hypertensive patients with a prevalence that increases with increasing age (27% of patients under 60 years of age vs 35% of patients over 60 years of age). A small study by Streeten et al. *(23)* found that there was a high prevalence of Hashimoto's in the hypothyroid patients. In fact, a large number of patients (50%–80%) with subclinical hypothyroidism have positive antibodies against thyroid peroxidase (TPO) *(22)*, the hormone involved in iodide organification and thus thyroid hormone synthesis. However, there are multiple other causes of subclinical hypothyroidism; patients affected include those with treated hyperthyroidism and patients on medications that modulate thyroid function (lithium, amiodarone, and α-interferon) and other autoimmune forms of thyroiditis *(22)*.

Hyperthyroidism is more common in women, affecting 2% of women vs 0.2% of men. The prevalence of hypertension in patients with hyperthyroidism is not really known but is estimated at about 25%. A study by Saito and Saruta *(6)* examined retrospectively 446 patients with untreated hyperthyroidism and hypertension and compared them to 549 control patients who were euthyroid, although with a goiter. They found a significantly higher prevalence of hypertension (>160/95 mmHg) in hyperthyroid patients younger than 49 years. Thus, hyperthyroidism, in contrast to hypothyroidism, tends to affect younger patients *(24)*, so is not discussed here in as much detail as hypothyroidism. The three most common causes of hyperthyroidism are Graves' disease, toxic multinodular goiter, and nodular goiter.

Patients with advanced clinical hyper- or hypothyroidism have characteristic features, which suggest the diagnosis. Patients with hypothyroidism may present with nonpitting edema (myxedema), dry skin, and psychomotor retardation. Patients with Grave's hyperthyroidism have a diffusely enlarged thyroid gland and can present with weight loss, can have protuberance of their eyes (exophthalmos) related to autoimmune involvement of the retro-orbital muscles and lid lag (Fig. 3).

Management

Approximately one-third of those patients with concurrent high BP and hypothyroidism become normotensive when they become euthyroid after treatment with thyroid hormone. Most of the patients who do not have an improvement in BP tend to be older *(23,25)*. Thus, the older patients may have other causes of hypertension besides hypothyroidism. However, these studies did not stratify responders vs nonresponders by the degree of severity of the hypothyroidism.

Similarly, when hyperthyroid patients were treated, systolic blood pressure (SBP) dropped as thyroid hormone levels dropped, although the improvement in BP was more common in patients younger than 49 years *(26)*.

Issues in Treatment

The effect of treatment of subclinical hypothyroidism on cholesterol values has been more carefully studied than the effects of treatment of thyroid hormone on BP. Thus, some insight may be gained by examining how thyroid hormone affects cholesterol metabolism because of applicability to thyroid hormone effects on BP. The effects of treatment of subclinical hypothyroidism with thyroid hormone on cholesterol values is controversial, with some studies showing no benefit in those patients with total cholesterol values below 240 mg/dL and others showing a small benefit if the total cholesterol value was above 240 mg/dL *(22)*. However, the key might be what the TSH value is, with probably no

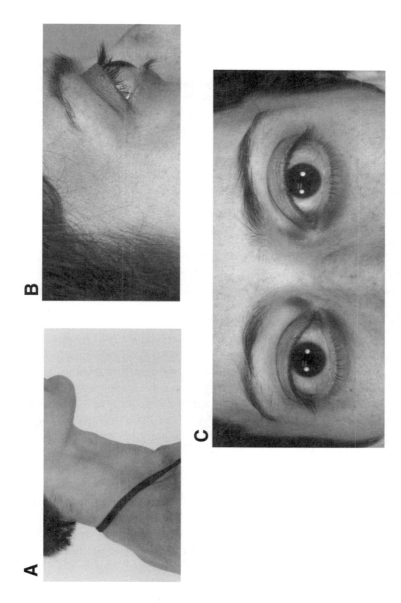

Fig. 3. Patient with Grave's disease demonstrating a diffuse enlargement of the thyroid gland (**A**). Patients with Grave's disease also have prominence of the eyes (exophthalmos) related to the autoimmune involvement of the retroorbital muscles of the eye (**B**), and this prominence of the eyes together with lid retraction leads to a characteristic "stare" (**C**).

benefit of thyroid hormone on cholesterol lowering if the TSH value is less than 10 mU/L *(20,22)*. Similarly, there might be no benefit of thyroid hormone replacement for normalization of BP if the TSH is only slightly increased. In addition, the benefit of thyroid hormone replacement needs to be balanced by the known potential complications of thyroid hormone overreplacement, such as osteoporosis and cardiac arrhythmias.

To address the natural history of subclinical hypothyroidism, Huber et al. *(21)* followed for an average of 10 years 82 women with subclinical hypothyroidism. Patients were divided into three groups according to the initial TSH value between 4 and 6 mU/L, between 6 and 12 mU/L, and greater than 12 mU/L. Anti-TPO antibodies and thyroid hormone levels in response to stimulation with thyrotropin-releasing hormone (TRH) were also measured. After 10 years, 68% of the patients remained subclinically hypothyroid, 28% of the patients became frankly hypothyroid (TSH >20 mU/L), and 4% of the patients had normalization of their TSH. No patient with mildly elevated TSH (4–6 mU/L) progressed to frank hypothyroidism. In fact, the 4% of patients who had normalization of their TSH value all had a low value (between 4 and 6 mU/L) at the beginning. Factors that were predictive of development of frank hypothyroidism were the presence of antibodies against TPO (anti-TPO or anti-microsomal antibodies; thyroid peroxidase is the enzyme involved in iodide organification in the thyroid follicle), a greater degree of TSH elevation (greater than 6 mU/L), and a suboptimal thyroid response to TRH stimulation.

Thus, it is possible that thyroid hormone replacement therapy may not be indicated in the hypertensive patient with TSH values less than 6 mU/L, negative anti-TPO antibodies, and no symptoms, although a patient with TSH values greater than 10 mU/L should probably be placed and maintained on thyroid hormone replacement irrespective of BP response because of other potential cardiovascular benefits.

A separate issue is the age at which patients should be screened for subclinical hypothyroidism. Because of the ease of testing for thyroid abnormalities, Cooper *(22)* suggested that all women older than 35 years should have TSH measured as an initial screening, and if normal, then the TSH should be rechecked every 5 years. Because of the lower prevalence of hypothyroidism in younger men, he recommended that screening not be done in men until age 65 years or older.

PRIMARY HYPERALDOSTERONISM

Aldosterone is the principal mineralocorticoid hormone produced by the outer glomerulosa layer of the adrenal cortex. Aldosterone is responsible for maintaining intravascular volume, along with antidiuretic hormone, by regulating sodium excretion in the kidneys and sweat glands. Aldosterone also affects serum potassium levels by having an impact on urinary potassium excretion. In vivo, the main regulators of aldosterone secretion appear to be Ang II and serum potassium levels *(27,28)*. Aldosterone overproduction is primary when caused by adrenal overproduction of aldosterone and secondary when other extra-adrenal factors are involved (e.g., renin overproduction, volume depletion, etc.).

Pathogenesis of the Hypertension

Because aldosterone, a mineralocorticoid hormone, leads to fluid retention, patients with primary hyperaldosteronism would be expected to have increased intravascular fluid volume. However, this does not seem always the case. A study by Bravo et al. *(29)* compared plasma volume in 80 patients with primary hyperaldosteronism to those of 70 patients with essential hypertension. Although 30% of patients did have an increase in their plasma volume, 25% of the patients with primary hyperaldosteronism had a low plasma volume, and there was considerable overlap with those patients with essential hypertension. However, patients with primary hyperaldosteronism and high BP respond to treatment with diuretics *(30),* suggesting that an increase in plasma volume is at least partially involved in the pathogenesis of the hypertension.

The potential contribution of aldosterone-mediated changes in TPR as a mechanism for BP elevation has also been studied. Wenting et al. *(31)* studied 10 patients with primary hyperaldosteronism (all with an adrenal adenoma) treated with spironolactone. When this medication was stopped, an increase in BP and blood volume could be observed after 2 weeks. However, at the end of 6 weeks blood volume and cardiac output remained increased in 5 of the 10 patients, but in the other 5 patients, blood volume and cardiac output returned to normal, and TPR remained elevated (36 ± 13% over control).

A subsequent study by Yamakado et al. *(32)* evaluated the acute effects of infusion of an aldosterone antagonist (canrenoate potassium) in BP response in patients with essential hypertension, renovascular hypertension, or primary aldosteronism. The study found that the drug had a significantly greater effect in reducing BP in patients with primary hyperaldosteronism than in the other study groups. This was related to a significant reduction in the TPR index, suggesting that aldosterone has a direct vasoconstrictive effect on the vasculature. Part of the mechanism involved in the development of high BP may be an effect of aldosterone on the sodium-potassium and sodium-hydrogen exchangers and on calcium transport *(33).*

Marked fluid retention is not usually observed in patients with primary hyperaldosteronism because they undergo what is called the "escape phenomenon": as aldosterone levels rise, there is marked initial fluid retention; after several days (1–2 weeks), there is a natriuresis, resulting in a drop in blood volume *(34)*. It is now thought that ANP is at least partially involved in the development of this escape phenomenon.

Nakamura et al. *(35)* stopped spironolactone treatment in five patients with primary aldosteronism related to an adrenal adenoma. Plasma volume, body weight, and BP increased gradually; however, by day 13 these patients developed a natriuresis that correlated with an increase of ANP levels (from 26 ± 4 to 195 ± 47 pg/mL, baseline vs day 3).

Patients with primary hyperaldosteronism in fact have significantly elevated levels of ANP. Although ANP is known to inhibit aldosterone secretion *(36,37)*, patients with primary hyperaldosteronism have elevated aldosterone values despite having elevated ANP levels. This has generally been attributed to a downregulation of ANP receptors in target tissues of patients with primary hyperaldosteronism *(38)*. Interestingly, if ANP is infused into patients with primary hyperaldosteronism to double circulating ANP levels, a natriuresis ensues; however, there is no drop in aldosterone levels, suggesting that ANP had lost its ability to inhibit aldosterone secretion from adrenal glomerulosa cells *(39)*.

In most studies of ANP's mechanism of action in muscle and kidney, ANP-mediated increases in cyclic guanosine monophosphate (cGMP) seem to account for all of ANP's effects. However, studies from our laboratory have found that, although ANP does increase cGMP in adrenal glomerulosa cells, changes in cyclic nucleotides do not solely account for ANP's inhibitory action on aldosterone secretion *(36,40,41)*, suggesting that ANP action in the adrenal is intrinsically different from ANP action in other tissues.

We have demonstrated that ANP modulates calcium channel activity in the adrenal glomerulosa cells, but the quantitative contribution of this effect to inhibition of aldosterone secretion is unclear *(42–46)*. Finally, although ANP receptor expression on the adrenal gland in primary hyperaldosteronism is altered, whether the signaling pathways involved in ANP action in the adrenal glomerulosa cell are also altered remains to be determined.

Prevalence

Primary hyperaldosteronism was first described by Conn in 1955 in a patient with an aldosterone-producing adenoma *(47)* whose hypertension improved after surgical removal of the adrenal adenoma. At that time, Conn felt that the prevalence of this condition could be as high as 20% in the hypertensive population, spurring extensive research into this potentially curable form of hypertension. Since then, it has become clear that the prevalence of this condition is far less than the predicted 20%. Although adrenal adenomas are still the most common form of primary hyperaldosteronism (65%–75%), between 25% and 35% of patients have aldosterone secretion related to adrenal hyperplasia (idiopathic hyperaldosteronism); between 5 and 10% of patients have multiple benign tumors (bilateral cortical nodular hyperplasia), and other causes such as adrenal carcinoma and dexamethasone-suppressible hyperaldosteronism are uncommon (24,48).

Primary hyperaldosteronism related to an adrenal adenoma occurs between two and three times more commonly in women, and the peak incidence is between the third and fifth decades. There are no specific physical findings. Patients with severe hypokalemia may develop fatigue, muscle weakness, cramping, headaches, and palpitations (24). Aldosterone-producing tumors tend to be small (Fig. 4).

Estimates of the prevalence of primary hyperaldosteronism range between 0.03 and 2% of the hypertensive population. In the study by Anderson et al. (4), the screening test for primary hyperaldosteronism in their hypertensive population consisted of measurements of serum potassium, measurement of PRA and aldosterone after standing and ambulation for 1 hour, changes in BP in response to a 20-minute infusion of an Ang II antagonist (saralasin), or to enalaprilat. This was followed by infusion of 2 L of normal saline over a 3- to 4-hour period, at the end of which blood was drawn for aldosterone.

Using this protocol, the investigators (4) determined that 12% of patients with secondary hypertension (or 1.8% of the total hypertensive population) over the age of 50 years had primary hyperaldosteronism. This compared to 15% of the patients with secondary hypertension (or 1.2% of the total hypertensive population) between 18 and 49 years of age. What is interesting, however, is that in hypertensive patients between 18 and 49 years with primary aldosteronism the percentage of patients with adenomas vs hyperplasia did not change with age. In hypertensive patients with primary hyperaldosteronism who were older than 50 years, the number of patients with an adrenal adenoma as a percentage of the hypertensive population did not change with age (between 50 and 59 years of age, 0.6%; between 60 and 69 years of age, 0.5%; in patients older than 70 years, 0.7%). However, in those patients with adrenal hyperplasia as a cause of their primary hyperaldosteronism, their number as a percentage of the total hypertensive population decreased with

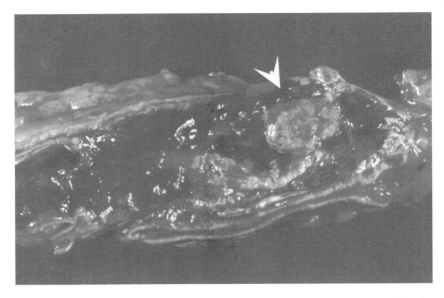

Fig. 4. Conn's syndrome. Adrenal aldosterone-producing tumors tend to be small (<1 cm) and have a high lipid content, which gives them the characteristic "canary yellow" appearance on sectioning.

age (between 50 and 59 years of age, 1.4%; between 60 and 69 years of age, 0.9%; in patients older than 70 years, 0.0%). Thus, an older patient presenting with primary hyperaldosteronism is more likely to have an adrenal adenoma than hyperplasia. In addition, if only patients with secondary hypertension with a diastolic blood pressure (DBP) of greater than 100 mmHg are screened, then the prevalence increases from 1.5% overall to 2.7% in those more severely hypertensive patients *(4)*.

It is possible that the prevalence of primary hyperaldosteronism is underestimated because of inadequate screening tests. Hiramatsu et al. *(49)* evaluated the use of simultaneously measuring both aldosterone and PRA and then expressing the results as the ratio of aldosterone to PRA (Aldo/PRA) as a screening tool for hyperaldosteronism in a hypertensive population. These investigators screened 348 patients and found 9 patients with elevated Aldo/PRA ratios subsequently confirmed to be true primary hyperaldosteronism, for a prevalence of 2.6% among this hypertensive population. In this study, patients with an aldosterone-producing adenoma had an Aldo/PRA ratio greater than 400, and patients with essential hypertension had ratio values less than 200, thus providing good discrimination between these hypertensive groups.

Gordon et al. *(50,51)* used the Aldo/PRA ratio to screen for primary hyperaldosteronism among patients recruited for antihypertensive drug trials and found a prevalence of close to 12%. They also used the Aldo/PRA ratio to screen patients referred to their hypertension clinic and among these patients found a prevalence of around 6.5%.

The utility of the Aldo/PRA ratio has been questioned by Montori et al. *(52)*. These investigators evaluated 221 African-American and 276 Caucasian patients with a diagnosis of essential hypertension between 1996 and 2000. They found that the Aldo/PRA ratio correlated with suppressed renin and did not add any value to the evaluation for primary hyperaldosteronism. They suggested, in fact, that further workup for primary hyperaldosteronism be done only in patients with both suppressed renin and elevated aldosterone and recommended that the Aldo/PRA ratio not be used in the evaluation of hypertensive patients.

Management

The presence of spontaneous hypokalemia in a hypertensive patient should always raise the possibility of primary hyperaldosteronism. As discussed, simultaneous aldosterone and PRA should be measured, and those patients with suppressed renin and elevated aldosterone should be evaluated further. An elevated Aldo/PRA ratio should be interpreted with caution and in the context of the patient under evaluation. The patient should be off angiotensin-converting enzyme inhibitors, β-blockers, calcium channel blockers, and diuretics for at least 2 weeks prior to the test. If they are on spironolactone, they should be off the medication for at least 6 weeks. The α-blockers do not interfere with this measurement. A positive screening test should be confirmed by a 24-hour urine aldosterone collection after 3 days of salt loading. A 24-hour aldosterone secretion rate above 14 μg with a urine sodium above 200 mEq/L is diagnostic. An elevated 18-hydroxycorticosterone value (>100 ng/dL) has also been suggested as helpful in distinguishing adrenal adenomas from hyperplasia.

Imaging studies are helpful to document the presence of an adrenal tumor, and a computed tomographic (CT) scanning or magnetic resonance imaging (MRI) is equally sensitive. If these studies are still equivocal, a bilateral adrenal vein catheterization with sampling of aldosterone and cortisol after a Cortrosyn (synthetic adrenocorticotropic hormone [ACTH]) stimulation test is the diagnostic procedure of choice.

In cases of adrenal adenoma, surgery is the preferred treatment if the patient has difficult-to-control hypertension or severe and persistent hypokalemia. Removal of the adrenal adenoma improves hypokalemia in all patients and eliminates the need for antihypertensive medication in 60 to 70% of patients. A worse outcome, inasmuch as persistent hypertension after surgery, is more common in older patients *(53)*. All patients, however, have improvement in their BP control. The BP response to spironolactone preoperatively is a good predictor of BP response to unilateral adrenalectomy. If the patient has adrenal hyperplasia, surgery is of no benefit, and medical treatment includes 100 mg per day of spironolactone initially, which can be increased to 400 mg per day as needed for BP control, or 5 mg per day of amiloride initially *(54–57)*.

Issues in Treatment

The major issue in the evaluation of a patient with hypertension for the possible diagnosis of primary hyperaldosteronism is patient selection, which patients should be screened and worked up. Part of the problem is that up to 40% of patients with essential hypertension have suppressed renin (particularly in older patients), which may remain relatively suppressed (<2 ng/mL per hour) even with stimulation in 15% to 20% of patients. In addition, up to 67% of patients with primary hyperaldosteronism may be normokalemic at presentation *(51)*. Thus, distinguishing patients with essential hypertension from those with primary hyperaldosteronism may be difficult, especially if they are otherwise asymptomatic. As outlined by Kaplan in an editorial in the *(58)*, if a patient is normokalemic and has a BP that is easily controlled by antihypertensive medications, then it may not be appropriate to perform an extensive workup for hyperaldosteronism or subject the patient to surgery. However, patients with persistent hypokalemia or difficult-to-control hypertension would benefit from an evaluation for primary hyperaldosteronism and possible surgery.

CUSHING'S SYNDROME

Cushing's (or hypercortisolism) is an unusual disease with a calculated incidence of 1 case per 100,000–500,000 population. The two main causes of hypercortisolism are either ACTH dependent or ACTH independent. Hypercortisolism secondary to an ACTH-secreting pituitary tumor (60%–70% of patients) is termed *Cushing's disease*. *Cushing's syndrome* is ACTH independent and refers to any condition resulting in exposure to high levels of glucocorticoids, such as adrenal adenomas (about 15% of patients), carcinomas, or exogenous administration *(24,59,60)*.

Interestingly, even though frank Cushing's syndrome is rare, the advent and widespread use of abdominal imaging techniques such as CT scan or MRI have resulted in detection of more incidental adrenal masses.

Workup of these patients frequently reveals that they have autonomous cortisol production, as assessed by the failure to suppress cortisol production after dexamethasone administration. Nonsuppressible cortisol is the most frequent endocrine abnormality found in these incidentally discovered adrenal masses. This condition has been termed *subclinical Cushing's syndrome (60)*. The prevalence of subclinical Cushing's in these incidental adrenal masses varies between 5% and 20%, depending on the study, with a calculated prevalence of about 78 cases per 100,000 population *(60)*. Thus, this condition is much more common than Cushing's disease. These patients with subclinical Cushing's have a higher incidence of high BP, obesity, and diabetes mellitus than the control population, although they do not have the classical clinical features of Cushing's *(60)*. There are no prospective studies to evaluate the best way to manage these patients, but these data suggest that cortisol hypersecretion, as a cause of hypertension, is probably more common than previously thought.

Full-blown clinical Cushing's has very characteristic clinical features (Fig. 5), including weight gain, fat accumulation in the face (moon facies) and back (buffalo hump), excessive hair growth (hirsutism), acne, and increased pigmentation (in Cushing's disease).

Pathogenesis of the Hypertension

The pathogenesis of an elevated BP in patients with Cushing's is poorly understood and multifactorial. In a study by Pirpiris et al. *(61)*, administration of 10 or 50 mg of cortisol orally for 5 days to six normal volunteers resulted in a 19% increase in cardiac output. In addition, steroids increase the hepatic production of angiotensinogen to almost two times higher, although renin levels are not elevated *(62,63)*.

A study by Heaney et al. *(64)* infused increasing concentrations of noradrenaline into eight patients with Cushing's disease and normal subjects. These investigators found that the change in mean arterial pressure compared to baseline was much greater in patients with Cushing's than in normal subjects (22 ± 4 vs 13 ± 2.4 mmHg, respectively), suggesting that patients with Cushing's have increased catecholamine sensitivity.

A number of investigators have also found that, in patients with Cushing's, there is a decrease in the production or activity of a number of hormones that oppose the hypertensive effect of cortisol. In patients with Cushing's, there is a decrease in the urinary excretion of prostaglandin E2 and of kallikrein, two known vasodilators *(62,65)*. In addition, cortisol inhibits the inducible nitric oxide synthase in endothelial cells, suggesting that part of cortisol's hypertensive mechanism may be to promote unopposed vasoconstriction *(66)*.

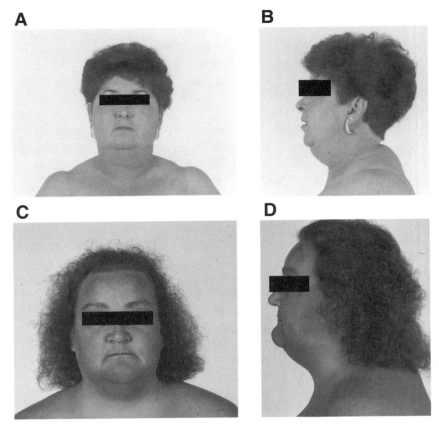

Fig. 5. Hypercortisolism. Patients with increased production of cortisol have characteristic "moon facies," dorsal fat pads, and buffalo hump (**A and B**). Patients with cortisol hypersecretion from a pituitary tumor (Cushing's disease) may also have increased pigmentation, male pattern baldness, and hirsutism (**C and D**).

Prevalence

The prevalence of Cushing's in a hypertensive population is quite low. In the Anderson et al. *(4)* study, the prevalence of Cushing's in the hypertensive population decreased with increasing age. There was a prevalence of 9% of the patients younger than 50 years of age with secondary hypertension; in patients older than 50 years, there was a prevalence of 2%. However, the converse is not true; in patients with Cushing's, the prevalence of hypertension is high, between 70% and 80%

(24). In fact, the presence of hypertension is a finding that helps discriminate patients with obesity and Cushingoid features (for whom there is a 20% prevalence of hypertension) vs patients with true Cushing's *(67)*.

Although the prevalence of hypertension is generally high in all patients with Cushing's irrespective of the etiology, in the case of Cushing's associated with exogenous steroid use, the prevalence of hypertension is only about 20% *(65)*. The severity of the hypertension in Cushing's tends to be mild; in fact, in one series a DBP greater than 100 mmHg tended to decrease the likelihood of Cushing's as the cause of the elevated BP (odds ratio of 0.7) *(4)*.

Management

For patients with Cushingoid features, a 24-hour collection for urinary free cortisol is the best screening test. For patients with an incidental adrenal mass, the best screening test to assess for autonomy of cortisol production is an overnight dexamethasone suppression test in which 1–3 mg of dexamethasone is administered at 11 PM and a serum cortisol is measured the next morning at 8 AM *(37,60)*. Reincke *(60)* has advocated the use of the higher dexamethasone dose (3 mg) because a potential adrenal source is already recognized; thus, this higher dose decreases the number of false-positive results. A postsuppression cortisol value of less than 3 μg/dL is normal and disproves cortisol hypersecretion. If the cortisol value is higher then 3 μg/dL, a high-dose (8 mg) dexamethasone suppression test is performed next.

The major issue is what to do with those patients with nonsuppressible cortisol production and an incidental adrenal mass. One author *(60)* proposed that patients with nonsuppressible cortisol production who are truly asymptomatic (no hypertension or stigmata of Cushing's) can be followed with serial 6-month or yearly testing of cortisol. There are no data on what to do if the patient has subclinical Cushing's and is not completely asymptomatic. The benefits of unilateral adrenalectomy in these patients need to be determined on a case-by-case basis by the patient's clinician.

PHEOCHROMOCYTOMA

Pheochromocytomas are tumors that arise from the chromaffin cells and produce an excess of catecholamines, usually norepinephrine. About half the patients have sustained hypertension, and half have paroxysmal hypertension. In patients with paroxysmal hypertension, symptomatology varied from once every month to multiple times per day and the "attacks" lasted anywhere from between 30 seconds and 1 week *(68)*.

Patients with pheochromocytoma usually are evaluated because of marked symptomatology. The combined presence of symptoms of headaches, diaphoresis, and palpitations had a sensitivity of 89% and a specificity of 67% in distinguishing patients with pheochromocytoma from patients with essential hypertension. Some of the characteristic features of pheochromocytoma are highlighted by the mnemonic device of "rules of 10," which rounds the true incidence of some of the features to 10%: 10% of pheochromocytomas are malignant, 10% are bilateral, 10% are extraadrenal, 10% are familial, and 10% occur in children. In the case of malignant pheochromocytoma, 30%–40% may be extra-adrenal *(37)*.

Pathogenesis of the Hypertension

Patients with pheochromocytomas have an increase in their TPR and increased heart rate, but cardiac output is unchanged *(68,69)*. Pheochromocytomas secrete norepinephrine predominantly. Norepinephrine activates α1-receptors on vascular smooth muscle to produce vasoconstriction with an increase in both DBP and SBP. Tumors that produce epinephrine predominantly can only be present in the adrenal gland or the organ of Zuckerkandl because these are the only tissues with the necessary enzymes for conversion of norepinephrine to epinephrine. Because epinephrine is relatively selective for β-receptors, which increase heart rate (β1) or induce smooth muscle relaxation (β2), a patient with a pheochromocytoma that secretes epinephrine predominantly can present with episodes of hypotension or alternating episodes of hypotension and hypertension.

Prevalence

Of all the endocrine causes of secondary hypertension, pheochromocytoma appears to be the one with the lowest prevalence. In the Anderson et al. *(4)* series, it only accounted for 0.3% of the cases of hypertension. The prevalence seems to be equally distributed among the age groups, accounting for 3% of the cases of secondary hypertension in both patients between 18 and 49 years of age and those 50 years and older and equally distributed between men and women. An autopsy series also demonstrated a 0.3% prevalence of patients with pheochromocytoma *(70)*. The diagnosis of pheochromocytoma is usually considered in patients with episodic or paroxysmal hypertension with the clinical triad of headaches (present in 35% of patients), diaphoresis (present in 34% of patients), and palpitations (present in 22% of patients), but this diagnosis is frequently missed.

Management

In an autopsy series from the Mayo clinic, 54 patients were identified as having a pheochromocytoma at autopsy between 1928 and 1977 *(70)*. In 41 of the 54 patients, the diagnosis of pheochromocytoma had not been entertained prior to their death. Of the 41 patients, 22 (54%) had an elevated BP. Of concern was that 11 of these 41 patients (27%) with "silent" pheochromocytoma died from a hypertensive or hypotensive crisis during or after surgery for unrelated conditions.

In a more recent autopsy series involving 32 cases of pheochromocytoma at the Henry Ford Hospital *(71)* and with the advent of widespread use of imaging techniques such as abdominal MRI or CT scans, the number of clinically unsuspected pheochromocytomas had dropped to 18%. Nevertheless, these authors still had 7 patients present with symptoms only at the time of an unrelated surgery. Thus, it is important to keep a high index of suspicion for pheochromocytoma in patients with essential hypertension who are under evaluation for surgery.

Issues in Treatment

Screening tests for pheochromocytoma should be ordered even if there is a low clinical suspicion; however, not all patients with hypertension need to be screened. Because pheochromocytomas are rare, screening of all hypertensive patients would result in a number of false-positive results. Typical screening tests include a 24-hour urine collection for two of three tests: urinary free catecholamines, vanillylmandelic acid (VMA), or metanephrines. Mildly elevated catecholamines are usually secondary to other causes besides pheochromocytomas. The finding of 1.5- to 2-fold higher than the upper limit of normal urinary catecholamines or metanephrines is highly suggestive of pheochromocytomas *(72)*. Plasma catecholamines and plasma metanephrines have also been proposed to be more sensitive for detection of pheochromocytomas. Plasma-free metanephrines have a sensitivity of 99% and a specificity of 90% in the diagnosis of pheochromocytoma, but their use remains limited *(33)*. Pheochromocytomas tend to be large (about 5-cm) tumors, in which the catecholamines are metabolized and could result in low urinary-free catecholamines but elevated VMA and metanephrines; small tumors could result in elevated levels of urinary-free catecholamines with normal levels of VMA or metanephrines.

Once the biochemical diagnosis of pheochromocytoma is made, imaging techniques (abdominal MRI or CT scan) can be used. However, because of the high prevalence of incidentally discovered adrenal masses (in which Cushing's is a more common endocrine abnormality, as discussed in the section on Cushing's syndrome), one should not proceed directly to imaging techniques. Nuclear imaging is also helpful, particularly use of meta-iodobenzylguanidine, which is taken up by the tumor. Most recently, 6-[18F]-fluorodopamine (a dopamine analog) with positron emission tomography scanning has been found to be very sensitive for detection of pheochromocytomas *(33)*. The treatment of pheochromocytomas is surgical removal, which can be performed laparoscopically *(73,74)*.

CONCLUSION

Four endocrine conditions, hyper- and hypothyroidism, primary hyperaldosteronism, Cushing's, and pheochromocytomas, can result in a reversible form of arterial hypertension. These conditions taken together account for 5.2% of the hypertensive population and 52% of the patients with secondary hypertension. Thus, every clinician should keep these four conditions in mind when evaluating hypertensive patients. All four of these conditions can present in a subclinical form and carry a diagnosis of essential hypertension, and a high index of suspicion by the clinician is required for appropriate treatment of these patients.

In two of these conditions (hypothyroidism and primary aldosteronism), screening and treatment are controversial. In subclinical Cushing's, the most appropriate treatment is still not well defined; in pheochromocytoma, the treatment is well defined, but it is frequently missed and presents catastrophically with a death during surgery for an unrelated condition. Screening for these conditions is easy and generally cheap. Further workup would depend on the results of the initial screening tests. Missing these endocrine diagnoses could be unfortunate for some of these conditions and disastrous in others. Above all, it is clear that the incidence of secondary hypertension increases with age, so the clinician's index of suspicion needs to be the highest with the older hypertensive population.

ACKNOWLEDGMENTS

I thank Dr. Edward Chin for providing the photographs of the patients with hypercortisolism and hyperthyroidism. My work is supported in part by funding from the National Institutes of Health (NIDDH 2 ul DN 58680).

REFERENCES

1. Burt VL, Cutler JA, Higgins M, et al. Trends in the prevalence, awareness, treatment, and control of hypertension in the adult US population. Data from the health examination surveys, 1960 to 1991. *Hypertension* 1995;26:60–69.

2. Perloff D. Hypertension in women. *Cardiovasc Clin* 1989;19:207–241.
3. Danielson M, Dammstrom B. The prevalence of secondary and curable hypertension. *Acta Med Scand* 1981;209:451-455.
4. Anderson GH Jr, Blakeman N, Streeten DH. The effect of age on prevalence of secondary forms of hypertension in 4429 consecutively referred patients. *J Hypertens* 1994;12:609–615.
5. Haynes R. Thyroid and antithyroid drugs. In: Taylor P, ed. *The Pharmacological Basis of Therapeutics*. 8th ed. Elmsford, NY: Pergamon Press; 1990:1361–1383.
6. Saito I, Saruta T. Hypertension in thyroid disorders. *Endocrinol Metab Clin North Am* 1994;23:379–386.
7. Coulombe P, Dussault JH, Letarte J, Simmard SJ. Catecholamines metabolism in thyroid diseases. I. Epinephrine secretion rate in hyperthyroidism and hypothyroidism. *J Clin Endocrinol Metab* 1976;42:125–131.
8. Coulombe P, Dussault JH, Walker P. Plasma catecholamine concentrations in hyperthyroidism and hypothyroidism. *Metabolism* 1976;25:973–979.
9. Diekman MJ, Harms MP, Endert E, Wieling W, Wiersinga WM. Endocrine factors related to changes in total peripheral vascular resistance after treatment of thyrotoxic and hypothyroid patients. *Eur J Endocrinol* 2001;144:339–346.
10. Cho Y, Somer BG, Amatya A. Natriuretic peptides and their therapeutic potential. *Heart Dis* 1999;1:305–328.
11. Cowie MR, Mendez GF. BNP and congestive heart failure. *Prog Cardiovasc Dis* 2002;44:293–321.
12. McMurray J, Pfeffer MA. New therapeutic options in congestive heart failure: Part I. *Circulation* 2002;105:2099–2106.
13. Gardner DG, Gertz BJ, Hane S. Thyroid hormone increases rat atrial natriuretic peptide messenger ribonucleic acid accumulation in vivo and in vitro. *Mol Endocrinol* 1987;1:260–265.
14. Rolandi E, Santaniello B, Bagnasco M, et al. Thyroid hormones and atrial natriuretic hormone secretion: study in hyper- and hypothyroid patients. *Acta Endocrinol (Copenh)* 1992;127:23–26.
15. Bernstein R, Midtbo K, Urdal P, et al. Serum N-terminal pro-atrial natriuretic factor 1-98 before and during thyroxine replacement therapy in severe hypothyroidism. *Thyroid* 1997;7:415–419.
16. Kohno M, Murakawa K, Yasunari K, Nishizawa Y, Morii H, Takeda T. Circulating atrial natriuretic peptides in hyperthyroidism and hypothyroidism. *Am J Med* 1987;83:648–652.
17. Kohno M, Horio T, Yasunari K, et al. Stimulation of brain natriuretic peptide release from the heart by thyroid hormone. *Metabolism* 1993;42:1059–1064.
18. Ojamaa K, Klein I, Sabet A, Steinberg SF. Changes in adenylyl cyclase isoforms as a mechanism for thyroid hormone modulation of cardiac β-adrenergic receptor responsiveness. *Metabolism* 2000;49:275–279.
19. Everett AW, Umeda PK, Sinha AM, Rabinowitz M, Zak R. Expression of myosin heavy chains during thyroid hormone-induced cardiac growth. *Fed Proc* 1986;45: 2568–2572.
20. Kong WM, Sheikh MH, Lumb PJ, et al. A 6-month randomized trial of thyroxine treatment in women with mild subclinical hypothyroidism. *Am J Med* 2002;112: 348–354.
21. Huber G, Staub JJ, Meier C, et al. Prospective study of the spontaneous course of subclinical hypothyroidism: prognostic value of thyrotropin, thyroid reserve, and thyroid antibodies. *J Clin Endocrinol Metab* 2002;87:3221–3226.

22. Cooper DS. Clinical practice. Subclinical hypothyroidism. *N Engl J Med* 2001;345:260–265.
23. Streeten DH, Anderson GH Jr, Howland T, Chiang R, Smulyan H. Effects of thyroid function on blood pressure. Recognition of hypothyroid hypertension. *Hypertension* 1988;11:78–83.
24. Akpunonu BE, Mulrow PJ, Hoffman EA. Secondary hypertension: evaluation and treatment [published erratum appears in *Dis Mon* 1997;43:62]. *Dis Mon 1996*;42: 609–722.
25. Dluhy RG. Uncommon forms of secondary hypertension in older patients. *Am J Hypertens* 1998;11(3 pt 2):52S–56S.
26. Saito I, Ito K, Saruta T. The effect of age on blood pressure in hyperthyroidism. *J Am Geriatr Soc* 1985;33:19–22.
27. Barrett PQ, Bollag WB, Isales CM, McCarthy RT, Rasmussen H. Role of calcium in angiotensin II-mediated aldosterone secretion. *Endocr Rev* 1989;10:1–22.
28. Rasmussen H, Isales CM, Calle R, et al. Diacylglycerol production, Ca2+ influx, and protein kinase C activation in sustained cellular responses. *Endocr Rev* 1995;16:649–681.
29. Bravo EL, Tarazi RC, Dustan HP, et al. The changing clinical spectrum of primary aldosteronism. *Am J Med* 1983;74:641–651.
30. Bravo EL, Fouad-Tarazi FM, Tarazi RC, Pohl M, Gifford RW, Vidt DG. Clinical implications of primary aldosteronism with resistant hypertension. *Hypertension* 1988;11(2 pt 2):I207–I211.
31. Wenting GJ, Man in 't Veld AJ, Derkx FH, Schalekamp MA. Recurrence of hypertension in primary aldosteronism after discontinuation of spironolactone. Time course of changes in cardiac output and body fluid volumes. *Clin Exp Hypertens A* 1982;4(9–10):1727–1748.
32. Yamakado M, Nagano M, Umezu M, Tagawa H, Kiyose H, Tanaka S. Extrarenal role of aldosterone in the regulation of blood pressure. *Am J Hypertens* 1988;1(3 pt 1):276–279.
33. Pacak K, Koch CA, Eisenhofer G. Current approaches and new advances in endocrine hypertension. *Trends Endocrinol Metab* 2002;13:96–97.
34. Field M, Giebisch G. Physiologic actions of aldosterone in the kidney. In: Brenner B, ed. *Hypertension: Pathophysiology, Diagnosis and Management*. New York: Raven Press; 1990:1273–1285.
35. Nakamura T, Ichikawa S, Sakamaki T, et al. Role of atrial natriuretic peptide in mineralocorticoid escape phenomenon in patients with primary aldosteronism. *Proc Soc Exp Biol Med* 1987;185:448–454.
36. Isales CM, Bollag WB, Kiernan LC, Barrett PQ. Effect of ANP on sustained aldosterone secretion stimulated by angiotensin II. *Am J Physiol* 1989;256(Cell Physiol 25):C89–C95.
37. Mulrow PJ, Takagi M, Takagi M, Franco-Saenz R. Inhibitors of aldosterone secretion. *J Steroid Biochem* 1987;27:941–946.
38. Tunny TJ, Gordon RD, Klemm SA, Stowasser M. Reduced renal extraction of atrial natriuretic peptide in primary aldosteronism. *Hypertension* 1995;26:624–627.
39. Pedrinelli R, Panarace G, Spessot M, et al. Low dose atrial natriuretic factor in primary aldosteronism: renal, hemodynamic, and vascular effects. *Hypertension* 1989;14:156–163.
40. Barrett PQ, Zawalich K, Isales CM. Role of cGMP in the inhibitory action of atrial natriuretic peptide on aldosterone secretion stimulated by angiotensin II. In: Brenner B, Laragh J, eds. *Biologically Active Atrial Peptides*. New York: Raven Press; 1987:269–271.

41. Barrett PQ, Isales CM. The role of cyclic nucleotides in atrial natriuretic peptide-mediated inhibition of aldosterone secretion. *Endocrinology* 1988;122:799–808.
42. Isales CM, Lewicki JA, Nee JJ, Barrett PQ. ANP-(7-23) stimulates a DHP-sensitive Ca^{2+} conductance and reduces cellular cAMP via a cGMP-independent mechanism. *Am J Physiol* 1992;263(2 pt 1):c334–c342.
43. Barrett PQ, Isales CM, Bollag WB, McCarthy RT. Ca^{2+} channels and aldosterone secretion: modulation by K+ and atrial natriuretic peptide. *Am J Physiol* 1991;261(4 pt 2):f706–f719.
44. Barrett PQ, Isales CM, Bollag WB, McCarthy RT. Modulation of Ca^{2+} channels by atrial natriuretic peptide in the bovine adrenal glomerulosa cell. *Can J Physiol Pharmacol* 1991;69:1553–1560.
45. Barrett PQ, Ertel EA, Smith MM, Nee JJ, Cohen CJ. Voltage-gated calcium currents have two opposing effects on the secretion of aldosterone. *Am J Physiol* 1995;268(4 pt 1):c985–c992.
46. McCarthy RT, Isales CM, Bollag WB, Rasmussen H, Barrett PQ. Atrial natriuretic peptide differentially modulates T- and L-type calcium channels. *Am J Physiol* 1990;258(3 pt 2):f473–f478.
47. Conn J. Primary aldosteronism: a new clinical syndrome. *J Lab Clin Med* 1955;45:661–664.
48. Drury PL. Disorders of mineralocorticoid activity. *Clin Endocrinol Metab* 1985;14:175–202.
49. Hiramatsu K, Yamada T, Yukimura Y, et al. A screening test to identify aldosterone-producing adenoma by measuring plasma renin activity. Results in hypertensive patients. *Arch Intern Med* 1981;141:1589–1593.
50. Gordon RD, Ziesak MD, Tunny TJ, Stowasser M, Klemm SA. Evidence that primary aldosteronism may not be uncommon: 12% incidence among antihypertensive drug trial volunteers. *Clin Exp Pharmacol Physiol* 1993;20:296–298.
51. Gordon RD, Klemm SA, Stowasser M, Tunny TJ, Storie WJ, Rutherford JC. How common is primary aldosteronism? Is it the most frequent cause of curable hypertension? *J Hypertens Suppl* 1993;11(suppl 5):S310–S311.
52. Montori VM, Schwartz GL, Chapman AB, Boerwinkle E, Turner ST. Validity of the aldosterone-renin ratio used to screen for primary aldosteronism. *Mayo Clin Proc* 2001;76:877–882.
53. Obara T, Ito Y, Okamoto T, et al. Risk factors associated with postoperative persistent hypertension in patients with primary aldosteronism. *Surgery* 1992;112:987–993.
54. Noth RH, Biglieri EG. Primary hyperaldosteronism. *Med Clin North Am* 1988;72:1117–1131.
55. Biglieri E, Irony I, Kater C. Adrenocortical forms of human hypertension. In: Brenner B, ed. *Hypertension: Pathophysiology, Diagnosis and Management.* New York: Raven Press; 1990:1609–1638.
56. Bravo EL. Primary aldosteronism. Issues in diagnosis and management. *Endocrinol Metab Clin North Am* 1994;23:271–283.
57. Bravo EL. Medical management of primary hyperaldosteronism. *Curr Hypertens Rep* 2001;3:406–409.
58. Kaplan NM. Caution about the overdiagnosis of primary aldosteronism. *Mayo Clin Proc* 2001;76:875–876.
59. Kirk LF Jr, Hash RB, Katner HP, Jones T. Cushing's disease: clinical manifestations and diagnostic evaluation. *Am Fam Physician* 2000;62:1119–1127, 1133–1134.
60. Reincke M. Subclinical Cushing's syndrome. *Endocrinol Metab Clin North Am* 2000;29:43–56.

61. Pirpiris M, Yeung S, Dewar E, Jennings GL, Whitworth JA. Hydrocortisone-induced hypertension in men. The role of cardiac output. *Am J Hypertens* 1993;6:287–294.
62. Saruta T, Suzuki H, Handa M, Igarashi Y, Kondo K, Senba S. Multiple factors contribute to the pathogenesis of hypertension in Cushing's syndrome. *J Clin Endocrinol Metab* 1986;62:275–279.
63. Klett C, Ganten D, Hellmann W, et al. Regulation of hepatic angiotensinogen synthesis and secretion by steroid hormones. *Endocrinology* 1992;130:3660–3668.
64. Heaney AP, Hunter SJ, Sheridan B, Brew Atkinson A. Increased pressor response to noradrenaline in pituitary dependent Cushing's syndrome. *Clin Endocrinol (Oxf)* 1999;51:293–299.
65. Danese RD, Aron DC. Cushing's syndrome and hypertension. *Endocrinol Metab Clin North Am* 1994;23:299–324.
66. Radomski MW, Palmer RM, Moncada S. Glucocorticoids inhibit the expression of an inducible, but not the constitutive, nitric oxide synthase in vascular endothelial cells. *Proc Natl Acad Sci USA* 1990;87:10,043–10,047.
67. Ross EJ, Linch DC. Cushing's syndrome—killing disease: discriminatory value of signs and symptoms aiding early diagnosis. *Lancet* 1982;2:646–649.
68. Gifford RW Jr, Manger WM, Bravo EL. Pheochromocytoma. *Endocrinol Metab Clin North Am* 1994;23:387–404.
69. Levenson JA, Safar ME, London GM, Simon AC. Haemodynamics in patients with phaeochromocytoma. *Clin Sci (Lond)* 1980;58:349–356.
70. Sutton MG, Sheps SG, Lie JT. Prevalence of clinically unsuspected pheochromocytoma. Review of a 50-year autopsy series. *Mayo Clin Proc* 1981;56:354–360.
71. Krane NK. Clinically unsuspected pheochromocytomas. Experience at Henry Ford Hospital and a review of the literature. *Arch Intern Med* 1986;146:54–57.
72. Stein PP, Black HR. A simplified diagnostic approach to pheochromocytoma. A review of the literature and report of one institution's experience. *Medicine (Baltimore)* 1991;70:46–66.
73. Kercher KW, Park A, Matthews BD, Rolband G, Sing RF, Heniford BT. Laparoscopic adrenalectomy for pheochromocytoma. *Surg Endosc* 2002;16:100–102.
74. MacGillivray DC, Whalen GF, Malchoff CD, Oppenheim DS, Shichman SJ. Laparoscopic resection of large adrenal tumors. *Ann Surg Oncol* 2002;9:480–485.

11 Diagnosis and Management of Hypertensive Renal and Renovascular Disease in the Elderly

Wanpen Vongpatanasin, MD and Ronald G. Victor, MD

CONTENTS

INTRODUCTION

The prevalence of both renal parenchymal and renovascular hypertension (RVH) increases sharply with age, making these the two most common causes of secondary hypertension in the elderly *(1)*. The main causes of renal parenchymal disease in the elderly are diabetes mellitus and hypertension *(2)*; the main contributor to RVH is atherosclerosis.

Because the prognosis of patients with end-stage renal disease (ESRD) over the age of 60 years is extremely poor, tight control of blood pressure (BP) is essential in preventing renal disease progression. Antihypertensive medications that block the renin–angiotensin–aldosterone system (RAAS) appear to have renoprotective effects beyond BP lowering and should be first-line therapy. The target goal BP for elderly patients with renal parenchymal disease from diabetes mellitus (DM) or primary

From: *Clinical Hypertension and Vascular Diseases: Hypertension in the Elderly*
Edited by: L. M. Prisant © Humana Press Inc., Totowa, NJ

glomerulopathy with proteinuria greater than 1 g per day is now set at below 130/80 mmHg.

The diagnosis of RVH should be considered in patients with generalized atherosclerosis, resistant hypertension, abdominal systolic/diastolic bruit, azotemia that is unexplained or induced by treatment with an angiotensin-converting enzyme (ACE) inhibitor or angiotensin-receptor blocker (ARB), recurrent flash pulmonary edema, or discrepancy in kidney sizes. Because clinical responses to both percutaneous intervention and vascular surgery for RVH are highly variable, revascularization should be considered only in patients with (a) bilateral renal artery stenosis or stenosis of the unilateral functioning kidney, (b) rapid decline in renal function, (c) resistant hypertension despite three or more antihypertensive medications, or (d) recurrent pulmonary edema.

RENAL PARENCHYMAL DISEASE

Epidemiology

Renal insufficiency constitutes a common cause of secondary hypertension, second only to RVH. In the United States, at least 30% of nondiabetic persons over the age of 60 years have some degree of renal impairment (3). Elderly hypertensives are more susceptible to develop renal insufficiency and ESRD than younger individuals (4,5). Of hypertensive patients older than 60 years with normal renal function, 10% develop elevated serum creatinine within 1 year, whereas only 5% of hypertensive patients aged 50 to 59 and 2% of those aged 30 ot 49 develop hypertension-related renal insufficiency (5).

It is clear that ESRD has now become a geriatric disease. The mean age of patients who enter a dialysis program increased from 58 in 1990 to 61 in 1999 (6). During the d 1990s, the rate of increase in incidence of dialysis slowed in all other age groups except in the elderly (age 65 years or older), for whom the rate of rise has been exponential (Fig. 1). DM and hypertension are two major causes of ESRD in the elderly; glomerulonephritis and cystic disease of the kidney are less frequent (Fig. 2). Elderly patients who develop ESRD have a poor prognosis, with average life expectancy of only 3 years and an annual mortality rate of 34% (6). Cardiovascular disease is the most common cause of death, accounting for 40 to 60% of the mortality rate (6,7).

Pathogenesis

Aging is inevitably associated with loss of nephron mass. In normotensive individuals, the number of normally functioning glomeruli decreases with age (8), and the glomerular filtration rate (GFR) declines at

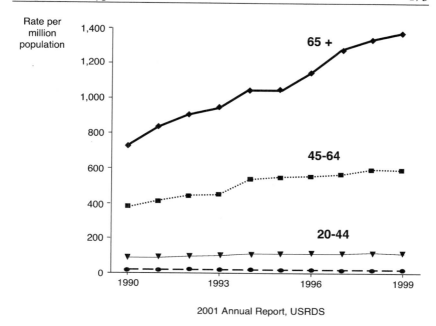

2001 Annual Report, USRDS

Fig. 1. Temporal trend in incidence of dialysis (per million population) in different age group. (From ref. 6.)

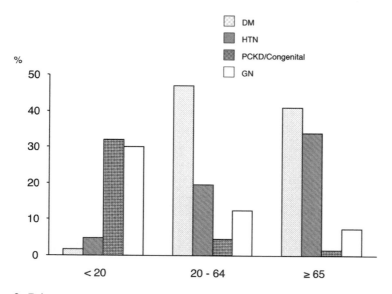

Fig. 2. Primary causes (%) of end-stage renal disease among different age populations in the United States. DM, diabetes mellitus; GN, glomerulonephritis; HTN, hypertension; PCKD, polycystic kidney disease. (From ref. 6.)

the average rate of 1 mL/minute/1.73 m^2 per year *(9)*. In untreated hypertensives, this rate is accelerated 10-fold *(10)*.

Renal parenchymal hypertension traditionally has been viewed as largely volume-dependent because of the failing kidney's inability to excrete salt and water. However, in the overwhelming majority of patients, the main hemodynamic fault is increased systemic vascular resistance with an inappropriately "normal" cardiac output. This suggests either impaired vasodilator mechanisms or augmented vasoconstrictor mechanisms. Among these is activation of the RAAS.

Plasma renin activity is inappropriately normal or mildly elevated despite an expanded plasma volume and a reduced nephron mass *(11)*. The interaction of angiotensin II (Ang II) with angiotensin subtype I (AT_1)receptor accelerates numerous cellular processes that contribute to hypertension. These include aldosterone release, peripheral vasoconstriction, and production of superoxide anion and reactive oxygen species that inactivate nitric oxide (NO) and impair endothelial function.

Other potential pathogenetic mechanisms include overactivity of the sympathetic nervous system, caused by either activation of central AT_1I receptors and/or uremic metabolites acting on excitatory renal afferents in the failing kidneys *(12)*. Asymmetric dimethylarginine, a putative endogenous inhibitor of nitric oxide synthase normally cleared by the kidney, accumulates excessively in the plasma of patients with ESRD. The resultant NO inhibitor may contribute to both hypertension and mortality in patients with ESRD *(7)*.

Diagnosis

Evaluation of elderly patients with renal parenchymal disease should include urinalysis to detect proteinuria or hematuria. Renal sonography should be performed to exclude urinary tract obstruction, to exclude adult polycystic kidney disease, and to determine kidney size. Renal insufficiency should be considered when there is proteinuria by dipstick or when the serum creatinine level is 1.4 mg/dL or higher for hypertensive men and 1.2 mg/dL or higher for hypertensive women. However, renal function at a given serum creatinine level is usually much lower in the elderly than in younger individuals because of decreased muscle mass that accompanies aging. Thus, the diagnosis of renal insufficiency should be confirmed by demonstration of creatinine clearance below 60 mL/minute or urinary protein excretion above 200 mg/24 hours. A 24-hour urine creatinine collection is less reliable than calculated creatinine clearance, using Cockcroft-Gault equations, in estimating GFR because of day-to-day variation in creatinine excretion and collection errors frequently found in this population *(13)*. The urinary clearance of [125]Iiodothalamate is considered to be a gold standard in measurement of GFR but is not readily available in most clinical facilities.

Treatment

In patients with mild or moderate renal insufficiency, stringent BP control is imperative to slow the progression to ESRD because untreated hypertensives have a rate of loss in GFR that is 10 times faster than for normotensive individuals (10). ACE inhibitors have been shown to reduce the rate of decline in GFR in diabetic or nondiabetic chronic nephropathy with mild-to-moderate severity (14,15). Among African Americans with hypertensive nephrosclerosis, the ACE inhibitor ramipril was found in the African American Study of Kidney Disease (AASK) trial to be superior to both the dihydropyridine-calcium channel blocker amlodipine and the β-blocker metoprolol in preventing the decline in GFR, ESRD, and death (16). Of note, excellent and comparable control of hypertension was achieved in all three arms of the study. In hypertensive patients with type 2 diabetic nephropathy, ARBs or ACE inhibitors are now first-line therapy because of the results of three large trials (17–19). ACE inhibitors remain first-line therapy for type 1 DM (14) because there are no data on renoprotective effects of ARB-based therapy in this population. Elderly patients with systolic hypertension and mild renal insufficiency (serum creatinine 1.4–2.4 mg/dL) should be treated with thiazide diuretics because they derive even more benefit in terms of cardiovascular prevention than those with normal renal function (20). The target BP in elderly hypertensives with renal insufficiency is still controversial. The Seventh Report of the Joint National Committee on Prevention, Detection, Evaluation, and Treatment of High Blood Pressure (21) recommended a BP goal of 130/80 mmHg for patients with chronic kidney diseases. The recommendation was largely based on results from *post hoc* analysis of the Modification of Diet in Renal Disease (MDRD) Study (22). The MDRD study demonstrated that treatment of hypertension to achieve a lower target BP goal (≤125/75 mmHg for patients 60 years of age or younger and ≤130/80 for patients 61 years or older) is associated with slower decline in GFR *only* in patients with proteinuria of 1 g per day or above. More recently, however, the AASK *failed* to demonstrate that, for patients with hypertensive renal disease, a lower BP goal (mean arterial pressure [MAP] of 92 or less or BP of 125/75 mmHg or less) was any better than the higher BP goal (MAP of 102–107 or BP of 130/85 to 140/90) in terms of renoprotection (16). The difference in the results of the two studies may be related to patients' characteristics. Although the MDRD study patients were mainly Caucasians with primary glomerular disease and polycystic kidney disease, the

AASK study participants all were African Americans with hypertensive nephrosclerosis. For diabetic patients with hypertension, the Hypertension Optimal Treatment study demonstrated a dramatic cardiovascular benefit of achieving a target diastolic blood pressure goal of less than 80 mmHg *(23)*. Taken together, the existing data support the goal BP of less than 130/80 mmHg for elderly patients with DM or primary glomerular disease with proteinuria above 1 g per day and the BP goal of less than 140/90 mmHg for those with hypertensive nephrosclerosis with nonnephrotic range proteinuria. In patients with far-advanced renal insufficiency, hypertension often becomes difficult to treat and may require either intensive medical regimen including loop diuretics, potent vasodilators, and central sympatholytics or initiation of chronic hemodialysis as the only effective way to reduce plasma volume. The target BP for chronic dialysis patients is even more controversial. Although some prospective *(24)* and retrospective studies *(25)* showed the positive correlation between BP and mortality, others showed no association *(26)* or even the inverse correlation *(27)*. The largest prospective study in hemodialysis patients *(28)* suggested a U-shaped curve correlation between systolic blood pressure (SBP) and mortality. The cardiovascular mortality was increased when SBP was less than 110 or above 180 mmHg. The precise mechanism by which patients with BP above or below this range experience increased mortality is not known. Patients with very low SBP may have occult left ventricular dysfunction; those with high systolic pressure may have increased arterial stiffness, which predisposes to left ventricular hypertrophy and increased cardiovascular mortality *(29,30)*. Randomized prospective studies are needed to determine if therapy that aims to improve arterial stiffness and maintain SBP in a specific range will translate into improved long-term outcome.

RENOVASCULAR HYPERTENSION

Definition and Epidemiology

RVH is the most common cause of secondary hypertension in the elderly, accounting for 5 to 7% of hypertension in patients over the age of 60 years (Fig. 3) *(1)*. Atherosclerosis is the major form of renal artery pathology in the elderly because fibromuscular dysplasia is seen predominantly in young adults. The incidence of atherosclerotic RVH is increasing in the United States, reflecting the increased life expectancy and the aging of our population. According to the US Renal Data System database, the incidence of ESRD related to renovascular diseases has doubled over the past decade (from 2.9 to 6.1 per million per year), rising at a faster rate than ESRD related to such other causes as DM *(31)* (Fig. 4).

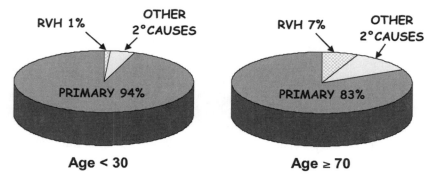

Fig. 3. Effects of age on prevalence of renovascular hypertension (%) among patients referred to hypertension clinic. (Data adapted from ref. *1*.)

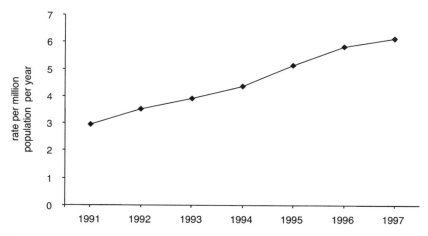

Fig. 4. Adjusted incidence rate of end-stage renal disease caused by renovascular disease. (Reprinted with permission from ref. *31*.)

It is estimated that 15 to 20% of elderly patients who enter a dialysis program have atherosclerotic renal artery stenosis as a contributing factor *(32,33)*. The prevalence of RVH is thought to be lower in African Americans than Caucasians *(34,35)*. However, this is an incorrect notion based on the captopril renogram. Angiographic studies have not confirmed such an ethnic difference *(36,37)*.

Atherosclerotic renovascular disease may lead to deterioration in renal function, *ischemic nephropathy*. Chronic underperfusion is thought to be the main mechanism leading to renal atrophy. Because renal dysfunction and atrophy are less common with fibromuscular dysplasia than atherosclerotic renal artery stenosis, additional mechanisms such as atheroembolism or damage in contralateral kidney from long-standing hypertension *(38,39)* may contribute to renal dysfunction in the elderly with renovascular disease.

It is important to emphasize that all patients with renal artery stenosis do not develop hypertension or renal dysfunction. Between 15 and 30% of patients undergoing abdominal aortogram or coronary angiogram were reported to have incidental renovascular disease. Only half of these patients have hypertension or renal dysfunction *(40,41)*. One-third of elderly patients with congestive heart failure were found to have stenotic renal artery disease, but only one-third of these had hypertension *(42)*. Thus, renal artery stenosis should not be used synonymously with RVH or ischemic nephropathy.

Natural History and Prognosis

In the, elderly atherosclerotic renal artery stenosis tends to progress over time. The 3-year incidence of renal atrophy is 10 to 20% *(43)*, doubling of serum creatinine is 15% *(44)*, and progression to ESRD is 7–10% *(44–46)*. Patients with more severe disease are more susceptible to have ipsilateral renal atrophy, but those with high SBP are also at increased risk of renal atrophy in both ipsilateral and contralateral kidneys independent of severity of stenosis *(43)*. Thus, the presence of renal artery stenosis does not necessarily protect the kidney against harmful effects of systemic hypertension. Because renal function is influenced by many factors other than renal perfusion, it is usually difficult to show a correlation between the severity of the renal artery lesion with either baseline renal function or the subsequent decline in renal function *(46,47)*.

Once renal dysfunction develops, the prognosis of elderly patients with renovascular disease is poor. Death rates increase from 5% per year in those with preserved renal function to 15–20% per year in those with severe renal failure *(46)*. Elderly patients who develop ESRD have a very poor prognosis, with a 2-year survival rate of 50% *(45)* and a 10-year survival rate of only 5% *(33)*. The major causes of death in these patients are myocardial infarction, stroke, and congestive heart failure *(44,46)*, reflecting generalized atherosclerosis in the coronary, carotid, and peripheral vascular beds *(48)*, respectively.

Pathogenesis

Analogous to human unilateral RVH, animals with the two-kidney, one-clip model of Goldblatt hypertension have early high levels of plasma renin. Increased production of renin from the ischemic kidney leads to increased production of Ang II and aldosterone, causing increased BP. Exposure of the contralateral kidney to high BP over time leads to glomerular hypertrophy, hyperfiltration, and pressure natriuresis (49). Thus, the animals maintain a high-renin state with normal extracellular volume. Other factors that contribute to the development of this hypertension include Ang II-stimulated release of vasoconstrictor prostaglandins (50) and reactive oxygen species (51), resulting in impairment in endothelium-dependent vasodilation, and stimulated central sympathetic outflow by an action of Ang II in the central nervous system (52).

In the late phase of Goldblatt hypertension, the contralateral kidneys develop glomerular fibrosis and irreversible renal injury. Reduction in GFR in both ipsilateral and contralateral kidneys leads to an expanded plasma volume, which suppresses plasma renin activity. Removal of the clip leads to resolution of hypertension early on. In the late stages, however, hypertension persists despite removal of the clip and resolves only after removal of the contralateral kidney, indicating that contralateral kidney damage from long-standing hypertension is important in maintenance of hypertension (53).

Analogous to the clinical condition of unilateral stenosis of a solitary functioning kidney or bilateral RVH, animals with a one-kidney, one-clip model of Goldblatt hypertension have an expanded plasma volume with normal or low plasma renin levels. ACE inhibitors and ARB have minimal effect on BP in this low-renin condition (54,55).

Diagnosis

Angiography is considered the gold standard for diagnosing renal artery stenosis. The minimal degree of stenosis that reduces renal perfusion in humans is not known, but in dogs a diameter stenosis above 70% is needed to decrease renal blood flow and increase the systemic arterial pressure (56). Because there are currently no clinical tests that can precisely assess the functional significance of a given stenosis, the diagnosis of RVH still relies heavily on clinical presentation expo facto and the BP response to revascularization. However, such reliance may still lead to inaccurate interpretation because lack of BP responses to revascularization may occur in some patients with RVH who develop irreversible contralateral or ipsilateral renal parenchymal injury.

CAPTOPRIL RENAL SCINTIGRAPHY

Renal perfusion can be assessed by radionuclide imaging study before and 1 to 2 hours after administration of oral captopril or intravenous enalaprilat. The radiopharmaceuticals commonly used in this test are technetium-99m (^{99m}Tc) diethylenediaminepentaacetic acid (DTPA) and ^{99m}Tc mercaptoacetyltriglycine (MAG$_3$). DTPA is purely filtered by the glomerulus; therefore, renal uptake of DTPA is proportional to the GFR. MAG$_3$ is cleared mostly by the proximal tubules, and its renal uptake provides an estimate of renal plasma flow. In the presence of RVH, the uptake and clearance of radiopharmaceuticals are normal at baseline but become significantly reduced after captopril, which antagonizes the action of Ang II at the efferent arterioles, causing an acute fall in renal perfusion distal to stenosis.

Meta-analysis *(57)* and a large-scale, single-center experience *(58)* indicated that the test has a low-to-moderate sensitivity of 65 to 75% with a high specificity of 90% in detecting renal artery stenosis. The test is less accurate in patients with renal insufficiency and bilateral renal artery stenosis. It is reportedly less reliable in low-renin hypertension *(37)*, which is common in the elderly *(38)*. In many observational studies, positive captopril renal scintigraphy is reported to be highly predictive of successful control of hypertension after revascularization with a positive predictive value of 90 to 100% *(59–62)*.

However, data from prospective randomized studies challenge this concept. One study of patients with ostial atherosclerotic renal artery stenosis and positive captopril renography showed that the hypertension control was improved in only one-half of patients undergoing renal angioplasty or stenting *(63)*. The Dutch Renal Artery Stenosis Interventional Cooperative (DRASTIC) study *(64)* demonstrated that, in the group of patients who were randomized to receive angioplasty, the presence of an abnormal captopril renogram did not predict BP response over the 12 months of follow-up. There were no differences in either BP or doses of antihypertensive medication between patients with normal scintigraphy vs those with abnormal scintigraphy at entry (Fig. 5).

DUPLEX DOPPLER ULTRASONOGRAPHY

Detection of renal blood flow velocity by Doppler sonography is another technique often employed to detect renal artery stenosis. The abdominal aorta is usually imaged first, and the peak systolic velocities (PSVs) are measured from the origin, proximal, middle, and distal segments of each renal artery. Acceleration of velocity normally occurs at the stenotic site, and the Doppler signal distal to high-grade stenosis appears dampened with low velocity, so-called tardus and parvus. The presence of a renal artery PSV of 180 cm/second or above and the ratio of the PSV of the renal artery to the suprarenal abdominal aorta of 3.5 or higher indicates severe stenosis of 60% or greater *(65)*. The procedure is time consuming and highly dependent on the skill of the sonographer.

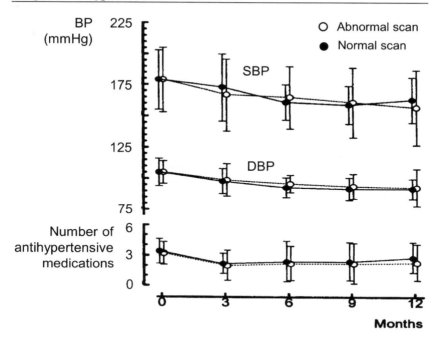

Fig. 5. Failure of captopril renography in predicting blood pressure (BP) response to percutaneous renal angioplasty in the DRASTIC study *(64)*. The systolic BP, diastolic BP, and number of antihypertensive medications were identical among the group of patients with or without abnormal scan prior to intervention. (Reprinted with permission from ref. *64*.)

Bowel gas and abdominal obesity are the major limiting factors for a successful study. It also has limited usefulness in diagnosis of the accessory vessel or branch vessel disease *(38)*. Overall sensitivity and specificity of the test are approximately 80 to 90%.

Duplex Doppler sonography may have both prognostic and diagnostic value. One recent study indicated that a high renal resistance index (1 − End diastolic velocity/Peak systolic velocity) × 100 ≥ 80 is a reliable predictor of unsuccessful outcome after revascularization (Fig. 6) *(66)*. A resistance index of 80 or above is indicative of irreversible renal parenchymal disease *(67)*. The resistance index of the contralateral kidney is often even higher than that of the kidney with renal artery stenosis *(39)* and may also be predictive of the clinical response to revascularization.

RENAL VEIN RENIN

The renal vein renin test is based on the premise that ischemic kidneys produce excessive renin, and renin production from the contralateral

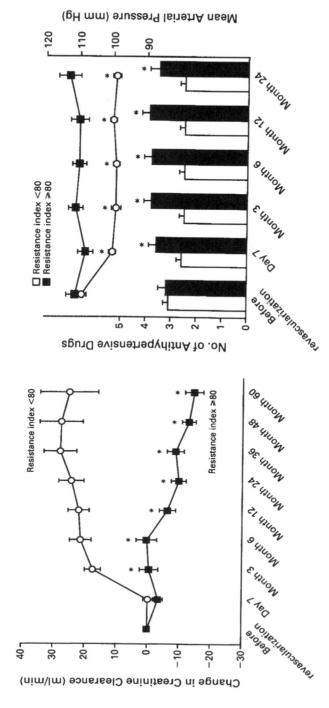

Fig. 6. Change in creatinine clearance (left) and number of antihypertensive medications and mean arterial pressure (right) before and 60 months after renal revascularization in patients with high resistance index ($\Re{\geq}80$) and low index (<80) at baseline. (Reprinted with permission from ref. 66.)

kidney is suppressed. The test is considered positive when the renal vein renin ratio from ischemic to nonischemic kidney is more than 1.5:1 or 2:1. However, the test is almost never used any more for the following reasons. It is invasive and cumbersome with low sensitivity (60–80%) and specificity (55–65%). Furthermore, there can be lateralization in patients with primary hypertension *(68)*.

MAGNETIC RESONANCE ANGIOGRAPHY

The noninvasive procedure of magnetic resonance angiography (MRA) allows visualization of renal arteries without exposure to iodinated contrast and thus can be performed safely in patients with renal insufficiency or those with contrast dye allergy. MRA is suitable for detection of stenosis in the ostium and proximal portion of renal arteries, which are found in the majority of patients with atherosclerotic renal artery stenosis. It has limitation in detecting subtler stenoses in the distal main renal arteries or intrarenal branches *(69)*. Overall sensitivity and specificity of the gadolinium-enhanced three-dimensional MRA is between 90 and 100% *(57)*.

SPIRAL COMPUTED TOMOGRAPHIC ANGIOGRAPHY

The spiral computed tomographic (CT) angiography test also provides direct visualization of renal vessels with high spatial resolution. However, administration of nephrotoxic contrast agents during the test limits its safety in patients with chronic renal insufficiency. Accessory and main renal arteries can be imaged with high accuracy *(70)*. Sensitivity and specificity of spiral CT angiography are comparable to that of gadolinium-enhanced MRA but are superior to non-gadolinium-enhanced MRA, captopril renal scintigraphy, and Duplex Doppler ultrasonography in diagnosing renal artery stenosis (Fig. 7). In our institution, CT angiography has become the procedure of choice because of the local expertise of our radiologists.

Management

MEDICAL THERAPY

Unilateral Renovascular Hypertension. In experimented animals with high-renin Goldblatt hypertension, treatment with ACE inhibitors or ARBs consistently reduces systemic arterial pressure and intra-glomerular pressure while increasing GFR, urine flow, and sodium excretion in the unclipped kidney *(71,72)*. Thus, antagonism of effects of Ang II by these medications can attenuate glomerular sclerosis and tubulo-interstitial injury in the unclipped kidney and prevent the serum creatinine rise in the chronic phase of hypertension *(49)*. The effect of ACE

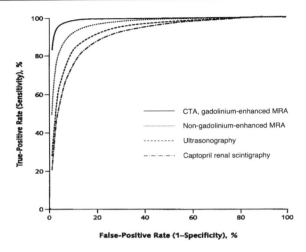

Fig. 7. Summary receiver-operating characteristic curves comparing captopril renal scintigraphy, ultrasonography, non-gadolinium-enhanced magnetic resonance angiography (MRA), and computed tomographic angiography (CTA) and gadolinium-enhanced MRA in the diagnosis of renal artery stenosis. (Reprinted with permission from ref. *57.*)

inhibitors or ARBs on the clipped kidney, however, is much more variable, depending on the dose and magnitude of BP reduction. At low doses, GFR of the clipped kidney is well maintained *(73,74)*, but at high doses, excessive reduction in BP is accompanied by a deleterious reduction in GFR and urine flow *(72)*.

Although these experimental findings initially raised concern about the safety of long-term ACE inhibitor use in patients with renal artery stenosis, ACE inhibitors did not increase incidence of renal atrophy in a prospective study by Caps and colleagues *(43)*. In addition, one retrospective study by Chabova et al. *(44)* demonstrated the safety of ACE inhibitor use in elderly hypertensive patients with atherosclerotic renal artery stenosis who were managed without revascularization. After an average follow-up of 39 months, renal function was stable in 85% of patients and worsened in 15% with no change in BP. However, the need for antihypertensive medications increased from 1.6 to 1.9 drugs.

ACE inhibitors not only exert beneficial effects on renal structure and function, but also cause regression of left ventricular and aortic hypertrophy *(75,76)* and improve survival in the rat model better than other antihypertensive drugs compared with diuretics or hydralazine. Improved survival of patients with renovascular disease treated with ACE inhibitors has also been reported in a prospective study by Losito and colleagues *(77)*.

Bilateral Renovascular Hypertension. Medical therapy has a limited role in this clinical condition, and most patients require revascularization. Reduction of BP even into normal but not below normal range causes a significant reduction in renal plasma flow *(78)*. Nearly all patients with bilateral disease or unilateral disease involving a solitary functioning kidney developed a significant increase in serum creatinine with an ACE inhibitor *(63)* and between 6 and 30% of these patients developed acute renal failure *(79–81)*.

PERCUTANEOUS INTERVENTION

Percutaneous intervention is the revascularization procedure developed to improve BP control while preserving renal function with less morbidity and mortality than surgical revascularization. In most nonrandomized studies, the procedural success of percutaneous transluminal renal angioplasty (PTRA) is more favorable in young patients with fibromuscular dysplasia (FMD) than in older patients with atherosclerotic renal artery stenosis (90–100% vs 60–70%, respectively) *(82)*. The hypertension cure rates are also much higher in patients with FMD than in those with atherosclerotic renal artery stenosis (30–60% vs 0–29%). In addition, a significant proportion of the latter patients experienced no improvement or even deterioration of global renal function as assessed by creatinine clearance or individual kidney function as assessed by nuclear imaging study, despite successful revascularization *(83,84)*. This was probably related to frequent atheroembolism and associated hypertensive nephrosclerosis in elderly patients with atherosclerosis.

Therefore, although PTRA is the treatment of choice in patients with FMD, the role of percutaneous intervention in those with atherosclerotic RVH is still evolving. Most of the published studies of PTRA in the elderly were retrospective with incomplete follow-up and an inadequate control group. Outcomes of studies are less well defined and relied on single measurement of office BP or serum creatinine and thus were subjected to observational bias and regression to the mean *(85)*.

Randomized Studies of PTRA vs Medical Therapy. Three randomized prospective studies compared effects of PTRA vs medical therapy in hypertensive patients with atherosclerotic renal artery stenosis. The results of these studies are summarized in Table 1.

The Scottish and Newcastle Renal Artery Stenosis Collaborative Group *(86)* randomly assigned 55 hypertensive patients with renal artery stenosis (for whom BP cannot be controlled despite two antihypertensive medications) to PTRA vs continued medical therapy. Patients over the age of 75 years and those with serum creatinine above 5 mg/dL were

Table 1
Randomized Studies Comparing Effects of Angioplasty vs Medical Therapy in Patients With Atherosclerotic Renovascular Hypertension

Study	Year	N	Follow-up duration (months)	% Crossover	Quantity of medication at follow-up		Reduction in SBP/DBP from baseline (mmHg)		Δ Renal function from baseline		Cr p*	Drug p*	BP p*
Webster (86)	1998	55	12	0	Medical Rx	2.7 drugs	Medical Rx	OBP 8/1	Medical Rx	Scr +0.04 mg/dLd	NS	0.014	
					PTRA	2.3 drugs*	PTRA		PTRA				
							Unilateral stenosis	OBP 2/2	Unilateral stenosis	Scr +0.08 mg/dL			
							Bilateral stenosis	OBP 34/11*	Bilateral stenosis	Scr +0.1 mg/dL		<0.005	
EMMA (87)	1998	49	6	28	Medical Rx	1.78 DDD units	Medical Rx	ABP 8/5	Medical Rx	CrCL +0.6 mL/min	NS	0.009	NS
					PTRA	1 DDD units*	PTRA	ABP 12/10	PTRA	CrCL +3.6 mL/min			
DRASTIC (88)	2000	106	12	44	Medical Rx	2.4 drugs	Medical Rx	OBP 17/7	Medical Rx	CrCL +2 mL/min	NS	0.002	NS
					PTRA	1.9 drugs*	PTRA	OBP 19/11	PTRA	CrCL +3 mL/min			

ABP, ambulatory blood pressure; BP, blood pressure; DBP, diastolic blood pressure; DDD, defined daily dose; EMMA, Essai Multicentrique Medicaments vs Angioplastie; NS, not significant; OBP, office blood pressure; Rx, therapy; SBP, systolic blood pressure; PTRA, percutaneous transluminal renal angioplasty.

*p < 0.05 compared with medical therapy.

excluded from the study. There was no crossover between the two groups. A benefit of angioplasty on BP control was seen mainly in the group with bilateral renal artery stenosis. There was no benefit on BP control in the unilateral artery stenosis patients treated with PTRA compared with those treated with medical therapy. There was no difference in renal function in either unilateral or bilateral renal artery stenosis patients treated with PTRA compared with those treated medically.

The Essai Multicentrique Medicaments vs Angioplastie Study Group randomly assigned 49 patients with unilateral renal artery stenosis, mild-to-moderate hypertension, and positive captopril renography or elevated renal vein renin ratio to PTRA vs medical therapy *(87)*. All patients had a creatinine clearance above 50 mL/minute. During the study, 28% of patients treated with medical therapy were crossed over to the PTRA because of refractory hypertension. Periprocedural complications, mainly related to groin hematoma, occurred in 26% of patients undergoing PTRA. At 6-month follow-up, there was no difference in 24-hour ambulatory BP or renal function between the two treatment groups, but the patients treated with medical therapy alone required more antihypertensive medications than those treated with angioplasty.

The DRASTIC study *(88)* is the most recent randomized study of 106 difficult-to-treat hypertensive patients with atherosclerotic renal artery stenosis and positive renal captopril renography. The study excluded patients older than 75 years, those with a serum creatinine above 2.3 mg/dL, and those with kidney size below 8 cm. During the study, 44% of patients randomly assigned to medical therapy were crossed over to PTRA because of uncontrolled hypertension or progressive azotemia. Restenosis occurred in 48% of the patients randomly assigned to PTRA. Based on intention-to-treat analysis, there was no difference in office BP or creatinine clearance between the two groups at 12-month follow-up, but the angioplasty group required less antihypertensive medication than the drug-therapy group.

Taken together, the data from these three trials indicate that PTRA rarely cures hypertension. Most patients continue to require antihypertensive medications. However, BP is easier to control than with medical therapy alone with no difference in renal function. High restenosis rates after angioplasty may be responsible for these modest results and thus should be avoidable by stent placement. It is therefore disappointing that, to date, both nonrandomized and randomized studies have not suggested greater clinical benefit of stenting over PTRA.

Studies of Renal Artery Stenting. Stenting now has replaced angioplasty for percutaneous revascularization of atherosclerotic renal artery stenosis because of its ability to prevent elastic recoil seen commonly in the ostial or proximal location of the artery. Meta-analysis of 14 renal arterial stent studies indicated that renal stenting can cure hypertension in 20% of the patients and improve BP control in 49% *(89)*. However, 4 of 14 studies defined *cure* as SBP below 150–160 mmHg. Renal function was improved in 30% of patients, unchanged in 38%, and worsened in 32% *(89)*.

When stenting was directly compared with PTRA in a randomized prospective study *(63)*, stenting was associated with higher technical success (88 vs 57%) and less restenosis (14 vs 48%). No difference in BP control or renal outcome was demonstrated at follow-up. Failure to demonstrate improvement in renal function despite the higher patency rates in the stent group may be related to contrast nephropathy, hypertensive nephrosclerosis, or distal embolization during procedure. However, the presence of rapid decline in renal function before stenting *(90,91)* or angioplasty *(92)* is associated with a favorable response on renal failure progression after procedure. This is possibly related to the amount of viable nephron mass at risk, which may be salvaged by percutaneous intervention.

SURGICAL REVASCULARIZATION

Surgical revascularization of renal arteries can be achieved using three techniques: endarterectomy, aortorenal bypass, or extra-anatomic bypass. Endarterectomy is suitable for patients with focal disease or those who also require aortic replacement *(93)*. Aortorenal bypass can be performed with autologous or prosthetic conduits and was shown to have excellent long-term results. Extra-anatomic bypass such as hepatorenal or splenorenal bypass grafting avoids aortic clamping and direct operation on diseased aorta.

Long-term results of all these surgical techniques are comparable, with 5-year patency of 80 to 90% *(93–95)*. However, operative mortality is 20% in patients over the age of 65 years *(93,95,96)*. Surgical revascularization offers comparable clinical results to percutaneous revascularization in terms of BP responses *(93,97)*, but the cost of surgery is much higher *(98)*. Renal function was improved in 30 to 60% of patients, unchanged in 30 to 50%, and worsened in 10 to 30% *(96,99,100)*.

The presence of atheroembolism *(101)* or elevated renal resistance index by duplex Doppler ultrasonography *(102)* predicts poor long-term outcome after surgery. In one study, patients with a rapid decline in renal function (GFR decreased more than 5 mL per minute each week) derived more benefit from surgical revascularization in terms of preventing further decline in GFR than those with slower decline in renal function *(99)*.

For these reasons, surgery should be considered in elderly patients only when the renal function deteriorates on medical therapy and for whom the lesions are not suitable for percutaneous intervention.

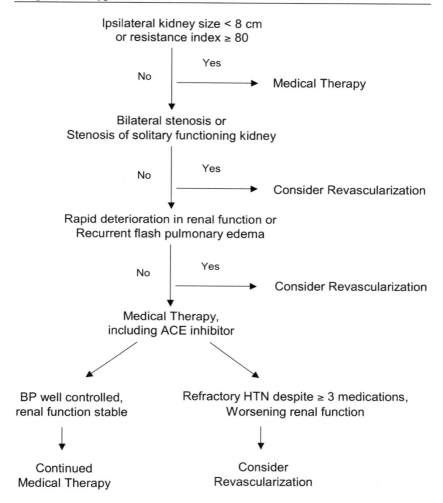

Fig. 8. Algorithm in management of patients with hypertension and atherosclerotic renovascular disease. ACE, angiotensin-converting enzyme; BP, blood pressure; HTN, hypertension.

Recommendations

Treatment of elderly patients with RVH needs to be highly individualized, with a careful assessment of comorbid diseases and benefit vs risk from revascularization. Our algorithm, based on the current knowledge base, is shown in Fig. 8.

The approach to the patients with suspected RVH begins with an accurate assessment of kidney size (by plain abdominal radiography, ultrasonography, MRI, or CT angiography). A unilateral atrophic kidney (<8 cm) suggests irreversible renal parenchymal disease that is not amendable to revascularization. In the absence of atrophic kidneys, a Doppler study showing a resistance index of 80 units or more also is indicative of irreversible renal disease. Such patients should be treated medically. In contrast, revascularization should be considered for patients with (a) bilateral stenoses or stenoses of solitary functioning kidney, (b) rapid deterioration in renal function, or (c) recurrent flash pulmonary edema. In the absence of these clinical features, medical therapy of hypertension should be initiated with an ACE inhibitor and additional classes of antihypertensives as needed. Revascularization should be considered if hypertension cannot be adequately controlled with three or more medications of different classes, including ACE inhibitors and diuretics.

In the future, the ability to predict the likelihood of success may be improved with novel imaging modalities developed to assess viability of renal tissue and the pattern of intrarenal perfusion, which may elucidate mechanism of renal injury *(103)*. To minimize the risk of revascularization, a distal protection device is under development to reduce the risk of atheroembolism during stent placement *(104)*. It remains to be seen if better selection criteria, more rigorous control of BP with a combined antihypertensive regimen, and the new interventional technique to prevent distal embolization will improve long-term outcome in these patients.

REFERENCES

1. Anderson GH Jr, Blakeman N, Streeten DH. The effect of age on prevalence of secondary forms of hypertension in 4429 consecutively referred patients. *J Hypertens* 1994;12:609–615.
2. Faubert PF, Porush JG. Chronic renal failure. In: Faubert PF, Porush JG, eds. *Renal Disease in the Elderly.* 2nd ed. New York: Marcel Dekker; 1998:310–311.
3. Clase CM, Garg AX, Kiberd BA. Prevalence of low glomerular filtration rate in nondiabetic Americans: Third National Health and Nutrition Examination Survey (NHANES III). *J Am Soc Nephrol* 2002;13:1338–1349.
4. Shulman NB, Ford CE, Hall WD, et al. Prognostic value of serum creatinine and effect of treatment of hypertension on renal function. Results from the Hypertension Detection and Follow-up Program. The Hypertension Detection and Follow-up Program Cooperative Group. *Hypertension* 1989;13(5 suppl):I80–I93.
5. Perneger TV, Nieto FJ, Whelton PK, et al. A prospective study of blood pressure and serum creatinine. Results from the "Clue" Study and the ARIC Study. *JAMA* 1993;269:488–493.
6. US Renal Data System. USRDS 2001 Annual Data Report. Bethesda, MD: The National Institutes of Health, National Institute of Diabetes and Digestive and Kidney Diseases; 2001.
7. Zoccali C, Bode-Boger S, Mallamaci F, et al. Plasma concentration of asymmetrical dimethylarginine and mortality in patients with end-stage renal disease: a prospective study. *Lancet* 2001;358:2113–2117.

8. McLachlan MS. The ageing kidney. *Lancet* 1978;2:143–145.
9. Lindeman RD, Tobin J, Shock NW. Longitudinal studies on the rate of decline in renal function with age. *J Am Geriatr Soc* 1985;33:278–285.
10. Bakris GL, Williams M, Dworkin L, et al. Preserving renal function in adults with hypertension and diabetes: a consensus approach. National Kidney Foundation Hypertension and Diabetes Executive Committees Working Group. *Am J Kidney Dis* 2000;36:646–661.
11. Tuncel M, Augustyniak R, Zhang W, et al. Sympathetic nervous system function in renal hypertension. *Curr Hypertens Rep* 2002;4:229–236.
12. Converse RLJ, Jacobsen TN, Toto RD, et al. Sympathetic overactivity in patients with chronic renal failure. *N Engl J Med* 1992;327:1912–1918.
13. National Kidney Foundation. Evaluation of laboratory measurements for clinical assessment of kidney disease. *Am J Kidney Dis* 2002;39:S76–S110.
14. Lewis EJ, Hunsicker LG, Bain RP, et al. The effect of angiotensin-converting-enzyme inhibition on diabetic nephropathy. *N Engl J Med* 1993;329:1456–1462.
15. Ruggenenti P, Perna A, Gherardi G, et al. Renoprotective properties of ACE-inhibition in non-diabetic nephropathies with non-nephrotic proteinuria. *Lancet* 1999;354:359–364.
16. Wright JT Jr, Bakris GL, Greene T, et al. Effect of blood pressure lowering and antihypertensive drug class on progression of hypertensive kidney disease: Results from the AASK trial. *JAMA* 2002;288:2421–2431.
17. Brenner BM, Cooper ME, de Zeeuw D, et al. Effects of losartan on renal and cardiovascular outcomes in patients with type 2 diabetes and nephropathy. *N Engl J Med* 2001;345:861–869.
18. Lewis EJ, Hunsicker LG, Clarke WR, et al. Renoprotective effect of the angiotensin-receptor antagonist irbesartan in patients with nephropathy due to type 2 diabetes. *N Engl J Med* 2001;345:851–860.
19. Barnett AH, Bain SC, Barter P, et al; Diabetics Exposed to Telmisartan and Enalapril Study Group. Angiotensin-receptor blockade versus converting-enzyme inhibition type 2 diabetes and nephropathy. *N Engl J Med* 2004;351:1952–1961.
20. Pahor M, Shorr RI, Somes GW, et al. Diuretic-based treatment and cardiovascular events in patients with mild renal dysfunction enrolled in the Systolic Hypertension in the Elderly Program. *Arch Intern Med* 1998;158:1340–1345.
21. Joint National Committee on Prevention, Detection, Evaluation, and Treatment of High Blood Pressure. The Seventh Report of the Joint National Committee on Prevention, Detection, Evaluation, and Treatment of High Blood Pressure. *JAMA* 2003;289:2560–2572.
22. The Modification of Diet in Renal Disease Study Group. Blood pressure control, proteinuria, and the progression of renal disease. *Ann Intern Med* 1995;123:754–762.
23. Hansson L, Zanchetti A, Carruthers SG, et al. Effects of intensive blood-pressure lowering and low-dose aspirin in patients with hypertension: principal results of the Hypertension Optimal Treatment (HOT) randomised trial. HOT Study Group. *Lancet* 1998;351:1755–1762.
24. Merkus MP, Jager KJ, Dekker FW, et al. Predictors of poor outcome in chronic dialysis patients: The Netherlands Cooperative Study on the Adequacy of Dialysis. The NECOSAD Study Group. *Am J Kidney Dis* 2000;35:69–79.
25. Charra B, Calemard E, Ruffet M, et al. Survival as an index of adequacy of dialysis. *Kidney Int* 1992;41:1286–1291.
26. Salem MM. Hypertension in the haemodialysis population: any relationship to 2-years survival? *Nephrol Dial Transplant* 1999;14:125–128.
27. Foley RN, Parfrey PS, Harnett JD, et al. Impact of hypertension on cardiomyopathy, morbidity and mortality in end-stage renal disease. *Kidney Int* 1996;49:1379–1385.

28. Zager PG, Nikolic J, Brown RH, et al. "U" curve association of blood pressure and mortality in hemodialysis patients. *Kidney Int* 1998;54:561–569.
29. Blacher J, Guerin AP, Pannier B, et al. Impact of aortic stiffness on survival in end-stage renal disease. *Circulation* 1999;99:2434–2439.
30. Klassen PS, Lowrie EG, Reddan DN, et al. Association between pulse pressure and mortality in patients undergoing maintenance hemodialysis. *JAMA* 2002;287: 1548–1555.
31. Fatica RA, Port FK, Young E. Incidence trends and mortality in end-stage renal disease attributed to renovascular disease in the United States. *Am J Kidney Dis* 2001;37:1184–1190.
32. Scoble JE, Maher ER, Hamilton G, et al. Atherosclerotic renovascular disease causing renal impairment—a case for treatment. *Clin Nephrol* 1989;31:119–122.
33. Mailloux LU, Napolitano B, Bellucci AG, et al. Renal vascular disease causing end-stage renal disease, incidence, clinical correlates, and outcomes: a 20-year clinical experience. *Am J Kidney Dis* 1994;24:622–629.
34. Davis BA, Crook JE, Vestal RE, et al. Prevalence of renovascular hypertension in patients with grade III or IV hypertensive retinopathy. *N Engl J Med* 1979;301: 1273–1276.
35. Appel RG, Bleyer AJ, Reavis S, et al. Renovascular disease in older patients beginning renal replacement therapy. *Kidney Int* 1995;48:171–176.
36. Svetkey LP, Kadir S, Dunnick NR, et al. Similar prevalence of renovascular hypertension in selected blacks and whites. *Hypertension* 1991;17:678–683.
37. Emovon OE, Klotman PE, Dunnick NR, et al. Renovascular hypertension in blacks. *Am J Hypertens* 1996;9:18–23.
38. Safian RD, Textor SC. Renal-artery stenosis. *N Engl J Med* 2001;344:431–442.
39. Tullis MJ, Zierler RE, Caps MT, et al. Clinical evidence of contralateral renal parenchymal injury in patients with unilateral atherosclerotic renal artery stenosis. *Ann Vasc Surg* 1998;12:122–127.
40. Harding MB, Smith LR, Himmelstein SI, et al. Renal artery stenosis: prevalence and associated risk factors in patients undergoing routine cardiac catheterization. *J Am Soc Nephrol* 1992;2:1608–1616.
41. Choudhri AH, Cleland JG, Rowlands PC, et al. Unsuspected renal artery stenosis in peripheral vascular disease. *BMJ* 1990;301:1197–1198.
42. MacDowall P, Kalra PA, O'Donoghue DJ, et al. Risk of morbidity from renovascular disease in elderly patients with congestive cardiac failure. *Lancet* 1998;352:13–16.
43. Caps MT, Zierler R, Polissar NL, et al. Risk of atrophy in kidneys with atherosclerotic renal artery stenosis. *Kidney Int* 1998;53:735–742.
44. Chabova V, Schirger A, Stanson AW, et al. Outcomes of atherosclerotic renal artery stenosis managed without revascularization. *Mayo Clin Proc* 2000;75:437–444.
45. Baboolal K, Evans C, Moore RH. Incidence of end-stage renal disease in medically treated patients with severe bilateral atherosclerotic renovascular disease. *Am J Kidney Dis* 1998;31:971–977.
46. Wright JR, Shurrab AE, Cheung C, et al. A prospective study of the determinants of renal functional outcome and mortality in atherosclerotic renovascular disease. *Am J Kidney Dis* 2002;39:1153–1161.
47. Suresh M, Laboi P, Mamtora H, et al. Relationship of renal dysfunction to proximal arterial disease severity in atherosclerotic renovascular disease. *Nephrol Dial Transplant* 2000;15:631–636.
48. Zierler RE, Bergelin RO, Polissar NL, et al. Carotid and lower extremity arterial disease in patients with renal artery sclerosis. *Arch Intern Med* 1998;158:761–767.

49. Kobayashi S, Ishida A, Moriya H, et al. Angiotensin II receptor blockade limits kidney injury in two-kidney, one-clip Goldblatt hypertensive rats with special reference to phenotypic changes. *J Lab Clin Med* 1999;133:134–143.

50. Wilcox CS, Cardozo J, Welch WJ. AT_1 and TxA2/PGH2 receptors maintain hypertension throughout 2K, 1C Goldblatt hypertension in the rat. *Am J Physiol* 1996;271:R891–R896.

51. Higashi Y, Sasaki S, Nakagawa K, et al. Endothelial function and oxidative stress in renovascular hypertension. *N Engl J Med* 2002;346:1954–1962.

52. Bergamaschi C, Campos RR, Schor N, et al. Role of the rostral ventrolateral medulla in maintenance of blood pressure in rats with Goldblatt hypertension. *Hypertension* 1995;26:1117–1120.

53. Floyer MA. The effect of nephrectomy and adrenalectomy upon the blood pressure in hypertensive and normotensive rats. *Clin Sci* 1951;10:405–421.

54. Brunner HR, Kirshman JD, Sealey JE, et al. Hypertension of renal origin: evidence for two different mechanisms. *Science* 1971;174:1344–1346.

55. Gavras H, Brunner HR, Thurston H, et al. Reciprocation of renin dependency with sodium volume dependency in renal hypertension. *Science* 1975;188:1316–1317.

56. Imanishi M, Akabane S, Takamiya M, et al. Critical degree of renal arterial stenosis that causes hypertension in dogs. *Angiology* 1992:833–842.

57. Vasbinder GB, Nelemans PJ, Kessels AG, et al. Diagnostic tests for renal artery stenosis in patients suspected of having renovascular hypertension: a meta-analysis. *Ann Intern Med* 2001;135:401–411.

58. van Jaarsveld BC, Krijnen P, Derkx FH, et al. The place of renal scintigraphy in the diagnosis of renal artery stenosis. Fifteen years of clinical experience. *Arch Intern Med* 1997;157:1226–1234.

59. Fommei E, Ghione S, Hilson AJ, et al. Captopril radionuclide test in renovascular hypertension: a European multicentre study. European Multicentre Study Group. *Eur J Nucl Med* 1993;20:617–623.

60. Meier GH, Sumpio B, Black HR, et al. Captopril renal scintigraphy—an advance in the detection and treatment of renovascular hypertension. *J Vasc Surg* 1990;11:770–776.

61. Setaro JF, Chen CC, Hoffer PB, et al. Captopril renography in the diagnosis of renal artery stenosis and the prediction of improvement with revascularization. The Yale Vascular Center experience. *Am J Hypertens* 1991;4:698S–705S.

62. Dondi M, Fanti S, De Fabritiis A, et al. Prognostic value of captopril renal scintigraphy in renovascular hypertension. *J Nucl Med* 1992;33:2040–2044.

63. van de Ven PJ, Beutler JJ, Kaatee R, et al. Angiotensin converting enzyme inhibitor-induced renal dysfunction in atherosclerotic renovascular disease. *Kidney Int* 1998;53:986–993.

64. van Jaarsveld BC, Krijnen P. Prospective studies of diagnosis and intervention: the Dutch experience. *Semin Nephrol* 2000;20:463–473.

65. Caps MT, Perissinotto C, Zierler RE, et al. Prospective study of atherosclerotic disease progression in the renal artery. *Circulation* 1998;98:2866–2872.

66. Radermacher J, Chavan A, Bleck J, et al. Use of Doppler ultrasonography to predict the outcome of therapy for renal-artery stenosis. *N Engl J Med* 2001;344:410-7.

67. Mostbeck GH, Kain R, Mallek R, et al. Duplex Doppler sonography in renal parenchymal disease. *J Ultrasound Med* 1991;10:189–194.

68. Roubidoux MA, Dunnick NR, Klotman PE, et al. Renal vein renins: inability to predict response to revascularization in patients with hypertension. *Radiology* 1991;178:819–822.

69. Marcos HB, Choyke PL. Magnetic resonance angiography of the kidney. *Semin Nephrol* 2000;20:450–455.
70. Halpern EJ, Nazarian LN, Wechsler RJ, et al. US, CT, and MR evaluation of accessory renal arteries and proximal renal arterial branches. *Acad Radiol* 1999;6:299–304.
71. Cervenka L, Navar LG. Renal responses of the nonclipped kidney of two-kidney/ one-clip Goldblatt hypertensive rats to type 1 angiotensin II receptor blockade with candesartan. *J Am Soc Nephrol* 1999;10(suppl 11):S197–S201.
72. Huang WC, Ploth DW, Bell PD, et al. Bilateral renal function responses to converting enzyme inhibitor (SQ 20,881) in two-kidney, one clip Goldblatt hypertensive rats. *Hypertension* 1981;3:285–293.
73. al-Qattan KK, Johns EJ. A comparison of the actions of cilazapril in normal, dietary sodium-depleted and two-kidney, one clip Goldblatt hypertensive anaesthetised rats. *J Hypertens* 1992;10:423–429.
74. Frei U, Schindler R, Matthies C, et al. Glomerular hemodynamics of the clipped kidney: effects of captopril and diltiazem. *J Pharmacol Exp Ther* 1992;263:938–942.
75. Dussaillant GR, Gonzalez H, Cespedes C, et al. Regression of left ventricular hypertrophy in experimental renovascular hypertension: diastolic dysfunction depends more on myocardial collagen than it does on myocardial mass. *J Hypertens* 1996;14:1117–1123.
76. Levy BI, Michel JB, Salzmann JL, et al. Effects of chronic inhibition of converting enzyme on mechanical and structural properties of arteries in rat renovascular hypertension. *Circ Res* 1988;63:227–239.
77. Losito A, Gaburri M, Errico R, et al. Survival of patients with renovascular disease and ACE inhibition. *Clin Nephrol* 1999;52:339–343.
78. Textor SC, Novick AC, Tarazi RC, et al. Critical perfusion pressure for renal function in patients with bilateral atherosclerotic renal vascular disease. *Ann Intern Med* 1985;102:308–314.
79. Hollenberg NK. The treatment of renovascular hypertension: surgery, angioplasty, and medical therapy with converting-enzyme inhibitors. *Am J Kidney Dis* 1987;10(1 suppl 1):52–60.
80. Franklin SS, Smith RD. Comparison of effects of enalapril plus hydrochlorothiazide vs standard triple therapy on renal function in renovascular hypertension. *Am J Med* 1985;79:14–23.
81. Jackson B, Matthews PG, McGrath BP, et al. Angiotensin converting enzyme inhibition in renovascular hypertension: frequency of reversible renal failure. *Lancet* 1984;1:225–226.
82. Bloch MJ, Pickering T. Renal vascular disease: medical management, angioplasty, and stenting. *Semin Nephrol* 2000;20:474–488.
83. Mikhail A, Cook GJ, Reidy J, et al. Progressive renal dysfunction despite successful renal artery angioplasty in a single kidney. *Lancet* 1997;349:926.
84. Farmer CK, Reidy J, Kalra PA, et al. Individual kidney function before and after renal angioplasty. *Lancet* 1998;352:288–289.
85. Brawn LA, Ramsay LE. Is "improvement" real with percutaneous transluminal angioplasty in the management of renovascular hypertension? *Lancet* 1987;2: 1313–1316.
86. Webster J, Marshall F, Abdalla M, et al. Randomised comparison of percutaneous angioplasty vs continued medical therapy for hypertensive patients with atheromatous renal artery stenosis. Scottish and Newcastle Renal Artery Stenosis Collaborative Group. *J Hum Hypertens* 1998;12:329–335.

87. Plouin PF, Chatellier G, Darne B, et al. Blood pressure outcome of angioplasty in atherosclerotic renal artery stenosis: a randomized trial. Essai Multicentrique Medicaments vs Angioplastie (EMMA) Study Group. *Hypertension* 1998;31:823–829.

88. van Jaarsveld BC, Krijnen P, Pieterman H, et al. The effect of balloon angioplasty on hypertension in atherosclerotic renal-artery stenosis. Dutch Renal Artery Stenosis Intervention Cooperative Study Group. *N Engl J Med* 2000;342:1007–1014.

89. Leertouwer TC, Gussenhoven EJ, Bosch JL, et al. Stent placement for renal arterial stenosis: where do we stand? A meta-analysis. *Radiology* 2000;216:78–85.

90. Watson PS, Hadjipetrou P, Cox SV, et al. Effect of renal artery stenting on renal function and size in patients with atherosclerotic renovascular disease. *Circulation* 2000;102:1671–1677.

91. Beutler JJ, Van Ampting JM, Van De Ven PJ, et al. Long-term effects of arterial stenting on kidney function for patients with ostial atherosclerotic renal artery stenosis and renal insufficiency. *J Am Soc Nephrol* 2001;12:1475–1481.

92. Muray S, Martin M, Amoedo ML, et al. Rapid decline in renal function reflects reversibility and predicts the outcome after angioplasty in renal artery stenosis. *Am J Kidney Dis* 2002;39:60–66.

93. Erdoes LS, Berman SS, Hunter GC, et al. Comparative analysis of percutaneous transluminal angioplasty and operation for renal revascularization. *Am J Kidney Dis* 1996;27:496–503.

94. Cambria RP, Brewster DC, L'Italien GJ, et al. The durability of different reconstructive techniques for atherosclerotic renal artery disease. *J Vasc Surg* 1994;20:76–87.

95. Lawrie GM, Morris GCJ, Glaeser DH, et al. Renovascular reconstruction: factors affecting long-term prognosis in 919 patients followed up to 31 years. *Am J Cardiol* 1989;63:1085–1092.

96. Lamawansa MD, Bell R, House AK. Short-term and long-term outcome following renovascular reconstruction. *Cardiovasc Surg* 1995;3:50–55.

97. Weibull H, Bergqvist D, Bergentz SE, et al. Percutaneous transluminal renal angioplasty vs surgical reconstruction of atherosclerotic renal artery stenosis: a prospective randomized study. *J Vasc Surg* 1993;18:841–852.

98. Xue F, Bettmann MA, Langdon DR, et al. Outcome and cost comparison of percutaneous transluminal renal angioplasty, renal arterial stent placement, and renal arterial bypass grafting. *Radiology* 1999;212:378–384.

99. Dean RH, Tribble RW, Hansen KJ, et al. Evolution of renal insufficiency in ischemic nephropathy. *Ann Surg* 1991;213:446–455.

100. Cherr GS, Hansen KJ, Craven TE, et al. Surgical management of atherosclerotic renovascular disease. *J Vasc Surg* 2002;35:236–245.

101. Krishnamurthi V, Novick AC, Myles JL. Atheroembolic renal disease: effect on morbidity and survival after revascularization for atherosclerotic renal artery stenosis. *J Urol* 1999;161:1093–1096.

102. Frauchiger B, Zierler R, Bergelin RO, et al. Prognostic significance of intrarenal resistance indices in patients with renal artery interventions: a preliminary duplex sonographic study. *Cardiovasc Surg* 1996;4:324–330.

103. Romero JC, Lerman LO. Novel noninvasive techniques for studying renal function in man. *Semin Nephrol* 2000;20:456–462.

104. Henry M, Klonaris C, Henry I, et al. Protected renal stenting with the PercuSurge GuardWire device. *J Endovasc Ther* 2001;8:227–237

12 Heart Failure in the Older Hypertensive Patient

L. Michael Prisant, MD, FACC, FACP,
Carolyn Landolfo, MD, FACC,
John Thornton, MD, FACC,
and Vincent J. B. Robinson, MBBS, FACC

CONTENTS

EPIDEMIOLOGY

Overview

The prevalence of heart failure is 4,900,000 and is rising *(1)*. The prevalence of heart failure progressively increases with aging (Fig. 1). The incidence is 550,000 and approaches 10 per 1000 people after age 65 years. The annual rate for new and recurrent heart events is displayed in Fig. 2. Data from the Framingham Heart Study suggest that the incidence of heart failure has declined in women, but not men *(2)*. At age 40 years, the lifetime risk of developing heart failure is about 20%. Mortality from heart failure is grim, with 20% of patients dying within 1 year (Fig. 3).

From: *Clinical Hypertension and Vascular Diseases: Hypertension in the Elderly*
Edited by: L. M. Prisant © Humana Press Inc., Totowa, NJ

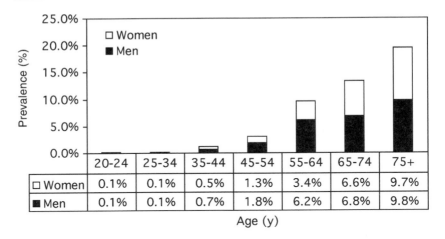

	20-24	25-34	35-44	45-54	55-64	65-74	75+
□ Women	0.1%	0.1%	0.5%	1.3%	3.4%	6.6%	9.7%
■ Men	0.1%	0.1%	0.7%	1.8%	6.2%	6.8%	9.8%

Age (y)

Fig. 1. Prevalence of heart failure by age and gender. The prevalence of heart failure progressively increases with aging in both men and women. (Data from ref. *1*.)

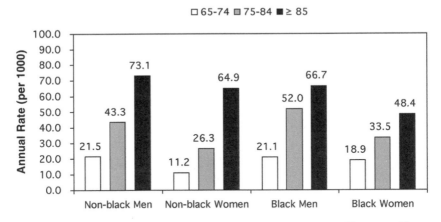

Fig. 2. Annual rates of new and recurrent heart failure events. The rate of heart failure events progressively increases with each decade. (Data from ref. *1*.)

Hypertension is antecedent in 75% of heart failure cases *(1,3)*. Among patients who developed heart failure in the Framingham Study, hypertension with or without coronary disease preceded the development in 70% of men and 77% of women. Although less common, electrocardiographic left ventricular hypertrophy (LVH) is the most potent predictor of heart failure in both younger and older men and women. It is a more potent predictor than diabetes or hypertension. Thus, the population-

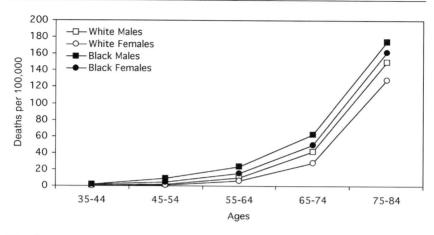

Fig. 3. Death rates for heart failure by age, race, and sex, 1999. Mortality from heart failure sharply increases at 65 years and older. Mortality is higher for males than females and blacks than whites. (Data from ref. *6*.)

attributable risk of hypertension for heart failure is 39% for men and 59% for women *(4,5)*. This compares to the population-attributable risk of myocardial infarction (MI) for heart failure, which is 34% for men and 13% for women.

The direct and indirect cost of managing patients with heart failure is $24.3 billion each year. There are 999,000 hospital discharges with heart failure each year. Figure 4 shows that the hospitalization rate for the elderly has tripled since 1971 *(6)*. Over the last 20 years, better treatment of hypertension has been associated with considerable reduction in the hospital case fatality rate for heart failure (Fig. 5) *(6)*. Overall survival appears to be improving in men and women *(2)*.

Observations of the Cardiovascular Health Study

The Cardiovascular Health Study is a prospective population-based study of 5888 men and women 65 years or older that has provided important information on heart failure in the elderly *(7,8)*. The prevalence of confirmed heart failure was 8.8% of the 4842 subjects who underwent a protocol evaluation *(8)*. The clinical features most often present in patients with heart failure are displayed in Fig. 6. With increasing age and serum creatinine, the prevalence increased. Echocardiographic features associated with heart failure included increased left atrial size and left ventricular diastolic dimensions. Normal systolic function was present in 55% of patients with heart failure and was more common in women (67%) than men (42%, $p < 0.001$).

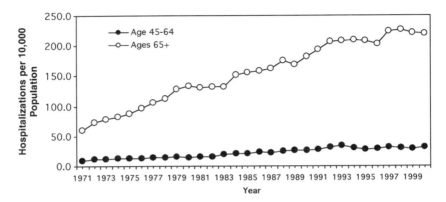

Fig. 4. Hospitalization rates for heart failure. Hospitalization rate for the elderly has tripled since 1971. (Data from ref. 6.)

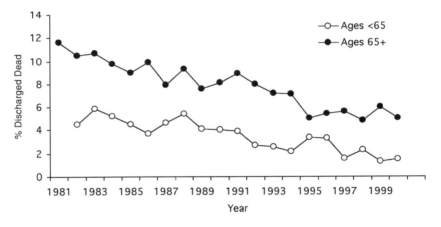

Fig. 5. Heart failure hospital case-fatality rates. The heart failure hospital deaths have declined since 1981. (Data from ref. 6.)

From the cohort of 2671 subjects who did not have atrial fibrillation, heart disease, or heart failure at baseline, 170 persons (6.2%) developed heart failure after 5.2 years (7). Patients who developed heart failure were more likely to be older, male, diabetic, and hypertensive and weigh more. MI was a precipitating factor in 18% of cases of heart failure. At the time of hospitalization, 57% of subjects had an echocardiographic ejection fraction (EF) 45% or greater. Depressed echocardiographic systolic function and abnormalities of Doppler diastolic filling were predictive of heart failure.

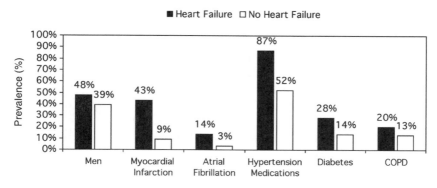

Fig. 6. Associations of heart failure in the elderly. In the Cardiovascular Health Study (*n* = 4842), heart failure (*n* = 425) was more likely to occur with the variables displayed. COPD, chronic obstructive pulmonary disease. (Data from ref. *8.*)

Outcomes on heart failure (Fig. 7) have been reported for the Cardiovascular Health Study *(9)*. Patients without heart failure but with an impaired or borderline EF had a higher mortality rate ($p < 0.001$) than normal persons. Patients with heart failure and a normal EF had a higher mortality than patients without heart failure and a normal EF ($p < 0.001$). The highest mortality rate was seen with heart failure and an abnormal EF. The all-cause mortality rate was 16 and 45% in patients without and with heart failure, respectively, after a median follow-up of 6.4 years ($p < 0.001$). Because 63% of patients with heart failure had a normal EF, the potential impact for a mortality intervention would be greatest for this group.

CARDIOVASCULAR SYSTEM IN THE OLDER PATIENT

There are a number of age-related changes that occur in the cardiovascular system in older patients that increase the likelihood of the development of heart failure *(10)*. In varying amounts, morphological modifications of the myocardium include myocyte enlargement; tubular dilatation; lipofuscin deposition (brown atrophy); loss of myocytes and sinus node cells; increased fibrous tissue, fat, and amyloid deposition; and calcification of mitral annulus and aortic valve. The vasculature can be altered by both atherosclerosis and arteriosclerosis.

These changes result in alterations in cardiovascular function *(10)*. Because there is less distensibility of the aorta, cardiac workload increases, and exercise duration and peak oxygen consumption diminish *(11)*. Because the ventricle is less distensible owing to hypertrophy and

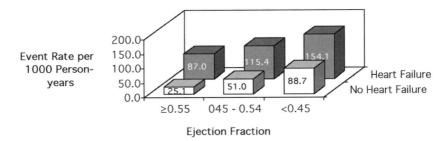

Fig. 7. All-cause mortality event rate in elderly based on heart failure and ejection fraction. In the Cardiovascular Health Study, patients without heart failure but with an impaired or borderline ejection fraction had a higher mortality rate ($p < 0.001$). Patients with heart failure and a normal ejection fraction had a higher mortality than patients without heart failure and a normal ejection fraction ($p < 0.001$). The highest mortality rate was seen with heart failure and an abnormal ejection fraction. (Data from ref. 9.)

fibrosis, early relaxation of the muscle declines, resulting in diastolic filling abnormalities and the critical need for normal atrial contractility. The β-receptor density and peripheral vasodilator capacity fall with aging. Exercise-induced augmentation of heart rate diminishes. Thus, cardiac output at rest and during physical activity in older patients is lower than in younger persons.

CLINICAL OVERVIEW AND DIAGNOSIS

Clinical Assessment

There are difficulties with the clinical diagnosis of the heart failure syndrome in the elderly (12). Because of a sedentary lifestyle, no symptoms or nonspecific symptoms, including cough, fatigue, weakness, anorexia, or confusion, may be reported rather than the classic symptoms of exertional dyspnea, orthopnea, and paroxysmal nocturnal dyspnea. An S_3 gallop and elevated jugular venous pressure have prognostic significance in heart failure (13) but may not be present.

Once a diagnosis is made, then the etiology and precipitating causes must be determined. Correctable causes of heart failure, such as ischemic heart disease, uncontrolled hypertension, aortic stenosis, hypothyroidism, hyperthyroidism, anemia, alcoholism, and rhythm disturbances, must be determined because the etiology will drive overall management and treatment. Acute precipitating causes include cardiac ischemia; severe hypertension; rhythm disturbances; excess sodium intake; use of nonsteroidal anti-inflammatory drugs (NSAIDs), calcium antago-

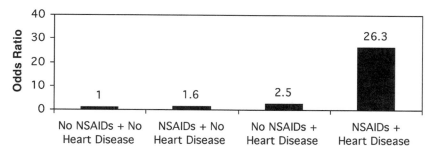

Fig. 8. Nonsteroidal anti-inflammatory drugs (NSAIDs) and risk of heart failure admissions. The use of nonaspirin NSAIDs in elderly patients with heart disease was strongly associated with the first admission for heart failure. (Data from ref. *15*.)

nists, and anti-arrhythmic drugs; pulmonary infections; and poor adherence to therapy *(14,15)*. NSAIDs, including cyclooxygenase 2 inhibitors, represent a potent factor for exacerbation of heart failure in the elderly and may be responsible for 19% of heart failure admissions (Fig. 8) *(15)*. In addition, these drugs attenuate the blood pressure (BP)-lowering effect of most antihypertensive drugs.

Differences Between Depressed and Normal Ejection Heart Failure

A study of 147 older subjects compared 60 patients with systolic heart failure (EF 35% or less), 59 patients with diastolic heart failure (EF 50% or greater), and 28 controls using a combination of echocardiography, exercise testing for anaerobic ventilatory threshold, neurohormones, and quality of life *(16)*. For most measures in this study, the age-matched control group fared better. The left ventricular diastolic and systolic chamber sizes were smaller, septal and posterior walls were thicker, and early deceleration time was greater for those with diastolic heart failure compared to the subjects with diastolic heart failure. The peak exercise systolic and diastolic blood pressures (DBPs) and duration of exercise were less for systolic than diastolic heart failure; however, there was no difference in ventilatory anaerobic threshold and peak lactate level. The 6-minute walk distance was similar for diastolic and systolic heart failure, but both were significantly less than for the control patients. Plasma norepinephrine levels, brain natriuretic peptide (BNP), and C-terminal peptide levels were significantly lower in the control group than in either heart failure group (Fig. 9). The natriuretic peptide levels were higher for systolic heart failure than for diastolic heart failure. Quality

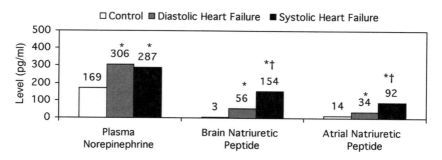

Fig. 9. Neuroendocrine activation in heart failure and controls. Systolic and diastolic heart failure have higher levels of plasma norepinephrine and brain and C-terminal atrial natriuretic peptide levels than controls (*$p \leq 0.02$). Brain and C-terminal atrial natriuretic peptide levels are higher in systolic heart failure than diastolic heart failure (†$p < 0.05$). (Data from ref. *16*.)

of life was more diminished with both systolic and diastolic heart failure, but was worse with systolic failure.

Diagnosis

The distinction between systolic and diastolic heart failure is difficult on clinical grounds *(17)*. M-mode, two-dimensional, and Doppler echocardiography have been advocated for all elderly patients with heart failure *(18)*. Most clinicians use a modification of the criteria for *definite* diastolic heart failure proposed by Vasan and Levy: (a) clinical evidence of heart failure, as evidenced by symptoms, signs, chest X-ray, and a response to diuretics; (b) left ventricular EF 50% or greater within 72 hours of the heart failure event; and (c) abnormal left ventricular relaxation, filling, or distensibility indices on cardiac catheterization *(19)*. The third criterion is difficult to implement; therefore, the diagnosis is usually *probable* diastolic heart failure. It is important to understand that diastolic heart failure is a heterogeneous syndrome, but hypertension and ischemic heart disease are common causes.

Role of Echocardiography

The prevalence and severity of diastolic dysfunction increase with aging (Fig. 10) *(20)*. Two-dimensional and Doppler echocardiographic techniques are likely to assist in the diagnosis and clinical management of elderly patients presenting with heart failure. Assessment of ventricular chamber sizes, wall thickness, and EF is useful in distinguishing systolic vs primary diastolic heart failure. Detection of abnormal regional wall motion may indicate an ischemic etiology of heart failure. The use of

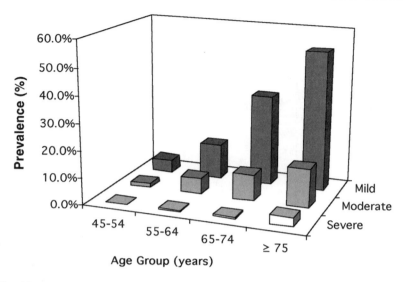

Fig. 10. Prevalence of diastolic dysfunction by severity and age. The prevalence of diastolic dysfunction increases with increasing age. (Data from ref. *20*.)

a Doppler mitral inflow pattern *alone* is inadequate for the assessment of diastolic function *(21)*.

Comprehensive evaluation of diastolic function (Table 1) using Doppler assessment of mitral valve inflow and pulmonary venous patterns and Doppler tissue imaging is an essential part of the examination of patients presenting with heart failure, particularly in the elderly population *(20)*. Recognition of the classification of Doppler-derived mitral inflow patterns has important implications for determining the severity of diastolic dysfunction and for assessing prognosis (Table 1). Although the majority of "normal" elderly subjects will have an abnormal Doppler filling pattern (i.e., impaired relaxation) that occurs as part of the aging process and may not lead to clinical heart failure, mitral inflow patterns reported as "pseudonormal" or "restrictive" in this population are indicative of abnormalities in compliance and typically reflect higher left atrial pressures. Patients with restrictive diastolic filling have a significantly worse prognosis, particularly in the setting of concomitant systolic dysfunction. With complete assessment of diastolic parameters, most patients with systolic heart failure will have diastolic dysfunction. Echocardiographic examination of the valvular structures is also a requisite component of the evaluation of the elderly patient with heart failure, specifically looking for aortic stenosis and mitral regurgitation.

Table 1
Doppler Criteria for Diastolic Dysfunction

	Normal	Mild: impaired relaxation	Moderate: pseudonormal	Severe: reversible restrictive	Severe: fixed restrictive
Mitral inflow	0.75 < E/A < 1.5, DT > 140 ms	E/A ≤ 0.75	0.75 < E/A < 1.5, DT > 140 ms	E/A > 1.5, DT < 140 ms	E/A > 1.5, DT < 140 ms
Peak valsalva mitral inflow	Δ E/A < 0.05	Δ E/A < 0.05	Δ E/A ≥ 0.05	Δ E/A ≥ 0.05	Δ E/A ≥ 0.05
Doppler tissue mitral annular motion	E/e' < 10	E/e' < 10	E/e' ≥ 10	E/e' ≥ 10	E/e' ≥ 10
Pulmonary venous flow	S ≥ D, ARdur < Adur	S > D, ARdur < Adur	S < D or ARdur > Adur + 30 ms	S < D or ARdur > Adur + 30 ms	S < D or ARdur > Adur + 30ms
LV relaxation	Normal	Impaired	Impaired	Impaired	Impaired
LV compliance	Normal	Normal to ↓	↓↓	↓↓↓	↓↓↓
Atrial pressure	Normal	Normal	↑↑	↑↑	↑↑↑

Mitral inflow measurements: E, peak early filling velocity; A, atrial contraction velocity; Adur, duration of A; DT, mitral deceleration time.
Mitral annular measurements: e', early diastolic motion velocity.
Pulmonary venous flow measurements: S, systolic flow velocity; D, diastolic flow velocity; ARdur, duration of pulmonary venous atrial reversal flow. (Modified from ref. 20.)

Brain Natriuretic Peptide

The use of BNP levels requires specific knowledge of assay-, age-, and gender-specific bounds *(22)*. As shown in Fig. 9, the average level of BNP is lower with diastolic heart failure than with systolic heart failure, but there is considerable overlap for individual patients *(16)*. BNP levels may be useful for monitoring the effectiveness of treatment and determining prognosis *(23–27)*.

TREATMENT

Overview of Trials of Systolic Dysfunction

The treatment of heart failure has evolved from the old view of augmenting myocardial contractility to blocking the renin–angiotensin–aldosterone system (RAAS). If the prospective heart failure trials (Table 2) are examined and postinfarction left ventricular dysfunction trials are excluded, then the following can be concluded:

1. Enalapril reduces mortality and decreases hospitalization rates *(28–30)*.
2. Higher doses (32.5–35.0 mg daily) of lisinopril compared to lower doses (2.5–5.0 mg daily) of lisinopril reduce hospitalization rates *(31)*.
3. Bisoprolol *(32)*, carvedilol *(33)*, and metoprolol succinate *(34)* (but not metoprolol tartrate) *(35)* reduce total mortality in combination with angiotensin-converting (ACE) inhibitors.
4. Spironolactone reduces mortality in combination with ACE inhibitors *(36)*.
5. Candesartan reduces total and cardiovascular mortality and reduces heart failure hospitalizations alone or in combination with ACE inhibitors and β-blockers *(37)*.

The applicability of the randomized, controlled trials (RCTs) of heart failure in older patients is uncertain. Few trials *(38,39)* were designed as heart failure trials of older persons, but the average age of study participants was generally 60 years or older (Table 1). Elderly patients in these heart failure trials are poorly documented *(40)*. Few RCTs showed an exact breakdown of results for patients aged 60 years or older. In fact, some RCTs did not include older patients.

Limitations of Current Trials

Whether current guidelines for heart failure are applicable to older patients is questionable *(41)*. Most RCTs enrolled patients on the basis of systolic dysfunction rather than diastolic dysfunction *(42)*. Thus, the report that concluded that most hospitalized older patients could not have been enrolled in the published trials of heart failure is not surprising

Table 2
Major Placebo-Controlled Clinical Trial of Heart Failure

Trial	n	Study drug	Duration (years)	Heart failure class	Mean age (years)	% Male	Baseline % ACE inhibitor	Baseline % β-blocker	Placebo mortality, %	Absolute mortality difference, %	NNT
CONSENSUS	253	Enalapril	0.5	IV = 100%	70–71	70–71	—	2–4	43.6	–17.7	5.6
SOLVD-Treatment	2569	Enalapril	3.4	I = 11%, II = 57%, III = 30%, IV = 2%	61	80	—	7.0–8.3	39.7	–4.5	22.2
SOLVD-Prevention	4228	Enalapril	3.1	I = 67%, II = 33%	59.1	89	—	24	15.8	–1.0	100
RALES	1663	Spironolactone	2	III = 71%, IV = 29%	65	73	94–95	10–11	46	–11	9.1
US Carvedilol	1094	Carvedilol	0.5	II = 53%, III = 44%, IV = 3%	58	77	95	—	7.8	–4.6	21.7
CIBIS-II	2647	Bisoprolol	1.3	III = 83%, IV = 17%	61	81	96	—	17.3	–5.5	18.2
MERIT-HF	3991	Metoprolol succinate	1.0	II = 41%, III = 55%, IV = 4%	64	77	89	—	11.0	–3.8	26.3
COPERNICUS	2289	Carvedilol	0.87	IV = 100%	63	80	97	—	18.5	–7.1	14.1

BEST	2708	Bucindolol	2	III = 92%, IV = 8%	60	78	91	—	33	–3.0	33.3
Val-HeFT	5010	Valsartan	1.9	II = 62%, III = 36%, IV = 2%	63	80	93	35	19.4	+0.3	—
CHARM	7601	Candesartan	3.1	II = 45%, III = 52%, IV = 3%	66	68	41	55	25	–2	50

ACE, angiotensin-converting enzyme; NNT, number needed to treat to benefit one patient; BEST, β-Blocker Evaluation Survival Trial; CHARM, Candesartan in Heart Failure Assessment of Reduction in Mortality and Morbidity; CIBIS-II, Cardiac Insufficiency Bisoprolol Study II; CONSENSUS, Cooperative North Scandinavian Enalapril Survival Study; COPERNICUS, Carvedilol Prospective Randomized Cumulative Survival Study; MERIT, Metoprolol CR/XL Randomized Intervention Trial in Heart Failure; RALES, Randomized Aldactone Evaluation Study; SOLVD, Study of Left Ventricular Dysfunction; Val-HeFT, Valsartan Heart Failure Trial.

(43). Of older patients 65 years or older who were hospitalized for heart failure, only 17% could have been enrolled in the Study of Left Ventricular Dysfunction *(29)*, 13% in Metoprolol CR/XL Randomized Intervention Trial in Heart Failure *(34)*, and 25% in Randomized Aldactone Evaluation Study *(36)*.

Despite these limitations, specific outcome trials are reviewed. Data that are relevant to older patients are highlighted when available.

ACE Inhibitors

Angiotensin (Ang) II is a potent direct vasoconstrictor that augments cardiac output by amplifying sympathetic activity, increases thirst and antidiuretic hormone secretion, stimulates the adrenal cortex to release aldosterone, and acts on the kidney to increase sodium reabsorption *(44)*. Ang II directly reduces renin release. Ang II possesses potent cellular growth properties, resulting in vascular and cardiac hypertrophy. Many tissues and organs can produce Ang II independent of the classic circulating system.

ACE inhibitors work by inhibiting ACE or kininase II *(45)*. In heart failure, ACE inhibitors decrease systemic vascular resistance, pulmonary wedge pressure, and both end-systolic and end-diastolic left ventricular volume. Thus, stroke volume and cardiac output improve. In addition, there are favorable neurohormonal changes.

ACE inhibitors are proven therapy for the treatment of heart failure and are recommended for all asymptomatic and symptomatic patients with heart failure unless contraindicated *(46)*. The ACE inhibitor captopril improved mean exercise time by 28 seconds compared to digoxin and by 47 seconds compared to placebo in a multicenter, double-blind trial of 300 patients with mild-to-moderate heart failure *(47)*. The Cooperative North Scandinavian Enalapril Survival Study (CONSENSUS) proved that enalapril dosed up to 20 mg twice daily reduced all-cause mortality 31% after 1 year compared to placebo in 253 patients with class IV heart failure treated in a double-blind fashion *(28)*. Heart failure was less likely to progress among enalapril-treated participants.

The Studies of Left Ventricular Dysfunction in symptomatic and asymptomatic patients extended the results of CONSENSUS by examining classes I through III heart failure patients *(29,30)*. In both studies, patients with an EF 35% or less received placebo or enalapril dosed 2.5–20 mg daily. After 41.4 months, the symptomatic patients ($n = 2569$) treated with enalapril had a 4.5% lower mortality than those receiving placebo ($p < 0.0036$) *(29)*. The asymptomatic patients ($n = 4228$) were followed for 37.4 months, but treatment with enalapril did not reduced all-cause mortality *(30)*. However, there was a 37% reduction in the development of heart failure and a 36% reduction in first hospitalization for heart failure with enalapril.

The Assessment of Treatment With Lisinopril and Survival study assigned patients with an EF of 30% or lower to low-dose or high-dose lisinopril to examine safety, mortality, and hospitalization in heart failure *(31)*. Although this trial did not observe any reduction in all-cause mortality with the higher dose of treatment, there was a 24% reduction in heart failure hospitalizations ($p = 0.002$). The rate for stopping medication was similar with each group.

Each of the ACE inhibitor trials provided essentially no data on elderly patients. A meta-analysis of 27 heart failure trials examined total mortality by various subgroups treated with ACE inhibitors or placebo *(48)*. This analysis observed a significant reduction in total mortality of 19% for 3510 patients older than 60 years and a 28% reduction for the 3021 patients 60 years or younger. The composite end point of total mortality or hospitalization was reduced by 29% in younger patients and 21% in older patients. In a cohort of 554 elderly patients with heart failure and systolic dysfunction, patients who received the recommended dose of an ACE inhibitor, according to current guidelines, had a significant decline in mortality compared to the patients receiving low doses of an ACE inhibitor *(49)*. High doses did not reduce readmissions for heart failure. In an analysis of a hospital registry of 2906 older patients with heart failure, treatment with an ACE inhibitor was associated with improved survival and quality of life if the EF was 40 to 49% *(50)*. Among patients with an EF 50% or higher, functional heart failure class improved, but mortality and heart failure re-admissions were not reduced.

Thus, there appears to be a benefit in using high-dose ACE inhibitors in older patients with systolic heart failure. For diastolic heart failure, symptoms and exercise duration are improved *(51)*.

β-*Blockers*

Progression of heart failure is caused by sympathetic activation. β-Blockers are standard therapy for heart failure. β-Blockers were believed to improve heart failure symptoms more than 20 years ago *(52)*. To test this hypothesis, the Metoprolol in Dilated Cardiomyopathy study examined 383 subjects with idiopathic dilated cardiomyopathy and an EF less than 40% *(53)*. The majority of patients in this trial had class II to III heart failure. Most of the subjects were treated with ACE inhibitors. Metoprolol tartrate was gradually increased from 10 mg daily to as high as 150 mg daily, as tolerated. Although there was no reduction in mortality in metoprolol-treated patients, fewer patients receiving metoprolol tartrate underwent heart transplantation. Left ventricular EF increased by 12% in metoprolol-treated patients compared to 6% in placebo-treated patients. Also, an improvement in exercise time and heart failure class was documented. Thus, the results of this trial initiated the large outcome trials of β-blockers for systolic heart failure *(54)*.

Bisoprolol is an ultraselective β_1-blocker without α_1-blocking characteristics. The Cardiac Insufficiency Bisoprolol Study II randomly assigned, using a randomized, double–blind design, 2647 patients with symptomatic heart failure with an EF 35% or less *(32)*. Bisoprolol was initiated at 1.25 mg once daily and titrated to 10 mg once daily. Most patients received concomitant therapy with an ACE inhibitor. After an average follow-up of 1.3 years, the study was prematurely terminated because of a significant reduction in all-cause mortality (17.3% in placebo-treated patients vs 11.8% in bisoprolol-treated patients, $p < 0.0001$). Other benefits included fewer cardiovascular deaths ($p = 0.0049$), fewer hospitalizations for heart failure ($p = 0.0006$), fewer sudden deaths ($p = 0.0011$), and fewer episodes of ventricular tachycardia and fibrillation ($p = 0.006$). Approximately 20% of the subjects were 71 years or older *(55)*. This group had a 32% relative reduction in total mortality and a 50% reduction in progression of heart failure. Bisoprolol did not reduce sudden death in this group.

In the Metoprolol CR/XL Randomized Intervention Trial in Congestive Heart Failure, controlled release/extended release metoprolol succinate was tested in 3991 patients with an EF 40% or less with class II to IV heart failure *(34)*. Conducted as a double-blind, RCT, metoprolol succinate controlled release/extended release was titrated from 12.5 to 200 mg once daily over 8 weeks. The average follow-up period was 1 year, and the trial was stopped early because of mortality benefit. The overall mortality was 11.0% in the placebo group and 7.2% in the metoprolol succinate group ($p = 0.0062$). In addition, there was a 38% reduction in cardiovascular mortality ($p = 0.00003$) and 41% reduction in sudden death ($p = 0.0002$). Also, there were fewer hospitalizations owing to heart failure or cardiovascular causes. Among the 153 study participants who were 69.4 years or older, total mortality was significantly reduced.

Carvedilol is a nonselective β-blocker with α-blocking and antioxidant properties. The US Carvedilol Heart Failure Study, a composite of four separate protocols, enrolled 1094 patients with class II to III heart failure with an EF of 35% or less *(56)*. Of the subjects, 95% received concomitant ACE inhibitors. The patients who could tolerate 6.25 mg of carvedilol twice daily for 2 weeks ultimately were enrolled in the double-blind portion of this trial. Although the trial was not designed as a mortality study, the overall mortality was 7.8% in the placebo group and 3.2% in the carvedilol group, for an absolute reduction in mortality of

4.6% ($p < 0.001$). There was also a 5.5% absolute reduction in the risk of hospitalization. The most common side effect experienced by carvedilol-assigned patients was dizziness in 33% of patients compared to 20% of placebo-assigned patients.

Using a double-blind trial design, the Carvedilol Prospective Randomized Cumulative Survival Study randomly assigned 2289 patients with severe heart failure *(33)*. Placebo or carvedilol 6.25 mg twice daily titrated to 25 mg twice daily was given. The trial was stopped after 10.4 months because of a beneficial reduction in total mortality with active treatment (18.5% placebo vs 11.4% carvedilol, $p = 0.0014$). A significant reduction in mortality was seen in the subgroup of patients 65 years or older.

In the Carvedilol or Metoprolol European Trial, 3029 patients with class II to IV heart failure were titrated to a target of 25 mg carvedilol twice daily or 50 mg metoprolol tartrate twice daily using a randomized, double-blind design *(35)*. After 58 months, the all-cause mortality was 6% lower in the carvedilol group ($p = 0.0017$). Heart rate was significantly lower with carvedilol during the first 16 months of the study, and systolic blood pressure was lower with carvedilol. Among patients 65 years or older, the relative reduction in mortality was 16%. This trial emphasized that metoprolol tartrate should not be used for heart failure.

Bucindolol is a nonselective β-blocker with mild vasodilating characteristics. The Beta Blocker Evaluation Survival Trial (BEST) studied class III to IV heart failure patients with an ejection fraction 35% of less *(57)*. Bucindolol dosed 3–100 mg twice daily or placebo was given to 2708 patients for an average follow-up of 2 years. Approximately 56% of the study population were 60 years or older. For the entire cohort, mortality was reduced 12.5% but not statistically decreased with bucindolol. For subjects 65 years or older, there was no survival advantage with bucindolol ($p = 0.31$) *(58)*.

Current guidelines recommend β-blockers for asymptomatic or symptomatic heart failure for stable patients with or without a previous MI *(46)*. In a long-term care facility, 477 men and women older than age 60 years with a prior MI and an EF 40% or less received β-blockers, ACE inhibitors, both, or neither *(59)*. The combination of β-blockers and ACE inhibitors was the most effective strategy for reducing coronary events and heart failure in this nonrandomized study. An observational study of 11,942 elderly patients from Alberta, Canada, with heart failure reported 36 and 45% reduction in all-cause mortality with high-dose β-blocker and ACE inhibitor use, respectively *(60)*. Heart failure hospitalizations decreased 29% over 21 months with β-blockers and 11% with ACE inhibitors.

Thus, β-blockers should be used in patients with systolic heart failure. Care must be taken to titrate the medication every 2 weeks while carefully assessing heart rate, fluid retention, and BP. The results of these trials argue against a "class effect" of β-blockers for heart failure. Thus, only bisoprolol, metoprolol succinate, and carvedilol should be prescribed instead of metoprolol tartrate or atenolol.

Angiotensin Receptor Blockers

Ang II receptors are distributed in the brain, heart, kidney, adrenal gland, and blood vessels (61). Although the role of Ang II is to defend the body acutely against hemorrhage or dehydration, the chronic effects of stimulation are ventricular and vascular hypertrophy. Angiotensin-receptor blockers (ARBs) block the type I angiotensin II (AT_1) receptor. Once the AT_1 receptor is blocked, plasma renin, Ang I, and Ang II increase. There are other Ang II receptor subtypes, but the AT_2 receptor is present during fetal development (62). The AT_2 receptor may mediate apoptosis and tissue remodeling. Stimulation of AT_2 receptors from blockade of the AT_1 receptor increases nitric oxide production and afferent arteriolar dilatation. CONSENSUS documented a significant positive correlation between mortality and levels of Ang II ($p < 0.05$) in patients treated with placebo (63). Because of the powerful predictive implications of angiotensin II on heart failure mortality, it was anticipated that the targeted blockade of Ang II would be even more effective in reducing overall mortality than the ACE inhibitors. The Evaluation of Losartan in the Elderly (ELITE) randomly assigned 722 patients 65 years or older to losartan or captopril (39). Using a randomized, double-blind design, patients with class II to IV heart failure with an EF of 40% or less received losartan titrated to 50 mg once daily or captopril titrated to 50 mg three times a day for 48 weeks. This was a tolerability rather than a mortality trial: the primary end point was an increase in serum creatinine 0.3 mg/dL or greater. There was no difference between losartan and captopril for increases in serum creatinine. The secondary composite end point was death and/or hospital admission for heart failure. The result was 9.4% for losartan-treated patients and 13.2% for captopril-treated patients ($p = 0.075$). Although there was no reduction in hospital admissions for heart failure, total mortality was lower with losartan than captopril (4.8 vs 8.7%, $p = 0.035$) because of a reduction in sudden cardiac death. There were fewer adverse events among losartan-treated patients (12.2%) vs captopril-treated patients (20.8%, $p \leq 0.002$).

ELITE-II was designed as a double-blind, randomized trial to assess all-cause mortality *(38)*. This study enrolled 3152 patients 60 years or older with symptomatic heart failure (class II to IV) with an EF 40% or less. Captopril and losartan were dosed the same as in the ELITE study. After a mean follow-up of 555 days, there was no difference in mortality between the captopril (15.9%) and losartan (17.7%, $p = 0.16$) arms. There was no difference in the rate of sudden death or heart failure hospitalizations. Captopril was superior to losartan among patients receiving β-blockers. Losartan was better tolerated than captopril (9.4 vs 14.5%, $p < 0.001$). ELITE-II has been criticized for failing to use higher doses of losartan because other outcome trials using 100 mg of losartan were successful in achieving the primary end points *(64–66)*.

The Valsartan Heart Failure Trial (Val-HeFT) was designed to compare the long-term effect of 160 mg valsartan or placebo dosed twice daily on morbidity, mortality, and quality of life *(67)*. This multicenter, double-blind, placebo-controlled trial enrolled 5010 patients with class II to IV heart failure *(68)*. The primary end point of all-cause mortality was 19.7% in the valsartan group and 19.4% in the placebo group ($p = 0.80$). Among the 366 patients not receiving an ACE inhibitor, mortality was reduced significantly by 9.8% ($p = 0.017$) *(69)*. The combined end point of mortality and heart failure morbidity was significantly decreased because of the reduction of heart failure hospitalizations in the valsartan group compared to placebo (13.8 vs 18.2%, $p < 0.001$). The combined end point for the 2350 elderly patients 65 years or older was reduced but not significantly.

The Candesartan in Heart Failure Assessment of Reduction in Mortality and Morbidity (CHARM) program definitively answered the question regarding whether an ARB is effective for patients with heart failure *(37)*. This randomized, double-blind trial had three components investigated in patients with heart failure. The study examined patients with an EF 40% or less (a) receiving ACE inhibitors (CHARM-Added, $n = 2548$) or (b) not receiving ACE inhibitors (CHARM-Alternative, $n = 2028$), and (c) patients with an EF greater than 40% (CHARM-Preserved, $n = 3023$) *(42,70,71)*. The median follow-up for the overall trial was 37.7 months. For the entire study, total ($p = 0.032$) and cardiovascular ($p = 0.006$) mortality were significantly reduced *(37)*. Hospital admissions for heart failure were reduced by 4.3%. The composite end point of cardiovascular death or first admission for heart failure significantly favored candesartan-assigned participants who were 65 years or older, which comprised 57% of the entire cohort.

In the CHARM-Added population, cardiovascular death was reduced by 3.6% ($p = 0.021$) and heart failure hospitalizations by 3.8% ($p = 0.018$) *(70)*. Candesartan reduced the composite end point in the presence of concomitant β-blocker therapy. Candesartan-treated patients were more likely to experience an increase in creatinine (7.8 vs 4.1%, $p = 0.0001$) and hyperkalemia (3.4% vs 0.7%, $p < 0.0001$). In the CHARM-Alternative cohort, cardiovascular death was reduced by 3.2% ($p = 0.02$) and heart failure hospitalizations by 7.8% ($p < 0.0001$) *(71)*. The 17% relative reduction in total mortality was significant ($p = 0.033$) after covariate adjustment. The greatest percentage (26.7%) of study participants 75 years or older was in the CHARM-Preserved cohort *(42)*. Heart failure hospitalizations were reduced by 2.4% ($p = 0.041$).

Current heart failure guidelines view ARBs as appropriate therapy for patients who cannot be given an ACE inhibitor because of cough or angioneurotic edema *(46)*. The addition of an ARB to an ACE inhibitor was considered controversial. The results of CHARM should alter those recommendations.

Aldosterone Antagonists

Like Ang II, aldosterone is a potent predictor of mortality in patients with heart failure. The Randomized Aldactone Evaluation Study enrolled 1663 patients with predominantly class III to IV heart failure *(36)*. There were 822 patients randomly assigned to receive 25 mg spironolactone daily and 841 to placebo. Concomitant therapy with ACE inhibitors was used in 95% of patients, but only 10 to 11% received β-blockers. All-cause mortality was the primary end point. After an average follow-up period of 24 months, the study was discontinued prematurely. The death rate in the placebo group was 45.9% compared to 34.5% in the spirono-lactone group ($p < 0.001$). The benefit was similar for patients younger than 67 years and those 67 years or older.

Spironolactone-assigned patients were less likely to have progression of heart failure (15.4 vs 22.5%, $p < 0.001$) and sudden death (10.0 vs 13.1%, $p = 0.02$). Furthermore, these subjects were less likely to be hospitalized for worsening heart failure ($p < 0.001$). Surprisingly, serious hyperkalemia did not occur commonly in the spironolactone patients. However, there was a greater rate of gynecomastia and breast pain in men, but they were not more likely to discontinue the study drug because of adverse events.

Eplerenone, a selective aldosterone-receptor antagonist should be associated with fewer side effects because it has a lower affinity for the androgen and progestin receptors compared with spironolactone. In a double-blind, placebo-controlled study evaluating the effect of eplerenone among 3313 patients with acute MI complicated by left ventricular dysfunction and heart failure, 25–50 mg eplerenone per day reduced mortality by 15% ($p = 0.008$) *(72)*.

Current guidelines favor the limited use of spironolactone for class IV systolic heart failure with preserved renal function and normal potassium concentrations *(73,74)*. However, multiple reports have alerted physicians that serious hyperkalemia may occur in older patients with heart failure treated with ACE inhibitors and spironolactone *(75,76)*. Common features that promote hyperkalemia in older patients include concomitant NSAIDs, renal insufficiency, diabetes with type IV renal tubular acidosis, and volume depletion.

Vasodilators

Two trials have been published regarding the combination of hydralazine and isosorbide dinitrate *(77,78)*. The first Veterans Administration Cooperative Vasodilator-Heart Failure Trial (V-HeFT I) compared placebo, 2.5–5 mg prazosin dosed four times daily, or 20–40 mg dosed isosorbide dinitrate four times daily with 37.5–75 mg hydralazine dosed four times daily *(77)*. The 642 men with chronic heart failure in this study received background therapy with digoxin and diuretics before they were assigned, using a randomized, double-blind trial design, to study medications. After 2.3 years, mortality was reduced with a combination of hydralazine and isosorbide dinitrate but not prazosin. Of 623 study participants, 13% had a radionuclide ventricular EF of 45% or greater *(79)*. In this preserved systolic function group, the annual mortality of the patients receiving combined vasodilators was lower than for the placebo group (5.3 vs 9.0%, not significant).

V-HeFT II compared the hydralazine and isosorbide dinitrate combination with 5 to 10 mg enalapril dosed twice daily *(78)*. This trial enrolled 804 men and followed them for an average of 2.5 years. After 2 years, the mortality was lower in the enalapril group (18 vs 25%, $p = 0.016$). Overall mortality was 32.8% among patients assigned to enalapril and 38.2% for the combination of hydralazine and isosorbide dinitrate-hydralazine ($p = 0.08$). There were fewer sudden deaths for the enalapril group. However, EF and exercise tolerance improved more with the combined vasodilators.

In a separate analysis of the V-HeFT I and II trials, there were 105 (16.3%) patients older than 65 years in V-HeFT I and 225 (28.0%) in V-HeFT II *(80)*. For the older patients in V-HeFT I, neither prazosin ($p = 0.60$) nor the combined vasodilators ($p = 0.98$) was superior to placebo for survival. In fact, prazosin was associated with a 67% higher mortality for ages 61 to 65 years and a 28% higher mortality above age 65 years compared with placebo. In V-HeFT II, there was no difference in mortality for older patients treated with enalapril or hydralazine-isosorbide dinitrate ($p = 0.69$). In these studies, age was not an independent determinant of survival.

The combination of hydralazine and isosorbide dinitrate is only recommended for patients who cannot take ACE inhibitors because of renal insufficiency or hypotension (46). There are no recommendations for their use as alternatives to ACE inhibitors or in combination with ARBs or ACE inhibitors. However, based on a *post hoc* analysis, there appears to be an advantage for using hydralazine and isosorbide for the reduction of heart failure mortality for African Americans, and this hypothesis is now under testing in the African American Heart Failure Trial (81,82).

Digitalis

The Digitalis Investigators Group (DIG) trial studied whether digoxin added to diuretics and ACE inhibitors would reduce mortality in patients with heart failure (83). There were 7788 persons with heart failure enrolled in this randomized, double-blind, placebo-controlled study: 69.3% of the study population were 60 years or older, and 12.7% of study patients had an EF greater than 45% (84). There was no reduction in total mortality. Mortality caused by worsening heart failure was reduced 12% ($p = 0.06$), and heart failure hospitalizations were reduced 28% ($p < 0.001$) (83). Two *post hoc* analyses of the DIG trial have raised issues of concern: (a) digoxin therapy is associated with an increased risk of all-cause mortality among women, but not men, with heart failure and depressed left ventricular systolic function, and (b) the optimum serum digoxin concentrations for men are in the range 0.5–0.8 ng/mL because levels greater than 0.8 ng/mL are associated with increased mortality (85,86).

Increasing age was associated with increasing mortality and heart failure hospitalizations (Fig. 11). There was no interaction between age and digoxin treatment for either mortality or heart failure hospitalization. The older DIG study participants did not experience a significant increase in digoxin toxicity compared to placebo. Although digoxin is considered detrimental to patients with preserved systolic function, this was not apparent in terms of all-cause mortality (Fig. 11).

Digoxin is recommended for the treatment of symptomatic left ventricular systolic dysfunction (46). The role of digoxin for preserved systolic function to minimize heart failure symptoms remains controversial, but does not appear hazardous when tested prospectively.

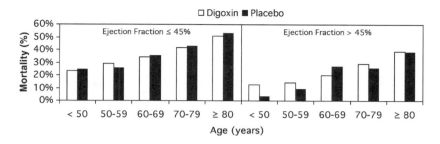

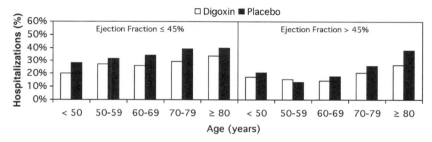

Fig. 11. Effect of digoxin on mortality and heart failure hospitalizations by age and ejection fraction. There was no benefit or hazard of digoxin use in reducing mortality in patients with systolic dysfunction or preserved ejection fraction (upper panel). Digoxin reduced heart failure hospitalizations in patients with systolic dysfunction or preserved ejection fraction (lower panel). (Data from ref. *84.*)

New Trials in the Elderly

There are several trials in progress that focus on heart failure in the elderly *(87,88)*. The Perindopril for Elderly People With Chronic Heart Failure trial enrolled patients 70 years or older with an EF 40% or greater to placebo or perindopril for a minimum of 1 year *(88)*. The primary outcome is total mortality and heart failure hospitalization. Enrollment was closed with just over 800 patients recruited in June 2003 and should continue for a further 18 months.

The Study of the Effects of Nebivolol Intervention on Outcomes and Rehospitalization in Seniors With Heart Failure is a randomized, double-blind, parallel-group trial that will enroll 2000 patients 70 years or older with heart failure and with or without systolic dysfunction *(87)*. Placebo or nebivolol 1.25 mg titrated to 10 mg will be given for up to 29 months. The primary outcome of this trial is death or cardiovascular hospital admission.

The Irbesartan in Heart Failure With Preserved Systolic Function study will randomly assign 3600 patients who are 60 years or older with class II to IV heart failure and an EF of 45% or greater. Hospitalization for heart failure within the previous 6 months or current heart failure symptoms and corroborative evidence by electrocardiography, chest X-ray, or echocardiography are required for enrollment. The trial will be conducted as a randomized, double-blind, placebo-controlled, parallel-group design. The primary composite outcome will be all-cause mortality and cardiovascular hospitalization. Patients will be followed for 48 months. Secondary outcome measures include (a) all-cause mortality; (b) cardiovascular death, which will be analyzed as the time to the first event; (c) combined cardiovascular death and nonfatal myocardial infarction and stroke; (d) combined heart failure mortality and heart failure hospitalization; (e) quality of life; (f) improvement in heart failure class; and (g) improvement in BNP levels.

Issues for Diastolic Heart Failure Management

Predictors of 1-year mortality in 683 patients 70 years or older with heart failure was similar for normal and abnormal heart failure: systolic blood pressure, blood urea nitrogen, and the Activities of Daily Living (ADL) Scale *(89)*. Heart failure class was an additional factor for preserved systolic function, and serum albumin and male gender were factors for systolic dysfunction.

There are four recommendations in the management of preserved EF heart failure: (a) manage BP, (b) control tachycardia, (c) reduce pulmonary congestion, and (d) improve myocardial ischemia *(46)*. There are scanty data on outcomes. The CHARM-Preserved trial provided the best data available. The Irbesartan in Heart Failure With Preserved Systolic Function, Perindopril for Elderly People With Chronic Heart Failure, and Study of the Effects of Nebivolol Intervention on Outcomes and Rehospitalization in Seniors With Heart Failure trials will support and extend knowledge of treatment.

β-Blockers and the nondihydropyridine calcium channel blockers potentially slow the heart and treat ischemia. A prospective study of 158 elderly patients with preserved systolic function heart failure and a prior MI was conducted to assess outcome of adding propranolol adjunctive therapy or placebo to treatment with ACE inhibitors and diuretics *(90)*. Propranolol was associated with a reduction in total mortality and nonfatal MI rate. In a blinded crossover study, verapamil was shown to improve the peak filling rate and exercise duration in elderly patients with heart failure and preserved systolic function *(91)*. Verapamil improves exercise duration decreased pulse wave velocity in elderly patients *(92)*. Losartan increased exercise duration in subjects with diastolic dysfunction *(93)*. ACE inhibitors are usually recommended also, but not all trials show an improvement in exercise duration *(94)*.

ADHERENCE

There are many reasons that contribute to nonadherence to treatment of heart failure. However, among elderly patients with heart failure, the rate appears to be especially high *(95)*. Among 7247 New Jersey Medicaid recipients 65 years or older who received a new prescription for digoxin, 19% of the cohort did not refill their initial prescription. Also, medication was not taken on average for 111 days over the period of a year. However, among patients receiving multiple medications for heart failure, the average number of missed days of medication was 56 days. In addition, a prior hospitalization or an age of 85 years or older was associated with more adherence to therapy *(95)*.

A nurse-directed, multidisciplinary approach appears to be more effective *(96)*. In a randomized prospective trial, 282 subjects 70 years or older who were hospitalized for heart failure were assigned to conventional therapy or a comprehensive individualized education, which included information on disease, diet, medications, discharge planning, and follow-up. The intervention group had fewer heart failure admissions within 90 days after discharge compared to the control group (24 vs 54%, $p = 0.04$). In addition, there was more improvement in quality of life and cost savings in the special intervention group.

PREVENTION

Systolic and pulse pressures confer the greatest risk for the development of heart failure *(97)*. The treatment of heart failure is expensive. Prevention offers a rational long-term approach to avoid the impairment in lifestyle and increased mortality and morbidity of heart failure. Current heart failure guidelines highlight the identification of patients at high risk for heart failure *(46)*. This includes systemic hypertension, diabetes mellitus, coronary artery disease, and alcohol abuse. The recommended approach includes the treatment of hypertension and lipids, smoking cessation, exercise, avoidance of alcohol and illicit drugs, and use of ACE inhibitors in high-risk patients. Weight reduction should be included because there is a graded risk of heart failure with increasing body mass index *(98)*.

The clinical trials of hypertension have provided the best-documented evidence in the reduction of heart failure *(99–103)*. Diuretics alone or in combination with β-blockers prevented heart failure *(101,103)*. ACE inhibitors were more effective than calcium channel blockers *(104)*. Diuretics were associated with lower rates of heart failure than amlodipine or the α_1-blocker doxazosin *(102,103,105)*. The increasing use of antihypertensive medications and the decline in left ventricular hypertrophy *(106)* are likely to be associated with lower rates of heart failure if the benefits are not offset by the increasing incidence of obesity and diabetes mellitus.

SUMMARY

Diastolic heart failure occurs in about 50% of older persons and is most often associated with female gender, systemic hypertension, and left ventricular hypertrophy. Nonpharmacological therapy with sodium restriction, exercise, and weight reduction are required. Strict control of blood pressure, diabetes, and lipids is likely to benefit the patient. Maintaining a sinus rhythm is vital. Candesartan benefits both systolic and diastolic heart failure. β-Blockers reduce mortality from ischemic heart disease and systolic heart failure, control the ventricular response in atrial fibrillation, reduce mortality in combination with diuretics in hypertensive patients, and increase the diastolic filling time. The assessment and treatment of heart failure in the elderly is a challenge with insufficient tools for diagnosis and trials that may not be totally relevant.

REFERENCES

1. American Heart Association. Heart and Stroke Statistics—2003 Update Dallas, TX: American Heart Association; 2002.
2. Levy D, Kenchaiah S, Larson MG, et al. Long-term trends in the incidence of and survival with heart failure. *N Engl J Med* 2002;347:1397–1402.
3. Ho KK, Pinsky JL, Kannel WB, Levy D. The epidemiology of heart failure: the Framingham Study. *J Am Coll Cardiol* 1993;22(4 suppl A):6A–13A.
4. Levy D, Larson MG, Vasan RS, Kannel WB, Ho KK. The progression from hypertension to congestive heart failure. *JAMA* 1996;275:1557–1562.
5. Kannel WB. Vital epidemiologic clues in heart failure. *J Clin Epidemiol* 2000;53: 229–235.
6. Morbidity and mortality: 2002 Chart Book on cardiovascular, lung, and blood diseases. US Department of Health and Human Services. National Institutes of Health; 2002:90. Available at: http://www.nhlbi.nih.gov/resources/docs/cht-book.htm. October 22, 2003
7. Aurigemma GP, Gottdiener JS, Shemanski L, Gardin J, Kitzman D. Predictive value of systolic and diastolic function for incident congestive heart failure in the elderly: the cardiovascular health study. *J Am Coll Cardiol* 2001;37:1042–1048.
8. Kitzman DW, Gardin JM, Gottdiener JS, et al. Importance of heart failure with preserved systolic function in patients > or = 65 years of age. CHS Research Group. Cardiovascular Health Study. *Am J Cardiol* 2001;87:413–419.
9. Gottdiener JS, McClelland RL, Marshall R, et al. Outcome of congestive heart failure in elderly persons: influence of left ventricular systolic function. The Cardiovascular Health Study. *Ann Intern Med* 2002;137:631–639.

10. Wei JY. Age and the cardiovascular system. *N Engl J Med* 1992;327:1735–1739.
11. Hundley WG, Kitzman DW, Morgan TM, et al. Cardiac cycle-dependent changes in aortic area and distensibility are reduced in older patients with isolated diastolic heart failure and correlate with exercise intolerance. *J Am Coll Cardiol* 2001;38:796–802.
12. Tresch DD. Signs and symptoms of heart failure in elderly patients. *Am J Geriatr Cardiol* 1996;5:27–33.
13. Drazner MH, Rame JE, Stevenson LW, Dries DL. Prognostic importance of elevated jugular venous pressure and a third heart sound in patients with heart failure. *N Engl J Med* 2001;345:574–581.
14. Tsuyuki RT, McKelvie RS, Arnold JM, et al. Acute precipitants of congestive heart failure exacerbations. *Arch Intern Med* 2001;161:2337–2342.
15. Page J, Henry D. Consumption of NSAIDs and the development of congestive heart failure in elderly patients: an underrecognized public health problem. *Arch Intern Med* 2000;160:777–784.
16. Kitzman DW, Little WC, Brubaker PH, et al. Pathophysiological characterization of isolated diastolic heart failure in comparison to systolic heart failure. *JAMA* 2002;288:2144–2150.
17. Tresch DD, McGough MF. Heart failure with normal systolic function: a common disorder in older people. *J Am Geriatr Soc* 1995;43:1035–1042.
18. Aronow WS. Echocardiography should be performed in all elderly patients with congestive heart failure. *J Am Geriatr Soc* 1994;42:1300–1302.
19. Vasan RS, Levy D. Defining diastolic heart failure: a call for standardized diagnostic criteria. *Circulation* 2000;101:2118–2121.
20. Redfield MM, Jacobsen SJ, Burnett JC Jr, Mahoney DW, Bailey KR, Rodeheffer RJ. Burden of systolic and diastolic ventricular dysfunction in the community: appreciating the scope of the heart failure epidemic. *JAMA* 2003;289:194–202.
21. Yamamoto K, Wilson DJ, Canzanello VJ, Redfield MM. Left ventricular diastolic dysfunction in patients with hypertension and preserved systolic function. *Mayo Clin Proc* 2000;75:148–155.
22. Redfield MM, Rodeheffer RJ, Jacobsen SJ, Mahoney DW, Bailey KR, Burnett JC Jr. Plasma brain natriuretic peptide concentration: impact of age and gender. *J Am Coll Cardiol* 2002;40:976–982.
23. Latini R, Masson S, Anand I, et al. Effects of valsartan on circulating brain natriuretic peptide and norepinephrine in symptomatic chronic heart failure: the Valsartan Heart Failure Trial (Val-HeFT). *Circulation* 2002;106:2454–2458.
24. Tsutamoto T, Wada A, Maeda K, et al. Attenuation of compensation of endogenous cardiac natriuretic peptide system in chronic heart failure: prognostic role of plasma brain natriuretic peptide concentration in patients with chronic symptomatic left ventricular dysfunction. *Circulation* 1997;96:509–516.
25. Maeda K, Tsutamoto T, Wada A, et al. High levels of plasma brain natriuretic peptide and interleukin-6 after optimized treatment for heart failure are independent risk factors for morbidity and mortality in patients with congestive heart failure. *J Am Coll Cardiol* 2000;36:1587–1593.
26. Koglin J, Pehlivanli S, Schwaiblmair M, Vogeser M, Cremer P, vonScheidt W. Role of brain natriuretic peptide in risk stratification of patients with congestive heart failure. *J Am Coll Cardiol* 2001;38:1934–1941.
27. Stanek B, Frey B, Hulsmann M, et al. Prognostic evaluation of neurohumoral plasma levels before and during beta-blocker therapy in advanced left ventricular dysfunction. *J Am Coll Cardiol* 2001;38:436–442.
28. Effects of enalapril on mortality in severe congestive heart failure. Results of the Cooperative North Scandinavian Enalapril Survival Study (CONSENSUS). The CONSENSUS Trial Study Group. *N Engl J Med* 1987;316:1429–1435.

29. Effect of enalapril on survival in patients with reduced left ventricular ejection fractions and congestive heart failure. The SOLVD Investigators. *N Engl J Med* 1991;325:293–302.

30. Effect of enalapril on mortality and the development of heart failure in asymptomatic patients with reduced left ventricular ejection fractions. The SOLVD Investigators. *N Engl J Med* 1992;327:685–691.

31. Packer M, Poole-Wilson PA, Armstrong PW, et al. Comparative effects of low and high doses of the angiotensin-converting enzyme inhibitor, lisinopril, on morbidity and mortality in chronic heart failure. ATLAS Study Group. *Circulation* 1999;100: 2312–2318.

32. The Cardiac Insufficiency Bisoprolol Study II (CIBIS-II): a randomised trial. *Lancet* 1999;353:9–13.

33. Packer M, Coats AJ, Fowler MB, et al. Effect of carvedilol on survival in severe chronic heart failure. *N Engl J Med* 2001;344:1651–1658.

34. Effect of metoprolol CR/XL in chronic heart failure: Metoprolol CR/XL Randomised Intervention Trial in Congestive Heart Failure (MERIT-HF). *Lancet* 1999;353:2001–2007.

35. Poole-Wilson PA, Swedberg K, Cleland JG, et al. Comparison of carvedilol and metoprolol on clinical outcomes in patients with chronic heart failure in the Carvedilol Or Metoprolol European Trial (COMET): randomised controlled trial. *Lancet* 2003;362:7–13.

36. Pitt B, Zannad F, Remme WJ, et al. The effect of spironolactone on morbidity and mortality in patients with severe heart failure. Randomized Aldactone Evaluation Study Investigators. *N Engl J Med* 1999;341:709–717.

37. Pfeffer MA, Swedberg K, Granger CB, et al. Effects of candesartan on mortality and morbidity in patients with chronic heart failure: the CHARM-Overall programme. *Lancet* 2003;362:759–766.

38. Pitt B, Poole-Wilson PA, Segal R, et al. Effect of losartan compared with captopril on mortality in patients with symptomatic heart failure: randomised trial—the Losartan Heart Failure Survival Study ELITE II. *Lancet* 2000;355:1582–1587.

39. Pitt B, Segal R, Martinez FA, et al. Randomised trial of losartan vs captopril in patients over 65 with heart failure (Evaluation of Losartan in the Elderly Study, ELITE). *Lancet* 1997;349:747–752.

40. Heiat A, Gross CP, Krumholz HM. Representation of the elderly, women, and minorities in heart failure clinical trials. *Arch Intern Med* 2002;162:1682–1688.

41. Ahmed A. American College of Cardiology/American Heart Association Chronic Heart Failure Evaluation and Management guidelines: relevance to the geriatric practice. *J Am Geriatr Soc* 2003;51:123–126.

42. Yusuf S, Pfeffer MA, Swedberg K, et al. Effects of candesartan in patients with chronic heart failure and preserved left-ventricular ejection fraction: the CHARM-Preserved Trial. *Lancet* 2003;362:777–781.

43. Masoudi FA, Havranek EP, Wolfe P, et al. Most hospitalized older persons do not meet the enrollment criteria for clinical trials in heart failure. *Am Heart J* 2003;146:250–257.

44. Williams GH. Converting-enzyme inhibitors in the treatment of hypertension. *N Engl J Med* 1988;319:1517–1525.

45. Deedwania PC. Angiotensin-converting enzyme inhibitors in congestive heart failure. *Arch Intern Med* 1990;150:1798–1805.

46. Hunt SA, Baker DW, Chin MH, et al. ACC/AHA guidelines for the evaluation and management of chronic heart failure in the adult: executive summary. A report of the American College of Cardiology/American Heart Association Task Force on

Practice Guidelines (Committee to Revise the 1995 Guidelines for the Evaluation and Management of Heart Failure). *J Am Coll Cardiol* 2001;38:2101–2113.

47. Comparative effects of therapy with captopril and digoxin in patients with mild to moderate heart failure. The Captopril-Digoxin Multicenter Research Group. *JAMA* 1988;259:539–544.

48. Garg R, Yusuf S. Overview of randomized trials of angiotensin-converting enzyme inhibitors on mortality and morbidity in patients with heart failure. Collaborative Group on ACE Inhibitor Trials [published erratum appears in *JAMA* 1995;274:462]. *JAMA* 1995;273:1450–1456.

49. Chen YT, Wang Y, Radford MJ, Krumholz HM. Angiotensin-converting enzyme inhibitor dosages in elderly patients with heart failure. *Am Heart J* 2001;141:410–417.

50. Philbin EF, Rocco TA Jr, Lindenmuth NW, Ulrich K, Jenkins PL. Systolic vs diastolic heart failure in community practice: clinical features, outcomes, and the use of angiotensin-converting enzyme inhibitors. *Am J Med* 2000;109:605–613.

51. Aronow WS, Kronzon I. Effect of enalapril on congestive heart failure treated with diuretics in elderly patients with prior myocardial infarction and normal left ventricular ejection fraction. *Am J Cardiol* 1993;71:602–604.

52. Waagstein F, Hjalmarson A, Swedberg K, Wallentin I. Beta blockade in congestive cardiomyopathy. *Lancet* 1981;2:1115–1116.

53. Waagstein F, Bristow MR, Swedberg K, et al. Beneficial effects of metoprolol in idiopathic dilated cardiomyopathy. Metoprolol in Dilated Cardiomyopathy (MDC) Trial Study Group. *Lancet* 1993;342:1441–1446.

54. Hash TW, Prisant LM. β-Blocker use in systolic heart failure and dilated cardiomyopathy. *J Clin Pharmacol* 1997;37:7–19.

55. Erdmann E, Lechat P, Verkenne P, Wiemann H. Results from post-hoc analyses of the CIBIS II trial: effect of bisoprolol in high-risk patient groups with chronic heart failure. *Eur J Heart Fail* 2001;3:469–479.

56. Packer M, Bristow MR, Cohn JN, et al. The effect of carvedilol on morbidity and mortality in patients with chronic heart failure. US Carvedilol Heart Failure Study Group. *N Engl J Med* 1996;334:1349–1355.

57. A trial of the beta-blocker bucindolol in patients with advanced chronic heart failure. *N Engl J Med* 2001;344:1659–1667.

58. Aranda JM, Krause-Steinrauf HJ, Greenberg BH, et al. Comparison of the beta blocker bucindolol in younger vs older patients with heart failure. *Am J Cardiol* 2002;89:1322–1326.

59. Aronow WS, Ahn C, Kronzon I. Effect of β blockers alone, of angiotensin-converting enzyme inhibitors alone, and of β blockers plus angiotensin-converting enzyme inhibitors on new coronary events and on congestive heart failure in older persons with healed myocardial infarcts and asymptomatic left ventricular systolic dysfunction. *Am J Cardiol* 2001;88:1298–1300.

60. Sin DD, McAlister FA. The effects of β-blockers on morbidity and mortality in a population-based cohort of 11,942 elderly patients with heart failure. *Am J Med* 2002;113:650–656.

61. Goodfriend TL, Elliott ME, Catt KJ. Angiotensin receptors and their antagonists. *N Engl J Med* 1996;334:1649–1654.

62. Burnier M, Brunner HR. Angiotensin II receptor antagonists. *Lancet* 2000;355:637–645.

63. Swedberg K, Eneroth P, Kjekshus J, Wilhelmsen L. Hormones regulating cardiovascular function in patients with severe congestive heart failure and their relation to mortality. CONSENSUS Trial Study Group. *Circulation* 1990;82:1730–1736.

64. Brenner BM, Cooper ME, de Zeeuw D, et al. Effects of losartan on renal and cardiovascular outcomes in patients with type 2 diabetes and nephropathy. *N Engl J Med* 2001;345:861–869.

65. Lindholm LH, Ibsen H, Dahlof B, et al. Cardiovascular morbidity and mortality in patients with diabetes in the Losartan Intervention for Endpoint reduction in hypertension study (LIFE): a randomised trial against atenolol. *Lancet* 2002;359:1004–1010.

66. Dahlof B, Devereux RB, Kjeldsen SE, et al. Cardiovascular morbidity and mortality in the Losartan Intervention for Endpoint reduction in hypertension study (LIFE): a randomised trial against atenolol. *Lancet* 2002;359:995–1003.

67. Cohn JN, Tognoni G, Glazer RD, Spormann D, Hester A. Rationale and design of the Valsartan Heart Failure Trial: a large multinational trial to assess the effects of valsartan, an angiotensin- receptor blocker, on morbidity and mortality in chronic congestive heart failure. *J Card Fail* 1999;5:155–160.

68. Cohn JN, Tognoni G. A randomized trial of the angiotensin-receptor blocker valsartan in chronic heart failure. *N Engl J Med* 2001;345:1667–1675.

69. Maggioni AP, Anand I, Gottlieb SO, Latini R, Tognoni G, Cohn JN. Effects of valsartan on morbidity and mortality in patients with heart failure not receiving angiotensin-converting enzyme inhibitors. *J Am Coll Cardiol* 2002;40:1414–1421.

70. McMurray JJ, Ostergren J, Swedberg K, et al. Effects of candesartan in patients with chronic heart failure and reduced left-ventricular systolic function taking angiotensin-converting-enzyme inhibitors: the CHARM-Added trial. *Lancet* 2003;362:767–771.

71. Granger CB, McMurray JJ, Yusuf S, et al. Effects of candesartan in patients with chronic heart failure and reduced left-ventricular systolic function intolerant to angiotensin-converting-enzyme inhibitors: the CHARM-Alternative trial. *Lancet* 2003;362:772–776.

72. Pitt B, Remme W, Zannad F, et al. Eplerenone, a selective aldosterone blocker, in patients with left ventricular dysfunction after myocardial infarction. *N Engl J Med* 2003;348:1309–1321.

73. Duprez DA, De Buyzere ML, Rietzschel ER, et al. Inverse relationship between aldosterone and large artery compliance in chronically treated heart failure patients. *Eur Heart J* 1998;19:1371–1376.

74. Weber KT. Aldosterone in congestive heart failure. *N Engl J Med* 2001;345:1689–1697.

75. Schepkens H, Vanholder R, Billiouw JM, Lameire N. Life-threatening hyperkalemia during combined therapy with angiotensin-converting enzyme inhibitors and spironolactone: an analysis of 25 cases. *Am J Med* 2001;110:438–441.

76. Obialo CI, Ofili EO, Mirza T. Hyperkalemia in congestive heart failure patients aged 63 to 85 years with subclinical renal disease. *Am J Cardiol* 2002;90:663–665.

77. Cohn JN, Archibald DG, Ziesche S, et al. Effect of vasodilator therapy on mortality in chronic congestive heart failure. Results of a Veterans Administration Cooperative Study. *N Engl J Med* 1986;314:1547–1552.

78. Cohn JN, Johnson G, Ziesche S, et al. A comparison of enalapril with hydralazine-isosorbide dinitrate in the treatment of chronic congestive heart failure. *N Engl J Med* 1991;325:303–310.

79. Cohn JN, Johnson G. Heart failure with normal ejection fraction. The V-HeFT Study. Veterans Administration Cooperative Study Group. *Circulation* 1990;81(2 suppl):III48–III53.

80. Hughes CV, Wong M, Johnson G, Cohn JN. Influence of age on mechanisms and prognosis of heart failure. The V-HeFT VA Cooperative Studies Group. *Circulation* 1993;87(6 suppl):VI111–VI117.

81. Carson P, Ziesche S, Johnson G, Cohn JN. Racial differences in response to therapy for heart failure: analysis of the vasodilator-heart failure trials. Vasodilator-Heart Failure Trial Study Group. *J Card Fail* 1999;5:178–187.

82. Franciosa JA, Taylor AL, Cohn JN, et al. African-American Heart Failure Trial (A-HeFT): rationale, design, and methodology. *J Card Fail* 2002;8:128–135.

83. The effect of digoxin on mortality and morbidity in patients with heart failure. The Digitalis Investigation Group. *N Engl J Med* 1997;336:525–533.

84. Rich MW, McSherry F, Williford WO, Yusuf S. Effect of age on mortality, hospitalizations and response to digoxin in patients with heart failure: the DIG study. *J Am Coll Cardiol* 2001;38:806–813.

85. Rathore SS, Wang Y, Krumholz HM. Sex-based differences in the effect of digoxin for the treatment of heart failure. *N Engl J Med* 2002;347:1403–1411.

86. Rathore SS, Curtis JP, Wang Y, Bristow MR, Krumholz HM. Association of serum digoxin concentration and outcomes in patients with heart failure. *JAMA* 2003;289: 871–878.

87. Shibata MC, Flather MD, Bohm M, et al. Study of the Effects of Nebivolol Intervention on Outcomes and Rehospitalisation in Seniors with Heart Failure (SENIORS). Rationale and design. *Int J Cardiol* 2002;86:77–85.

88. Cleland JG, Tendera M, Adamus J, et al. Perindopril for elderly people with chronic heart failure: the PEP-CHF study. The PEP investigators. *Eur J Heart Fail* 1999;1:211–217.

89. Pernenkil R, Vinson JM, Shah AS, Beckham V, Wittenberg C, Rich MW. Course and prognosis in patients > or = 70 years of age with congestive heart failure and normal vs abnormal left ventricular ejection fraction. *Am J Cardiol* 1997;79:216–219.

90. Aronow WS, Ahn C, Kronzon I. Effect of propranolol vs no propranolol on total mortality plus nonfatal myocardial infarction in older patients with prior myocardial infarction, congestive heart failure, and left ventricular ejection fraction > or = 40% treated with diuretics plus angiotensin-converting enzyme inhibitors. *Am J Cardiol* 1997;80:207–209.

91. Setaro JF, Zaret BL, Schulman DS, Black HR, Soufer R. Usefulness of verapamil for congestive heart failure associated with abnormal left ventricular diastolic filling and normal left ventricular systolic performance. *Am J Cardiol* 1990;66:981–986.

92. Chen CH, Nakayama M, Talbot M, et al. Verapamil acutely reduces ventricular-vascular stiffening and improves aerobic exercise performance in elderly individuals. *J Am Coll Cardiol* 1999;33:1602–1609.

93. Warner JG Jr, Metzger DC, Kitzman DW, Wesley DJ, Little WC. Losartan improves exercise tolerance in patients with diastolic dysfunction and a hypertensive response to exercise. *J Am Coll Cardiol* 1999;33:1567–1572.

94. Zi M, Carmichael N, Lye M. The effect of quinapril on functional status of elderly patients with diastolic heart failure. *Cardiovasc Drugs Ther* 2003;17:133–139.

95. Monane M, Bohn RL, Gurwitz JH, Glynn RJ, Avorn J. Noncompliance with congestive heart failure therapy in the elderly. *Arch Intern Med* 1994;154:433–437.

96. Rich MW, Beckham V, Wittenberg C, Leven CL, Freedland KE, Carney RM. A multidisciplinary intervention to prevent the readmission of elderly patients with congestive heart failure. *N Engl J Med* 1995;333:1190–1195.

97. Haider AW, Larson MG, Franklin SS, Levy D. Systolic blood pressure, diastolic blood pressure, and pulse pressure as predictors of risk for congestive heart failure in the Framingham Heart Study. *Ann Intern Med* 2003;138:10–16.

98. Kenchaiah S, Evans JC, Levy D, et al. Obesity and the risk of heart failure. *N Engl J Med* 2002;347:305–313.

99. Amery A, Birkenhäger W, Brixko P, et al. Mortality and morbidity results from the European Working Party on High Blood Pressure in the Elderly trial. *Lancet* 1985;1:1349–1354.

100. Kostis JB, Davis BR, Cutler J, et al. Prevention of heart failure by antihypertensive drug treatment in older persons with isolated systolic hypertension. SHEP Cooperative Research Group. *JAMA* 1997;278:212–216.

101. Dahlöf B, Lindholm LH, Hansson L, Scherstén B, Ekbom T, Wester PO. Morbidity and mortality in the Swedish Trial in Old Patients With Hypertension (STOP-Hypertension). *Lancet* 1991;338:1281–1285.

102. Major cardiovascular events in hypertensive patients randomized to doxazosin vs chlorthalidone: the antihypertensive and lipid-lowering treatment to prevent heart attack trial (ALLHAT). ALLHAT Collaborative Research Group. *JAMA* 2000;283:1967–1975.

103. Major outcomes in high-risk hypertensive patients randomized to angiotensin-converting enzyme inhibitor or calcium channel blocker vs diuretic: the Antihypertensive and Lipid-Lowering Treatment to Prevent Heart Attack Trial (ALLHAT). *JAMA* 2002;288:2981–2997.

104. Hansson L, Lindholm LH, Ekbom T, et al. Randomised trial of old and new antihypertensive drugs in elderly patients: cardiovascular mortality and morbidity the Swedish Trial in Old Patients With Hypertension-2 study. *Lancet* 1999;354:1751–1756.

105. Diuretic vs α-blocker as first-step antihypertensive therapy: final results from the Antihypertensive and Lipid-Lowering Treatment to Prevent Heart Attack Trial (ALLHAT). *Hypertension* 2003;42:239–246.

106. Mosterd A, D'Agostino RB, Silbershatz H, et al.. Trends in the prevalence of hypertension, antihypertensive therapy, and left ventricular hypertrophy from 1950 to 1989. *N Engl J Med* 1999;340:1221–1227.

13 Ischemic Heart Disease in the Older Hypertensive Patient

Evaluation and Management

Jan Laws Houghton, MD

Contents

INTRODUCTION

Ischemic heart disease (IHD) is characterized by an imbalance between myocardial blood flow supply and metabolic demand. In Westernized society, this is found principally in the setting of atherosclerotic coronary artery disease (CAD), also known as coronary heart disease (CHD), but is also present in other disease states commonly found in the hypertensive elderly patient, including valvular heart disease, dilated cardiomyopathy, atrial fibrillation (AF), metabolic disorders such as hypothyroidism, left ventricular hypertrophy (LVH), and diastolic dysfunction. In patients with CAD, supply is limited by the degree of luminal narrowing in epicardial coronary vessels. In those with hypertension with or without LVH, excess demand is present owing to increases in wall stress and in metabolic demands of the hypertrophied myocardium. In both of these disorders, there is associated endothelial dysfunction in

From: *Clinical Hypertension and Vascular Diseases: Hypertension in the Elderly*
Edited by: L. M. Prisant © Humana Press Inc., Totowa, NJ

the coronary microvasculature, which can also limit supply to the myocardium (1). When CAD and hypertension with or without LVH coexist, both supply and demand are adversely affected, thus worsening the degree of expected ischemia.

In our society, about 50% of men and women ultimately die of cardiovascular disease (CVD) (2). CHD is the leading cause of morbidity and mortality among the elderly. Of all CHD deaths on a yearly basis, 85% occur in those aged 65 years and older (3). In the Framingham cohort, among hypertensive subjects aged 65 to 89 years, approximately 50% of both men and women had a history of CVD, including angina pectoris and myocardial infarction (MI) (4). This review of IHD in the elderly hypertensive patient discusses current recommendations for evaluation and management of coronary risk factors, subclinical CHD, chronic stable angina, and the spectrum of acute coronary syndromes (ACS), which includes unstable angina (UA), non-ST-segment elevation MI (NSTEMI), and ST-segment elevation MI (STEMI). In the spirit of evidence-based medicine, whenever possible, studies in elderly patients have been utilized for recommendations.

However, elderly people and women have been underrepresented in randomized clinical trials. Between 1966 and 1990, published trial enrollment of patients aged 75 years and older averaged 2% (5). This increased to 9% during 1991 through 2000. Similarly, among women, enrollment rose slightly from 20% to 25%. Both represent significant underenrollment when compared with prevalence of disease. For this reason, recommendations are extrapolated from randomized clinical trial data observed in younger patients when necessary. In addition, registry and observational databases, which often contain a wealth of information regarding patients of all ages, are used to support certain recommendations. Finally, although *geriatric* is a term generally used to define those 65 years and older, further age partitioning is frequently seen in the literature; for example, the youngest-old are defined as those between 65 and 74 years. If clinically important, any differences across "old age" are addressed.

RISK FACTORS IN THE ELDERLY

The elderly continue to comprise a larger and larger segment of the American population as people live longer and the birth rate drops. In the 2000 US Census, nearly 35 million Americans aged 65 years and older (12.4%) were counted (6). By the middle of the 21st century, it is projected this group will number 80 million or 20% of the total population. As the geriatric population grows, an important and controversial issue

Table 1
Guide to Primary Prevention of Cardiovascular Disease and Stroke in Adults

Risk intervention	Goal
Smoking	Complete cessation; no exposure to second-hand smoke.
Hypertension	Blood pressure <140/90 mmHg; <135/85 if CRI or CHF present; <130/80 if diabetes present
Hypercholesterolemia	Primary goal: LDL-C <160 mg/dL, if one or less risk factor; <130 mg/dL if two or more risk factors and 10-year CHD risk <20%; and <100 mg/dL if two or more risk factors and 10-year CHD risk ≥20% or presence of DM or PVD Secondary goal: Non-HDL-C Other targets: TG >150 mg/dL, HDL-C <40 mg/dL in men and <50 in women
Diabetes	Near-normal fasting plasma glucose (<110 mg/dL) and HbA_{1c} < 7%
Physical activity	At least 30 minutes of moderately intense physical activity on most days; may need physician clearance to initiate exercise program (exercise stress test?)
Weight management	Achieve and maintain desirable weight (BMI 18.5–24.9 kg/m^2); when BMI ≥25, waist circumference at the iliac crest ≤40 inches in men and ≤35 inches in women.
Diet	Match energy intake with energy needs; saturated fat <10% of calories, cholesterol <300 mg/day, salt <6 g/day

BMI, body mass index; CHD, coronary heart disease; CHF, congestive heart failure; CRI, chronic renal insufficiency; HbA_{1c}, indicator of glycosylated hemoglobin; HDL-C, high-density lipoprotein cholesterol; LDL-C, low-density lipoprotein cholesterol; non-HDL-C, total cholesterol minus HDL-C; TG, triglycerides. (Adapted from ref. 7.)

is the need for treatment of coronary risk factors in the elderly. Consensus statements have been issued for prevention of cardiac morbidity and mortality in patients with and without known CHD (7,8). Table 1 details recommendations issued for primary prevention of CVD and stroke in adults (7). These are based on investigations performed primarily in nonelderly patients but are presumed suitable for all adults.

Current life expectancy in the United States at the time of birth is 79.8 years in women and 74.4 years in men (9). Once a person achieves the age of 80 years, it is estimated that the individual is likely to survive an additional 8 years. However, living longer is not equivalent to aging better. Women, as a group, live on average 5 years longer than men, but they spend twice as much time disabled before death (10). Thus, the focus in the elderly must be not only treatment, but also prevention as a way to enhance quality of life.

Recent research suggests that coronary artery plaque rupture is correlated with a low-grade inflammatory state related to the presence of one or more uncontrolled risk factors (11). Vascular inflammation and increased risk of a coronary event are predicted by an elevated high-sensitivity C-reactive protein (hs-CRP) level. As demonstrated in a follow-up to the Air Force/Texas Coronary Atherosclerosis Prevention Study, a randomized primary prevention clinical trial performed in 5742 patients (aged 45–73 years), lovastatin was effective in reducing the risk of acute coronary events not only in subjects with elevated low-density lipoprotein cholesterol (LDL-C) level regardless of hs-CRP level but also in those with low LDL-C and high hs-CRP (12).

One argument against treating risk factors in the elderly is that the cumulative effect of decades of exposure cannot be significantly countered at such a late stage. This line of thinking concludes that the risk–benefit ratio does not support the use of potentially toxic drugs in the elderly. However, if treatment of risk factors were also likely to stabilize atherosclerotic coronary artery plaques in the elderly, then such treatment would shift the balance away from the vulnerable plaque, lessening the likelihood of rupture and ACS. Because ACS is more lethal among the elderly and particularly so among those 80 years and older (13), substantial benefit from efforts aimed at plaque stabilization are to be expected. Coronary mortality has been declining in the general population, including the elderly, since 1970 (14). This generalized benefit suggests that advances in medical interventions or therapies are potentially responsible for the observed improved prognosis among all subsets of the population.

The coronary risk factor profile overall worsens with age, although tobacco use and obesity decline in the elderly (15). Definite hypertension is present in nearly 50% of men and in 60% of women aged 75 years and older from the Framingham cohort. Among those 65 to 74 years, the corresponding numbers are 38% and 48%, respectively. Isolated systolic hypertension (ISH) is the predominant form of hypertension among the elderly. The risk of MI associated with ISH is increased two- to threefold among the elderly. CHD is the most common cardiovascular outcome of hypertension in Framingham study subjects aged 65–94 years, outnumbering stroke, peripheral vascular disease (PVD), and congestive heart failure (CHF) (4). Hypertension may be, but generally is not, an isolated risk factor among the elderly, found in less than 20%.

Other major risk factors tend to cluster with hypertension in increasing proportion based on presence and degree of central obesity, conferring greater risk of an adverse cardiovascular event. Two or more additional risk factors occur in 50% of people with hypertension. This association of risk factors is called the *metabolic* or *insulin resistance syndrome*, which is characterized by hypertension, central obesity, type 2 diabetes mellitus (DM), and dyslipidemia *(16)*. The last is characterized by elevated triglyceride fraction, depressed high-density lipoprotein cholesterol (HDL-C) fraction, and accumulation of atherogenic, small, dense LDL-C particles. This syndrome is promoted by visceral adiposity and, as such, has been increasingly seen in all segments of the general population, including children, in association with doubling of obesity prevalence over the past decade.

A recently popularized concept is risk equivalence *(17)*. The most powerful predictor of future major cardiovascular events over the succeeding 10 years is current clinical presence of atherosclerosis in coronary and noncoronary beds. Thus, PVD, symptomatic carotid artery disease, and abdominal aortic aneurysm (AAA) are considered risk equivalent to known CHD. This was shown to hold true for subjects 65 years or older in the Cardiovascular Health Study, a longitudinal study that included more than 6000 elderly men and women *(18)*. Interestingly, this relationship held even for subclinical CHD. Type 2 DM is now classified as a potent risk equivalent for CHD.

Using the preceding line of thinking, the National Cholesterol Education Program Adult Treatment Panel III (ATP-III) guidelines for treatment of lipids recommended lowering LDL-C below 100 mg/dL in patients (a) with known CHD; (b) in risk-equivalent disease processes, including PVD, symptomatic carotid artery disease, AAA, and DM; and (c) in patients with multiple coronary risk factors that confer a 10-year CHD risk greater than 20% *(17)*. These guidelines went on to recommend calculation of 10-year risk using gender-specific multivariable scoring instruments derived from prospective Framingham Study data in all subjects with two or more risk factors (Fig. 1). Using age (20–79 years), systolic blood pressure (treated or untreated), total cholesterol, HDL-C, and smoking status, the 10-year predicted CHD risk (%) is derived. A 10-year risk less than 10% is considered low risk, 10–20% confers intermediate or moderate risk, and greater than 20% is high risk, mandating aggressive primary prevention. *A priori*, those with a history of CHD, PVD, symptomatic carotid artery disease, AAA, or DM are considered to have risk equivalence for CAD and require aggressive primary/secondary prevention.

Another concept promoted by the ATP-III guidelines is assessment of the total burden of disease. Global risk assessment recognizes the importance of nontraditional risk factors, which include *life habit risk factors* (obesity, physical inactivity, atherogenic diet) and *emerging risk factors* (hs-CRP, homocysteine, lipoprotein[a], fibrinogen, and subclinical

Estimate of 10 – Year Risk of CHD for Men and Women (Framingham Point Scores)

Age (y)	Points M	Points F
20-34	-9	-7
35-39	-4	-3
40-44	0	0
45-49	3	3
50-54	6	6
55-59	8	8
60-64	10	10
65-69	11	12
70-74	12	14
74-79	13	16

TCHOL (mg/dl)	Points Age 20-39y M	Age 20-39y F	Age 40-49y M	Age 40-49y F	Age 50-59y M	Age 50-59y F	Age 60-69y M	Age 60-69y F	Age 70-79y M	Age 70-79y F
<160	0	0	0	0	0	0	0	0	0	0
160-199	4	4	3	3	2	2	1	1	0	1
200-239	7	8	5	6	3	4	1	2	0	1
240-279	9	11	6	8	4	5	2	3	1	2
≥280	11	13	8	10	5	7	3	4	1	2

Tobacco	Points Age 20-39y M	Age 20-39y F	Age 40-49y M	Age 40-49y F	Age 50-59y M	Age 50-59y F	Age 60-69y M	Age 60-69y F	Age 70-79y M	Age 70-79y F
Nonsmoker	0	0	0	0	0	0	0	0	0	0
Smoker	8	9	5	7	3	4	1	2	1	1

HDLC (mg/dl)	Points M F
≥60	-1
50-59	0
40-49	1
<40	2

SBP (mmHg)	Points Untreated M	Untreated F	Treated M	Treated F
<120	0	0	0	0
120-129	0	1	1	3
130-139	1	2	2	4
140-159	1	3	2	5
≥160	2	4	3	6

Point Total and 10-Year Risk, %

M		F	
<0	<1	<9	<1
0	1	9	1
1	1	10	1
2	1	11	1
3	1	12	1
4	1	13	2
5	2	14	2
6	2	15	3
7	3	16	4
8	4	17	5
9	5	18	6
10	6	19	8
11	8	20	11
12	10	21	14
13	12	22	17
14	16	23	22
15	20	24	27
16	25	≥25	≥30
≥17	≥30		
Total	Male % Risk	Total	Female % Risk

Fig. 1. Multivariable Framingham scoring tool developed for estimation of 10-year risk of coronary heart disease. BP, blood pressure; HDL, high-density lipoprotein. (Adapted from ref. *17*.)

CVD) *(19)*. Although the nontraditional risk factors do not modify the LDL-C goal, they can be used in concert with traditional risk factors to guide the intensity of risk-reduction therapy.

SUBCLINICAL CARDIOVASCULAR DISEASE

Because subclinical CVD was found to be an important predictor of future cardiac events among the elderly in the Cardiovascular Health Study, it is appropriate to consider whether detection of subclinical CHD and of the related risk equivalents PVD, symptomatic carotid artery disease, AAA, and DM is indicated. This would allow targeted therapy of those most at risk for future cardiovascular events. More than 40% of men and women in the Cardiovascular Health Study were demonstrated to have subclinical CVD *(18)*. In the elderly, more than 30% of all MIs are unrecognized. This is especially common in men with DM and in both men and women with hypertension *(15)*. Among the latter, an astounding one of two MIs is clinically silent or unrecognized. Elderly patients, especially women, are more likely to describe symptoms atypical for the diagnosis of coronary ischemia when presenting with angina or an ACS. The most common anginal equivalent symptom in elderly women is exertional or rest dyspnea.

Thus, diagnosis of subclinical CVD requires more than historical information offered by the patient. One suggested approach is to perform noninvasive screening tests, which are specific for different vascular beds. In many cases, the physical exam may suggest the suspected diagnosis and the indicated screening test. For example, after auscultation of a femoral artery bruit, measurement of the ankle–brachial blood pressure ratio, if 0.9 or less, is highly suggestive of significant PVD and is associated with a threefold higher rate of CHD death, MI, and vascular death *(20)*.

In elderly patients with dyspnea, performance of an electrocardiogram (ECG) may yield findings diagnostic for previous MI. Likewise, performance of a two-dimensional echocardiogram allows visualization of myocardial wall motion abnormalities secondary to previous non-Q-wave as well as Q-wave MI. The only clue suggesting left ventricular dysfunction may be a soft systolic murmur secondary to mitral regurgitation, a frequent finding after inferior or posterior MI. Significant carotid artery stenosis is usually diagnosed after auscultation of a classic bruit or after a patient presents with symptoms consistent with transient ischemic attack. Carotid ultrasonography can be used to quantitate internal carotid artery luminal stenosis and intima-media thickness, both indicators of atherosclerotic burden.

Treatment of subclinical CVD in healthy elderly people is supported by observational databases. Both the ankle–brachial blood pressure ratio and carotid artery intima-media thickness have been shown to predict CVD in the elderly independently of traditional cardiac risk factors *(20)*. Although many feel screening for subclinical disease may be an appropriate use of resources in a healthy elderly population, recommendation of this approach by a consensus panel awaits results of randomized clinical trials.

CHRONIC ANGINA

Patients with chronic stable angina represent the majority of cardiology outpatient and inpatient visits. It is estimated that for every patient with an acute MI who survives to hospital admission, 30 people have a history of chronic stable angina *(21)*. In 1999, there were 550,000 patients in the United States (60% were 65 years and older) hospitalized for acute MI, but more than 16 million people, the majority geriatric, required treatment for chronic angina.

In 1995, using a Medicare diagnosis and payment database, chronic IHD was the diagnosis in 95% of elderly patients hospitalized with the diagnosis of CAD and undergoing cardiac catheterization during the same admission *(21)*. In that same year, the prevalence of chronic IHD in people 65 years and older was 83 per 1000 men and 90 per 1000 women *(22)*. This increased to 217 per 1000 men and 129 per 1000 women among those 75 years and older. At autopsy, nearly 50% of women and 80% of men demonstrate significant obstructive CAD *(23)*.

An important challenge is diagnosis of CHD in the elderly, for whom atypical symptoms predominate, most commonly dyspnea and CHF. It is hypothesized that these presentations are related to an exaggerated rise in left ventricular mean and end-diastolic pressures during ischemia, mediated through reduction in left ventricular compliance in association with LVH *(24)*. The increased frequency of angina equivalent symptoms in addition to predominance of NSTEMI infarcts may in large part explain the underdiagnosis of CAD in the elderly, especially among women, for whom acute MI eludes diagnosis in 50% of cases. After diagnosis of IHD or MI, studies have shown decreased use of proven beneficial therapies in the elderly, such as aspirin, β-blocking drugs, and angiotensin-converting enzyme (ACE) inhibitors *(25)*.

Just as in younger patients, a key goal in geriatric patients with chronic angina is secondary prevention measures. Table 2 details recommendations for secondary prevention of CVD and events in patients with established coronary and other vascular disease. Three of the classical Framingham risk factors deserve special attention. Those considered

Table 2
Guide to Secondary Prevention of Cardiovascular Disease and Stroke in Adults With Coronary and Other Vascular Disease

Risk intervention	Goal
Smoking	Complete cessation; no exposure to second-hand smoke
Hypertension	Blood pressure <140/90 mmHg; <135/85 if CRI or CHF present; <130/80 if diabetes present
Hypercholesterolemia	Primary goal: LDL-C <100 mg/dL
	Secondary goal: If TG ≥200 mg/dL, then non-HDL-C should be <130 mg/dL; if TG 200–499 mg/dL, consider fibrate or niacin after LDL-C lowering; if TG ≥500, consider fibrate or niacin before LDL-C lowering
	Other targets: TG >150 mg/dL, HDL-C <40 in men and <50 in women
Diabetes	Near-normal fasting plasma glucose (<110 mg/dL) and HbA_{1c} <7%.
Physical activity	At least 30 minutes of exercise daily using exercise stress testing to guide recommended intensity; medically supervised programs are indicated in higher risk patients
Weight management	Achieve and maintain desirable weight (BMI 18.5–24.9 kg/m^2); when BMI ≥25, waist circumference at the iliac crest ≤40 inches in men and ≤35 inches in women
Diet	Match energy intake with energy needs; saturated fats <7% of total calories, total fat 25–35%; carbohydrates 50–60%; protein 15%; dietary fiber 20–30 g/day; cholesterol <200 mg/day; salt <4g/day

See Table 1 for definitions of abbreviations. (Adapted from ref. 8.)

essential to secondary prevention in the geriatric age group are hypertension, tobacco, and lipid management. The Systolic Hypertension in the Elderly Program was the first trial to investigate the treatment of systolic hypertension in those 60 years and older (mean age 71 years) (26). After 5 years, the active treatment group had reduced incidence of cardiovascular events, stroke, and CHF.

The Systolic Hypertension in Europe trial found that active treatment in older adults led to a 42% reduction in stroke and 26% reduction in cardiac events after 2 years (27). A parallel study, the Systolic Hypertension in China trial, found that treatment of systolic hypertension reduced stroke by 38%, cardiovascular mortality by 58%, and all cardiovascular events by 37% (28). A meta-analysis of eight trials contributing nearly

16,000 patients over the age of 60 years with ISH found a treatment advantage resulting in 30% reduction in stroke and 26% reduction in cardiovascular events *(29)*.

Results of the International Verapamil-Trandolapril Study, a randomized controlled trial (RCT) in hypertensive patients with stable CAD, were reported *(30)*. This trial included a significant percentage of elderly, female, and diabetic patients. The purpose was to compare death, nonfatal MI, and nonfatal stroke, as well as other measures of clinical efficacy, in those randomly assigned to treatment with verapamil sustained release or atenolol. Trandolapril and/or hydrochlorothiazide were added to achieve blood pressure goals recommended by the Sixth Report of the Joint National Committee on the Prevention, Detection, Evaluation, and Treatment of High Blood Pressure *(30a)*. After a follow-up period of 2 to 5 years, the study found that a calcium antagonist strategy with an ACE inhibitor was as effective clinically as a β-blocker with diuretic strategy. All major outcome trials of hypertension in the elderly are reviewed in Chapter 7 (*see* Table 4).

Patients with IHD who cease tobacco use accrue significant cardiovascular benefits within 1 year, including up to 25% reduction in mortality after MI. Even greater risk reduction is seen after 1 year with continuing tobacco abstinence *(31)*. The benefit in risk reduction extends to all age groups, including the geriatric population.

Most secondary prevention trials testing lipid lowering had upper age limits and enrolled predominantly younger patients. However, significant numbers of elderly patients were included in some studies and are available for subgroup analysis, testing the effect of age. Furthermore, trials typically lasted 5 to 6 years, extending the experience of statin use well into the eighth decade. The Scandinavian Simvastatin Survival Study enrolled patients with CAD and hypercholesterolemia and with an upper age limit of 70 years *(32)*. Of the 4444 men and women randomly assigned to placebo or simvastatin, 1021 between 65 and 70 years of age were enrolled. Cholesterol lowering with simvastatin produced similar relative risk reduction (34%) for major coronary events in patients 65 years and older when compared with those younger than 65 years. The absolute risk reduction for all-cause and for CHD mortality was significantly greater among simvastatin-treated older patients.

In the Cholesterol and Recurrent Events (CARE) trial, 4159 men and women with a history of MI and mild to moderate hypercholesterolemia were enrolled, providing age was below 75 years *(33)*. Pravastatin and placebo were randomly administered, and follow-up was performed at a median of 5 years. Of 1283 patients aged 65–75 years, major coronary events were reduced by 32% compared with 19% in those younger than

65 years. CHD mortality was decreased by 45% in the elderly group and by 11% in those younger than 65 years old.

The Long Term Intervention With Pravastatin in Ischemic Disease study enrolled 9014 patients with a previous history of ACS and a wide range of total cholesterol levels (155–271 mg/dL) for randomization to pravastatin or placebo *(34)*. There were 3514 patients enrolled between the ages of 65 and 75 years, the oldest age allowed. Among those on pravastatin, death from CHD was reduced by 22% in those younger than 65 years and by 23% in those older than 65 years after a follow-up period of 6 years. The combined end point of cardiac death and nonfatal MI was reduced by 22% in those younger than 65 years and by 21% in those older than 65 years.

The Prospective Pravastatin Pooling Project was devised in 1992 to pool data from three large pravastatin trials with similar designs but with enrollment of patients with differing degrees of risk for coronary events *(35)*. These trials included the West of Scotland Coronary Prevention Study, CARE study, and Long Term Intervention With Pravastatin in Ischemic Disease study. Using this large database, which includes 19,768 patients, and after stratifying by age (<55, 55–64, 65–75 years), there is a consistent reduction in risk of CHD death and MI, ranging between 21% and 32%. For those in the oldest decade, the percentage reduction in risk was 26%.

Because of the paucity of randomized clinical trial data in patients older than 75 years, several recently completed trials were designed to redress this deficiency. The Heart Protection Study enrolled 9515 patients older than 65 years of age at baseline (46% of the study population) *(36)*. After the 5-year treatment period, simvastatin reduced coronary and vascular events similarly in older and younger patients with a history of CVD, diabetes, or treated hypertension *(37)*. Risk of heart attack and stroke was reduced by more than 20% in both high-risk and lower risk patients on active treatment. The benefit of treatment was shared by women, patients with diabetes, and the elderly (over 70 years).

The Prospective Study of Pravastatin in the Elderly at Risk was designed to study pravastatin vs placebo in an older cohort (recruitment ages 70–82 years) with proven vascular disease of any kind or risk factors for vascular disease *(38)*. The primary end point of the study was combination of CHD death, MI, and stroke. Pravastatin reduced the primary end point by 15% after an average follow-up of 3.2 years. This reduction was driven by a nearly 20% reduction in coronary events *(39)*.

The National Cholesterol Education Program ATP-III evidence-based clinical guidelines for treatment of hypercholesterolemia specify that age is no barrier to treatment *(17)*. Data acquired since the last treatment guide was published in 1993 show that elderly at-risk patients up to age 78 years demonstrated similar benefit in risk reduction after LDL-C lowering, as did those younger than 65 years in both primary and secondary prevention trials.

A secondary goal after treatment of LDL-C lowering recommended by ATP-III is treatment of the metabolic syndrome in both primary and secondary prevention. As in younger patients, medical management of this syndrome in geriatric patients is inextricably connected to weight loss, exercise, and treatment of hypertriglyceridemia, low HDL-C, and insulin resistance. Exercise as a secondary prevention tool is complicated in the geriatric population by greater prevalence of osteoporosis, arthritis, pulmonary disease, PVD, poor vision, lack of social support, lack of a safe convenient environment conducive to ambulation, and dementia. Furthermore, devising an exercise prescription for an elderly patient with chronic IHD is often complicated by the atypical nature of anginal symptoms in the elderly. However, some studies have suggested an inverse relationship between physical activity and mortality among healthy older people with the diagnosis of CHD. In the British Regional Heart Study, light-to-moderate activity was associated with reduced mortality during 5-year follow-up in 5934 men (mean age 63 years) with CHD *(23)*.

To date, the most promising approach in older patients appears to be recommendation of frequent low-impact exercise, especially walking, combined with nutritional counseling. An optimal setting is found in formal cardiac rehabilitation programs, in which there is the potential also for socialization in a supportive environment. Unfortunately, insurance coverage for such programs in the elderly is limited, and the logistics of participation may deter a significant number.

The goals of pharmacological therapy and revascularization procedures in patients with chronic angina are twofold: first to prevent MI and death, and thus prolong life, and second to alleviate symptoms and reduce ischemia, thereby improving quality of life. Among the elderly, the emphasis is frequently shifted to quality of life. Of necessity, many of these recommendations are extrapolated from trials performed in a general population of patients with CAD. Aspirin and β-blocking drugs are indicated as first-line therapy, if tolerated.

Two studies in patients with stable angina showed a greater than 30% reduction in risk of adverse cardiovascular events attributable to aspirin usage *(40)*. Aspirin has been shown to protect against future vascular events in all subgroups of patients, including the elderly. Low-to-medium dosed (75–325 mg per day) aspirin is as effective as high-dose antiplatelet therapy and with fewer complications.

For those patients intolerant of aspirin, clopidogrel (75 mg per day) is a proven alternative *(41)*. β-Blockers have been shown to improve prognosis in ACS. In chronic angina, β-blockers effectively delay ischemia, leading to improvement in exercise duration *(21)*. In patients with conduction system disease, β-blockers may not be tolerated because of bradycardia or heart block.

Additional proven medical therapies in chronic angina are lipid-lowering agents, nitrates, and calcium antagonist drugs. As discussed, both the Scandinavian Simvastatin Survival Study and CARE studies demonstrated reduction in mortality and coronary event rates in patients with CAD treated with cholesterol-lowering medications. Nitrates improve both demand and supply ischemia and exert antiplatelet effects in patients with stable angina *(21)*. As anti-ischemic therapy, the combination of β-blockers and nitrates is more effective than either alone *(42)*. Randomized trials have shown that calcium antagonists are as effective as β-blockers in chronic angina *(21)*. Nitrates or β-blockers in combination with calcium antagonists produce greater anti-anginal efficacy than the individual components in stable angina. Heart rate-modulating calcium antagonists are relatively contraindicated in the setting of conduction disease and decompensated heart failure *(21)*. Randomized clinical trials have shown that hormone replacement therapy is not indicated for primary or secondary prevention of CHD in postmenopausal women *(43–45)*.

At clinical presentation, the elderly are more likely to have multivessel CAD, left main artery disease, moderate-to-severe target lesion calcification, and smaller reference diameter. In addition to beneficial medical therapies, percutaneous coronary interventions (PCIs) are offered less frequently to elderly patients *(46)*. When performed, studies suggest that initial angiographic success is comparable to that observed in younger patients after PCI when stents are employed. In addition, clinical restenosis rates are similar. However, there is an excess of periprocedural MI, hospital death, and bleeding complications among the elderly, particularly among women and octogenarians.

A pooled analysis of six multicenter stent trials, which included 301 (4.9%) patients 80 years and older, found an angiographic success rate equal to 97%, in-hospital mortality equal to 1.3%, and 1-year mortality equal to 5.7% *(47)*. Bleeding complications were present in 5%. Although angiographic success rate was similar among the remaining patients younger than 80 years old, mortality and bleeding complication rates were significantly better. Periprocedural MI was similar but higher than expected among the aged and nonaged groups, 9.6% vs 7.6%. This was attributed to greater use of rotational atherectomy prior to stenting, a procedure more commonly used during the study time period (1995–1999), and to complete ascertainment of cardiac enzyme data.

Other studies reported periprocedural MI rates between 0.4 and 2.2% among older patients *(48)*. Restenosis rates were similar among the aged and nonaged groups, 11.2% vs 11.9%. A single-center observational study examined stent procedure outcomes in 1238 patients undergoing procedures between January 1995 and October 1996 *(49)*. This cohort included 564 patients younger than 65 years old, 221 between 65 and 75 years, and 122 older than 75 years. At 6 months, event-free survival was 94.5%, 90.5%, and 89.3%, respectively (not significant). Death occurred, respectively, in 0.4, 0.5, and 1.6%; MI in 1.2, 2.3, and 1.6%; and target vessel revascularization in 4.3, 8.6, and 7.4% (not significant).

When employed in the elderly, especially in those older than 75 years or in those with significant comorbidities, PCI is often used as a palliative measure. Thus, culprit lesion intervention is performed in conjunction with ancillary antianginal medication as an alternative to coronary artery bypass grafting (CABG) surgery. Although this type of revascularization is considered incomplete, it is often an acceptable alternative with lower short-term morbidity and mortality.

CABG surgery is performed in the elderly for significant left main disease and/or severe three-vessel disease. Other accepted indications are multivessel (two or more vessels) disease with depressed left ventricular ejection fraction (40% or lower) or in the setting of the comorbidity diabetes *(21)*. However, with the recent introduction of sirolimus- and paclitaxel-coated stents, restenosis rates are now less than 5%, even among diabetics. Thus, PCI is assuming an increasing role in multivessel coronary revascularization.

In 1998, of all CABG procedures 21% were performed in patients 75 years or older. Despite this, there are few data from randomized clinical trials regarding this age group. Perioperative morbidity and mortality rise with age and are currently estimated to be less than 5% among patients 70 years or older. From the database of the Society of Thoracic Surgeons (1995–1996), a 4.7% mortality rate was described for octogenarians *(50)*. However, there was an excess of postoperative AF, stroke, and protracted hospitalization.

One recent review of clinical registry data, which included more than 161,000 CABG procedures performed between 1993 and 1998, found mortality rates of 5% to 8% in those 80 years and older when compared with 2% to 3% in those 60 years and younger *(51)*. In patients 75 years or older, there was a 3% to 6% risk of permanently disabling stroke or coma. In addition, less-overt but significant cognitive impairment was reported in up to 50% of elderly post-CABG patients *(52)*.

Despite the higher acute risk of CABG, one observational study found a 3-year survival rate of 77% in those 80 years and older treated with elective CABG vs 54% in those treated medically *(53)*. However, this may reflect a selection bias, with healthier patients selected for surgery. There appears to be no argument that elderly patients who survive CABG in the absence of major stroke report an improved quality of life with relief of symptoms and enhanced functional status.

ACUTE CORONARY SYNDROMES

Acute MI is underdiagnosed in the elderly. It is estimated that one-third of all MIs in those over 65 years are unrecognized as such *(54)*. This is particularly true in elderly hypertensive women, for whom up to 50% of MIs are unappreciated. Approximately 60% of all acute MIs occur in those 65 years and older, and 30% are in those 75 years or older *(55)*. One manifestation of acute MI, sudden cardiac death, increases with age *(56)*. Without treatment after acute MI, the mortality rate is 25% in those 75 years or older.

The term ACS has replaced many of the older terms used in the setting of suspected acute MI *(57,58)*. Included under this umbrella are UA, the closely related NSTEMI, and STEMI. Between 1991 and 2000, only 9% of patients enrolled in randomized clinical trials investigating ACS were 75 years and older *(6)*. Thus, many recommendations of necessity are supported by study results from younger patients. The diagnosis of ACS is often assigned at the time of emergency department triage so that the patient with anginal chest pain or with an anginal equivalent can be moved rapidly through a clinical pathway, which emphasizes immediate monitoring of the heart rhythm and performance and interpretation of a 12-lead ECG within 10 minutes (Figs. 2 and 3). Based on the ECG, patients with evidence of STEMI can be identified rapidly and urgent reperfusion measures undertaken, if appropriate. Those without ST elevation are classified as having UA/NSTEMI and treated accordingly.

UA/NSTEMI occurs after coronary plaque disruption leads to intracoronary formation of thrombus and platelet aggregation. It is believed that this process results in partial but not total occlusion of the vessel, although there are circumstances for which excellent collateral formation may forestall transmural infarction even in the setting of total occlusion of the vessel. UA and NSTEMI are closely related conditions but differ in severity. The distinction is made based on detection of myocardial damage using biomarkers such as troponin I, troponin T, and creatine kinase-MB *(57)*. In UA, there is no biomarker evidence of myocardial necrosis and transient or no ST segment and T-wave changes.

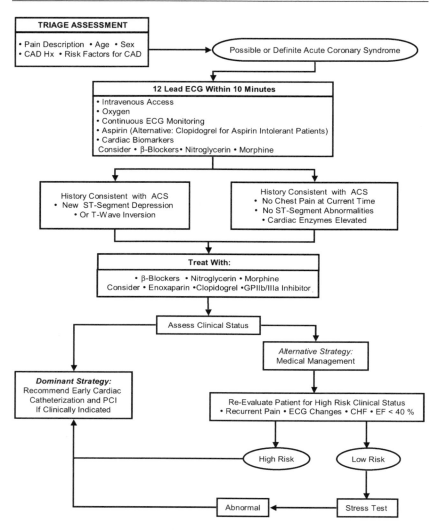

Fig. 2. Treatment guidelines for management of unstable angina and non-ST segment elevation myocardial infarction. ACS, acute coronary syndromes; CAD, coronary artery disease; CHF, congestive heart failure; ECG, electrocardiogram; Hx, history; PCI, percutaneous coronary intervention. (Adapted from ref. 57.)

In NSTEMI, biomarker evidence of myocardial necrosis is present, and ST segment depressions with evolutionary T-wave changes usually occur. The two conditions are grouped together because the initial evaluation and treatment are similar.

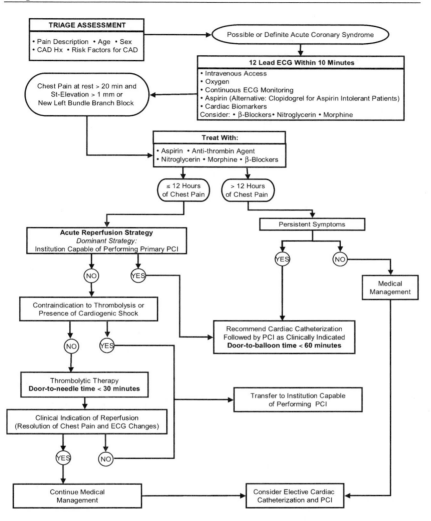

Fig. 3. Treatment guidelines for management of ST segment elevation myocardial infarction. CAD, coronary artery disease; ECG, electrocardiogram; Hx, history; PCI, percutaneous coronary intervention. (Adapted from ref. *58*.)

When presenting with ACS, the elderly are likely to exhibit atypical symptoms, including dyspnea, worsening heart failure, weakness, and confusion. Silent ischemia is more common among the elderly. They are more likely to have had a previous MI and harbor a greater atherosclerotic burden together with increased prevalence of comorbid diseases. In the Thrombolysis in Myocardial Infarction (TIMI) III registry, 25% of more than 3300 patients with UA or NSTEMI were 75 years or older

(59). Elderly patients in this registry were less likely to receive β-blockers and heparin and markedly less likely to undergo coronary angiography and revascularization, although angiography documented more extensive disease. The approximate relative risks of mortality and recurrent MI at 6 weeks were four times and two times that of younger patients, respectively.

Data from large clinical trials in ACS have shown that the highest risk of cardiac death is at the time of presentation *(60)*. For survivors, the risk declines thereafter, so that by 2 months, mortality rates equal the level present in patients with chronic stable angina. For this reason, a strategy for initial evaluation and management is essential.

Patients triaged with ACS but with normal or unchanged ECG and initially normal cardiac biomarkers can be observed in a chest pain or telemetry unit. Repeat ECG and cardiac biomarkers are obtained 6 to 12 hours after presentation. If negative, fast-track stress testing is performed.

Patients with enzyme or ECG abnormalities are admitted for aggressive antithrombotic and antiplatelet therapies (Fig. 2). In the absence of a contraindication, all such patients are treated with aspirin, clopidogrel, a β-blocker, antithrombin therapy, and a glycoprotein IIb/IIIa inhibitor *(57)*. Enoxaparin is preferable to unfractionated heparin as antithrombin therapy *(61)*. On this regimen, coronary angiography and PCI are frequently performed early, although there is a camp favoring a period of medical stabilization for 12 to 24 hours prior to angiography. This approach is described as the *early invasive strategy*. An alternative approach to routine angiography is the *early conservative strategy*, for which angiography is performed in those with recurrent ischemia or with a markedly positive stress test despite medical therapy *(62)*. In the TIMI IIIB study, there was a benefit in those patients 65 years and older who were treated with an early invasive strategy employing coronary angiography and PCI *(63)*. These patients had a lower incidence of death and reinfarction at 42 days. However, in the Veterans Affairs Non-Q-Wave Infarction Strategies in Hospital Trial, a more contemporary study, there was no benefit among the elderly of an early invasive strategy *(62)*.

Following angiography, a revascularization decision (PCI or CABG) can be made. It has been shown that an initial diagnosis of UA, when compared with chronic angina, does not influence survival 5 years after PCI or CABG *(64)*. Thus, the goals of revascularization in the elderly with UA/NSTEMI are similar to those with chronic angina. Indications were addressed in the preceding section. Implicit in the revascularization decision equation is the higher adverse event rate among the elderly. However, revascularization can be performed safely in many and should be considered despite chronological age.

Untreated STEMI is a lethal disease. Mortality increases with the number of ECG leads exhibiting ST segment elevation *(65)*. Approximately one-half of patients with acute MI die within the first hour, not surviving to hospitalization. Many presenting with STEMI delay seeking care for at least 2 hours, and some wait 12 hours or longer. After 12 hours, acute reperfusion therapy is generally of little benefit *(66)*. Because of time acuity, diagnosis and treatment of STEMI requires a structured approach (Fig. 3).

Following the ACS pathways, ECG is obtained within 10 minutes of emergency department entry for the complaint of ischemic chest pain. In the elderly, there should be a greater level of suspicion in those with atypical complaints such as dyspnea. After confirmation of ST segment elevation (>0.1 mV in two contiguous leads) or the diagnostic equivalent, new left bundle branch block, urgent revascularization is immediately performed, unless contraindicated, providing elapsed time from onset is less than 12 hours *(58)*.

Revascularization options currently include thrombolytic therapy and primary PCI. CABG is no longer performed routinely for acute treatment of MI. The temporal goal when using thrombolytic therapy follows the philosophy of "door-to-needle time" as 30 minutes or less. Similarly, for primary PCI, the temporal goal is a "door-to-ballooning time" window of 60 minutes. Rescue PCI refers to those who clinically fail thrombolytic therapy and then undergo PCI. Pooled data from nine trials of thrombolytic therapy vs control for acute MI showed a highly significant reduction in 35-day mortality (9.6% vs 11.5%), which in follow-up translated to improved long-term survival *(67)*.

Thrombolytic therapy is recommended (class I indication) for the treatment of acute STEMI in those younger than 75 years *(58)*. For those 75 years or older, thrombolytic therapy receives a class IIa indication. There may be decreased benefit with the use of thrombolytic therapy in those 75 years or older, but the consensus currently is that the absolute reduction in mortality supports its use unless contraindicated. It is preferable, however, that the patient be transferred expeditiously to a center with a primary angioplasty program if possible.

One dreaded complication of thrombolytic therapy is intracranial hemorrhage, which occurs more frequently among the elderly (age >65 years) *(68)*. Other clinical variables predictive of increased risk of stroke are weight less than 70 kg, hypertension, and use of alteplase. Risk of stroke increases with the number of predictive clinical variables present. Contraindications to thrombolytic therapy include active or potential bleeding sources, recent trauma or major surgery, known intracranial pathology, aortic dissection, severe hypertension ($\geq$180/110 mmHg), and bleeding diathesis *(58)*.

Thrombolytic therapy or PCI is performed for acute STEMI based on availability of 24-hour catheterization and/or PCI availability. It is estimated that 20% of US hospitals have cardiac catheterization laboratories to perform percutaneous revascularization or angioplasty for acute STEMI (58). Not all laboratories have engaged in full-time primary PCI programs because of the resources and staff commitment required. A meta-analysis of 10 randomized trials (2606 patients) comparing primary PCI vs intravenous thrombolysis for acute STEMI found 30-day mortality rates of 4.4% and 6.5% ($p = 0.02$), respectively (69). Primary PCI is a class I recommendation as an alternative to thrombolytic therapy in patients with acute STEMI (58). It is a class IIa recommendation in those who have a contraindication to thrombolytic therapy.

It is generally acknowledged that primary PCI is innately superior to thrombolytic therapy based on prevalence of TIMI III grade flow in the infarct-related artery after the alternative therapies (>90% vs <60%). In the Global Utilization of Streptokinase and t-PA for Occluded Coronary Arteries study, a trial comparing four regimens of thrombolytic therapy, the overall mortality rate was 7%, but 30-day mortality rates were 9.5%, 19.6%, and 30.3% in those 65–74 years, 74–85 years, and over 85 years (70). By way of comparison, primary PCI trials have shown a mortality rate of approximately 10% in patients older than 75 years (71). Both Global Utilization of Streptokinase and t-PA for Occluded Coronary Arteries IIb and the Primary Angioplasty in Myocardial Infarction I trials showed improved outcomes in older patients receiving primary PCI vs thrombolytic therapy (72,73).

The American College of Cardiology/National Cardiovascular Data Registry reported the results of 8828 PCI procedures performed from 1998 to 2000 in octogenarians (74). Among this group, in-hospital mortality was 1.35% in those without recent MI within 1 week. However, when performed within 6 hours of MI, there was a 10-fold increase in mortality to 13.8%. In the SHOCK (Should We Emergently Revascularize Occluded Coronary Arteries for Cardiogenic Shock) trial, patients older than 75 years undergoing emergency PCI for cardiogenic shock had a 41% higher mortality than those receiving aggressive medical therapy, including the use of intra-aortic balloon pump (75). Definitive recommendations for treatment of acute MI await randomized clinical trials in the elderly.

CONCLUSIONS

Hypertension is a major contributor to LVH, IHD, AF, and heart failure in older patients. Poorly controlled hypertension worsens symptoms of chronic angina and alters prognosis in ACS. Elderly patients of all ages benefit from medical therapies routinely accorded to younger patients for treatment of ischemia and for primary and secondary prevention of CHD. Implementation of some therapies may be impractical in elderly patients with comorbid diseases such as advanced cognitive disorders. When performed in suitable elderly patients, elective revascularization procedures such as CABG and PCI are effective with acceptable, although higher, complication rates.

There is insufficient RCT data in elderly patients with ACS to strongly recommend a single approach. However, available information from registries, observational studies, and subset analyses from RCTs suggests the following. Elderly patients younger than 75 years with ACS can be effectively managed in the same way as recommended by existing consensus statements with minimal increase in mortality and complication rates. Many patients older than 75 years with UA/NSTEMI can be managed using an early conservative strategy, allowing a period of medical therapy and stabilization prior to further risk assessment and invasive procedures. Some, with high-risk presentations, may benefit from an early invasive strategy.

Patients aged 80 years and older presenting with STEMI exhibit markedly increased mortality after thrombolytic therapy or primary PCI performed within 6 hours when compared with younger patients. Those older than 75 years with cardiogenic shock have a particularly high mortality when treated with primary PCI, which exceeds that demonstrated in similar patients treated with aggressive medical therapy and an intra-aortic balloon pump. Thus, many patients over age 80 and those over age 75 years presenting with cardiogenic shock will benefit from a period of medical stabilization prior to revascularization procedures. However, the risk–benefit ratio should be addressed prior to implementing a treatment plan in each patient over age 80 years presenting with STEMI and in those over age 75 years with cardiogenic shock.

REFERENCES

1. Treasure CB, Klein L, Vita JA, et al. Hypertension and left ventricular hypertrophy are associated with impaired endothelium-mediated relaxation in human coronary resistance vessels. *Circulation* 1993;87:86–93.
2. American Heart Association. 1998 Heart and Stroke Facts: Statistical Update. Dallas, TX: American Heart Association; 1998.
3. American Heart Association. 2001 Heart and Stroke Statistical Update. Dallas, TX: American Heart Association; 2000.
4. O'Donnell CJ, Kannel WB. Epidemiologic appraisal of hypertension as coronary risk factor in the elderly. *Am J Geriatr Cardiol* 2002;11:86–92.
5. Lee PY, Alexander KP, Hammill BG, et al. Representation of elderly persons and women in published randomized trials of acute coronary syndromes. *JAMA* 2001;286:708–713.

6. Hertzel L, Smith A. The 65 Years and Over Population: 2000 US Census Bureau. Washington DC, US Department of Commerce, Economics and Statistics Administration; 2001.
7. Pearson TA, Blair SN, Daniels SR, et al. Guidelines for primary prevention of cardiovascular disease and stroke: 2002 update. *Circulation* 2002;106:388–391.
8. Smith SC, Blair SN, Bonow RO, et al. AHA/ACC Guidelines for preventing heart attack and death in patients with atherosclerotic cardiovascular disease: 2001 update. *Circulation* 2001;104:1577–1579.
9. Arias E, Smith BL. Deaths: Preliminary Data for 2001. National vital statistics reports. Vol. 51, no. 5. Hyattsville, MD: National Center for Health Statistics; 2003.
10. LaCroix AZ, Newton KM, Leveille SG, et al. Healthy aging: a women's issue. *West J Med* 1997;167:220–232.
11. Ross R. Atherosclerosis—an inflammatory disease. *N Engl J Med* 1999;340:115–126.
12. Ridker PM, Rifai N, Clearfield M, et al. for the Air Force/Texas Coronary Atherosclerosis Prevention Study Investigators. Measurement of C-reactive protein for the targeting of statin therapy in the primary prevention of acute coronary events. *N Engl J Med* 2001;344:1959–1965.
13. Maggioni AP, Maseri A, Fresco C, et al. Age-related increase in mortality among patients with first myocardial infarctions treated with thrombolysis: the Investigators of GISSI-2. *N Engl J Med* 1993;329:1442–1448.
14. Kannel WB. Prevalence, incidence, and mortality of coronary heart disease. In: Fuster V, Ross R, Topol EJ, eds. *Atherosclerosis and Coronary Artery Disease.* Philadelphia, PA: Lippincott-Raven Publishers; 1996:13–21.
15. Kannel WB. Coronary heart disease risk factors in the elderly. *Am J Geriatr Cardiol* 2002;11:101–107.
16. Kannel WB, Wilson PWF, Silbershatz H, et al. Epidemiology of risk factor clustering in elevated blood pressure. In Gotto AH Jr, ed. *Multiple Risk Factors in Cardiovascular Disease: Strategies of Prevention of Coronary Heart Disease, Cardiac Failure.* Dordrecht, The Netherlands: Kluwer Academic; 1998:325–333.
17. Expert Panel on Detection, Evaluation, and Treatment of High Blood Cholesterol in Adults. Executive Summary of the Third Report of the National Cholesterol Education Program (NCEP) Expert Panel on detection, evaluation, and treatment of high blood cholesterol in adults (Adult Treatment Panel III). *JAMA* 2001;285:2486–2497.
18. Kuller L, Fischer L, McClelland R, et al. Differences in prevalence of and risk factors for subclinical vascular disease among black and white participants in the Cardiovascular Health Study. *Arterioscl Thromb Vasc Biol* 1998;18:283–293.
19. Greenland P, Abrams J, Aurigemma GP, et al. Prevention Conference V. Beyond secondary prevention: identifying the high-risk patient for primary prevention. Noninvasive tests of atherosclerotic burden. *Circulation* 2000;101:e16–e22.
20. O'Leary DH, Polak JF, Kronmal RA, et al. Carotid-artery intima and media thickness as a risk factor for myocardial infarction and stroke in older adults: Cardiovascular Health Study. *N Engl J Med* 1999;340:14–22.
21. Gibbons RJ, Chatterjee K, Daley J, et al. ACC/AHA/ACP-ASIM guidelines for the management of patients with chronic stable angina: a report of the American College of Cardiology/American Heart Association Task Force on Practice Guidelines. (Committee on Management of Patients with Chronic Stable Angina). *J Am Coll Cardiol* 1999;33:2092–2197.
22. National Center for Health Statistics. Current Estimates From the National Health Interview Survey, 1995. Hyattsville, MD: US Dept of Health and Human Services, Centers for Disease Control and Prevention; 1998. DHS publication (PHS) 98-1527.

23. Williams MA, Fleg JL, Ades PA, et al. Secondary prevention of coronary heart disease in the elderly (with emphasis on patients ≥ 75 years of age). *Circulation* 2002;105:1735–1751.
24. Lernfelt B, Wikstrand J, Svanborg A, et al. Aging and left ventricular function in elderly healthy people. *Am J Cardiol* 1991;68:547–549.
25. Krumholtz HM, Radford MJ, Wang Y, et al. National use and effectiveness of β-blockers for the treatment of elderly patients after acute myocardial infarction. *JAMA* 1998;280:623–629.
26. Systolic Hypertension in the Elderly Program Cooperative Research Group. Implications of the systolic hypertension in the elderly program. *Hypertension* 1993;21:335–343.
27. Staessen JA, Fagard R, Thijs L, et al. Randomized double-blind comparison of placebo and active treatment for older patients with isolated systolic hypertension. The Systolic Hypertension in Europe (Syst-Eur) Trial. *Lancet* 1997;350:757–764.
28. Liu L, Wang JC, Gong L, et al. Comparison of active treatment and placebo in older Chinese patients with isolated systolic hypertension. Systolic Hypertension in China (Syst-China) Collaborative Group. *J Hypertens* 1998;16:1823–1829.
29. Staessen JA, Gasowski J, Wang JC, et al. Risks of untreated and treated isolated systolic hypertension in the elderly: meta-analysis of outcome trials. *Lancet* 2000;355:865–872.
30. Pepine CJ, Handberg EM, Cooper-DeHoff RM, et al. A calcium antagonist vs a non-calcium antagonist hypertension treatment strategy for patients with coronary artery disease. The International Verapamil-Trandolapril Study (INVEST): a randomized controlled trial. *JAMA* 2003;290:2805–2816.
30a. The Joint National Committee. The Sixth Report of the Joint National Committee on Prevention, Detection, Evaluation, and Treatment of High Blood Pressure. Arch Intern Med 1997;157:2413–2445.
31. Gourlay SG, Benowitz NL. The benefits of stopping smoking and the role of nicotine replacement therapy in older patients. *Drugs Aging* 1996;9:8–23.
32. Miettinen TA, Pyorala K, Olsson AG, et al. Cholesterol-lowering therapy in women and elderly patients with myocardial infarction or angina pectoris: findings from the Scandinavian Simvastatin Survival Study Group (4S). *Circulation* 1997;96: 4211–4218.
33. Lewis SJ, Moye LA, Sacks FM, et al. Effect of pravastatin on cardiovascular events in older patients with myocardial infarction and cholesterol levels in the average range. Results of the Cholesterol and Recurrent Events (CARE) trial. *Ann Intern Med* 1998;129:681–689.
34. Hunt D, Young P, Simes J, et al. Benefits of pravastatin on cardiovascular events and mortality in older patients with coronary heart disease are equal to or exceed those seen in younger patients. Results from the LIPID trial. *Ann Intern Med* 2001;134:931–940.
35. Sacks FM, Tonkin AM, Shepherd J, et al. Effect of pravastatin on coronary disease events in subgroups defined by coronary risk factors: the Prospective Pravastatin Pooling Project. *Circulation* 2000;102:1893–1898.
36. Collins R, Peto R, Armitage J. MRC/BHF Heart Protection Study. Preliminary Results. *Int J Clin Prac* 2000;56:53–56.
37. Heart Protection Study Collaborative Group. MRC/BHF Heart Protection Study of cholesterol-lowering with simvastatin in 5963 people with diabetes: a randomized placebo-controlled trial. *Lancet* 2003;361:2005–2016.
38. Shepherd J, Blauw GJ, Murphy MB, et al. The design of a Prospective Study of Pravastatin in the Elderly at Risk (PROSPER). *Am J Cardiol* 1999;84:1192–1196.

39. Shepherd J, Blauw GJ, Murphy MB, et al. on behalf of the Prosper Study Group. Pravastatin in elderly individuals at risk of vascular disease (PROSPER): a randomized controlled trial. *Lancet* 2002;360:1623–1630.
40. Ridker PM, Manson JE, Gaziano JM, et al. Low-dose aspirin therapy for chronic stable angina. A randomized placebo-controlled clinical trial. *Ann Intern Med* 1991;114:835–839.
41. Caprie Steering Committee. A randomized, blinded trial of clopidogrel vs aspirin in patients at risk of ischemic events. (CAPRIE). *Lancet* 1996;348:1329–1339.
42. Waysbort J, Meshulam N, Brunner D. Isosorbide-5-mononitrate and atenolol in the treatment of stable exertional angina. *Cardiology* 1991;79(suppl 2):19–26.
43. Hulley S, Grady D, Bush T, et al. for the Heart and Estrogen/Progestin Replacement Study (HERS) Research Group. Randomized trial of estrogen plus progestin for secondary prevention of coronary heart disease in postmenopausal women. *JAMA* 1998;280:605–613.
44. Writing Group for the Women's Health Initiative Investigators. Risks and benefits of estrogen plus progestin in healthy postmenopausal women. Principal results from the Women's Health Initiative randomized controlled trial. *JAMA* 2002;288:321–333.
45. NHLBI Advisory for Physicians on the WHI Trial of Conjugated Equine Estrogens vs Placebo. Available at: www.nhlbi.nih.gov/whi/; March 2004. Accessed March 2004.
46. Peterson ED, Batchelor WB. Percutaneous intervention in the very elderly: weighing the risks and benefits. *Am Heart J* 1999;137:585–587.
47. Chauhan MS, Kuntz RE, Ho KL, et al. Coronary artery stenting in the aged. *J Am Coll Cardiol* 2001;37:856–862.
48. DeGregorio JD, Kobayashi Y, Albiero R, et al. Coronary artery stenting in the elderly: short-term outcome and long-term angiographic and clinical follow-up. *J Am Coll Cardiol* 1998;32:577–583.
49. Nasser TK, Fry E, Annan K, et al. Comparison of coronary artery stenting in patients < 65, 65–75, and > 75 years of age. *Am J Cardiol* 1997;80:998–1001.
50. Edwards FH, Carey JS, Grover FL, et al. Impact of gender on coronary bypass operative mortality. *Ann Thorac Surg* 1998;66:125–131.
51. Cheitlin MD, Gerstenblith G, Hazzard WR, et al. Do existing databases answer clinical questions about geriatric cardiovascular disease and stroke. *Am J Geriatr Cardiol* 2001;10:207–221.
52. Newman MF, Kirchner JL, Phillips-Bute B, et al. Longitudinal assessment of neurocognitive function after coronary artery bypass surgery. *N Engl J Med* 2001;344:395–402.
53. Ko W, Gold JP, Lazzaro R, et al. Survival analysis of octogenarian patients with coronary artery disease managed by elective coronary artery bypass surgery vs conventional medical treatment. *Circulation* 1992;86:II191–II197.
54. Kannel WB, Dannenberg AL, Abbott RO. Unrecognized myocardial infarction and hypertension. *Am Heart J* 1985;109:581–585.
55. Goldberg RJ, McCormick D, Gurwitz JH, et al. Age-related trends in short- and long-term survival after acute myocardial infarction: a 20-year population based perspective (1975–1995). *Am J Cardiol* 1998;82:1311–1317.
56. Zheng ZJ, Croft JB, Giles WH, Mensah GA. Sudden cardiac death in the United States, 1989 to 1998. *Circulation* 2001;104:2158–2163.
57. Braunwald E, Antman EM, Beasley JW, et al. ACC/AHA 2002 Guideline update for the management of patients with UA and non-ST-segment elevation myocardial infarction: a report of the American College of Cardiology/American Heart Association Task Force on Practice Guidelines (Committee on the Management

of Patients With Unstable Angina). 2002. Available at: http://www.acc.org/clinical/guidelines/unstable/unstable.pdf. Accessed March 2004.

58. Ryan TJ, Antman EM, Brooks NH, et al. ACC/AHA 1999 Guideline update for the management of patients with acute myocardial infarction: a report of the American College of Cardiology/American Heart Association Task Force on Practice Guidelines (Committee on the Management of Patients with Acute Myocardial Infarction). 1999. Available at: http://www.acc.org/clinical/guidelines/nov96/edits. Accessed March 2004.

59. Stone PH, Thompson B, Anderson HV, et al. Influence of race, sex, and age on management of UA and non-Q-wave myocardial infarction: the TIMI III registry. *JAMA* 1996;275:1104–1112.

60. PURSUIT Trial Investigators. Inhibition of platelet glycoprotein IIB/IIIA with eptifibatide in patients with acute coronary syndromes: receptor suppression using integrelin therapy. *N Engl J Med* 1998;339:436–443.

61. Antman EM, Cohen M, Radley D, et al. Assessment of the treatment effect of enoxaparin for UA/non-Q-wave myocardial infarction. TIMI IIB ESSENCE meta-analysis. *Circulation* 1999;100:1602–1608.

62. Boden WE, O'Rourke RA, Crawford MH, et al. Outcomes in patients with acute non-Q-wave myocardial infarction randomly assigned to an invasive as compared with a conservative management strategy. Veterans Affairs Non-Q-Wave Infarction Strategies in Hospital (VANQWISH) Trial Investigators. *N Engl J Med* 1998;338:1785–1792.

63. The TIMI IIIB Investigators. Effects of tissue plasminogen activator and a comparison of early invasive and conservative strategies in UA and non-Q wave myocardial infarction. *Circulation* 1994;89:1545–1556.

64. Jones RH, Kesler K, Phillips HR, et al. Long-term survival benefits of coronary artery bypass grafting and percutaneous transluminal angioplasty in patients with coronary artery disease. *J Thorac Cardiovasc Surg* 1996;111:1013–1025.

65. Mauri F, Gasparini M, Barbonaglia L, et al. Prognostic significance of the extent of myocardial injury in acute myocardial infarction treated by streptokinase (the GISSI trial). *Am J Cardiol* 1989;63:1291–1295.

66. National Heart, Lung, and Blood Institute. 9-1-1: Rapid Identification and Treatment of Acute Myocardial Infarction. Bethesda, MD: US Dept of Health and Human Services, Public Health Service, National Institutes of Health; May 1994. NIH publication 94-3302.

67. Fibrinolytic Therapy Trialists' (FTT) Collaborative Group. Indications for fibrinolytic therapy in suspected acute myocardial infarction: collaborative overview of early mortality and major morbidity results from all randomized trials of more than 1000 patients. *Lancet* 1994;343:311–322.

68. De Jaegere PP, Arnold AA, Balk AH, Simoons ML. Intracranial hemorrhage in association with thrombolytic therapy: incidence and clinical predictive factors. *J Am Coll Cardiol* 1992;19:289–294.

69. Weaver WD, Simes RJ, Betriu A, et al. Comparison of primary coronary angioplasty and intravenous thrombolytic therapy for acute myocardial infarction: a quantitative review. *JAMA* 1997;278:2093–2098.

70. The GUSTO Investigators. An international randomized trial comparing four thrombolytic strategies for acute myocardial infarction. *N Engl J Med* 1993;329:673–682.

71. DeGeare VS, Stone GW, Grines L, et al. Angiographic and clinical characteristics associated with increased in-hospital mortality in elderly patients with acute myocardial infarction undergoing percutaneous intervention (a pooled analysis of the Primary Angioplasty in Myocardial Infarction trials). *Am J Cardiol* 2000;86:30–34.

72. Holmes DR, White HD, Pieper KS, et al. Effect of age on outcome with primary angioplasty vs thrombolysis. *J Am Coll Cardiol* 1999;33:412–419.
73. Stone GW, Grines CL, Browne KF, et al. Predictors of in-hospital and 6-month outcome after acute myocardial infarction in the reperfusion era: the primary angioplasty in myocardial infarction (PAMI) trial. *J Am Coll Cardiol* 1995;25: 370–377.
74. Klein LW, Block P, Brindis RG, et al. on behalf of the ACC-NCDR Registry. Percutaneous coronary interventions in octogenarians in the American College of Cardiology-National Cardiovascular Data Registry: development of a nomogram predictive of in-hospital mortality. *J Am Coll Cardiol* 2002;40:394–402.
75. Hochman JS, Sleeper LA, Webb JG, et al. Early revascularization in acute myocardial infarction complicated by cardiogenic shock. Should We Emergently Revascularize Occluded Coronary Arteries for Cardiogenic Shock (SHOCK) investigators. *N Engl J Med* 1999;341:625–634.

14 Cerebrovascular Disease in the Elderly Hypertensive

Fenwick T. Nichols III, MD, FACP

CONTENTS

INTRODUCTION
OVERVIEW
STROKE SUBTYPES
HYPERTENSION AND DEMENTIA
CONCLUSIONS
REFERENCES

INTRODUCTION

The term *cerebrovascular disease* encompasses a variety of specific disease states that affect the cerebral blood vessels and cause focal dysfunction of the central nervous system (CNS) (i.e., stroke) *(1)*. In 1997, approximately 160,000 people in the United States died from a stroke, making it the third leading cause of death, ranking behind heart disease and cancer *(2)*. Although there are many different risk factors for cerebrovascular disease, hypertension is the single biggest risk factor for all mechanisms of stroke. According to data from the American Heart Association *(2)*, more than half the population over the age of 65 years is hypertensive. Over the age of 75 years, nearly 60% of white men, 71% of black men, 76% of white women, and 78% of black women have hypertension. Hypertension increases the risk of intracerebral hemorrhage, subarachnoid hemorrhage (SAH), large artery infarction, cardiac-source embolic stroke, small artery disease, and cognitive decline. In patients with other causes of cognitive impairment, stroke can cause further cognitive decline. Treatment of hypertension, particularly early, may decrease the risk of stroke and cognitive impairment.

From: *Clinical Hypertension and Vascular Diseases: Hypertension in the Elderly*
Edited by: L. M. Prisant © Humana Press Inc., Totowa, NJ

This chapter first briefly reviews the overall mechanisms of nontraumatic hemorrhagic and ischemic strokes plus the major risk factors for cerebrovascular disease, with particular emphasis on the role of hypertension and cardiac disease. Then, each type of stroke within the two major categories is discussed in more detail, focusing on pertinent current research reports of epidemiological data, underlying pathology and related risk factors, clinical presentations and complications, plus diagnostic and treatment guidelines. The complicated interrelationship between hypertension and the various stroke subtypes is also addressed. Finally, a special section is devoted to dementia and hypertension, especially the numerous recent studies of the effects of midlife hypertension on the development of late-life dementia.

OVERVIEW

A disease of the elderly, 72% of those who suffer a stroke are over the age of 65 years. The estimated annual stroke rates for ages 65 to 74, 75 to 84, and older than 85 years are displayed in Table 1. Table 2 displays the estimated prevalence of stroke for these age categories. Of the currently estimated 720,000 strokes that occur every year, about 500,000 are first-time events, and about 200,000 are recurrent. It is estimated that in the year 2000 there were about 4.7 million stroke survivors.

The stroke death rate varies depending on the mechanism and size of stroke. The lowest 30-day mortality rate (about 5–15%) is seen with lacunar infarction and the highest (30–50%) with intracerebral hemorrhages. Between 1970 and 1995, the stroke death rate fell almost 70%. Since 1995, the death rate from stroke has remained essentially unchanged. Part of this decline has been presumed to be secondary to treatment of hypertension, resulting in a reduced incidence of intracerebral hemorrhage. Another factor may be better medical management of stroke patients who require hospitalization. The advent of computed axial tomographic (CT) scanning and magnetic resonance imaging (MRI) has significantly improved the ability to correctly identify strokes, especially smaller nonfatal ones, and reduced the number of deaths previously incorrectly attributed to stroke. This combination may also have contributed to the decline in stroke mortality.

Overall, 20% to 30% of those who suffer a stroke will die within the following year. More than half will die within 8 years. About 25% of patients who have a stroke will have a second one within the next 5 years. Of the survivors, 15% to 30% will remain permanently disabled, and 20% will require long-term institutional care. Older patients are less likely to have good functional outcomes than younger patients.

Table 1
Estimated Annual Stroke Rate Per 1000 Population
by Race, Gender, and Age

	Age in years		
	65–74	75–84	>85
White men	14.4	24.6	27.9
Black men	11.9	17.5	40.8
White women	6.2	22.7	30.6
Black women	16.1	22.4	0.0

From ref. 2.

Table 2
The Prevalence of Stroke by Age and Gender
(Percentage of Population)

	Age, years		
	65–74	75–84	>85
Men	4.0	5.9	12.5
Women	2.7	5.8	10.7

From ref. 2.

Stroke Mechanisms

Stroke is a clinical phenomenon characterized by the relatively abrupt onset of focal neurological dysfunction attributable to vascular disease of the CNS. The two major categories of stroke are hemorrhagic (accounting for 15–20%) and ischemic (accounting for 80–85%). This chapter does not cover traumatic hemorrhage. The following discussion refers only to nontraumatic hemorrhagic stroke, which may be differentiated into intraparenchymal and subarachnoid. Intraparenchymal hemorrhage (IPH) frequently results from the rupture of small penetrating arteries, which leads to local tissue injury, distortion of adjacent brain tissue, and increased intracranial pressure. SAH, usually the result of rupture of Berry aneurysms around the base of the brain, may cause sudden death or delayed vasospasm and subsequent cerebral ischemia. Ischemic stroke results from obstruction of arterial flow by local atherothrombosis, embolization, small vessel occlusion, or a more global process such as hypotension from myocardial infarction (MI), arrhythmia, or other systemic process.

As with all illnesses, treatment of stroke should primarily be aimed at prevention. Once the stroke has developed, there are two objectives of treatment. One is evaluation for appropriate hyperacute intervention, and the other is evaluation and institution of long-term management to prevent recurrent stroke. For ischemic stroke, when treatment can be delivered within 3 hours of onset, tissue plasminogen activator used under appropriate circumstances can improve the likelihood of functional recovery at 3 months *(3)*. Once patients are beyond this 3-hour time window, they need to be evaluated for the cause of the stroke so that appropriate secondary prevention can be directed at the underlying mechanism.

Risk Factors

To decrease the risk of development of stroke, patients and physicians need to recognize and manage its risk factors *(4)*. It is also important to understand that the more risk factors a patient has, the greater is the risk of stroke *(5)*. Age, hypertension, cardiac disease of any type, cigarette smoking, diabetes mellitus (DM), lipid abnormalities, transient ischemic attacks (TIAs), and prior strokes are considered the major risk factors for stroke.

Stroke risk increases with age. Over the age of 55 years, the risk of stroke almost doubles for every 10-year increase in age *(6,7)*. Although generally regarded as a nonmodifiable factor, it is likely that much of the risk from increasing age is actually caused by the summation of injury from other risk factors over time.

Cardiac disease of any type increases stroke risk, partly because of shared risk factors (hypertension, lipid abnormalities, smoking) as well as the increased risk of cardiac source embolism (MI, atrial fibrillation [AF], valvular heart disease, congestive heart failure [CHF]).

Cigarette smoking increases the risk of stroke in a dose-dependent fashion: smoking two packs of cigarettes a day doubles the risk of stroke *(8)*. Within 2 to 5 years of smoking cessation, stroke risk returns to the level of someone who never smoked *(9,10)*.

Patients with DM have a three- to sixfold increase in stroke risk, mostly attributable to hypertension, which occurs in 40% to 70% of this population. Tight blood pressure (BP) control significantly reduces stroke risk for these individuals *(11)*. Although tight control of blood glucose appears to decrease the risk of diabetic microvascular complications (retinopathy, peripheral neuropathy), it does not appear to decrease stroke risk.

When lipid abnormalities are evaluated in relationship to all causes of stroke, there is no increased risk of stroke *(12)*. However, patients with low high-density lipoprotein cholesterol (HDL-C) and high low-density lipoprotein cholesterol (LDL-C) are at increased risk of large artery atherosclerosis and the development of carotid artery disease (CAD), as well as CAD with resultant cardiac source embolism. Statins have been shown to decrease future stroke risk in patients with CAD and elevated cholesterol *(13)*.

TIAs and prior stroke increase the risk of subsequent stroke. Overall, approximately 25% of patients who have suffered a stroke will have another one within the following 4 to 5 years. Patients who experience a TIA have a 15% risk of stroke within the following month and a 30% to 50% risk of stroke in the following 5 years *(14)*. The actual risk of stroke following a TIA is probably best predicted by the cause of the TIA. A high-grade carotid stenosis has an associated 20% to 35% risk of stroke in the following 2 years. The combination of AF, CHF, and hypertension carries about a 34% risk of developing a stroke over the following 2 years.

Other potential risk factors for stroke include race, family history, obesity, sedentary lifestyle, alcohol abuse, and homocystinemia.

Hypertension is a major risk factor for all types of stroke and is the single most modifiable variable for stroke prevention. Treatment of hypertension is effective for both primary and secondary stroke prevention *(15–22)*. There is a linear correlation between elevated BP and stroke risk. The Framingham Study data indicated that patients with hypertension had about a fourfold increase in risk of atherothrombotic cerebral infarction compared to normotensive patients. Their data indicated that, even in younger patients, systolic blood pressure (SBP) was as strong a predictor of stroke risk as diastolic blood pressure (DBP) or pulse pressure *(23,24)*. Higher stroke risk begins within the normal range of BP and progressively rises with increasing BP *(12,16)*. In some series, elevation of DBP appears to be a more important determinant of stroke risk for patients under the age of 65; over age 65 years, SBP elevation assumes increasing importance in determining stroke risk.

Although stroke incidence markedly increases in patients with SBPs greater than 160 mmHg, it should be noted that the majority of strokes occur in those with SBPs below this level. Although BP reduction only decreases stroke risk a small amount in a given year, the cumulative benefit appears much greater, with not only a decreased stroke risk but also a preservation of cognitive function (which is discussed later in this chapter). Treatment of elevated BP significantly reduces stroke risk. For a 6 mmHg reduction in DBP, there is a 42% risk reduction for the development of stroke *(16,17)*.

Isolated systolic hypertension becomes increasingly frequent with increasing age, occurring in approximately 20% of men and 30% of women over 80 years of age. Borderline systolic hypertension, defined as isolated SBP between 140 and 160 mmHg, has been shown to significantly increase stroke risk. One study found that borderline hypertension was associated with a 42% increase in stroke risk even after controlling for other identifiable risk factors *(25)*. Treatment of isolated systolic hypertension has been clearly demonstrated to reduce stroke risk. Both the Systolic Hypertension in the Elderly Program (SHEP) *(26)* and the Systolic Hypertension in Europe (Syst-Eur) study *(27)* have demonstrated a significant decrease in stroke risk when isolated systolic hypertension is treated. There was a 36% relative risk reduction of stroke in the SHEP treatment arm and a 42% relative risk reduction in that of Syst-Eur.

Left ventricular hypertrophy (LVH) is also a risk factor for stroke. LVH increases in prevalence with increasing age as well as with increasing BP. Many authors have thought that the increased stroke risk with LVH best correlated with the presence of hypertension (with LVH suggesting suboptimal BP control); others have thought that other variables such as minority race, obesity, or genetics might contribute to the association of LVH with stroke risk *(28,29)*.

STROKE SUBTYPES

Hemorrhagic Stroke

SUBARACHNOID HEMORRHAGE

The term *stroke* is used for the clinical phenomenon of abrupt onset focal neurological dysfunction secondary to either ischemia or hemorrhage involving vessels of the CNS (Fig. 1). About 10% of all strokes result from nontraumatic SAH. The age-specific incidence of SAH increases with increasing age *(6,30)*. Although there are a number of possible causes of blood leakage into the subarachnoid space (e.g., Berry aneurysms, mycotic aneurysms, arteriovenous malformations, coagulopathies, amyloid angiopathy), some patients have no identifiable etiology.

Most SAHs, however, arise from rupture of Berry aneurysms around the base of the brain *(31)*. The majority of Berry aneurysms occur at branch points in the internal carotid artery (ICA) distribution, particularly at the takeoff of the posterior communicating artery, the anterior communicating artery, and the middle cerebral artery (MCA) bifurcation. These aneurysms are most likely the result of congenital and acquired degenerative changes in the artery. Local hemodynamics also

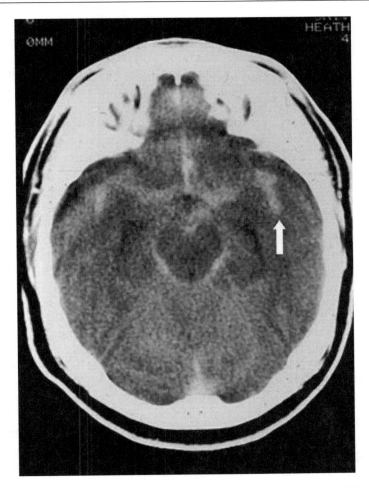

Fig. 1. Computed tomographic scan of brain showing a subarachnoid hemor-rhage. There is high density (blood) in the subarachnoid space around the upper brain stem and in the Sylvian fissures. The arrow points to blood in the left Sylvian fissure. Patient had a posterior communicating artery aneurysm that ruptured.

plays a role. It has been noted that patients with anatomic variants of the circle of Willis who have increased volume flow through the anterior or posterior communicators have a higher incidence of aneurysms than those with a normal circle of Willis. Risk factors for SAH include cigarette smoking, hypertension, alcohol abuse, and family history of SAH *(32)*.

The usual clinical presentation of SAH is the abrupt onset of head-ache, usually described as the worst headache of the patient's life. There may be sudden loss of consciousness at the time of onset. Of these patients, 15% to 30% die at the onset of hemorrhage. Another 30% die in the first 30 days after the presenting hemorrhage. A number of complications from SAH contribute to its high mortality, including early rebleeding, hydrocephalus, vasospasm, hyponatremia, seizures, and cardiac arrhythmias.

In general, for patients in reasonable clinical condition, early surgical clipping or possibly coiling of the aneurysm is appropriate to minimize the risk of rebleeding. Most patients with SAH receive nimodipine to decrease the risk of symptomatic vasospasm. The greater the volume of subarachnoid blood, the greater is the risk of developing symptomatic vasospasm. Vasospasm tends to begin about day 3, peak around days 7 to 10, and begin to resolve about day 14. In those patients who do develop symptomatic vasospasm, treatment is usually hypervolemic hemodilution with induced hypertension (triple H therapy); balloon angioplasty of the vasospastic vessels has been used for those who fail triple H therapy.

Intraparenchymal Hemorrhage

IPH accounts for approximately 10% of strokes. Hypertension is the most common cause of IPH, accounting for 60 to 80% of nontraumatic IPHs (32). Hypertension damages small penetrating end arteries that arise from the MCA stem (the lenticulostriates), the posterior cerebral (thalamoperforates), and the basilar (pontine penetrators). Hypertensive injury to these small arterioles, which has been variously referred to as segmental disorganization, fibrinoid necrosis, or hyaline arterionecrosis (33), usually develops over a number of years; however, acute increases in BP may occasionally cause rupture of these same vessels. Hypertensive IPHs tend to occur in the putamen (~50%), the thalamus (about 10%), pons (about 10%), and cerebellum (about 10%). The best treatment is primary prevention by treatment of the hypertension.

Surgical treatment for the putamenal, thalamic, and pontine IPHs improves survival but generally does not improve functional outcome. However, hemorrhage into the cerebellum is a potentially life-threatening emergency, and neurosurgical intervention may be lifesaving. One series found that 26% of IPHs enlarged within the first few hours, and that by 24 hours after onset, 38% had increased in size (34). Although the cause of this size increase has not been clearly determined, it does not appear to be related to the degree of hypertension. However, most stroke physicians recommend reducing the BP by at least 20% in patients who have elevated BP with a clinical picture consistent with hypertensive hemorrhages.

Hypertensive IPHs occur when very small vessels bleed, so they are low-pressure hemorrhages with relatively slow expansion, unlike the high-pressure hemorrhage of SAH. The clinical presentation tends to be a relatively rapid onset (over seconds to minutes) focal neurological deficit. In hypertensive hemorrhage, if the bleeding extends beyond the original site, it tends to track along the white matter and may rupture into the ventricular system. Hypertensive IPH almost never extends through the cortex, so the presence of hemorrhage crossing the cortex suggests a nonhypertensive etiology, such as coagulopathy, amyloid angiopathy, local vascular abnormality, or trauma. IPH causes CNS dysfunction by local tissue destruction and by distortion of adjacent tissue initially by the hematoma and later by hemorrhage-associated edema. To date, no controlled randomized trials have demonstrated that any therapy, including BP control, decreases the risk of hypertensive IPH enlargement.

Occasionally, IPH occurs in association with anticoagulation, particularly in patients on warfarin. In these cases, the hemorrhage may have a slowly progressive expansion, taking place over many hours to days. Treatment requires reversal of the anticoagulation (by either vitamin K or fresh frozen plasma), with surgical intervention occasionally necessary after reversal of the anticoagulation.

Cerebral amyloid angiopathy (CAA) is a disease of the aging population. It generally begins to appear after the age of 60 years and increases in frequency with increasing age. This amyloid is not that seen with systemic amyloidosis, but it is similar to that seen in the senile plaques of Alzheimer's disease (AD). There is no significant correlation between the severity of AD and the presence of CAA; it has been noted that some patients with severe pathological changes of AD do not have amyloid angiopathy; others with minimal AD pathology have significant amyloid deposition in the cerebral vessels.

In amyloid angiopathy, there is deposition of amyloid material in the walls of cerebral cortical arterioles, in the meninges, in the cortical arterioles, and in the medullary penetrating arterioles. This deposition is thought to make these arterioles stiff and noncompliant. In addition, some pathological series have reported an inflammatory component in the media that could predispose to vessel weakening and increased risk of rupture.

Patients with CAA may have IPH (Fig. 2) that occurs in the absence of recognized head trauma or other precipitating events. CAA-associated hemorrhages also frequently recur. Unlike hypertensive IPHs, these hemorrhages are frequently large and lobar in location, and they usually extend through the cortex into the subadjacent white matter. They may also extend into the subarachnoid space, and some may even extend deep

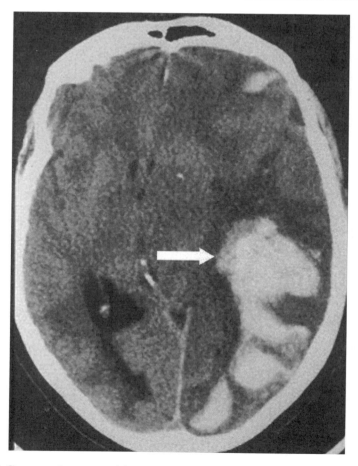

Fig. 2. Computed tomographic scan of brain showing a hemorrhage from amyloid angiopathy. Arrow indicates large area of high density in left posterior temporal, parietal, and occipital lobes, with smaller area in left frontal lobe. Significant mass effect with shift of the midline from left to right.

into the ventricular system. In typical cases, the age of the patient, the lobar location of the hemorrhages, as well as the extension into the cortex and subarachnoid space distinguish CAA hemorrhages from hypertensive hemorrhages (35). However, in a number of cases the neuroimaging is not specific, and it is only after a repeated lobar hemorrhage that the diagnosis becomes more apparent. There is no specific treatment other than symptomatic management. CAA hemorrhage does not appear to be related to hypertension; however, there does appear to be an association between CAA with small deep infarctions and lowered BP. This is discussed later in this chapter.

Other causes for IPH include arteriovenous malformation, mycotic aneurysm, venous infarction, hemorrhagic conversion of an ischemic infarction, coagulopathy, bleeding into tumors, and unrecognized trauma.

Ischemic Stroke

Ischemic injury results from inadequate delivery of blood to the parenchyma, usually caused by atherosclerotic narrowing, superimposed thrombus on atherosclerotic narrowing, embolism, hypercoagulable states, vasculitis, or hypotension. Most series attempt to classify ischemic strokes into several categories: lacunar, large artery atherothrombotic, cardiac source embolism, other defined cause, and cryptogenic (or infarction of undefined cause).

LARGE ARTERY ATHEROSCLEROTIC DISEASE

Extracranial cerebral artery atherosclerosis accounts for about 10% of all strokes. It most commonly occurs in the origin of the ICA, at the level of the common carotid artery bifurcation. The bifurcation is located near the angle of the jaw, at about the level of the third and fourth cervical vertebrae. Bruits are frequently heard at this level when there is local stenosis.

The major risk factors for carotid bifurcation atherosclerosis are the same as those for coronary artery disease: hypertension, low HDL-C, elevated LDL-C, cigarette smoking, and DM. White males are more likely to develop stenosis at this site than white females. Approximately 90% to 95% of symptomatic large cerebral artery atherosclerosis in whites is located at the common carotid bifurcation, with the remainder located in the intracranial arteries, primarily the distal internal carotid and proximal MCA. An estimated 20% of patients with peripheral arterial disease (PAD) will have a stroke caused by carotid artery disease. About 25% of patients with symptomatic ICA stenosis will have symptomatic CAD, with another 25% having asymptomatic CAD (36).

Atherosclerosis may cause cerebral ischemia by two mechanisms: (a) the stenosis may become severe enough, either by increasing plaque size or superimposed clot, to restrict flow and produce distal hypoperfusion, and (b) atherosclerotic-related material may embolize and lodge distally, obstructing flow. The embolic material can originate from plaque rupture, resulting in a cholesterol embolism. Also, the irregular surface of the plaque, particularly under the high-shear stress associated with significant stenosis, may promote either platelet fibrin aggregation or red clot formation; this material may then embolize distally. Clot formation and embolization are more likely to occur with more severe stenosis.

Patients with severe ICA stenosis or occlusion do not always develop a stroke. Collateral flow may provide adequate perfusion to the ICA territory to prevent the occurrence of symptomatic ischemia. The major collateral pathways are across the circle of Willis via the anterior and posterior communicating arteries. Other potential sources of collateral flow are from branches of the external carotid through the ophthalmic artery to the distal ICA and via end-to-end connections between the distal branches of the major intracranial arteries (middle cerebral, anterior cerebral, and posterior cerebral), referred to as leptomeningeal collaterals.

At least 50% of patients with stroke secondary to large artery atherostenosis report a TIA prior to the development of infarction. The territory supplied by the affected artery determines TIA symptoms. Because the ophthalmic artery arises from the ICA, ocular TIAs caused by ICA stenosis are ipsilateral to the stenotic artery and usually consist of amaurosis fugax (also referred to as transient monocular blindness). Patients with amaurosis fugax usually describe the sensation of "a shade descending over one eye." There is no associated pain or other symptom. The visual loss usually lasts 3 to 5 minutes and then resolves, much like fog disappearing in the morning. Rarely, small embolic-appearing material may be seen on funduscopic exam during or after the symptoms (37). The cerebral symptoms of ICA territory TIAs most typically consist of contralateral weakness and/or numbness of the lower face and distal arm, with associated dysarthria. More severe episodes of ischemia may result in weakness and/or numbness of the contralateral face, arm, and leg, with accompanying language disturbance (dominant hemisphere) or nondominant behavioral syndrome, depending on which hemisphere is affected (38,39).

Based on the results of the North American Symptomatic Carotid Endarterectomy Trial, the currently recommended treatment for symptomatic patients with greater than 70% stenosis of the ICA origin is carotid endarterectomy (40,41). In this trial, patients with greater than 70% stenosis who had experienced a TIA or minor stroke were randomly assigned to best medical therapy vs carotid endarterectomy plus best medical therapy. After a 2-year follow-up, the stroke rate in the best medical treatment arm was 26%, whereas it was only 9% in the surgical arm. Carotid endarterectomy can be safely performed in appropriately selected very elderly patients (42). Several trials are under way to evaluate the potential role of carotid angioplasty and/or stenting in the management of ICA origin stenosis.

A racial difference exists in the location of symptomatic cerebral arterial stenosis *(43)*. Although whites have the majority of their symptomatic stenosis in the origin of the ICA, African-Americans and Asians have 30% to 50% of their symptomatic large artery disease located intracranially. Intracranial arterial stenosis is also seen more frequently in Asians and African-Americans, patients with poorly controlled hypertension, and patients with DM. The distal ICA is the most frequent site of intracranial arterial stenosis, followed by the proximal middle cerebral, the distal vertebrals, and the basilar. Atherosclerosis only rarely affects the anterior and posterior cerebral arteries *(44)*. The best treatment for intracranial arterial stenosis is not yet known. Aggressive management of associated risk factors coupled with antiplatelet therapy or anticoagulation is the usual first line of therapy.

EMBOLIC STROKES

Embolic infarcts account for 15% to 30% of all strokes. This wide range of estimates partly reflects the variations among various research studies' definitions of embolic stroke. Studies that have used radiographic criteria for embolism have found a higher frequency of embolic strokes; those that required proof of a definite embolic source have reported a lower incidence. The heart is the most frequently identified source of embolic stroke, with AF accounting for approximately 50% of cardiac source embolism. CAD, which accounts for another 25%, may produce embolism in several ways: acute MI can cause embolism by either the formation of thrombus on necrotic endomyocardium or triggering atrial arrhythmias; later, ventricular aneurysms (a late effect of MI) may also be a source for embolic particles. Prosthetic valves contribute up to 10% of cardiac source emboli. Other cardiac causes of embolism include dilated cardiomyopathy, mitral annulus calcification, aortic valve calcification, endocarditis, atrial myxoma, and paradoxical embolism through a right-to-left cardiac shunt.

AF is the most studied of these cardiac stroke risk factors. The prevalence of AF increases with increasing age. Present in approximately 0.5% of the population under the age of 60 years, it increases to more than 9% over 80 years of age. Hypertension, because of its high prevalence in the elderly, appears to be the single most important risk factor for the development of AF *(45,46)*. Diabetes also increases the risk of AF. AF's attributable risk for stroke increases with increasing age. Between 50 and 59 years, there is a 1.5% attributable risk to AF; however, this increases to a 23.5% attributable risk in the population over 80 years. Among patients with AF, there is a 3–5% per year cumulative risk of embolic stroke. AF, when combined with CHF, hypertension, and prior embolic event, increases the risk of embolic stroke to 17% per year.

Warfarin therapy, with an international normalized ratio of 2 to 3, decreases stroke risk by 70 to 80% (47,48).

Another potential cause for cerebral embolism is aortic arch atheroma with superimposed clot. Autopsy studies, as well as transesophageal echocardiogram studies, have documented the frequent finding of aortic arch atheroma. There appears to be an increased risk of stroke associated with the presence of large thick plaques, especially those with a mobile component (thrombus) that may embolize and result in stroke. The actual incidence of embolism from aortic arch plaque is not clear, but those patients who have strong clinical and imaging evidence of embolic stroke should be considered for transesophageal echocardiogram to evaluate the aortic arch (49,50).

LACUNAR INFARCTIONS

Lacunar infarctions (51) account for about 20% of all strokes (Fig. 3). They are usually the result of hypertensive injury to the penetrating arteries of the brain, particularly in the basal ganglia, internal capsule, thalamus, pons, and corona radiata. Many of these areas are the same sites where hypertensive hemorrhage may occur. The major risk factor for lacunar strokes is hypertension. In the presence of hypertension, diabetes and cigarette smoking appear to increase the risk of developing lacunes as well.

Fisher (51) defined lacunes as small deep infarctions, less than 1.5 cc in volume, attributable to occlusion of a penetrating artery that arises from a large cerebral artery. In general, these arterioles are 100 to 400 µm in diameter and arise from much larger conduit arteries, namely, the middle cerebral, posterior cerebral, and basilar. Lacunes have only rarely been described in the white matter above the ventricles. The medullary penetrators that arise from the cortical arteries supply this area of white matter, referred to as the centrum semiovale. Other unusual causes of small deep infarctions include embolism, with the embolic material obstructing the origin of a single penetrator and resulting in a lacunar-size infarction. More frequently, emboli will block the larger artery that gives rise to the penetrator, resulting in infarction in the territory of a number of penetrators; these infarctions are much larger than the typical lacune and strongly suggest occlusion of the parent vessel. Lacunar-size infarctions have also been described in cases of vasculitis, chronic meningitis with secondary vasculitis, hypercoagulable states, and polycythemia.

Prior to high-resolution neuroimaging, lacunes were diagnosed clinically. Several well-described clinical syndromes have been defined, including pure motor hemiparesis, pure sensory stroke, and ataxic hemiparesis. These strokes may have a variable onset, with some beginning

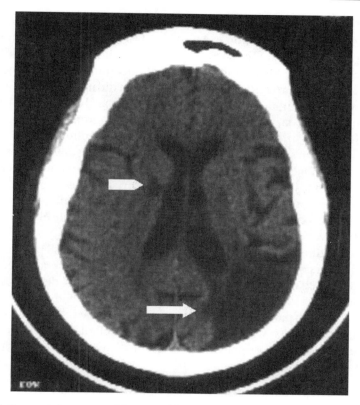

Fig. 3. Computed tomographic scan of brain with the large block arrow pointing to a large area of old infarction in the left parietal lobe with evidence of volume loss with dilation of the adjacent sulci and the ipsilateral ventricle. The smaller pointed arrow is indicates a lacune in the white matter adjacent to the right lateral ventricle.

relatively suddenly, and up to 30% have a stuttering onset over a maximum 36-hour period *(52,53)*. Because these strokes are small and located deep within the brain, they are unlikely to be associated with aphasia, higher cortical dysfunction, visual field cuts, altered levels of consciousness, or headache; the presence of any of these suggests a larger volume of brain injury than that seen with lacunes.

Patients who suffer multiple lacunar strokes may develop the "lacunar state" or *état lacunaire*. In this situation, there are usually several lacunes, with bilateral brain involvement. The patient may have a nasal dysarthric voice, difficulty swallowing, short-stepped shuffling gait, emotional lability, and occasionally urinary incontinence. This phenomenon occurred much more frequently prior to the advent of antihypertensive therapy.

SILENT CEREBRAL INFARCTION

Silent cerebral infarction is a term used to describe the MRI finding of asymptomatic hyperintensities consistent with prior stroke with no clinical correlate. Most of these are small, deep infarctions. However, some are larger cortically based infarctions that did not involve the motor strip and had initial symptoms that were primarily behavioral (e.g., Wernicke aphasia, nondominant behavioral syndrome) and were not identified as a stroke. The definition of silent infarction is not entirely consistent from study to study, making exact comparisons between studies difficult. One group has reported that patients with silent infarcts and white matter lesions had a five times greater risk of developing a stroke over 4.2 years of follow-up than did those without silent infarcts. Although the relative risk was increased, it should be noted that the absolute risk was only 6% over the entire 4.2 years of follow-up (54).

The Cardiovascular Health Study, which assessed 5888 people older than 65 years, reported on a subset of 1433 patients who underwent two MRI scans separated by 5 years. Between the scans, 254 developed new MRI lesions (81% lacunes); only 11% of these lesions had clinical symptoms. Although participants were cognitively similar at the time of their initial exams, those who developed silent infarctions had a more rapid cognitive decline. Those patients who had greater white matter abnormalities on the initial scan were more likely to develop silent infarcts (55).

Treatment of Blood Pressure to Prevent Stroke

It has been well documented that treatment of hypertension decreases the risk of stroke. It appears that any class of medication that lowers BP will decrease stroke risk. Previous reviews (56) have demonstrated an approximately 40% risk reduction for a 6-mm decrease in DBP. This applied across all ranges of BP and occurred with all antihypertensive agents (57,58). Two large studies, SHEP and Syst-Eur, have shown that treatment of isolated systolic hypertension can decrease stroke risk by approximately 40% (26,59).

There is a great deal of interest in the possibility that specific antihypertensive agents or classes of antihypertensives might have greater benefit than others. The Antihypertensive and Lipid Lowering Treatment to Prevent Heart Attack Trial (18) has demonstrated that hydrochlorothiazide was as or more effective in lowering BP *and* reducing stroke risk than a calcium channel blocker (amlodipine) or an angiotensin-converting enzyme inhibitor (lisinopril). The Losartan Intervention for Endpoint reduction in hypertension trial compared losartan with atenolol in hypertensives with LVH and demonstrated a similar BP reduction for the two agents but a lower stroke event rate for losartan

(60). Studies such as the Losartan Intervention for Endpoint raise the hope of identifying an agent or class of agents that will offer benefits beyond simple BP reduction. This remains a very exciting research topic with promising, but inconclusive, data about the effects of different antihypertensives on stroke risk reduction.

A large overview *(16)* demonstrating that BP levels are directly and continuously associated with stroke risk and that lowering BP reduces stroke risk not only suggested that those at highest risk of stroke (particularly those with prior stroke) might benefit the most from lowering BP but also suggested that BP reduction in patients with what was previously labeled as "normal" BP might result in stroke risk reduction. Several studies evaluating patients with prior strokes have reported that lowering BP, even in patients with no documented hypertension, decreases stroke risk.

The Heart Outcomes Prevention Evaluation trial evaluated the treatment of patients older than 55 years who were at high risk for future cardiovascular events because of a history of prior CAD, cerebrovascular disease, or PAD or who had diabetes plus one additional risk factor. At baseline, the average age was 66 years, mean BP was 139/79 mmHg, and 46% of the subjects had hypertension. Patients were treated with ramipril (titrated to 10 mg) or placebo and followed for an average of 4.5 years. BP decreased 3.8/2.8 mmHg. There were 156 (3.4%) on ramipril who had a stroke vs 226 (4.9%) on placebo, a 30% relative risk reduction *(61,62)*.

Several authors attributed the benefit of ramipril to a nonhypertensive effect, such as improvement in endothelial function or anti-atherosclerotic effects. However, one group reported on 24-hour BPs in 38 patients with PAD who participated in the Heart Outcomes Prevention Evaluation trial. They found that the 24-hour ambulatory BP was reduced by 10/4 mmHg in patients on ramipril; this reduction occurred primarily at nighttime. It was these authors' suggestion that the reduction in stroke risk could be explained solely by the degree of BP reduction over the 24-hour period *(63)*.

The Perindopril Protection Against Recurrent Stroke Study (PROGRESS) *(19)* was another trial that looked at BP reduction with the angiotensin-converting enzyme inhibitor perindopril alone or in combination with indapamide, if needed, in 6105 hypertensive and nonhypertensive patients (entry BP 136/79 mmHg) who had suffered a stroke or TIA. Patients were enrolled an average of 8 months after their event, with a range of 2 to 22 months. Patients received standard care for secondary stroke prevention, including antiplatelet therapy. Patients already receiving antihypertensive medications continued them. About

14% of patients dropped out during the "run-in period" (before random-ization) because of medication side effects. Over 4 years of follow-up, active treatment reduced BP by 9/4 mmHg. There were 307 strokes (10%) in the treated group and 420 strokes (14%) in the placebo group. Those patients treated with perindopril alone had their BP reduced by 5/3 mmHg and had no discernible reduction in stroke. Those patients treated with the combination of perindopril and indapamide, received by 58% of patients, had a reduction in their BP of 12/5 mmHg and had a 43% relative risk reduction for stroke. For the combination therapy, there was a 42% risk reduction for hypertensives (93/948 vs 159/955) and a 44% risk reduction for nonhypertensive (57/822 vs 96/819). These reductions are what would be predicted based on the intensity of the BP lowering *(16)* and do not necessarily indicate a specific drug or class benefit.

These two studies strongly indicate that patients who have had a stroke should have their BP lowered, even if they are normotensive. At this time, it is not clear if the reduction in future stroke risk is drug/class specific or simply a reflection of the degree of lowered BP. It is also unclear to what extent BP should be lowered in the normotensive group.

HYPERTENSION AND DEMENTIA

With the reports that midlife hypertension is a risk factor for late-life dementia *(64–66)* and the demonstration that treatment of hypertension may lessen the risk of dementia *(62,67,68)*, there has been a great deal of interest in the concept of vascular dementia and the identification of those patients who might benefit from treatment *(69)*. A large number of studies investigating various aspects of the relationship of stroke, cog-nitive impairment, dementia, and hypertension are reported. There are a number of issues involved in dementia and vascular disease research that need to be understood to interpret the results of these studies. Any discus-sion of cognitive impairment and dementia proves challenging because nearly all aspects of dementia are subject to debate, including criteria for clinical, as well as pathological, diagnosis and subtyping of the demen-tia. This section provides the background information, summary of recent research findings, and discussion of current controversial issues necessary to interpret these findings.

Background

Dementia is defined as a decline in previously acquired cognitive abilities or skills. This means that the individual had at some point acquired a certain level of higher cognitive function and subsequently had a decline in or loss of that ability. Normal higher cognitive function is based on a complex neural network of interconnections for which subsets of various functions may be located in different parts of the brain. Some networks have overlapping functions, so that a specific area of the brain may participate in a number of different functions. As a result, isolated lesions may result in dysfunction of several different higher cortical systems; conversely, because of the overlapping networks, significant impairment of a single complex function usually requires relatively widespread disturbance of neural function *(70)*. The number and site of interconnections are the result of genetic as well as developmental/environmental factors. Some individuals are born with brains that have limited ability to develop complex interconnections, whereas others have the potential to develop and maintain generous synaptic connections. With normal aging, there is a gradual loss of neurons and of some specific cognitive abilities. Brains that had fewer connections initially will be less able to compensate for this normal neuronal and synaptic loss. Increased educational attainment has been found to reduce the risk of incident dementia, suggesting it may impart a neuronal reserve that delays the onset of clinical manifestations *(71)*.

Beyond normal aging, any process that causes additional loss of neurons and/or their connections in the brain may result in further loss of higher cognitive function. The effects of different insults to the CNS may be additive, so that processes as varied as head trauma, alcohol abuse, prior stroke, and neurodegenerative diseases may all contribute to the development of dementia. For this reason, many cases of dementia may actually be multifactorial, with greater or lesser contributions from different causes.

Dementia is primarily a disease of the elderly. As the population ages, the prevalence of dementia is increasing rapidly. In one frequently cited study *(72)*, it was estimated that 29.8% of patients over the age of 85 years were diagnosed as demented. Based on the Framingham data, the incidence of dementia is estimated to double every 5 years over the age of 65 years, increasing from 7.0/1000 for ages 65 to 69 to 118/1000 for ages 85 to 89 years *(73)*.

Dementia does not strike suddenly. In most cases, there is a gradual loss of function over time, usually many months to years. The loss may be so gradual that the family does not notice it until a stressful situation arises (such as a medical illness, spousal loss, or change in living environment), and the patient is unable to respond appropriately. With dementia, social skills tend to be preserved until very late in the course, so that patients may act socially appropriate even when they are mildly to moderately demented. Although families frequently report the patient has had a sudden change in cognitive ability at the time of some crisis, in retrospect, it is usually clear that the patient had been gradually losing the ability to handle tasks that were previously a part of his or her normal daily activities (e.g., such as handling the checkbook, driving, shopping, going to social functions).

Dementia that develops in patients with more educational attainment may be more difficult to identify. Even though by clinical history they are clearly no longer functioning at their previous level, they initially tend to score within the normal range on neuropsychological testing. It is this initial subtle loss of function that is difficult to identify and makes early recognition of cognitive impairment challenging.

As noted, the diagnosis of dementia is based primarily on clinical history and examination. There are a number of potentially treatable processes (such as, but not limited to, hypothyroidism, vitamin B_{12} deficiency, thiamine deficiency, renal failure, liver failure, hypoxia, neurosyphilis, medication effects) that may cause dementia or may worsen a coexisting dementia. Occasionally, multifocal brain dysfunction can present with the clinical appearance of slow cognitive decline. Multiple brain lesions, particularly those that disrupt frontal pathways but spare the motor pathways, may present as cognitive decline without other associated findings. On rare occasions, multiple sclerosis or primary and metastatic brain tumors may present in this fashion. As part of the routine evaluation of patients with dementia, a workup with laboratory investigation (including comprehensive metabolic profile, complete blood count, B_{12} level, thyroid functions, and rapid plasma reagin), chest X-ray, and brain imaging is usually performed to identify any potential treatable causes or contributors to the dementing illness.

Unfortunately, the most common dementing illnesses, such as AD, frontotemporal dementias, and vascular dementias, do not have a specific blood test or neuroimaging procedure that makes the specific diagnosis of dementia and identifies its etiology. The diagnosis of these "primary dementias" is based on the clinical history and exam, with laboratory tests and neuroimaging usually "ruling out" other possible etiologies of cognitive impairment. Although specific neuropsychological test results, neuroimaging characteristics, and neuropathological findings can be helpful in differentiating the dementia subtypes, they must be used cautiously, with an understanding of their strengths and weaknesses.

As noted, there is some expected gradual loss of higher cognitive functioning with age. Researchers are attempting to define the limits of normal age-related changes and differentiate them from the cognitive decline of early dementia. A number of different terms, such as mild cognitive impairment *(74,75)*, aging-associated cognitive decline *(76)*, and cognitive impairment with no dementia *(77)*, have been developed to address those patients who show very mild cognitive deterioration but do not yet meet standard criteria for dementia. Numerous studies are under way in an attempt to define the exact relationship of these states of mild cognitive impairment to the future development of dementia.

When reading about cognitive impairment and dementia, it must be recognized that estimates of the incidence and prevalence of dementia are determined by the criteria used to make the diagnosis of dementia *(78)*. There are a number of different criteria that may be used to make this diagnosis.

The Canadian Study of Health and Aging studied a randomly selected population of 1879 men and women over the age of 65 years (mean age 80 years) and used an extensive neurological and neuropsychological evaluation *(79)*. Based on the data from this testing, patients were classified as having "no cognitive loss," "cognitive loss but no dementia," and "dementia." The authors classified the patients using six commonly accepted sets of criteria: those from the *DSM-III* (*Diagnostic and Statistical Manual of Mental Disorders, Third Edition*), the *DSM-III-Revised*, the *DSM-IV*, ICD-9 (*International Classification of Diseases, Ninth Revision*), ICD-10, and the Cambridge Examination for Mental Disorders of the Elderly (CAMDEX). The frequency of the diagnosis of dementia was as follows: *DSM-III*, 29.1%; *DSM-III-R*, 17.3%; *DSM-IV*, 13.7%; *ICD-9*, 5.0%; CAMDEX, 4.9%; and *ICD-10*, 3.1%, an almost 10-fold difference between the lowest and the highest estimated prevalences. Only 20 patients from the entire sample met dementia criteria for all six classifications, indicating that the classification schema tended to identify different patients as having dementia *(79)*. This finding has caused some concern about the validity of comparisons between studies using different criteria for the diagnosis of dementia.

Not only the identification of dementia is somewhat problematic, but also the issue of separating dementing illnesses into various subtypes (AD, vascular, mixed, other defined, other ill defined) is challenging. Few subtypes of dementia can be accurately classified during life. Most classifications identify AD as the most common form of dementia, followed by either vascular dementia or mixed dementia. Most series state that about 80% of dementias are AD, 10% multi-infarct, and 10% "other." When patients clinically diagnosed as having AD in life undergo autopsy, the diagnosis is typically confirmed in 60 to 80% of cases *(80)*. As with the general diagnosis of dementia, the clinical criteria used to classify patients into subtypes of dementia for research purposes vary widely among studies.

Vascular Dementia

Although AD has received the most attention and been the target of most research, vascular dementia is beginning to be recognized as a potentially preventable cause of dementia and is becoming a topic of great interest. There has been a gradual evolution in the thinking about cerebrovascular disease causing dementia. Although the concept of arteriosclerotic dementia, which suggested that chronic ongoing hypoperfusion caused cognitive impairment, was popular early, it subsequently fell into disfavor. Stroke was not generally regarded as a common cause of dementia. Single strokes cause isolated dysfunction (such as aphasia, hemiparesis, nondominant behavioral syndromes), but do not usually cause global cognitive impairment (i.e., dementia). Multiple strokes, affecting different regions of the brain, can cumulatively cause a decline in higher cortical function, resulting in dementia.

Tomlinson et al. *(81)* observed that dementia was typically manifest from stroke only when the total volume of brain injured exceeded 100 cc, suggesting a threshold effect. However, it was recognized by others that cognitive impairment could result from small, well-placed strokes, indicating patients could have clinical dementia from single small lesions *(82)*. Hachinski and co-workers proposed the term *multi-infarct dementia* (MID) to identify those with repeated strokes who developed cognitive impairment. This was the basis for the Hachinski score, which has been used in a number of studies to identify those with vascular dementia *(83,84)*.

In a study of poststroke cognitive impairment, Tatemichi et al. *(85)* compared 227 patients (older than 60 years) at 3 months after their stroke with 240 stroke-free controls. Testing consisted of 17 scored items. They found that 35.2% of the poststroke patients and 3.8% of the controls had evidence of cognitive impairment, which most frequently affected memory, language, orientation, and attention. They noted that functional impairment was greater in those with cognitive impairment, with 55% of those having cognitive impairment requiring assistance compared to 32% of those with stroke but no cognitive impairment. They also reported that the risk of subsequent development of new-onset dementia was higher in patients who had had a stroke. They found that, at 52 months of follow-up, 34% of the stroke patients (older than 60 years) had developed dementia (*DSM-III-R* criteria) vs 10% of the stroke-free age-matched cohort *(86)*. Tatemichi et al. also demonstrated that the mortality rate was significantly greater (19.8 deaths per 100 years of follow-up) for those with dementia (diagnosed by *DSM-III-R* criteria) following stroke than for those without dementia (6.9 deaths per 100 years of follow up). This finding persisted even after adjusting the model for cardiac disease, severity of stroke (Barthel index), stroke type, and recurrent stroke *(87)*.

In an effort to focus more attention on the possible contribution of hypertensive injury to cognitive impairment through mechanisms other than clinically recognized stroke, Hachinski developed the term *vascular cognitive impairment* as a concept that includes all different degrees of intellectual decline associated with ischemic cerebrovascular disease *(88)*. A number of questions have been raised by vascular cognitive impairment research, particularly regarding identification and treatment, which are addressed here.

In an effort to differentiate multifocal discrete brain lesions (usually stroke) from diffuse degenerative brain disease (AD), most of the older criteria for vascular dementia required the identification of discrete focal neurological events (strokes or TIAs) and focal abnormalities on the neurological exam. Some required abnormalities on neuroimaging consistent with stroke. As with dementia in general, a number of different criteria have been proposed for the diagnosis of vascular dementia.

The five most commonly used criteria developed to make the diagnosis of vascular dementia are the National Institute of Neurological Disorders and Stroke–Association Internationale pour la Recherche et l'Enseignement en Neurosciences (NINDS-AIREN; *89)*, *ICD-10 (90)*, the Alzheimer's Disease Diagnostic and Treatment Centers (ADDTC; *91)*, *DSM-IV (92)*, and the Hachinski score *(93)*. One study directly compared these criteria in a classification of 167 elderly patients with probable dementia and found that the number of cases classified as vascular dementia differed significantly among the different guidelines. In this study, 45 were classified as vascular dementia by *DSM-IV* criteria, 23 by ADDTC, 21 by *ICD-10*, and 12 by NINDS-AIREN; only 5 cases met criteria for vascular dementia by all of the guidelines *(94)*. This pattern of variable criteria and classification schemes is similar to that seen with the diagnosis of dementia in general *(95)*.

There are efforts to develop newer classification schemes designed to identify those cases with isolated "subcortical" vascular dementia. Subcortical vascular dementia is thought to be primarily a small vessel disease, presumably from hypertensive injury. The hope is that the development of these criteria will allow clear identification of a group of patients, presumably with a common etiology, who might be entered into targeted therapeutic trials *(96)*.

Neuropsychological Testing

There are numerous neuropsychological tests that may be used in clinical practice to identify patients with dementia. Some of these instruments are more sensitive for memory disorders, some for executive function; some are heavily education dependent. Although an overlap in clinical deficits occurs, patients with AD tend to have more prominent memory deficits, whereas patients with subcortical dementia, the type that is more frequently seen with vascular dementia, tend to have more problems with mood and executive function. Tests that fail to evaluate executive function may fail to identify the cognitive impairment seen with subcortical dementias *(97)*.

Many studies have chosen to use a simple screening instrument, the Folstein Mini-Mental Status Exam (MMSE), to both identify and follow patients with dementia. This test is heavily education dependent, so that those normal individuals with higher education will score 30, and those who are normal but functionally illiterate will score about 21, a score that is classified as moderately demented in many studies *(98)*. In addition, the MMSE is heavily weighted toward assessment of memory and is much less sensitive to executive function deficits that are usually seen with subcortical white matter disease. As a result, the MMSE may fail to identify those patients with moderate cognitive impairment from multiple small deep infarctions.

Executive functions, including conceptual reasoning, inhibition of overlearned patterns of behavior, inhibition of responses to stimuli, mental flexibility, organizational ability, planning, regulation of working memory, and fluency of thought, may be better assessed by other instruments, such as the Stroop test *(99)*, card sorting *(100)*, and go-no go tests. The brief screening exams, such as the MMSE, have been used in a large number of trials because they offer easy and rapid testing; however, their sensitivity and specificity are less than ideal. Some researchers have chosen to use more detailed neuropsychological testing to identify and follow patients to minimize the risk of falsely classifying patients as normal or abnormal.

Neuroimaging

Many reports discuss the CT and/or MRI abnormalities used to make or corroborate the diagnosis of vascular dementia; however, because there are no well-defined universal criteria to describe lesions in the white matter, interpreting the similarities and differences in these neuroimaging data from different reports may be challenging *(101)*. With the advent of improved neuroimaging, initially with high-resolution CT scanners and later with MRI, previously unrecognized white matter abnormalities began to be identified. It rapidly became apparent that the relationship between high-signal white matter abnormalities and dementia is a complex one.

The MRI white matter high signals are not specific; they simply identify increased water content. A number of processes other than ischemia can produce these high-signal abnormalities, including infectious processes (such as abscess, acquired immunodeficiency syndrome encephalopathy, progressive multifocal encephalopathy), inflammation (such as multiple sclerosis), edema, metastatic disease, primary brain tumors, trauma, leukodystrophies (such as adrenoleukodystrophy, metachromatic leukodystrophy), sequelae of radiation or chemotherapy, Pick's disease, Wallerian degeneration, and vasculitis (from systemic vasculitis, chronic meningitis, or isolated CNS vasculitis). Simple identification of deep white matter changes does not make a diagnosis of vascular dementia or identify a specific pathology. The imaging findings need to be interpreted in light of the clinical picture. The variability in cause and location of these lesions may partly explain why different studies have drawn very different conclusions about the significance of these white matter lesions *(101)*.

There are several frequently seen MRI patterns of high-signal white matter abnormalities (Figs. 4–6): very small punctate lesions, slightly larger well-defined lesions, and larger more diffuse areas of hyperintensity frequently seen around the ventricular poles and along the ventricular walls (Figs. 5 and 6). The very small punctate lesions, 1 to 2 mm in diameter, are usually the dilation of the Virchow-Robin spaces and are thought to represent tissue rarefaction around penetrating arterioles that have become thickened and ectatic. Some reactive astrocytosis is usually seen in the perivascular region, and there may be accompanying serum protein leakage into the perivascular space. These changes have been referred to as *état crible*.

The larger, on the order of 3 to 10 mm, cavitary lesions usually represent lacunar infarctions. Rarely, these larger lesions can represent small hemorrhage residua (easily differentiated on MRI by the presence of hemosiderin rings), marked dilation of the Virchow-Robin space (usually seen in the inferior basal ganglia), or ventricular diverticula *(102)*.

There are several less-well-defined areas of high signal that may not represent ischemic injury. The high signal seen anterior to the frontal horns is normal, a result of tissue rarefaction in this area. The rims that may be seen along the lateral walls of the ventricles may simply represent breakdown of the ventricular lining with periventricular gliosis *(102)*. Other areas of white matter high-signal abnormality have been noted and variously described in different reports as periventricular, deep white matter hyperintensities, or subcortical hyperintensities; others have simply referred to them as white matter lesions. These abnormalities range from small discrete lesions to vaguely defined confluent areas. Hachinski et al. introduced the term *leukoaraiosis* to emphasize the heterogeneity of these high-signal lesions and to avoid any presumption about their etiology or pathological correlate *(103)*.

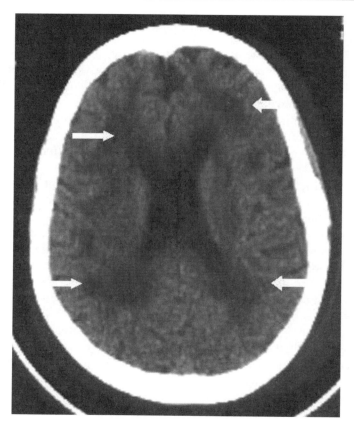

Fig. 4. Extensive leukoaraiosis in a computed tomographic scan of brain. Arrows point to areas of hypodensity of the white matter anterior and posterior to ventricles as well as in the white matter adjacent to the lateral aspects of the ventricles.

The presence of subcortical high-signal white matter lesions is most strongly associated with age. Many apparently normal elderly have white matter lesions *(104–107)*. Some reports have demonstrated a significant relationship between subcortical white matter hyperintensities and hypertension; others have not *(108,109)*. One report found a strong relationship between white matter lesions and the presence of uncontrolled hypertension, suggesting that the level of BP, particularly SBP, was related to the presence of these lesions *(110)*. The presence of white matter lesions does not strongly correlate with the presence of dementia or cognitive impairment.

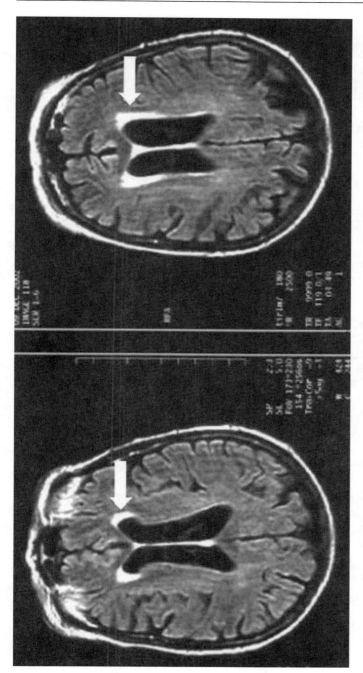

Fig. 5. Leukoaraiosis seen in magnetic resonance imaging of brain, fluid attenuated inversion recovery sequence. The left image arrow points to a "cap" in white matter adjacent to the anterior ventricles. The right image arrow points to a "rim" of high signal adjacent to body of lateral ventricles.

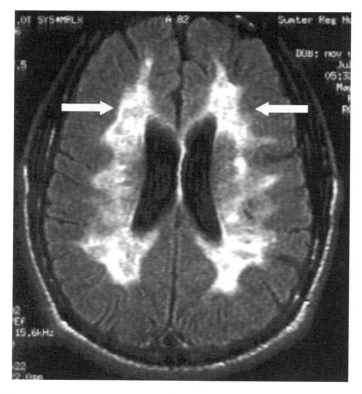

Fig. 6. Extensive leukoaraiosis shown in magnetic resonance imaging of brain with fluid attenuated inversion recovery sequence. Arrows point to areas of extensive confluent high signal in the white matter adjacent to lateral ventricles.

A number of studies have reported on the presence of these hyperintensities in relationship to hypertension, age, and cognitive function. Pathological examination of the more diffuse white matter hyperintensities has variously revealed myelin loss, myelin and axonal loss *(111–113)*, ischemic infarction *(114)*, diffuse decreased density of glial cells with accompanying vacuolation *(115)*, or "incomplete infarction" *(116-118)*. Brun and Englund *(116)* used the term *incomplete infarction* to describe areas of myelin and axon loss, with loss of oligodendroglia, associated with increased numbers of reactive astrocytes, but without cavitation or significant necrosis. This is thought to represent areas of repeated hypoperfusion presumably secondary to bouts of hypotension. Brun and Englund first described this phenomenon in the brains of patients with AD and noted that all of these patients had had low

BP, not high BP, suggesting that there was hypoperfusion in the territory of the medullary arteries. Other authors have noted a relationship between the occurrence of hypotension and the presence of dementia. Several studies have documented the decline in BP in elderly demented patients. It is not clear if the decline in BP is the cause of the cognitive decline or the result of the dementia (119–121).

The subcortical white matter could be vulnerable to several different types of vascular processes. Medullary penetrating arteries that arise from the cortical arterioles supply the white matter above the ventricles. With hypertensive injury, lipohyalinosis or thickening of the arterial wall of the penetrating arteries may develop. These arteries may then become less able to autoregulate blood flow and thus be unable to compensate for changes in BP. If the arterial walls of a single vessel became stenotic enough, there could be distal perfusion failure with resultant infarction. If the arteriole had impaired vasoreactivity, it would be unable to dilate in response to BP decreases, resulting in distal hypoperfusion with resultant neuronal and/or glial injury.

Amyloid angiopathy has also been associated with cerebral infarction. Amyloid angiopathy is caused by amyloid deposits in the small and medium-size vessels on the surface of the brain. Several authors have noted the presence of ischemic lesions in patients with amyloid angiopathy, and it has been proposed that the amyloid may cause occlusion or stiffening of these arterioles with loss of vasoreactivity, making the deep white matter susceptible to ischemia in the face of hypotension (122–125).

Moody and co-workers have suggested another possible mechanism for perfusion failure in the medullary artery territory(126,127). They demonstrated that, with increasing age, the medullary arteries lengthen and become more tortuous. Using a computer model, they suggested that the increase in length may raise the minimum BP necessary to perfuse the distal portions of these vessels (i.e., the periventricular white matter), raising another possible mechanism by which relative hypotension could result in ischemia in the deep white matter (126,127).

Okeda proposed an additional possible injury (128). In the event that the arterioles have lost the ability to autoregulate, there will be hypoperfusion in the case of hypotension, but there will be hyperperfusion with hypertension, and the delivery of high pressure blood flow into the distal medullary arteriole bed could result in fluid extravasation with local tissue injury (128).

Some MRI investigations of dementia, instead of focusing on white matter abnormalities, have focused more on cerebral volume loss, demonstrated by increased ventricular volume and decreased cortical gray matter volume. They have suggested that cortical atrophy is an index of disease severity for both AD and for subcortical vascular disease and is more strongly predictive of future decline than the presence of white matter changes, either focal (lacunar) or diffuse *(129)*.

Neuropathology

The pathological criteria used for dementia subtype classification may also significantly alter the percentages classified to each category. In some series using pathological data for dementia classification, the presence of a single stroke has been enough to classify the case as MID, but in others, multiple strokes in different areas of the brain were required for the classification of MID. This difference in classification schemas is reflected in the wide spread of percentage of cases of dementia, ranging from 10% to 60%, classified as vascular dementias in different series *(115)*.

Some pathologists routinely ignore small amounts of white matter ischemic injury, requiring large volumes of infarcted tissue to make the diagnosis; others require the presence of multiple cortical infarctions, and some focus on the presence of white matter abnormalities. There are authors who will only diagnosis vascular dementia in the absence of changes typical of AD; others may base their assessment on the preponderance of the pathological changes *(130–135)*. Some even suggest that AD is primarily a vascular disorder, and AD is simply part of the spectrum of vascular dementia *(136)*. Just as there are various etiologies for ischemic stroke, so there may be a spectrum of vascular diseases causing dementia, ranging from well-defined multiple cortical strokes to multiple lacunes to leukoaraiosis *(103)*, or a combination of these lesions. Vascular dementia may also cause an additive insult to the cognitive function of a patient already suffering from AD, a phenomenon that Munoz et al.'s study suggested could be a very frequent occurrence *(115)*.

Treatment of Hypertension to Prevent Cognitive Decline

Several trials have looked specifically at cognitive impairment (PROGRESS in a stroke population and Syst-Eur in a hypertensive population) to determine whether BP lowering could reduce the risk of dementia and/or cognitive decline. In the PROGRESS trial *(67)*, although there appeared to be some benefit to active treatment, most of the benefit appeared to be secondary to stroke reduction in the treated group. The "dementia with recurrent stroke" was reduced by about one-third, and the risk of cognitive decline with recurrent stroke was reduced by 34%. When the decline in MMSE scores was evaluated, there was a small difference between the active treatment arm (-0.05 ± 0.05 mean $\pm$ standard error) vs the placebo arm (0.19 ± 0.07) group.

The Syst-Eur study performed an extended follow-up of patients who had participated in the trial *(68)*. They used the MMSE to score patients and classified them by the *DSM-III-R* criteria. In follow-up of 2902 patients, they reported 64 incident cases of all-cause dementia (41 AD, 19 mixed or vascular), with 43 in the control group, 21 in the active treatment group, for a rate of 7.4 per 1000 patient-years for all-cause dementia in the control group and 3.3 in the active treatment group. It was not clear if this reduction simply represented a benefit from decreased BP or potentially a specific benefit of the calcium antagonist nitrendipine. They did not comment on the relationship between stroke and cognitive decline; therefore, no direct comparison to the PROGRESS observations can be made.

Data on risk factors for the development of dementia are frequently difficult to sort. In particular, information on hypertension may not be well defined. The definition of hypertension varies between many of the older studies and may not be specified in some. Readers of this text will be well aware of the issues surrounding identification of hypertension. There have been changes in the definition of hypertension over time, so that older studies used different criteria than newer ones.

The issue of how BP was measured is also important. A single BP measure at one point in time may not accurately represent the BP over time, with white-coat hypertension one example. Monitoring for 24 hours would provide better data than a single office BP measurement, and 24-hour mean BP was found in one study to be a strong predictor of risk for stroke *(137)*. To date, 24-hour BP monitoring has not been reported in any large studies on vascular dementia.

There are conflicting reports about the relationship of hypertension, its treatment, and its effect on cognition. Some reports demonstrated that reducing BP reduced the risk of dementia; others have failed to show such a relationship *(138)*. Other longitudinal studies have reported that there is a decline in BP that may precede or accompany the development of dementia, raising questions regarding what is cause and what is effect *(139)*. It is possible that initially hypertensive injury to small arteries triggers structural changes in the arterial walls that may result in ischemic injury to the brain. These structural changes in small arteries and arterioles may cause an impairment or loss of autoregulation; with a loss of autoregulation, hypotension may result in cerebral ischemia in the deep white matter. Amyloid angiopathy is another process that is frequently seen in the elderly that could impair the arterioles' ability to autoregulate.

As it becomes clear that hypertension may play a role in the development of dementia and that treatment of hypertension may decrease the risk of subsequent development of dementia, interest has focused on identification of those patients who would be most likely to benefit from early treatment.

CONCLUSIONS

Stroke is the third leading cause of death in the United States and is a leading cause of long-term disability. Hypertension is the most potent risk factor for future stroke development. Well-designed trials have demonstrated that reduction of BP dramatically decreases the risk of stroke. There is good data showing that almost all medications that reduce BP reduce stroke risk. There is also some data suggesting that different antihypertensive agents or classes may have greater benefits than others, but to date this has not been conclusively demonstrated. It appears that, in high-risk patients (i.e., those who have already suffered a stroke), lowering BP, even for nonhypertensives, reduces the risk of future stroke. Currently, it is not known to what extent pressure should be lowered or if specific antihypertensives may be more beneficial than others.

A strong association exists between hypertension and the development of cognitive impairment and dementia. The relationship between BP and dementia is complex, spanning the accumulated brain injury from multiple strokes to small blood vessel injuries with secondary effects on brain perfusion. It is apparent that antihypertensives can decrease stroke risk and its relative contribution to cognitive decline. There is exciting data that BP lowering can potentially decrease cognitive decline in other ways as well. It may be that early, aggressive management of BP will have a long-term benefit of lessening the risk of dementia.

REFERENCES

1. Barnett HJM, Mohr JP, Stein BM, Yatsu FM. *Stroke: Pathophysiology, Diagnosis, and Management.* New York: Churchill Livingstone; 1998.
2. American Heart Association. AHA Heart Disease and Stroke Statistics, 2003 Update. Dallas, TX: American Heart Association; 2002.
3. Adams HP Jr, Brott TG, Furlan AJ, et al. Guidelines for thrombolytic therapy for acute stroke: a supplement to the guidelines for the management of patients with acute ischemic stroke. A statement for healthcare professionals from a Special Writing Group of the Stroke Council, American Heart Association. *Stroke* 1996;27:1711–1718.
4. Goldstein LB, Adams R, Becker K, et al. Primary prevention of ischemic stroke: A statement for healthcare professionals from the Stroke Council of the American Heart Association. *Stroke* 2001;32:280–299.
5. Wolf PA, D'Agostino RB, Belanger AJ, Kannel WB. Probability of stroke: a risk profile from the Framingham Study. *Stroke* 1991;22:312–318.

6. Brown RD, Whisnant JP, Sicks JD, O'Fallon WM, Wiebers DO. Stroke incidence, prevalence, and survival: secular trends in Rochester, Minnesota, through 1989. *Stroke* 1996;27:373–380.

7. Wolf PA, D'Agostino RB, O'Neal MA, et al. Secular trends in stroke incidence and mortality. The Framingham Study. *Stroke* 1992;23:1551–1555.

8. Shinton R, Beevers G. Meta-analysis of relation between cigarette smoking and stroke. *BMJ* 1989;298:789–794.

9. Wolf PA, D'Agostino RB, Kannel WB, Bonita R, Belanger AJ. Cigarette smoking as a risk factor for stroke. The Framingham Study. *JAMA* 1988;259:1025–1029.

10. Wannamethee SG, Shaper AG, Whincup PH, Walker M. Smoking cessation and the risk of stroke in middle-aged men. *JAMA* 1995;274:155–160.

11. Tight blood pressure control and risk of macrovascular and microvascular complications in type 2 diabetes: UKPDS 38. UK Prospective Diabetes Study Group. *BMJ* 1998;317:703–713.

12. Cholesterol, diastolic blood pressure, and stroke: 13,000 strokes in 450,000 people in 45 prospective cohorts. Prospective studies collaboration. *Lancet* 1995;346: 1647–1653.

13. Blauw GJ, Lagaay AM, Smelt AH, Westendorp RG. Stroke, statins, and cholesterol. A meta-analysis of randomized, placebo-controlled, double-blind trials with HMG-CoA reductase inhibitors. *Stroke* 1997;28:946–950.

14. Hankey GJ. Long-term outcome after ischaemic stroke/transient ischaemic attack. *Cerebrovasc Dis* 2003;16(suppl 1):14–19.

15. Psaty BM, Lumley T, Furberg CD, et al. Health outcomes associated with various antihypertensive therapies used as first-line agents: a network meta-analysis. *JAMA* 2003;289:2534–2544.

16. MacMahon S, Peto R, Cutler J, et al. Blood pressure, stroke, and coronary heart disease. Part 1, prolonged differences in blood pressure: prospective observational studies corrected for the regression dilution bias. *Lancet* 1990;335:765–774.

17. Collins R, Peto R, MacMahon S, et al. Blood pressure, stroke, and coronary heart disease. Part 2, short-term reductions in blood pressure: overview of randomised drug trials in their epidemiological context. *Lancet* 1990;335:827–838.

18. Major outcomes in high-risk hypertensive patients randomized to angiotensin-converting enzyme inhibitor or calcium channel blocker vs diuretic: The Antihypertensive and Lipid-Lowering Treatment to Prevent Heart Attack Trial (ALLHAT). *JAMA* 2002;288:2981–2997.

19. Randomised trial of a perindopril-based blood-pressure-lowering regimen among 6105 individuals with previous stroke or transient ischaemic attack. *Lancet* 2001;358:1033–1041.

20. Gueyffier F, Boutitie F, Boissel JP, et al. Effect of antihypertensive drug treatment on cardiovascular outcomes in women and men. A meta-analysis of individual patient data from randomized, controlled trials. The INDANA Investigators. *Ann Intern Med* 1997;126:761–767.

21. Staessen JA, Gasowski J, Wang JG, et al. Risks of untreated and treated isolated systolic hypertension in the elderly: meta-analysis of outcome trials. *Lancet* 2000;355:865–872.

22. Celermajer DS. Clinical trials: evidence and unanswered questions—hypertension. *Cerebrovasc Dis* 2003;16(suppl 3):18–24.

23. Kannel WB, Dawber TR, Sorlie P, Wolf PA. Components of blood pressure and risk of atherothrombotic brain infarction: the Framingham study. *Stroke* 1976;7:327–331.

24. Kannel WB, Wolf PA, Verter J, McNamara PM. Epidemiologic assessment of the role of blood pressure in stroke: the Framingham Study. 1970. *JAMA* 1996;276: 1269–1278.

25. Sagie A, Larson MG, Levy D. The natural history of borderline isolated systolic hypertension. *N Engl J Med* 1993;329:1912–1917.
26. Prevention of stroke by antihypertensive drug treatment in older persons with isolated systolic hypertension. Final results of the Systolic Hypertension in the Elderly Program (SHEP). SHEP Cooperative Research Group. *JAMA* 1991;265:3255–3264.
27. Fagard RH, Staessen JA. Treatment of isolated systolic hypertension in the elderly: the Syst-Eur trial. Systolic Hypertension in Europe (Syst-Eur) Trial Investigators. *Clin Exp Hypertens* 1999;21:491–497.
28. Bikkina M, Levy D, Evans JC, et al. Left ventricular mass and risk of stroke in an elderly cohort. The Framingham Heart Study. *JAMA* 1994;272:33–36.
29. Benjamin EJ, Levy D. Why is left ventricular hypertrophy so predictive of morbidity and mortality? *Am J Med Sci* 1999;317:168–175.
30. Inagawa T. Trends in incidence and case fatality rates of aneurysmal subarachnoid hemorrhage in Izumo City, Japan, between 1980–1989 and 1990–1998. *Stroke* 2001;32:1499–1507.
31. Mayberg MR, Batjer HH, Dacey R, et al. Guidelines for the management of aneurysmal subarachnoid hemorrhage. A statement for healthcare professionals from a special writing group of the Stroke Council, American Heart Association. *Stroke* 1994;25:2315–2328.
32. Broderick JP, Adams HP Jr, Barsan W, et al. Guidelines for the management of spontaneous intracerebral hemorrhage: A statement for healthcare professionals from a special writing group of the Stroke Council, American Heart Association. *Stroke* 1999;30:905–915.
33. Fisher CM. Pathological observations in hypertensive cerebral hemorrhage. *J Neuropathol Exp Neurol* 1971;30:536–650.
34. Brott T, Broderick J, Kothari R, et al. Early hemorrhage growth in patients with intracerebral hemorrhage. *Stroke* 1997;28:1–5.
35. Lang EW, Ren Ya Z, Preul C, et al. Stroke pattern interpretation: the variability of hypertensive vs amyloid angiopathy hemorrhage. *Cerebrovasc Dis* 2001;12:121–130.
36. Adams RJ, Chimowitz MI, Alpert JS, et al. Coronary risk evaluation in patients with transient ischemic attack and ischemic stroke: a scientific statement for healthcare professionals from the Stroke Council and the Council on Clinical Cardiology of the American Heart Association/American Stroke Association. *Stroke* 2003;34:2310–2322.
37. Fisher CM. Observations of the fundus oculi in transient monocular blindness. *Neurology* 1959;9:333–347.
38. Albers GW, Hart RG, Lutsep HL, Newell DW, Sacco RL. AHA scientific statement. Supplement to the guidelines for the management of transient ischemic attacks: a statement from the Ad Hoc Committee on Guidelines for the Management of Transient Ischemic Attacks, Stroke Council, American Heart Association. *Stroke* 1999;30:2502–2511.
39. Culebras A, Kase CS, Masdeu JC, et al. Practice guidelines for the use of imaging in transient ischemic attacks and acute stroke. A report of the Stroke Council, American Heart Association. *Stroke* 1997;28:1480–1497.
40. Beneficial effect of carotid endarterectomy in symptomatic patients with high-grade carotid stenosis. North American Symptomatic Carotid Endarterectomy Trial Collaborators. *N Engl J Med* 1991;325:445–453.
41. Biller J, Feinberg WM, Castaldo JE, et al. Guidelines for carotid endarterectomy: a statement for healthcare professionals from a special writing group of the Stroke Council, American Heart Association. *Stroke* 1998;29:554–562.

42. Ommer A, Pillny M, Grabitz K, Sandmann W. Reconstructive surgery for carotid artery occlusive disease in the elderly—a high risk operation? *Cardiovasc Surg* 2001;9:552–558.

43. Caplan LR, Gorelick PB, Hier DB. Race, sex and occlusive cerebrovascular disease: a review. *Stroke* 1986;17:648–655.

44. Fisher CM, Gore I, Okabe N, White PD. Calcification of the carotid siphon. *Circulation* 1965;32:538–548.

45. Kannel WB, Wolf PA, Benjamin EJ, Levy D. Prevalence, incidence, prognosis, and predisposing conditions for atrial fibrillation: population-based estimates. *Am J Cardiol* 1998;82:2N–9N.

46. Healey JS, Connolly SJ. Atrial fibrillation: hypertension as a causative agent, risk factor for complications, and potential therapeutic target. *Am J Cardiol* 2003;91:9G–14G.

47. Risk factors for stroke and efficacy of antithrombotic therapy in atrial fibrillation. Analysis of pooled data from five randomized controlled trials. *Arch Intern Med* 1994;154:1449–1457.

48. Albers GW, Dalen JE, Laupacis A, Manning WJ, Petersen P, Singer DE. Antithrombotic therapy in atrial fibrillation. *Chest* 2001;119:194S–206S.

49. Amarenco P, Duyckaerts C, Tzourio C, Henin D, Bousser MG, Hauw JJ. The prevalence of ulcerated plaques in the aortic arch in patients with stroke. *N Engl J Med* 1992;326:221–225.

50. Amarenco P, Cohen A, Tzourio C, et al. Atherosclerotic disease of the aortic arch and the risk of ischemic stroke. *N Engl J Med* 1994;331:1474–1479.

51. Fisher CM. Lacunes: small, deep cerebral infarcts. *Neurology* 1965;15:774–784.

52. Fisher CM. Capsular infarcts: the underlying vascular lesions. *Arch Neurol* 1979;36:65–73.

53. Fisher CM. Lacunar strokes and infarcts: a review. *Neurology* 1982;32:871–876.

54. Vermeer SE, Hollander M, van Dijk EJ, Hofman A, Koudstaal PJ, Breteler MM. Silent brain infarcts and white matter lesions increase stroke risk in the general population: the Rotterdam Scan Study. *Stroke* 2003;34:1126–1129.

55. Longstreth WT Jr, Dulberg C, Manolio TA, et al. Incidence, manifestations, and predictors of brain infarcts defined by serial cranial magnetic resonance imaging in the elderly: the Cardiovascular Health Study. *Stroke* 2002;33:2376–2382.

56. MacMahon S, Rodgers A. Blood pressure, antihypertensive treatment and stroke risk. *J Hypertens Suppl* 1994;12:S5–S14.

57. MacMahon S. Blood pressure and the prevention of stroke. *J Hypertens Suppl* 1996;14:S39–S46.

58. Neal B, MacMahon S, Chapman N. Effects of ACE inhibitors, calcium antagonists, and other blood-pressure-lowering drugs: results of prospectively designed overviews of randomised trials. Blood Pressure Lowering Treatment Trialists' Collaboration. *Lancet* 2000;356:1955–1964.

59. Staessen JA, Fagard R, Thijs L, et al. Randomised double-blind comparison of placebo and active treatment for older patients with isolated systolic hypertension. The Systolic Hypertension in Europe (Syst-Eur) Trial Investigators. *Lancet* 1997;350:757–764.

60. Dahlof B, Devereux RB, Kjeldsen SE, et al. Cardiovascular morbidity and mortality in the Losartan Intervention for Endpoint reduction in hypertension study (LIFE): a randomised trial against atenolol. *Lancet* 2002;359:995–1003.

61. Yusuf S, Sleight P, Pogue J, Bosch J, Davies R, Dagenais G. Effects of an angiotensin-converting-enzyme inhibitor, ramipril, on cardiovascular events in high-risk patients. The Heart Outcomes Prevention Evaluation Study Investigators. *N Engl J Med* 2000;342:145–153.

62. Bosch J, Yusuf S, Pogue J, et al. Use of ramipril in preventing stroke: double blind randomised trial. *BMJ* 2002;324:699–702.
63. Svensson P, de Faire U, Sleight P, Yusuf S, Ostergren J. Comparative effects of ramipril on ambulatory and office blood pressures: a HOPE Substudy. *Hypertension* 2001;38:E28–E32.
64. Launer LJ, Masaki K, Petrovitch H, Foley D, Havlik RJ. The association between midlife blood pressure levels and late-life cognitive function. The Honolulu-Asia Aging Study. *JAMA* 1995;274:1846–1851.
65. Havlik RJ, Foley DJ, Sayer B, Masaki K, White L, Launer LJ. Variability in midlife systolic blood pressure is related to late-life brain white matter lesions: the Honolulu-Asia Aging study. *Stroke* 2002;33:26–30.
66. Glynn RJ, Beckett LA, Hebert LE, Morris MC, Scherr PA, Evans DA. Current and remote blood pressure and cognitive decline. *JAMA* 1999;281:438–445.
67. Tzourio C, Anderson C, Chapman N, et al. Effects of blood pressure lowering with perindopril and indapamide therapy on dementia and cognitive decline in patients with cerebrovascular disease. *Arch Intern Med* 2003;163:1069–1075.
68. Forette F, Seux ML, Staessen JA, et al. The prevention of dementia with antihypertensive treatment: new evidence from the Systolic Hypertension in Europe (Syst-Eur) study. *Arch Intern Med* 2002;162:2046–2052.
69. Manolio TA, Olson J, Longstreth WT. Hypertension and cognitive function: pathophysiologic effects of hypertension on the brain. *Curr Hypertens Rep* 2003;5:255–261.
70. Mesulam MM. Large-scale neurocognitive networks and distributed processing for attention, language, and memory. *Ann Neurol* 1990;28:597–613.
71. Stern Y, Gurland B, Tatemichi TK, Tang MX, Wilder D, Mayeux R. Influence of education and occupation on the incidence of Alzheimer's disease. *JAMA* 1994;271:1004–1010.
72. Skoog I, Nilsson L, Palmertz B, Andreasson LA, Svanborg A. A population-based study of dementia in 85-year-olds. *N Engl J Med* 1993;328:153–158.
73. Bachman DL, Wolf PA, Linn RT, et al. Incidence of dementia and probable Alzheimer's disease in a general population: the Framingham Study. *Neurology* 1993;43:515–519.
74. Petersen RC, Smith GE, Waring SC, Ivnik RJ, Tangalos EG, Kokmen E. Mild cognitive impairment: clinical characterization and outcome. *Arch Neurol* 1999;56:303–308.
75. Ritchie K, Touchon J. Mild cognitive impairment: conceptual basis and current nosological status. *Lancet* 2000;355:225–228.
76. Levy R. Aging-associated cognitive decline. Working Party of the International Psychogeriatric Association in collaboration with the World Health Organization. *Int Psychogeriatr* 1994;6:63–68.
77. Di Carlo A, Baldereschi M, Amaducci L, et al. Cognitive impairment without dementia in older people: prevalence, vascular risk factors, impact on disability. The Italian Longitudinal Study on Aging. *J Am Geriatr Soc* 2000;48:775–782.
78. Kukull WA, Ganguli M. Epidemiology of dementia: concepts and overview. *Neurol Clin* 2000;18:923–950.
79. Erkinjuntti T, Ostbye T, Steenhuis R, Hachinski V. The effect of different diagnostic criteria on the prevalence of dementia. *N Engl J Med* 1997;337:1667–1674.
80. Jellinger K, Danielczyk W, Fischer P, Gabriel E. Clinicopathological analysis of dementia disorders in the elderly. *J Neurol Sci* 1990;95:239–258.
81. Tomlinson BE, Blessed G, Roth M. Observations on the brains of demented old people. *J Neurol Sci* 1970;11:205–242.

82. Tatemichi TK, Desmond DW, Prohovnik I, et al. Confusion and memory loss from capsular genu infarction: a thalamocortical disconnection syndrome? *Neurology* 1992;42:1966–1979.
83. Hachinski VC, Lassen NA, Marshall J. Multi-infarct dementia. A cause of mental deterioration in the elderly. *Lancet* 1974;2:207–210.
84. Hachinski VC, Iliff LD, Zilhka E, et al. Cerebral blood flow in dementia. *Arch Neurol* 1975;32:632–637.
85. Tatemichi TK, Desmond DW, Stern Y, Paik M, Sano M, Bagiella E. Cognitive impairment after stroke: frequency, patterns, and relationship to functional abilities. *J Neurol Neurosurg Psychiatry* 1994;57:202–207.
86. Tatemichi TK, Paik M, Bagiella E, et al. Risk of dementia after stroke in a hospitalized cohort: results of a longitudinal study. *Neurology* 1994;44:1885–1891.
87. Tatemichi TK, Paik M, Bagiella E, Desmond DW, Pirro M, Hanzawa LK. Dementia after stroke is a predictor of long-term survival. *Stroke* 1994;25:1915–1919.
88. Hachinski V. Vascular dementia: a radical redefinition. *Dementia* 1994;5:130–132.
89. Roman GC, Tatemichi TK, Erkinjuntti T, et al. Vascular dementia: diagnostic criteria for research studies. Report of the NINDS-AIREN International Workshop. *Neurology* 1993;43:250–260.
90. Wetterling T, Kanitz RD, Borgis KJ. The ICD-10 criteria for vascular dementia. *Dementia* 1994;5:185–188.
91. Chui HC, Victoroff JI, Margolin D, Jagust W, Shankle R, Katzman R. Criteria for the diagnosis of ischemic vascular dementia proposed by the State of California Alzheimer's Disease Diagnostic and Treatment Centers. *Neurology* 1992;42:473–480.
92. Association AP. Diagnostic and Statistical Manual of Mental Disorders (DSM-IV). Washington, DC: American Psychiatric Association; 1994:143–147.
93. Rosen WG, Terry RD, Fuld PA, Katzman R, Peck A. Pathological verification of ischemic score in differentiation of dementias. *Ann Neurol* 1980;7:486–488.
94. Wetterling T, Kanitz RD, Borgis KJ. Comparison of different diagnostic criteria for vascular dementia (ADDTC, DSM-IV, ICD-10, NINDS-AIREN). *Stroke* 1996;27: 30–36.
95. Pohjasvaara T, Mantyla R, Ylikoski R, Kaste M, Erkinjuntti T. Comparison of different clinical criteria (DSM-III, ADDTC, ICD-10, NINDS-AIREN, DSM-IV) for the diagnosis of vascular dementia. National Institute of Neurological Disorders and Stroke-Association Internationale pour la Recherche et l'Enseignement en Neurosciences. *Stroke* 2000;31:2952–2957.
96. Erkinjuntti T, Inzitari D, Pantoni L, et al. Research criteria for subcortical vascular dementia in clinical trials. *J Neural Transm Suppl* 2000;59:23–30.
97. Cummings JL. Subcortical dementia. Neuropsychology, neuropsychiatry, and pathophysiology. *Br J Psychiatry* 1986;149:682–697.
98. Crum RM, Anthony JC, Bassett SS, Folstein MF. Population-based norms for the Mini-Mental State Examination by age and educational level. *JAMA* 1993;269:2386–2391.
99. Vendrell P, Junque C, Pujol J, Jurado MA, Molet J, Grafman J. The role of prefrontal regions in the Stroop task. *Neuropsychologia* 1995;33:341–352.
100. Delis DC, Squire LR, Bihrle A, Massman P. Componential analysis of problem-solving ability: performance of patients with frontal lobe damage and amnesic patients on a new sorting test. *Neuropsychologia* 1992;30:683–697.
101. Mantyla R, Erkinjuntti T, Salonen O, et al. Variable agreement between visual rating scales for white matter hyperintensities on MRI. Comparison of 13 rating scales in a poststroke cohort. *Stroke* 1997;28:1614–1623.

102. Chimowitz MI, Awad IA, Furlan AJ. Periventricular lesions on MRI. Facts and theories. *Stroke* 1989;20:963–967.
103. Hachinski VC, Potter P, Merskey H. Leuko-araiosis. *Arch Neurol* 1987;44:21–23.
104. Erkinjuntti T, Gao F, Lee DH, Eliasziw M, Merskey H, Hachinski VC. Lack of difference in brain hyperintensities between patients with early Alzheimer's disease and control subjects. *Arch Neurol* 1994;51:260–268.
105. Fazekas F. Magnetic resonance signal abnormalities in asymptomatic individuals: their incidence and functional correlates. *Eur Neurol* 1989;29:164–168.
106. Fazekas F, Schmidt R, Offenbacher H. Prevalence of white matter and periventricular magnetic resonance hyperintensities in asymptomatic volunteers. *J Neuroimaging* 1991;1:27–30.
107. Breteler MM, van Swieten JC, Bots ML, et al. Cerebral white matter lesions, vascular risk factors, and cognitive function in a population-based study: the Rotterdam Study. *Neurology* 1994;44:1246–1252.
108. de Leeuw FE, de Groot JC, Oudkerk M, et al. Hypertension and cerebral white matter lesions in a prospective cohort study. *Brain* 2002;125:765–772.
109. Longstreth WT Jr, Manolio TA, Arnold A, et al. Clinical correlates of white matter findings on cranial magnetic resonance imaging of 3301 elderly people. The Cardiovascular Health Study. *Stroke* 1996;27:1274–1282.
110. Liao D, Cooper L, Cai J, et al. Presence and severity of cerebral white matter lesions and hypertension, its treatment, and its control. The ARIC Study. Atherosclerosis Risk in Communities Study. *Stroke* 1996;27:2262–2270.
111. Leifer D, Buonanno FS, Richardson EP Jr. Clinicopathologic correlations of cranial magnetic resonance imaging of periventricular white matter. *Neurology* 1990;40:911–918.
112. Grafton ST, Sumi SM, Stimac GK, Alvord EC Jr, Shaw CM, Nochlin D. Comparison of postmortem magnetic resonance imaging and neuropathologic findings in the cerebral white matter. *Arch Neurol* 1991;48:293–298.
113. Chimowitz MI, Estes ML, Furlan AJ, Awad IA. Further observations on the pathology of subcortical lesions identified on magnetic resonance imaging. *Arch Neurol* 1992;49:747–752.
114. Marshall VG, Bradley WG Jr, Marshall CE, Bhoopat T, Rhodes RH. Deep white matter infarction: correlation of MR imaging and histopathologic findings. *Radiology* 1988;167:517–522.
115. Munoz DG, Hastak SM, Harper B, Lee D, Hachinski VC. Pathologic correlates of increased signals of the centrum ovale on magnetic resonance imaging. *Arch Neurol* 1993;50:492–497.
116. Brun A, Englund E. A white matter disorder in dementia of the Alzheimer type: a pathoanatomical study. *Ann Neurol* 1986;19:253–262.
117. Brun A. Pathology and pathophysiology of cerebrovascular dementia: pure subgroups of obstructive and hypoperfusive etiology. *Dementia* 1994;5:145–147.
118. Englund E. Neuropathology of white matter lesions in vascular cognitive impairment. *Cerebrovasc Dis* 2002;13(suppl 2):11–15.
119. Ruitenberg A, Skoog I, Ott A, et al. Blood pressure and risk of dementia: results from the Rotterdam study and the Gothenburg H-70 Study. *Dement Geriatr Cogn Disord* 2001;12:33–39.
120. Skoog I, Lernfelt B, Landahl S, et al. 15-year longitudinal study of blood pressure and dementia. *Lancet* 1996;347:1141–1145.
121. Qiu C, von Strauss E, Fastbom J, Winblad B, Fratiglioni L. Low blood pressure and risk of dementia in the Kungsholmen project: a 6-year follow-up study. *Arch Neurol* 2003;60:223–228.

122. Miklossy J. Cerebral hypoperfusion induces cortical watershed microinfarcts which may further aggravate cognitive decline in Alzheimer's disease. *Neurol Res* 2003;25:605–610.
123. Cadavid D, Mena H, Koeller K, Frommelt RA. Cerebral beta amyloid angiopathy is a risk factor for cerebral ischemic infarction. A case control study in human brain biopsies. *J Neuropathol Exp Neurol* 2000;59:768–773.
124. Olichney JM, Hansen LA, Lee JH, Hofstetter CR, Katzman R, Thal LJ. Relationship between severe amyloid angiopathy, apolipoprotein E genotype, and vascular lesions in Alzheimer's disease. *Ann NY Acad Sci* 2000;903:138–143.
125. Greenberg SM. Cerebral amyloid angiopathy and vessel dysfunction. *Cerebrovasc Dis* 2002;13(suppl 2):42–47.
126. Moody DM, Bell MA, Challa VR. Features of the cerebral vascular pattern that predict vulnerability to perfusion or oxygenation deficiency: an anatomic study. *AJNR Am J Neuroradiol* 1990;11:431–439.
127. Moody DM, Santamore WP, Bell MA. Does tortuosity in cerebral arterioles impair down-autoregulation in hypertensives and elderly normotensives? A hypothesis and computer model. *Clin Neurosurg* 1991;37:372–387.
128. Okeda R. Correlative morphometric studies of cerebral arteries in Binswanger's encephalopathy and hypertensive encephalopathy. *Acta Neuropathol (Berl)* 1973;26:23–43.
129. Mungas D, Reed BR, Jagust WJ, et al. Volumetric MRI predicts rate of cognitive decline related to AD and cerebrovascular disease. *Neurology* 2002;59:867–873.
130. Jellinger KA. Alzheimer disease and cerebrovascular pathology: an update. *J Neural Transm* 2002;109:813–836.
131. Jellinger KA. The pathology of ischemic-vascular dementia: an update. *J Neurol Sci* 2002;203–204:153–157.
132. Kalaria R. Similarities between Alzheimer's disease and vascular dementia. *J Neurol Sci* 2002;203–204:29–34.
133. Pantoni L, Palumbo V, Sarti C. Pathological lesions in vascular dementia. *Ann NY Acad Sci* 2002;977:279–291.
134. Olsson Y, Brun A, Englund E. Fundamental pathological lesions in vascular dementia. *Acta Neurol Scand Suppl* 1996;168:31–38.
135. Erkinjuntti T, Haltia M, Palo J, Sulkava R, Paetau A. Accuracy of the clinical diagnosis of vascular dementia: a prospective clinical and post-mortem neuropathological study. *J Neurol Neurosurg Psychiatry* 1988;51:1037–1044.
136. de la Torre JC. Alzheimer disease as a vascular disorder: nosological evidence. *Stroke* 2002;33:1152–1162.
137. Verdecchia P, Schillaci G, Reboldi G, Franklin SS, Porcellati C. Different prognostic impact of 24-hour mean blood pressure and pulse pressure on stroke and coronary artery disease in essential hypertension. *Circulation* 2001;103:2579–2584.
138. Scherr PA, Hebert LE, Smith LA, Evans DA. Relation of blood pressure to cognitive function in the elderly. *Am J Epidemiol* 1991;134:1303–1315.
139. Guo Z, Fratiglioni L, Winblad B, Viitanen M. Blood pressure and performance on the Mini-Mental State Examination in the very old. Cross-sectional and longitudinal data from the Kungsholmen Project. *Am J Epidemiol* 1997;145:1106–1113.

IV PHARMACOLOGICAL MANAGEMENT

15 Diuretics and β-Adrenergic Blockers in the Management of Hypertension in the Elderly

William C. Cushman, MD

INTRODUCTION

In the mid-20th century, it was becoming clear from epidemiological studies that elevated blood pressure (BP) was associated with increased risk of cardiovascular events. However, it was not feasible to conduct long-term morbidity trials to test whether lowering BP with medications would lower cardiovascular events until a class of medications was available that was safe and effective in long-term use in lowering BP, either alone or with other medications, and that was well tolerated. Thiazide-type diuretics, which became available in 1960, were that breakthrough class. Therefore, a series of clinical trials, beginning with the Veterans

From: *Clinical Hypertension and Vascular Diseases: Hypertension in the Elderly*
Edited by: L. M. Prisant © Humana Press Inc., Totowa, NJ

Administration (VA) Cooperative Study on treatment of hypertension in the 1960s *(1–3)*, was conducted with therapy based on thiazide-type diuretics and demonstrated that such antihypertensive therapy reduced strokes by 35–40%, myocardial infarction (MI) by 20–25%, and heart failure by more than 50% *(4,5)*.

There were fewer randomized controlled trials (RCTs) with β-adrenergic blockers than with thiazide-type diuretics *(5)*, the benefits were less consistent *(6)*, and none were conducted in the United States. However, until the late 1990s these were the only two classes of antihypertensive drugs tested as initial therapy in hypertension morbidity trials. Therefore, β-adrenergic blockers were added to diuretics as the other option for preferred initial therapy of hypertension in the 1984 US Joint National Committee (JNC) hypertension guidelines *(7,8)*. They were included with diuretics as preferred initial therapy in every JNC report since 1984 until 2003 (JNC 7), when diuretics were again given preference. In JNC 7, β-blockers, angiotensin-converting enzyme (ACE) inhibitors, calcium channel blockers (CCBs), and angiotensin-receptor blockers (ARBs) were all included as possible alternatives to the preferred diuretics for initial therapy because these classes had all also reduced cardiovascular events in large hypertension morbidity trials *(9)*.

Since diuretics and β-blockers were the only two classes recommended as initial therapy for many years and because some hypertension morbidity trials have permitted investigator choice of diuretic or β-blocker as initial therapy in one randomized treatment arm, these two classes are often considered together in discussions of antihypertensive treatment or in meta-analyses *(10)*. However, their mechanisms of antihypertensive action and pharmacodynamic effects appear as different as any two classes of antihypertensive agents. Nevertheless, because of the historical role of these two classes in demonstrating the benefits of treating hypertension, both are considered in their role in the management of hypertension in the elderly in this chapter. Table 1, adapted from JNC 7, provides a list of thiozide-type diuretics and β-blockers used in the United States with their recommended dosing ranges.

REDUCTION IN CARDIOVASCULAR EVENTS IN TRIALS

Placebo-Controlled Trials

The most important reason in choosing an antihypertensive agent as initial therapy in a patient is the experience of the drug in reducing cardiovascular events and/or mortality in large clinical trials. A number of placebo-controlled trials, and one with "usual care" as the comparison group, were completed with diuretics from the 1960s through the early

Table 1
Thiazide-Type Diuretics and β-Blockers

Class	Drug (trade name)	Usual dose range, mg/day	Usual daily frequency
Thiazide-type diuretics			
•	Chlorothiazide (Diuril)	125–500	1–2
•	Chlorthalidone (generic)	12.5–25	1
•	Hydrochlorothiazide (Microzide, HydroDIURIL*)	12.5–50	1
•	Polythiazide (Renese)	2–4	1
•	Indapamide (Lozol*)	1.25–2.5	1
•	Metolazone (Mykrox)	0.5–1.0	1
•	Metolazone (Zaroxolyn)	2.5–5	1
β-Blockers			
•	Atenolol (Tenormin*)	25–100	1
•	Betaxolol (Kerlone*)	5–20	1
•	Bisoprolol (Zebeta*)	2.5–10	1
•	Metoprolol (Lopressor*)	50–200	2
•	Metoprolol extended release (Toprol XL)	50–200	1
•	Nadolol (Corgard*)	40–120	1
•	Propranolol (Inderal*)	40–240	2
•	Propranolol long acting (Inderal LA*)	60–240	1
•	Timolol (Blocadren*)	20–40	2
β-Blockers with intrinsic sympathomimetic activity			
•	Acebutolol (Sectral*)	200–800	2
•	Penbutolol (Levatol)	10–40	1
•	Pindolol (generic)	10–40	2
Combined β-blockers and α-blockers			
•	Carvedilol (Coreg)	12.5–50	2
•	Labetalol (Normodyne, Trandate*)	200–800	2

*Available now or soon to become available in generic preparations. (Adapted from ref. 8, with modifications.)

1990s. Several placebo-controlled trials were conducted with β-blockers, although none of these were conducted in the United States.

Psaty et al. (5) summarized the results of 15 RCTs of thiazide-type diuretic-based therapy and four trials of β-blocker-based therapy compared with placebo (or usual care) in a meta-analysis of 48,220 participants. The thiazide-type diuretic trial analyses were divided into high-

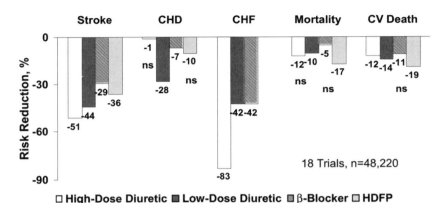

Fig. 1. Event reduction with low-dose or high-dose diuretic or β-blockers in placebo-controlled trials and in the Hypertension Detection and Follow-up Program (HDFP) *(5)*. Low-dose diuretic is the equivalent of 25 to 50 mg hydrochlorothiazide or 12.5 to 25 mg chlorthalidone. CHD, coronary heart disease; CHF, congestive heart failure; CV, cardiovascular.

or low-dose diuretic: low-dose trials used the equivalent of 12.5–25 mg of chlorthalidone or 25–50 mg of hydrochlorothiazide (HCTZ) and high-dose trials included doses higher than these. None of these trials used lower doses than those low doses for the usual titration steps. The earlier trials generally used "high"-dose diuretics and were conducted in mostly young and middle-aged populations, and the later trials used "low"-dose diuretics and were mostly in older hypertensive patients. Different dose ranges of diuretics were not compared by randomized assignment within the same trial.

High-dose thiazide-type diuretics significantly reduced strokes by 51%, heart failure by 83%, and cardiovascular mortality by 22%, although coronary heart disease (CHD) was not reduced (Fig. 1). Low-dose thiazide-type diuretics in older patients significantly reduced strokes by 34%, heart failure by 42%, cardiovascular mortality by 24%, all-cause mortality by 10%, and CHD by 28%. The absolute risk reduction was generally larger in elderly populations because of a higher cardiovascular event rate. In four trials, Psaty et al. reported that β-blockers significantly reduced strokes by 29% and heart failure by 42%, but neither CHD (–7%) nor mortality (–5%) were reduced significantly *(5)*.

Another meta-analysis limited to hypertension trials in the elderly reported that diuretics significantly reduced CHD (–21%), stroke (–36%), heart failure (–49%), and death (–12%) and β-blockers significantly reduced stroke (–31%) and heart failure (–43%), but not CHD or death

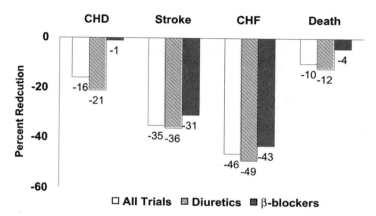

Fig. 2. Cardiovascular risk reduction with diuretics or β-blockers as first-line antihypertensive therapy in eight randomized controlled trials in older persons *(11)*. All reductions were significant (*p* < 0.05) except coronary heart disease (CHD) and death with β-blockers. CHF, congestive heart failure.

(Fig. 2) *(11)*. A subsequent systematic review by Messerli et al. of diuretics and β-blockers in elderly hypertensives concluded that diuretics significantly reduced strokes, CHD, mortality, and cardiovascular disease (CVD) mortality (including stroke and CHD mortality separately), but that β-blockers only reduced strokes *(12)*.

Comparison Between Thiazide-Type Diuretics and β-Blockers

In the British Medical Research Council (MRC) trial in mild hypertension in a younger hypertensive population (aged 35–64 years), active treatment with either the thiazide diuretic bendrofluazide or the β-blocker propranolol reduced strokes and overall CVD events compared with placebo, but the reduction in stroke rate on bendrofluazide was significantly greater than that on propranolol (*p* = 0.002) *(13)*. In the MRC trial of treatment of hypertension in older adults, both the β-blocker atenolol (50 mg) and HCTZ (25–50 mg) plus amiloride treatments reduced BP below the level in the placebo group *(6)*. Compared with the placebo group, actively treated subjects (diuretic and β-blocker groups combined) had a 25% reduction in stroke (*p* = 0.04), 19% reduction in coronary events (*p* = 0.08), and 17% reduction in all cardiovascular events (*p* = 0.03). After adjusting for baseline characteristics, the diuretic group had significantly reduced risks of stroke (–31%, *p* = 0.04), coronary events (–44%, *p* < 0.001), and all cardiovascular events (–35%, *p* < 0.001) compared with the placebo group. The β-blocker group showed no significant reductions in CVD events. As pointed out by Prisant *(14)*, there were limitations to this trial, such as the unblinded assignment of randomized therapy, the very low proportion of participants remaining on β-blocker (63% withdrawal or lost to follow-up), and an early difference in systolic BP reduction between the two active treatment arms. In addition, the dose of diuretic was consistent with prior trials, but the atenolol dose may have been too restricted. However, BP was reduced significantly more than placebo in the β-blocker arm, and regardless of the reasons, including poor persistence on assigned therapy, there were no CVD benefits demonstrated for the β-blocker.

In 2003, Psaty et al. *(15)* conducted a "network" meta-analysis comparing cardiovascular outcomes of various antihypertensive agents by combining direct and indirect comparisons from the evidence from 42 hypertension morbidity trials. Although the trials included were not restricted to the elderly, the majority of participants were elderly, and certainly the majority of events were in older patients. They confirmed a highly significant ($p \leq 0.002$ for each) reduction in CHD (–21%), strokes (–29%), heart failure (–49%), CVD (–24%), CVD mortality (–19%), and total mortality (–10%) for low-dose diuretics compared with placebo. Diuretics reduced CVD events significantly more (–11%) than β-blockers, and CHD (–13%), heart failure (–17%), and stroke (–10%) approached being significantly lower with diuretics.

Although β-blockers have been successful in reducing events in some clinical trials in the elderly, the evidence is not as consistent or as broad as with diuretics. In particular, perhaps surprisingly, β-blockers have appeared less effective in hypertension trials of the elderly in reducing CHD or mortality than thiazide-type diuretics have.

Comparison With Other Antihypertensive Drug Classes

Since 1998, the results of a number of trials comparing thiazide-type diuretics and/or β-blockers with other newer classes of antihypertensive agents have been published. These trials have been conducted predominantly in the elderly because they have more CVD events—otherwise, these relatively large long-term trials would have needed to be even larger and longer to have adequate power to detect potentially clinically meaningful differences. The primary results of these comparison trials are shown in Table 2. Most of these trials were designed as superiority trials: the hypothesis was that the newer antihypertensive agents were better at reducing the primary CVD outcome than diuretics and/or β-blockers.

The Captopril Prevention Program (CAPPP) demonstrated no superiority of captopril over diuretics and β-blockers, except in participants with diabetes mellitus *(16)*. In the Nordic Diltiazem (NORDIL) Study, the CCB diltiazem was not superior to diuretics and β-blockers for the primary outcome, combined fatal and nonfatal stroke, MI, and other

Table 2
Large Hypertension Trials Comparing Cerebrovascular Disease (CVD)
or CVD Mortality Between Diuretics and/or β-Blockers and Other
Antihypertensive Agents

Trial	Number	BPD	Outcomes
CAPPP	10,985	+3/+1	Captopril not superior to D/BB
NORDIL	10,881	+3/0	Diltiazem not superior to D/BB
CONVINCE	16,602	0/+1	Verapamil not superior to D/BB
STOP-2	6628	0/–1	Isradipine/felodipine not superior to D/BB
		0/0	ACEIs not superior to D/BB
INSIGHT	6592	0/0	Nifedipine GITS not superior to diuretic
LIFE	9193	+1/0	Losartan superior to atenolol
ANBP2	6083	+1/0	ACEIs not superior to diuretics
ALLHAT	42,418	–3/–1	Chlorthalidone superior to doxazosin
		–1/+1	Chlorthalidone superior to amlodipine (HF)
		–2/0	Chlorthalidone superior to lisinopril
INVEST	22,576	0/0	Verapamil (± trandolapril) equivalent to atenolol (± hydrochlorothiazide)

ACEIs, angiotensin-converting enzyme inhibitors; ALLHAT, Antihypertensive and Lipid Lowering Treatment to Prevent Heart Attack Trial *(24–26)*; ANBP2, Second Australian National Blood Pressure Study *(28)*; BPD, difference in blood pressure between regimens; CAPPP, Captopril Prevention Program *(16)*; CONVINCE, Controlled Onset Verapamil Investigation of Cardiovascular End Points trial *(18)*; D/BB, diuretics and/or β-blockers; GITS, gastrointestinal therapeutic system; HF, heart failure; INSIGHT, International Nifedipine GITS Study: Intervention as a Goal in Hypertension Treatment *(20)*; INVEST, International Verapamil-Trandolapril Study *(21)*; LIFE, Losartan Intervention for Endpoint Reduction in Hypertension study *(22)*; NORDIL, Nordic Diltiazem study *(17)*; STOP-2, Swedish Trial in Older Persons With Hypertension *(19)*.

CVD death (relative risk = 1.0) *(17)*. Stroke was less frequent with diltiazem ($p = 0.04$), although this was not the primary outcome and was only one of many outcome comparisons.

The Controlled Onset Verapamil Investigation of Cardiovascular End Points (CONVINCE) trial compared the nondihydropyridine CCB verapamil with diuretic or β-blocker (investigator choice prior to double-blind randomization) *(18)*. It was designed to be a noninferiority study, but was stopped early by the sponsoring pharmaceutical company for business reasons (the company was reportedly blinded to the ongoing results); the lack of difference between the regimens nevertheless nearly achieved the criterion to say the CCB was not inferior to the diuretic/β-blocker. However, the dose of the diuretic HCTZ (12.5–25 mg), although common in clinical practice in recent years, was lower than any of the placebo-controlled morbidity trials of diuretics.

In the Second Swedish Trial in Old Patients With Hypertension (STOP Hypertension-2), neither CCBs nor ACE inhibitors were superior to standard therapy with diuretics and/or β-blockers for the primary outcome, cardiovascular mortality, but MIs and heart failure were lower with ACE inhibitors than with CCBs *(19)*. These were only two of several secondary outcomes, so the investigators wrote this should not be taken as definitive evidence of a difference. However, the decreased benefit on heart failure with CCBs has been a recurrent observation.

In the International Nifedipine Gastrointestinal Therapeutic System Study: Intervention as a Goal in Hypertension Treatment (INSIGHT), nifedipine gastrointestinal therapeutic system (GITS) was not superior to the diuretic co-amilozide (25 mg HCTZ and 2.5 mg amiloride, one to two per day) for the primary combined cardiovascular outcome, although heart failure was twice as common ($p < 0.03$) and fatal MI was more than three times as frequent ($p < 0.02$) with nifedipine compared with the diuretic *(20)*. Although these were "primary outcomes" of the trial, they were not *the* primary outcome and are subject to multiple comparison limitations.

The International Verapamil-Trandolapril Study (INVEST) showed no difference in CVD events between the CCB verapamil and the β-blocker atenolol in hypertensive patients aged 50 years and older (mean 66 years) with coronary artery disease *(21)*. In the Losartan Intervention for Endpoint reduction in hypertension study (LIFE), the ARB losartan reduced the primary CVD outcome (mainly through effects on strokes) more than the β-blocker atenolol *(22)*. This was the first large hypertension trial to compare an ARB with another agent.

ANTIHYPERTENSIVE AND LIPID-LOWERING TREATMENT TO PREVENT HEART ATTACK TRIAL

The Antihypertensive and Lipid-Lowering Treatment to Prevent Heart Attack Trial (ALLHAT) compared clinical outcomes in 42,418 hypertensive participants 55 years or older (mean age 67 years) randomly assigned to receive initial double-blind treatment with a thiazide-type diuretic (chlorthalidone), an α_1-blocker (doxazosin), a CCB (amlodipine), or an ACE inhibitor (lisinopril) *(23)*. Except the drug classes tested or ARBs, other drugs were added as needed to control BP to less than 140/90 mmHg. The β-blocker atenolol was the most common drug added for BP control.

In 2000, the doxazosin arm was stopped early because it was associated with 25% more cardiovascular events and twice as much heart failure compared with the thiazide-type diuretic chlorthalidone and because the CHD primary outcome was so similar that it was very

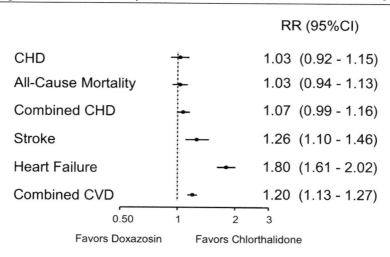

RR (95%CI)

		RR (95%CI)
CHD		1.03 (0.92 - 1.15)
All-Cause Mortality		1.03 (0.94 - 1.13)
Combined CHD		1.07 (0.99 - 1.16)
Stroke		1.26 (1.10 - 1.46)
Heart Failure		1.80 (1.61 - 2.02)
Combined CVD		1.20 (1.13 - 1.27)

0.50   1   2   3

Favors Doxazosin   Favors Chlorthalidone

Fig. 3. Relative risks (RRs) and 95% confidence intervals (CIs) of final cardiovascular outcome results comparing doxazosin with chlorthalidone in the Antihypertensive and Lipid-Lowering Treatment to Prevent Heart Attack Trial (ALLHAT) *(25)*. CHD, coronary heart disease; CVD, cardiovascular disease.

unlikely that any clinically meaningful or statistically significant difference in CHD would occur, even if the doxazosin arm was continued for several more years *(24,25)*. A subsequent report updated the results based on a more complete accounting of events that occurred prior to stopping the arm, which were an additional 9232 participant-years and 939 CVD events (Fig. 3) *(25)*. The doxazosin arm still had a higher risk of stroke (26%, $p = 0.03$), combined CVD (20%, $p < 0.001$), and heart failure (80%, $p < 0.001$) than the chlorthalidone arm; CHD and mortality were not different.

During a mean follow-up of 4.9 years, the incidence of the primary outcome (CHD death or nonfatal MI) and all-cause mortality was no different in the chlorthalidone, amlodipine, and lisinopril arms (Fig. 4) *(26)*. However, the rates of heart failure with amlodipine and lisinopril were significantly higher (by 38% and 19%, respectively) than with chlorthalidone in all participants and across all major groups, including age younger than 65 years and in the elderly (≥65 years), men and women, black and non-black participants, presence or absence of diabetes, and presence or absence of CHD. Participants in the lisinopril arm also had a significantly higher incidence of stroke and combined CVD events than participants receiving chlorthalidone. This is consistent with greater CVD benefits with the diuretic, although based on previous results

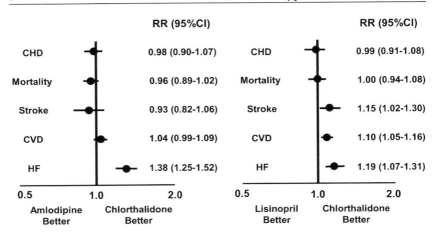

Fig. 4. Relative risks (RRs) and 95% confidence intervals (CIs) of cardiovascular outcomes results comparing amlodipine and lisinopril with chlorthalidone in the Antihypertensive and Lipid-Lowering Treatment to Prevent Heart Attack Trial (ALLHAT) *(26)*. CHD, coronary heart disease; CVD, cardiovascular disease; HF, heart failure.

with diuretics in placebo-controlled trials, the degree of difference suggests there would still be a net benefit for the ACE inhibitor and CCB if they were compared with no treatment. However, no cardiovascular outcome was reduced more with lisinopril or amlodipine than with chlorthalidone, either overall or in any major subgroup. Among blacks, the lisinopril group had significantly higher rates of stroke (40%), heart failure (32%), and combined CVD (19%) than the chlorthalidone group.

These observations support the initial use of diuretics over CCBs and ACE inhibitors as initial therapy in most older patients with hypertension, including those with diabetes mellitus or prior CHD. The data especially support the choice of diuretics over ACE inhibitors as initial therapy in black patients. However, the results of ALLHAT also suggest ACE inhibitors (in whites) or CCBs (in blacks) may be acceptable alternatives if a diuretic is contraindicated (rare) or not tolerated and preferred agents to add to a diuretic.

In ALLHAT, the chlorthalidone arm had fewer drug withdrawals and was more effective in controlling BP than the other three arms. After 5 years, BP was less than 140/90 mmHg in 68%, 66%, and 61% of the chlorthalidone, amlodipine, and lisinopril groups, respectively; participants were treated with an average of two drugs *(26,27)*. However, only 26% of participants had BP controlled on one drug, and only 49% were controlled on either one or two drugs after 5 years—at least 39% of participants received or would have required three or more drugs to control BP *(27)*. Therefore, most hypertensive patients will need at least two to three antihypertensive drugs to achieve adequate BP control. These data contributed to the JNC 7 recommendation to consider initiating antihypertensive therapy with two drugs if the systolic BP is 20 mmHg or greater above goal or the diastolic BP is 10 mmHg or greater above goal *(8,9)*.

SECOND AUSTRALIAN NATIONAL BLOOD PRESSURE STUDY

Several months after the primary results of ALLHAT were published, the effect of diuretics and ACE inhibitors on cardiovascular outcomes was also reported from the Second Australian National Blood Pressure Study (ANBP2) *(28)*. This open-label study randomly assigned 6083 elderly (aged 65–84 years) patients with hypertension to receive either a diuretic or an ACE inhibitor, with a median follow-up of 4.1 years. The rate of the primary composite end point (all cardiovascular events or death from any cause) was 11% lower in the ACE inhibitor arm, with a borderline statistical significance ($p = 0.05$). However, the reduction in events with an ACE inhibitor was noted only in men (relative risk reduction 17%), whereas no differences were observed among women (risk ratio 1.00). This is unusual because there are no important gender differences between drugs in most hypertension morbidity trials *(10)*. Furthermore, in the overall study population, there were no significant differences between the two groups in the incidence of any other outcomes, such as the first cardiovascular event ($p = 0.07$), CHD ($p = 0.16$), heart failure ($p = 0.33$), cerebrovascular events ($p = 0.35$), or stroke ($p = 0.91$). Failure to show a difference in time to first cardiovascular event is particularly important because this is the accepted analysis in almost all other cardiovascular or hypertension morbidity/mortality trials.

COMPARISON OF ALLHAT AND ANBP2

Several important factors may contribute to the apparent differences in the results of ALLHAT and ANBP2. There were four times as many participants in the diuretic and ACE inhibitor arms of ALLHAT ($n = 24,316$) as in ANBP2 ($n = 6083$), and the absolute number of cardiovascular events in ALLHAT was 5–10 times higher than in ANBP2, indicating greater statistical power and reliability for the ALLHAT results. By design, ALLHAT enrolled a substantial proportion of African-American and Hispanic patients. However, the largest racial/ethnic group in ALLHAT was still non-Hispanic whites (11,414 of the participants in the chlorthalidone and lisinopril arms), a subgroup nearly twice as large as the entire ANBP2 trial population, who were almost entirely (95%)

white non-Hispanics *(29,30)*. Some differences between ALLHAT and ANBP2 clearly do not appear to be related to racial and ethnic factors because the significantly higher incidence of heart failure with the ACE inhibitor compared with the diuretic seen in the overall population of ALLHAT was also evident in the white non-Hispanic cohort (15% higher, $p = 0.04$) *(29)*.

An important difference is the administration of randomly assigned drugs: ALLHAT was double blind, but ANBP was open label. This may have contributed to the higher proportion of patients who were receiving assigned therapy or drug from the same class at study end in ALLHAT than in ANBP2, both in the ACE inhibitor arm (73% vs 58%, respectively) and in the diuretic arm (81% vs 62%, respectively). In addition, investigators knowing which drug participants were assigned raises the potential for bias in the reporting of events (e.g., the rates of some outcomes might have been "expected" to be lower with the ACE inhibitor) *(29)*. BP control was also better at 5 years in ALLHAT (mean BP 135/ 75 vs 142/79 mmHg in ANBP2). Finally, whereas the higher heart failure incidence with the ACE inhibitor in ALLHAT was consistent across all major subgroups, including men and women, the apparent cardiovascular benefit of ACE inhibitors in ANBP2 was restricted to men.

Nevertheless, the results of the much smaller ANBP2 are consistent with those of ALLHAT if one compares the upper confidence limit for the relative risks in ANBP2 with the estimates of relative risk in ALLHAT *(29)*. In ALLHAT, the ACE inhibitor provided no advantage for any outcomes in white men or women, and the rates of heart failure in the ACE inhibitor group were higher than those in the diuretic group. Taken together, these considerations suggest that the results of ALLHAT can be translated into modern clinical practice with greater confidence and the totality of clinical trial evidence favors the diuretic.

META-ANALYSES OF CLASS COMPARISONS

A report by the Blood Pressure Lowering Treatment Trialists' Collaboration included meta-analyses to estimate the effects of strategies based on ACE inhibitors and calcium antagonists compared with diuretics and/or β-blockers as the comparator "drug" *(10)*. Unfortunately, a limitation in the meta-analysis is that they failed to use diuretics and β-blockers separately as the comparator groups. Although they reported that, in the comparisons of diuretic- or β-blocker-based regimens with other regimens, there was no evidence of heterogeneity for any outcome between trials that used diuretic alone, those that used β-blockers alone, or those that allowed the use of either as initial treatment, diuretic alone as a comparator may have led to somewhat different results, as was seen in ALLHAT and another meta-analysis *(15,26)*.

Nevertheless, the Blood Pressure Lowering Treatment Trialists' Collaboration reported that there were no differences in CHD, CVD, cardiovascular death, or total mortality among the three drug groups, ACE inhibitors, CCBs, or diuretics/β-blockers *(10)*. For stroke, there was a trend toward a greater risk reduction with regimens based on diuretics/β-blockers compared with regimens based on ACE inhibitors (9% [0–18], relative risk difference [confidence interval]) and trends toward greater reductions with regimens based on CCBs compared with those based on diuretics/β-blockers (7% [–1 to 14]) or with those based on ACE inhibitors (12% [1–25]). For heart failure, there was a nonsignificant trend toward a greater risk reduction with regimens based on diuretics/β-blockers compared with regimens based on ACE inhibitors (7% [–4 to 19]), but compared with regimens based on CCBs, diuretics/β-blockers (33% [21–47]) and ACE inhibitors (18% [8–27]) produced significantly greater reductions in heart failure.

In the Psaty et al. *(15)* "network" meta-analysis, which compared low-dose thiazide-type diuretic as the standard comparator group, "none of the other first-line treatment strategies—β-blockers, ACE inhibitors, CCBs, α_1-blockers, and ARBs—was significantly better than low-dose diuretics for any major CVD outcome. In 8 of the 30 between-drug comparisons, however, low-dose diuretics were significantly better than other treatments for the prevention of CVD health outcomes." Low-dose thiazide-type diuretics reduced CVD (6%, $p < 0.05$) and heart failure (26%, $p < 0.001$) more than CCBs and heart failure (12%, $p = 0.01$) and CVD (6%, $p = 0.04$) more than ACE inhibitors. They concluded, "This network meta-analysis provides compelling evidence that low-dose diuretics are the most effective first-line treatment for preventing the occurrence of CVD morbidity and mortality."

CLASS EFFECTS AND DOSAGE

A frequent practical question that arises is whether the benefits seen with a particular antihypertensive drug in a clinical trial can be generalized to other or all drugs in the same class. There is no clear consensus on when an observed benefit can be considered a class effect. In fact, unless a specific agent in the class has shown benefits on major clinical outcomes and long-term safety in large trials, one can never be sure if it will have the same effects and safety as those that have been tested. An often-overlooked issue is that, unless the same dose(s) of a medication is prescribed as used in one or more successful clinical trials, the same benefits (and safety) cannot be assumed to be achieved in practice.

For thiazide-type diuretics, a variety of different agents have been used in successful placebo-controlled trials. A meta-analysis of placebo-controlled trials using low-dose thiazide-type diuretics *(31)*, all of which were conducted in older hypertensive participants, has shown that the reduction in cardiovacsular events with regimens beginning with chlorthalidone *(32–34)* is similar to that of trials using nonchlorthalidone-based therapy, which included HCTZ/triamterine *(35)*, HCTZ/amiloride *(36)*, and indapamide *(37)*.

However, Carter et al. *(38)* reviewed the evidence that there are significant pharmacokinetic and pharmacodynamic differences between chlorthalidone and HCTZ: chlorthalidone is about 1.5 to 2 times as potent as HCTZ, and it has a much longer duration of action. Therefore, it is quite important to pay attention to the doses of each used in successful placebo-controlled trials. The dose range of chlorthalidone in low-dose trials, including the Systolic Hypertension in the Elderly Program (SHEP) *(32–34)* and ALLHAT *(23–26)* was 12.5–25 mg daily; the dose range for HCTZ in low-dose trials was 25–50 mg *(35,36)*. In previous trials, higher doses than these had reduced strokes and heart failure (but not CHD) at least as well as low doses, but lower doses than 25–50 mg HCTZ (or the equivalent) have never been adequately tested in a placebo-controlled morbidity trial. Unfortunately, some recent and ongoing morbidity trials have used 12.5–25 mg HCTZ as initial therapy in a randomized arm *(18,28)* or as add-on therapy *(22,39)* without any assurance that similar benefits were or will be seen as in previously successful thiazide-type diuretic trials.

For β-blockers, a variety of agents has been used repeatedly in morbidity trials, including propranolol, atenolol, and metoprolol, but the necessary doses are less clear. In the MRC trial in older adults, 50 mg atenolol was given, although that arm was not associated with significant benefit *(6)*. In STOP and STOP-2, 50 mg atenolol, 100 mg metoprolol, or 5 mg pindolol were given *(9,40)*. However, in more recent trials comparing β-blockers with other active treatments, atenolol was the usual β-blocker, and the usual dose was 50–100 mg *(18,21,22)*. There is very little information on the effects of β-blockers with intrinsic sympathomimetic activity, even though pindolol was one of several β-blockers used in the two STOP trials; however, the failure of such β-blockers to reduce CVD in patients post-MI also causes some concern about using them routinely in hypertension in the absence of definitive morbidity trial evidence *(41–43)*.

ANCILLARY ANTIHYPERTENSIVE THERAPY

In a number of clinical morbidity trials, either diuretics or β-blockers or both were used by investigator choice in one randomized arm as standard therapy or could be added to other initial drugs for BP control. Certainly, there are many diuretic and β-blocker combination products on the market that have proven antihypertensive efficacy *(8,9)*. In SHEP, 25 to 50 mg of atenolol or 0.05 to 0.1 mg of reserpine could be added for BP control in the actively treated group, 32% of whom were on atenolol and 8% on reserpine after an average of 4.5 years of follow-up; the addition of either did not substantially alter the risk ratios for chlorthalidone alone, although there was a trend for reserpine to reduce events more than atenolol with considerably larger risk reductions but large confidence intervals that included 1.0 *(44)*. The authors concluded that the CVD benefits in SHEP were based on lowering BP with a chlorthalidone-based regimen with no clear additional BP-independent effects attributable to atenolol or reserpine. In ALLHAT, 25–100 mg atenolol was the most common drug added to blinded therapy, although analyses of whether this affected outcomes have not been published *(45)*.

In ALLHAT, which had an older hypertensive population (age ≥55 years on entry, average 67 years), 66% of participants achieved BP control (<140/90 mmHg) at 5 years of follow-up with an average of two medications *(27)*. However, only 26% of participants were controlled on one drug, indicating that most older hypertensive patients will need two or more antihypertensive medications to control BP to less than 140/90 mmHg *(27,46)*. Furthermore, in ALLHAT only 49% of participants were controlled on one or two drugs, so a large proportion of hypertensive patients will require three or more antihypertensive medications to control BP *(27,46)*. Lower goals, such as are recommended for patients with diabetes or chronic kidney disease *(8,9)*, will require even more medications.

Although many combinations of antihypertensive medications are effective in lowering BP, regimens that include a diuretic are more effective in controlling BP than regimens not including a diuretic *(47)*. In ALLHAT, although the protocol called for additional medications to be added until BP was less than 140/90 mmHg, the chlorthalidone group reduced BP, especially systolic BP, more and achieved BP control more quickly than the other three arms and maintained superior BP control throughout the duration of the trial despite efforts to minimize BP differences: there were 68, 66, and 61% control rates at 5 years in the chlorthalidone, amlodipine, and lisinopril groups, respectively *(24,26,27,46)*.

Early control of BP has been hypothesized as a possible explanation for differences in outcomes in some clinical trials and has led to an increased emphasis on more rapid control of BP *(39,48)*. These kinds of data contributed to the JNC 7 recommendation to begin stage 2 hypertensive patients on two drugs as initial therapy *(8,9)*.

OTHER INDICATIONS FOR DIURETICS AND β-BLOCKERS

In addition to their benefits in improved BP control and reduction of CVD events in older patients with hypertension, both diuretics and β-blockers should also be included in regimens for any additional compelling indications, such as β-blockers post-MI or in certain forms of heart failure *(8,9)*. There are other indications or benefits that may also be considered for each, such as prevention or treatment of osteoporosis, renal lithiasis, or edema with diuretics and treatment of migraine or other headaches, arrhythmias, angina, and essential tremor with β-blockers. In the elderly, prevention of osteoporosis with thiazide-type diuretics has broad public health implications. For example, in a prospective population-based cohort study of 7891 elderly individuals, thiazide diuretic use for at least a year was associated with a statistically significant 54% lower risk of hip fracture *(49)*. This added value of preventing osteoporosis and hip fractures should be a further reason to increase the use of thiazide-type diuretics in addition to their unsurpassed cardiovascular benefits as antihypertensive agents.

SYMPTOMATIC ADVERSE EFFECTS

Both thiazide-type diuretics and β-blockers are generally well tolerated by the majority of elderly patients, and in double-blind studies are as well or better tolerated as other classes of antihypertensive agents *(50–53)*. In the VA Single-Drug Therapy Study, which compared HCTZ, atenolol, captopril, diltiazem, clonidine, and prazosin as monotherapy, HCTZ had the lowest withdrawal rate from adverse effects both short term (3%) and long term (1%), and atenolol was next-best tolerated (5% and 2% withdrawal rates, respectively) *(53)*. In ALLHAT, there were fewer withdrawals for drug intolerance from blinded therapy with chlorthalidone than with lisinopril, amlodipine, or doxazosin *(24,26)*.

Some reports have described a higher incidence of sexual dysfunction when thiazide-type diuretics, particularly at high doses, are used. In the Treatment of Mild Hypertension Study, participants randomly assigned to chlorthalidone reported a significantly higher incidence of erection problems through 24 months of the study; however, the incidence rate at 48 months was similar to placebo *(54)*. The VA Single-Drug Therapy

Study, which randomly assigned more patients, all of whom were men, to a thiazide diuretic did not find an increase in sexual dysfunction with the thiazide diuretic compared with other antihypertensive medications or placebo *(53)*. An even larger diuretic-treated (HCTZ 25–50 mg once or twice daily) cohort of elderly men (*n* = 690), the VA Treatment of Hypertension in the Elderly study, found no increase in sexual dysfunction on the thiazide diuretic, even with extensive "quality-of-life" testing. Although uncommon, thiazide diuretics may cause constipation, muscle cramps, urinary frequency, and sun sensitivity.

Although usually well tolerated, β-blockers are contraindicated in most patients with asthma, chronic obstructive lung disease, decompensated systolic dysfunction heart failure, greater than first-degree heart block, and sick sinus syndrome. They are reported to prolong hypoglycemia and mask the symptoms of hypoglycemia, but this has not been documented from clinical trials: in the United Kingdom Prospective Diabetes Study, there was no difference in episodes of hypoglycemia between participants randomized to atenolol or to captopril *(55)*.

METABOLIC EFFECTS

Both diuretics and β-blockers have been reported to worsen insulin resistance and have been associated with increased glucose levels and diabetes incidence in some clinical trials and observational studies *(56–58)*. However, thiazide-type diuretics reduce CVD events in patients with diabetes as well or better than other agents and reduce CVD events even in trials reporting a small absolute increase in diabetic levels of glucose. In ALLHAT, which had by far the largest group of patients with hypertension and diabetes studied in a clinical trial, chlorthalidone was unsurpassed in reducing CVD events and reduced heart failure significantly more than lisinopril or amlodipine in the diabetic subgroup *(26)*. The small differences in glucose levels in ALLHAT for the overall population, as well as in the diabetic subgroup, did not translate to higher CVD event rates for the chlorthalidone group over a 4- to 8-year period. In the United Kingdom Prospective Diabetes Study, the β-blocker atenolol reduced CVD and microvascular events as well as captopril *(55)*. Because ACE inhibitors and ARBs appear to have a beneficial effect on glucose, either could be added, if appropriate, for BP control or another compelling indication if glucose appears to increase on a thiazide diuretic or β-blocker.

There is evidence suggesting that the effect of thiazide diuretics on fasting glucose is linked to the potassium level *(59)*. Patients who maintain normal plasma and body levels of potassium rarely develop diabetes. In addition, restoration of low potassium levels through supplementation or withdrawal of the diuretic often leads to normalization of the glucose level. Thus, drug-induced diabetes appears to be more reversible than "naturally occurring" diabetes. Sustained weight loss and/or exercise will probably reverse any early tendency toward diabetes. However, one may consider withholding a diuretic or β-blocker for a short time in someone with elevated glucose while optimizing glycemic control with lifestyle or hypoglycemic medications if indicated, but the long-term cardiovascular benefits of a thiazide diuretic, and β-blocker if there is a compelling indication, should lead to reinstitution of one or both relatively soon.

There do not appear to be significant long-term effects on lipids or lipoproteins with either thiazide-type diuretics or at least cardioselective β-blockers (60). In ALLHAT, although serum cholesterol did not increase from baseline in any group, it was slightly lower in the CCB (1.6 mg/dL) and ACE inhibitor (2.2 mg/dL) groups than the diuretic group at 4 years (26). Thiazide-induced hypokalemia has been hypothesized to contribute to increased ventricular ectopy and possible sudden death, particularly with high doses of thiazides (61). In the SHEP trial, the positive benefits of diuretic therapy were not apparent in a retrospective analysis when serum potassium levels were below 3.5 mmol/L after 1 year of treatment (62). However, other studies have not demonstrated increased ventricular ectopy with diuretic-induced hypokalemia (63). Although rare, thiazide-type diuretics can cause or worsen hyponatremia, especially in frail elderly women or in combination with other drugs that can cause hyponatremia. Uric acid increases in many patients receiving a diuretic, but the increased incidence of gout is uncommon with current dosages of thiazides.

As with ACE inhibitors and ARBs, it is prudent to obtain creatinine, potassium, and sodium levels prior to (with other appropriate baseline laboratory tests) and within a month after initiating therapy with a thiazide-type diuretic. If levels are acceptable, then frequent monitoring is not necessary, and laboratory parameters may be monitored annually thereafter. Hypokalemia, which only occurs from thiazide diuretics in a minority of elderly patients, may be treated or offset with reduced salt intake, ACE inhibitor or ARB administration, potassium-sparing diuretic or aldosterone antagonist, or potassium supplementation or by reducing the dose of the thiazide diuretic if an appropriate dose level can be maintained.

ECONOMIC CONSIDERATIONS

Especially thiazide-type diuretics, but also many β-blockers, are less costly for the patient and/or the health care payer. Fischer and Avorn reported concerning an analysis showing that "adherence to evidence-based prescribing guidelines for hypertension could result in substantial savings in prescription costs for elderly patients with hypertension that would amount to savings of about $1.2 billion nationally" *(64)*. ALLHAT is conducting a cost-effectiveness analysis of the various treatment regimens, but it is likely the thiazide diuretic will be found to save considerably because events and hospitalizations were prevented more than with the other drugs, and the diuretic is certainly less costly. Another way to save patients drug costs and copayments and to improve the likelihood of controlling BP is to use one of the many combination products that include a thiazide-type diuretic or a β-blocker if it is less expensive than the drugs prescribed separately, which is often the case.

CONCLUSIONS

Reducing high BP reduces cardiovascular risk, but it does matter how it is lowered. Antihypertensive drugs vary in BP-lowering efficacy and can have BP-independent effects, as seen particularly with diuretics in the prevention of heart failure. Thiazide-type diuretics should be used as initial therapy for most patients with hypertension, especially the elderly, either alone or in combination with one of the other classes that have also been shown to reduce hypertensive complications in randomized outcome trials: β-blockers, ACE inhibitors, ARBs, and CCBs. Selection of one of these other agents as initial therapy is appropriate in the rare circumstance when a diuretic cannot be used or when a compelling indication is present that requires the use of another specific drug; however, in most cases when a compelling indication is present for another agent, a diuretic should also be used for optimal CVD benefit and BP control. Thiazide-type diuretics are particularly effective in reducing elevated systolic BP, the primary BP abnormality in the elderly. Both diuretics and β-blockers are underutilized in the treatment of hypertension: increased use of both is likely to save patients and payers of health care millions, if not billions, of dollars; improve BP control rates in the community; and most important, lead to further reductions in cardiovascular morbidity and mortality.

REFERENCES

1. Veterans Administration Cooperative Study Group on Antihypertensive Agents. Effect of treatment on morbidity in hypertension: results in patients with diastolic blood pressure averaging 115–129 mm Hg. *JAMA* 1967;202:116–122.
2. Veterans Administration Cooperative Study Group on Antihypertensive Agents. Effects of treatment on morbidity in hypertension II. Results in patients with diastolic blood pressure averaging 90 through 114 mm Hg. *JAMA* 1970;213:1143–1152.

3. Veterans Administration Cooperative Study Group on Antihypertensive Agents. Effects of treatment on morbidity in hypertension III. Influence of age, diastolic pressure, and prior cardiovascular disease: further analysis of side effects. *Circulation* 1972;45:991–1004.

4. Neal B, MacMahon S, Chapman N. Effects of ACE inhibitors, calcium antagonists, and other blood-pressure-lowering drugs: results of prospectively designed overviews of randomised trials. Blood Pressure Lowering Treatment Trialists' Collaboration. *Lancet* 2000;356:1955–1964.

5. Psaty BM, Smith NL, Siscovick DS, et al. Health outcomes associated with antihypertensive therapies used as first-line agents: a systematic review and meta-analysis. *JAMA* 1997;277:739–745.

6. Medical Research Council trial of treatment of hypertension in older adults: principal results. MRC Working Party. *BMJ* 1992;304:405–412.

7. The 1984 report of the Joint National Committee on Detection, Evaluation, and Treatment of High Blood Pressure. *Arch Intern Med* 1984;144:1045–1057.

8. Chobanian AV, Bakris GL, Black HR, et al. Seventh report of the Joint National Committee on Prevention, Detection, Evaluation, and Treatment of High Blood Pressure. *Hypertension* 2003;42:1206–1252.

9. Chobanian AV, Bakris GL, Black HR, et al. The seventh report of the Joint National Committee on Prevention, Detection, Evaluation, and Treatment of High Blood Pressure: the JNC 7 Report. *JAMA* 2003;289:2560–2571.

10. Blood Pressure Lowering Treatment Trialists' Collaboration. Effects of different blood-pressure-lowering regimens on major cardiovascular events: results of prospectively-designed overviews of randomised trials. *Lancet* 2003;362:1527–1535.

11. Cutler JA, Psaty BM, MacMahon S, Furberg CD. Public health issues in hypertension control: what has been learned from clinical trials. In Laragh JH, Brenner BM, eds. *Hypertension: Pathophysiology, Diagnosis, and Management.* 2nd ed. New York: Raven Press; 1995:253–279.

12. Messerli FH, Grossman E, Goldbourt U. Are β-blockers efficacious as first-line therapy for hypertension in the elderly? A systematic review. *JAMA* 1998;279:1903–1907.

13. Medical Research Council Working Party. MRC trial of treatment of mild hypertension: principal results. Medical Research Council Working Party. *BMJ* 1985;291:97–104.

14. Prisant LM. Should β—blockers be used in the treatment of hypertension in the elderly? *J Clin Hypertens* 2002;4:286–294.

15. Psaty BM, Lumley T, Furberg CD, et al. Health outcomes associated with various antihypertensive therapies used as first-line agents: a network meta-analysis. *JAMA* 2003;289:2534–2544.

16. Hansson L, Lindholm LH, Niskanen L, et al. for the Captopril Prevention Project (CAPPP) study group. Effect of angiotensin-converting-enzyme inhibition compared with conventional therapy on cardiovascular morbidity and mortality in hypertension. *Lancet* 1999;353:611–616.

17. Hansson L, Hedner T, Lund-Johansen P, et al. for the NORDIL Study Group. Randomized trial of calcium antagonist compared with diuretics and b-blockers on cardiovascular morbidity and mortality in hypertension: the Nordic Diltiazem (NORDIL) Study. *Lancet* 2000;356:359–365.

18. Black HR, Elliott WJ, Grandits G, et al. Principal results of the Controlled Onset Verapamil Investigation of Cardiovascular End Points (CONVINCE) trial. *JAMA* 2003;289:2073–2082.

19. Hansson L, Lindholm LH, Ekbom T, et al. Randomised trial of old and new antihypertensive drugs in elderly patients: cardiovascular mortality and morbidity: the Swedish Trial in Old Patients with Hypertension-2 study. *Lancet* 1999;354:1751–1756.

20. Brown MJ, Palmer CR, Castaigne A, et al. Morbidity and mortality in patients randomised to double-blind treatment with a long-acting calcium-channel blocker or diuretic in the International Nifedipine GITS study: Intervention as a Goal in Hypertension Treatment (INSIGHT). *Lancet* 2000;356:366–372.

21. Pepine CJ, Handberg EM, Cooper-DeHoff RM, et al. for the INVEST Investigators. A calcium antagonist vs a non-calcium antagonist hypertension treatment strategy for patients with coronary artery disease. The International Verapamil-Trandolapril Study (INVEST): a randomized controlled trial. *JAMA* 2003;290:2805–2816.

22. Dahlof B, Devereux RB, Kjeldsen SE, et al. Cardiovascular morbidity and mortality in the Losartan Intervention for Endpoint reduction in hypertension study (LIFE): a randomized trial against atenolol. *Lancet* 2002;359:995–1003.

23. Davis BR, Cutler JA, Gordon DJ, et al. Rationale and design for the Antihypertensive and Lipid Lowering Treatment to Prevent Heart Attack Trial (ALLHAT). *Am J Hypertens* 1996;9:342–360.

24. The ALLHAT Officers and Coordinators for the ALLHAT Collaborative Research Group. Major cardiovascular events in hypertensive patients randomized to doxazosin vs chlorthalidone: the Antihypertensive and Lipid-Lowering Treatment to Prevent Heart Attack Trial (ALLHAT). *JAMA* 2000;283:1967–1975.

25. ALLHAT Officers and Coordinators for the ALLHAT Collaborative Research Group. Diuretic vs α-blocker as first-step antihypertensive therapy. Final results from the Antihypertensive and Lipid-Lowering Treatment to Prevent Heart Attack Trial (ALLHAT). *Hypertension* 2003;42:239–246.

26. The ALLHAT Officers and Coordinators for the ALLHAT Collaborative Research Group. Major outcomes in high-risk hypertensive patients randomized to angiotensin-converting enzyme inhibitor or calcium channel blocker vs diuretic: the Antihypertensive and Lipid-Lowering Treatment to Prevent Heart Attack Trial (ALLHAT). *JAMA* 2002;288:2981–2997.

27. Cushman WC, Ford CE, Cutler JA, et al. for the ALLHAT Research Group. Success and predictors of blood pressure control in diverse North American settings: the Antihypertensive and Lipid-Lowering Treatment to Prevent Heart Attack Trial (ALLHAT). *J Clin Hypertens* 2002;4:393–404.

28. Wing LM, Reid CM, Ryan P, et al. A comparison of outcomes with angiotensin-converting–enzyme inhibitors and diuretics for hypertension in the elderly. *N Engl J Med* 2003;348:583–592.

29. Davis BR, Wright JT Jr, Cutler JA. Angiotensin-converting-enzyme inhibitors and diuretics for hypertension [Letter]. *N Engl J Med* 2003;349:91–92.

30. Wing LM, Reid CM, Jennings GL, for the ANBP2 Management Committee. Angiotensin-converting-enzyme inhibitors and diuretics for hypertension (Letter). *N Engl J Med* 2003;349:92–93.

31. Psaty BM, Lumley T, Furberg CD. Meta-analysis of health outcomes of chlorthalidone-based vs nonchlorthalidone-based low-dose diuretic therapies [Research letter]. *JAMA* 2004;292:43–44.

32. Perry MH Jr, Smith WM, McDonald RH, et al. Morbidity and mortality in the Systolic Hypertension in the Elderly Program (SHEP) pilot study. *Stroke* 1989;20:4–13.

33. SHEP Cooperative Research Group. Prevention of stroke by antihypertensive drug treatment in older persons with isolated systolic hypertension: final results of the Systolic Hypertension in the Elderly Program (SHEP). *JAMA* 1991;265:3255–3264.

34. Kostis JB, Davis BR, Cutler J, et al. Prevention of heart failure by antihypertensive drug treatment in older persons with isolated systolic hypertension. *JAMA* 1997;278:212–216.
35. Amery A, Birkenhager W, Brixko P, et al. Mortality and morbidity from the European Working Party on High Blood Pressure in the Elderly trial. *Lancet* 1985;1: 1349–1354.
36. Medical Research Council Working Party. Medical Research Council trial of treatment of hypertension in older adults: principal results. *BMJ* 1992;304:405–412.
37. PATS Collaborating Group. Post-stroke antihypertensive treatment study: a preliminary report. *Chin Med J (Engl)* 1995;108:710–717.
38. Carter BL, Ernst ME, Cohen JD. Hydrochlorothiazide vs chlorthalidone: evidence supporting their interchangeability. *Hypertension* 2004;43:4–9.
39. Julius S, Kjeldsen SE, Weber M, et al. Outcomes in hypertensive patients at high cardiovascular risk treated with regimens based on valsartan or amlodipine: the VALUE randomised trial. *Lancet* 2004;363:2022–2031.
40. Dahlöf B, Lindholm LH, Hansson L, Schersten B, Ekbom T, Wester PO. Morbidity and mortality in the Swedish trial in Old Patients with Hypertension (STOP-Hypertension). *Lancet* 1991;338:1281–1285.
41. Frishman WH, Furberg CD, Friedewald WT. β-Adrenergic blockade for survivors of acute myocardial infarction. *N Engl J Med* 1984;310:830–837.
42. Hjalmarson A, Olsson G. Myocardial infarction. Effects of β-blockade. *Circulation* 1991;84(6 suppl):VI101–VI107.
43. Gheorghiade M, Goldstein S. β-Blockers in the post-myocardial infarction patient. *Circulation* 2002;106:394–398.
44. Kostis JB, Berge KG, Davis BR, Hawkins CM, Probstfield J. Effect of atenolol and reserpine on selected events in the Systolic Hypertension in the Elderly Program (SHEP). *Am J Hypertens* 1995;8:1147–1153.
45. Davis BR, Cutler JA, Furberg CD, et al. Relationship of antihypertensive treatment regimens and change in blood pressure to risk for heart failure in hypertensive patients randomly assigned to doxazosin or chlorthalidone: further analyses from the Antihypertensive and Lipid-Lowering treatment to prevent Heart Attack Trial. *Ann Intern Med* 2002;137:313–320.
46. Cushman WC, Ford CE, Einhorn P, et al. Blood pressure control by randomized drug group in ALLHAT (Abstract). *Am J Hypertens* 2004;17:5(part 2):30A.
47. Materson BJ, Reda DJ, Cushman WC, Henderson WG, for the Department of Veterans Affairs Cooperative Study Group on Antihypertensive Agents: Results of combination antihypertensive therapy after failure of each of the components. *J Hum Hypertens* 1995;9:791–796.
48. Weber MA, Julius S, Kjeldsen SE, et al. Blood pressure dependent and independent effects of antihypertensive treatment on clinical events in the VALUE Trial. *Lancet* 2004;363:2049–2051.
49. Schoofs MW, van der Klift M, Hofman A, et al. Thiazide diuretics and the risk for hip fracture. *Ann Intern Med* 2003;139:476–482.
50. Materson BJ, Cushman WC, Goldstein G, et al. for the Department of Veterans Affairs Cooperative Study Group on Antihypertensive Agents. Treatment of hypertension in the elderly. I. Blood pressure and clinical changes. Results of a Department of Veterans Affairs Cooperative Study. *Hypertension* 1990;15:348–360.
51. Goldstein G, Materson BJ, Cushman WC, et al. for the Department of Veterans Affairs Cooperative Study Group on Antihypertensive Agents. Treatment of hypertension in the elderly. II. Cognitive and behavioral function. Results of a Department of Veterans Affairs Cooperative Study. *Hypertension* 1990;15:361–369.

52. Cushman WC, Khatri I, Materson BJ, et al. for the Department of Veterans Affairs Cooperative Study Group on Antihypertensive Agents. Treatment of hypertension in the elderly. III. Response of isolated systolic hypertension to various doses of hydrochlorothiazide: results of a Department of Veterans Affairs Cooperative Study. *Arch Intern Med* 1991;151:1954–1960.

53. Materson BJ, Reda DJ, Cushman WC, et al. for the Department of Veterans Affairs Cooperative Study Group on Antihypertensive Agents. Single-drug therapy for hypertension in men: a comparison of six antihypertensive agents with placebo. *N Engl J Med* 1993;328:914–921.

54. Grimm RH Jr, Grandits GA, Prineas RJ, et al. Long-term effects on sexual function of five antihypertensive drugs and nutritional hygienic treatment in hypertensive men and women. Treatment of Mild Hypertension Study (TOMHS). *Hypertension* 1997;29:8–14.

55. UK Prospective Diabetes Study Group. Efficacy of atenolol and captopril in reducing risk of macrovascular and microvascular complications in type 2 diabetes: UKPDS 39. *BMJ* 1998;317:713–720.

56. Prisant LM, Carr AA. Antihypertensive drug therapy and insulin resistance. *Am J Hypertens* 1992;5:775–777.

57. Padwal R, Laupacis A. Antihypertensive therapy and incidence of type 2 diabetes: a systematic review. *Diabetes Care* 2004;27:247–255.

58. Verdecchia P, Reboldi G, Angeli F, et al. Adverse prognostic significance of new diabetes in treated hypertensive subjects. *Hypertension* 2004;43:963–969.

59. Amery A, Birkenhager W, Brixko P, et al. Glucose intolerance during diuretic therapy in elderly hypertensive patients. A second report from the European Working Party on High Blood Pressure in the Elderly (EWPHE). *Postgrad Med J* 1986;62:919–924.

60. Lakshman MR, Reda DJ, Materson BJ, Cushman WC, Freis ED, for the Department of Veterans Affairs Cooperative Study Group on Antihypertensive Agents. Diuretics and β-blockers do not have adverse effects at one year on plasma lipid and lipoprotein profiles in men with hypertension. *Arch Intern Med* 1999;159:551–558.

61. Siscovick DS, Raghunathan TE, Psaty BM, et al. Diuretic therapy for hypertension and the risk of primary cardiac arrest. *N Engl J Med* 1994;330;1852–1857.

62. Franse LV, Pahor M, Di Bari M, Somes GW, Cushman WC, Applegate WB. Hypokalemia associated with diuretic use and cardiovascular events in SHEP. *Hypertension* 2000;35:1025–1030.

63. Papademetriou V, Burris JF, Notargiacomo A, Fletcher RD, Freis ED. Thiazide therapy is not a cause of arrhythmia in patients with systemic hypertension. *Arch Intern Med* 1988;148:1272–1276.

64. Fischer MA, Avorn J. Economic implications of evidence-based prescribing for hypertension: can better care cost less? *JAMA* 2004;291:1850–1856.

16 Assessment of the Role of ACE Inhibitors in the Elderly

Domenic A. Sica, MD

CONTENTS

INTRODUCTION

In the treatment of hypertension and cardiovascular disease (CVD), multiple treatment strategies have come and gone over the last several decades. The stepped care approach was popular for some time. However, adopting a stepped care approach to the treatment of hypertension *per se* neglected the diverse individualized pathophysiology of hypertension. Its advocates appreciated the purity of a standardization of hypertension treatment; others were disenchanted with its rigid nature. Yet, the stepped care approach to hypertension therapy, with diuretics and/or β-blockers, was supported by strong outcomes data from numerous randomized controlled trials (RCTs) *(1)*.

From: *Clinical Hypertension and Vascular Diseases: Hypertension in the Elderly*
Edited by: L. M. Prisant © Humana Press Inc., Totowa, NJ

However, for the elderly hypertensive such debate was always less relevant, in part because of the overwhelming comorbid disease state burden and the ever-present need to individualize treatment regimens *(2)*. Into this arena entered angiotensin-converting enzyme (ACE) inhibitors. This drug class at first was viewed as an acceptable alternative to the treatment of hypertension in the elderly but soon was recognized as having unique end-organ protective effects. Now, in many instances the selection of an agent to treat hypertension in the elderly is predicated first on the end-organ protection aspect of their use, and the accompanying blood pressure (BP) reduction is viewed as a secondary benefit *(3)*. However, although there exists a growing advocacy for ACE inhibitor use in the elderly, in practice many elderly patients with appropriate indications for ACE inhibitor therapy may not routinely receive one of these compounds *(4)*.

This chapter discusses the pharmacology, mechanism of action, and response data for ACE inhibitors, particularly as relates to their use in the elderly. If necessary, the reader will be directed to sources that provide more comprehensive discussion on particular themes.

PHARMACOLOGY

The first orally active ACE inhibitor was the sulfhydryl-containing compound captopril, which was introduced in 1981. Subsequently, the more long-acting compound enalapril maleate became available. Enalapril, a prodrug requiring in vivo hepatic and intestinal wall esterolysis to yield the active diacid inhibitor enalaprilat, and lisinopril became available shortly thereafter. All orally administered ACE inhibitors are prodrugs with the exception of lisinopril and captopril *(5)*. Although it was originally thought that formation of the active diacid metabolite of an ACE inhibitor, such as enalapril, could be inhibited in the presence of hepatic impairment, as may develop in advanced congestive heart failure (CHF), this appears not to occur in a clinically relevant manner *(6)*.

ACE inhibitors are structurally heterogeneous, with the chemical structure of their binding ligand serving as a criterion for dividing ACE inhibitors into three groups: sulfhydryl, carboxyl, and phosphinyl containing. The purported advantages with sulfhydryl-containing ACE inhibitors, such as captopril, are to date clinically unsubstantiated. Likewise is the belief that the phosphinyl group, found on fosinopril, might favorably alter its myocardial penetration and thereby improve myocardial energetics *(7)*. However, the sulfhydryl group found on captopril is believed the cause of the more frequent skin rashes—usually maculopapular—and the dysgeusia seen with this compound *(8)*. The latter can prove particularly troubling in the elderly.

ACE inhibitors can be distinguished by differences in rate and extent of absorption, plasma protein binding, systemic half-life, and mode of disposition; however, they behave quite similarly in the way they lower BP (Table 1) *(5,9,10)*. Beyond the issue of frequency of dosing, seldom are any of these pharmacological differences sufficiently important to govern selection of an agent *(3,10)*. Two pharmacological considerations for the ACE inhibitors, route of systemic elimination and tissue binding, have generated considerable recent debate and deserve some comment in the context of the elderly *(11,12)*.

Route of Elimination

Ramipril, enalapril, fosinopril, trandolapril, and benazepril do not accumulate in the presence of chronic kidney disease (CKD), suggesting that these prodrugs either undergo intact biliary clearance or their conversion to an active diacid form is not influenced by CKD *(13–15)*. These ACE inhibitor prodrugs are marginally active, making their accumulation (or not) in CKD less pertinent. The absence of ACE inhibitor prodrug accumulation in CKD should not be viewed as the existence of a clinically relevant dual route of elimination for these drugs. The active diacid forms fosinoprilat and trandolaprilat are the only two ACE inhibitors that undergo combined renal and hepatic elimination *(14,15)*. For all other ACE inhibitors, systemic elimination is almost exclusively renal, with varying degrees of filtration and tubular secretion occurring *(11)*. ACE inhibitor accumulation generally begins early in the course of CKD; thus, elderly patients can be expected to experience ACE inhibitor accumulation either in relationship to their age-related decline in renal function or as the result of comorbid conditions that have a negative impact on renal function.

In the elderly patient with CKD, adverse effects from ACE inhibitor accumulation have yet to be identified. However, the longer drug concentrations remain elevated (once a response occurs), the more likely it is that BP will remain reduced. Thus, the major adverse effect of ACE inhibitor accumulation may be that of protracted hypotension and its organ-directed sequelae *(16)*.

Tissue Binding

The second unsettled pharmacological feature of ACE inhibitors is that of tissue binding *(12,17)*. The physicochemical differences among ACE inhibitors, including binding affinity, potency, lipophilicity, and depot effect, permit the arbitrary classification of ACE inhibitors accord-

Table 1

Angiotensin-Converting Enzyme Inhibitors: Dosage Strengths and Treatment Guidelines

Drug	Trade name	Usual total dose and/or range Hypertension (frequency day)	Usual total dose and/or range Heart failure (frequency day)	Comment	Fixed dose combination[a]
Benazepril	Lotensin®	20–40 (1)	Not FDA approved for heart failure	Lotensin HCT®	
Captopril	Capoten®	12.5–100 (2–3)	18.75–150 (3)	Generically available	Capozide®[b]
Enalapril	Vasotec®	5–40 (1–2)	5–40 (2)	Generic and intravenous	Vaseretic®
Fosinopril	Monopril®	10–40 (1)	10–40 (1)	Renal and hepatic elimination	Monopril-HCT
Lisinopril	Prinivil®, Zestril®	2.5–40 (1)	5–20 (1)	Generically available	Prinizide®, Zestoretic®
Moexipril	Univasc®	7.5–30 (1)	Not FDA approved for heart failure		Uniretic®
Perindopril	Aceon®	2–16 (1)	Not FDA approved for heart failure		
Quinapril	Accupril®	5–80 (1)	10–40 (1–2)		Accuretic®
Ramipril	Altace®	2.5–20 (1)	10 (2)	Indicated in high-risk vascular patients	
Trandolapril	Mavik®	1–8 (1)	1–4 (1)	Renal and hepatic elimination	Tarka®

[a]Fixed-dose combinations in this class typically contain a thiazide-like diuretic.
[b]Capozide is indicated for first-step treatment of hypertension.
FDA, Food and Drug Administration.

ing to affinity for tissue ACE *(12,18)*. The level of tissue ACE inhibition produced by an ACE inhibitor parallels both the inhibitor's binding affinity and the free inhibitor concentration contained within that tissue. The free inhibitor concentration represents a state of dynamic equilibrium between ACE inhibitor conveyed to tissues and residual ACE inhibitor released from tissues and returned to the bloodstream.

The quantity of ACE inhibitor shuttled to tissues is dictated by traditional pharmacological variables, including dose frequency/amount, absolute bioavailability, plasma half-life, and tissue penetration. When blood levels of an ACE inhibitor are high (typically in the first third to half of the dosing interval), tissue retention *per se* of an ACE inhibitor is not needed for functional ACE inhibition. However, toward the end of the dosing interval, as ACE inhibitor blood levels fall, two factors—inhibitor binding affinity and tissue retention—assume added importance in prolonging functional ACE inhibition.

The question arises whether the degree of tissue ACE inhibition may extend to differences in the efficacy of various ACE inhibitors. First, there appears to be little—beyond differences that may arise based on half-life considerations—to distinguish one ACE inhibitor from another as far as BP reduction is concerned. Moreover, in the elderly, even with early stages of CKD the accumulation and thereby prolonged half-life of most ACE inhibitors further reduces the chances of any intraclass differences in BP reduction.

Second, an alternative question is whether these drugs differ in their ability to provide end-organ protection in a BP-independent fashion, as was speculated in the Heart Outcomes Prevention Evaluation (HOPE) study *(19)*. In this regard, it should be noted that consistent improvement in endothelial function is reported with those ACE inhibitors with higher tissue ACE affinity, such as quinapril and ramipril. If improvement in endothelial dysfunction can be used as a surrogate for protection from end events, then it is possible that relevant intraclass differences exist among ACE inhibitors. Yet, there have been few direct head-to-head trials between ACE inhibitors, which have varying tissue affinity. When such comparisons have occurred, the results have not convincingly supported the claim of overall superiority for lipophilic ACE inhibitors *(20,21)*. Moreover, in the elderly relevant differences for BP-independent effects of the various ACE inhibitors are even less likely in the face of CKD-related ACE inhibitor accumulation.

Application of Pharmacological Differences

Because there is very little that truly separates one ACE inhibitor from another in the treatment of hypertension, the cost of an ACE inhibitor has assumed added importance *(22)*. For pricing to be a major selection factor is not unreasonable if ACE inhibitors were only used for the control of BP. ACE inhibitors, however, are also extensively used for their cardiorenal benefits, and therein only a limited number of ACE inhibitors have been studied for their ability to modify specific end-organ disease states. The term *class effect* has entered into the discussion of both of these facets of ACE inhibitor use, relevant to one and not the other.

Class effect is a phrase often invoked to legitimatize use of a less-costly ACE inhibitor when a higher priced agent in the class has been the one specifically studied in a disease state, such as CHF or diabetic nephropathy *(19,23–25)*. The concept of class effect may be best suited for application to the BP effects of ACE inhibitors, for which scant difference exists among the various ACE inhibitors.

Alternatively, the concept of class effect, already vague in its definition, becomes even more ambiguous when "true" dose equivalence for a non-BP end point, such as rate of progression to end-stage renal disease or survival in the setting of CHF, is being established between the various ACE inhibitors. Determining ACE inhibitor dose equivalence for disease state end points other than BP is further confused by differing dose frequency, titration attempts, and level of renal function *(26–31)*. The last is particular relevant to the elderly because senescence-related changes in renal function extend ACE inhibitor functional half-life and make it virtually impossible to determine equivalence for various ACE inhibitors.

A prudent action regarding the concept of ACE inhibitor class effect is to assume that the benefits of a particular ACE inhibitor apply primarily to the investigated indication, dose amount, dose frequency, and outcomes.

MECHANISM OF ACTION
AND HEMODYNAMIC EFFECTS

The locus of activity of ACE inhibitors within the renin–angiotensin–aldosterone (RAA) axis is at the pluripotent ACE, which catalyzes the conversion of angiotensin (Ang) I to Ang II and facilitates bradykinin degradation to various vasoactive peptides *(32)*. However potent an ACE inhibitor is in this regard, it still only manages to suppress the Ang-II generated by ACE *(19)*. Other pathways for Ang-II production (e.g., chymase and other tissue-based proteases) remain functional despite administration of an ACE inhibitor *(33)*. These alternative pathways represent the principal mode of Ang-II generation in myocardial and vascular tissue *(34,35)*. Interestingly, the long-term administration of an ACE inhibitor is marked by a gradual return of Ang-II to pretherapy levels. This phenomenon is termed *angiotensin escape* and is presumably caused by an upregulation in the capacity of these alternative pathways. Substrate for these alternative pathways at least partly comes from the increase in Ang-I levels when ACE inhibition disinhibits renin secretion from the juxtaglomerular apparatus *(35,36)*.

Because ACE inhibitors reduce Ang-II levels only on the order of weeks *(36,37)*, alternative mechanisms for their persistent BP-lowering effect need to be considered; these include an increase in the concentration of the vasodilator bradykinin *(38,39)*, which in turn stimulates the production of endothelium-derived relaxing factor and the release of prostacyclin. However, the exact contribution of prostaglandins to the antihypertensive effect of ACE inhibitors, particularly in the elderly, is still debated *(40)*.

Alternatively, it has been recognized for some time that nonsteroidal anti-inflammatory drugs blunt the BP-lowering effect of ACE inhibitors *(41)*. This phenomenon is more common in salt-sensitive hypertensives, as is the case with the elderly *(42)*. Low-dose aspirin (100 mg/day or less) has minimal effect on the BP reduction seen with ACE inhibition *(43)*. For example, in the Hypertension Optimal Treatment study, long-term, low-dose aspirin did not interfere with the BP-lowering effect of antihypertensive agents, including combinations with ACE inhibitors, in elderly subjects 65 years or older *(44)*. However, higher doses, generally above 236 mg/day, can blunt the antihypertensive response to an ACE inhibitor *(45)*.

A variable portion of ACE inhibitor effect is caused by a reduction in both central and peripheral sympathetic nervous system activity (Table 2) *(46,47)*. ACE inhibitors also preserve circulatory reflexes and baroreceptor function; thus, they do not reflexly increase heart rate when BP is lowered *(48)*. This last property explains why this drug class is seldom associated with postural hypotension and provides an important safety advantage in elderly subjects, who as a group are typically prone to orthostatic hypotension *(49)*. ACE inhibitors also improve endothelial function, facilitate vascular remodeling, and favorably alter the viscoelastic properties of blood vessels *(50,51)*. These vascular properties of ACE inhibitors are the likely explanation for the incremental reduction in BP with the long-term use of these drugs.

BLOOD PRESSURE-LOWERING EFFECT

Diuretics are still commonly employed as first-step therapy for hypertension, although increasingly ACE inhibitors are viewed as a suitable

Table 2
Predominant Hemodynamic Effects of Angiotensin-Converting Enzyme Inhibitors

Hemodynamic parameter	Effect	Clinical significance
Cardiovascular		
• Total peripheral resistance	Decreased	
• Mean arterial pressure	Decreased	
• Cardiac output	Increased or no change	These parameters contribute to a general decrease in systemic blood pressure
• Stroke volume	Increased	
• Preload and afterload	Decreased	
• Pulmonary artery pressure	Decreased	
• Right atrial pressure	Decreased	
• Diastolic dysfunction	Improved	
Renal		
• Renal blood flow	Usually increased	Contributes to the renoprotective effect of these agents
• Glomerular filtration rate	Variable, usually unchanged but may decrease in renal failure	
• Efferent arteriolar resistance	Decreased	
• Filtration fraction	Decreased	
Peripheral nervous system		
• Biosynthesis of noradrenaline	Decreased	Enhances blood pressure-lowering effect and resets baroreceptor function
• Reuptake of adrenaline	Inhibited	
• Circulating catecholamines	Decreased	

first-step alternative, particularly in light of the positive outcomes associated with their use in high-risk elderly patients (52,53). The enthusiasm for the use of ACE inhibitors is not purely a matter of efficacy because they have a pattern of efficacy comparable to (and no better than) most other drug classes, with response rates from 40 to 70% in stage I or II hypertension (54). Physician preference for these drugs in the elderly also derives from their favorable side-effect profile and their highly touted end-organ protection features in at-risk cardiac and renal patients. The latter is not based on the BP-lowering ability of these drugs but rather on proposed tissue-based anti-inflammatory and antiproliferative effects, which are probably class and not agent specific.

There are very few predictors of the BP response to ACE inhibitors, whether it be in the elderly or not. When hypertension is accompanied by significant activation of the RAA axis, such as in renal artery stenosis, the response to an ACE inhibitor can be immediate and profound *(55)*. In most other instances, there is a limited relationship between the pre- and the posttreatment plasma renin activity value—used as a marker of RAA axis activity—and the vasodepressor response to an ACE inhibitor. Certain patient types are presumed to be less responsive to ACE inhibitor monotherapy, including low-renin, salt-sensitive individuals such as the diabetic and African-American or elderly hypertensive *(56)*. The low-renin state characteristic of the elderly hypertensive differs from other low-renin forms of hypertension in that it develops not as a response to volume expansion but rather because of senescence-related changes in the activity of the axis *(57)*. The elderly generally respond well to ACE inhibitors at conventional doses *(58)*, although senescence-related renal failure that slows the elimination of these drugs complicates interpretation of dose-specific treatment successes.

All 10 ACE inhibitors marketed in the United States are currently approved by the Food and Drug Administration for the treatment of hypertension with several others available on a global basis (Table 3). The Seventh Report of the Joint National Committee on the Detection, Evaluation, and Treatment of High Blood Pressure (JNC 7), the World Health Organization/International Society of Hypertension, and the European Society of Hypertension/European Society of Cardiology now recognize ACE inhibitors as an option for first-line therapy in patients with essential hypertension, especially in those with a high coronary disease risk profile, diabetes with renal disease/proteinuria, or CHF or who are postmyocardial infarction (MI) *(59,60)*. Results from a number of head-to-head trials support the comparable antihypertensive efficacy and tolerability of the various ACE inhibitors *if* similar doses of the individual ACE inhibitors are given (Table 1). However, there are differences among the ACE inhibitors regarding the time to onset of effect or the time to maximum BP reduction, which may relate to the absorption characteristics of a compound.

Considerable dosing flexibility exists with the orally available ACE inhibitors, whereas enalaprilat is the lone ACE inhibitor available in an intravenous form *(3)*. ACE inhibitors labeled as "once-daily" vary in their ability to reduce BP for a full 24 hours, as defined by a trough:peak ratio greater than 50% *(61)*. Consequently, the dosing frequency for ACE inhibitors is arbitrary and should consider the fact that these drugs often lose their effect at the end of the dosing interval, thereby requiring a second dose. However, in the elderly, senescence-related changes in renal function (and reduced ACE inhibitor renal clearance) and/or giving a high dose may obviate a second ACE inhibitor dose during the 24-

Table 3
Food and Drug Administration-Approved Indications for Angiotensin-
Converting Enzyme Inhibitors

Drug	HTN	CHF	Diabetic nephropathy	High-risk patients without left ventricular dysfunction
Captopril	•	• (post-MI)[a]	•	
Benazepril	•			
Enalapril	•	•[b]		
Fosinopril	•	•		
Lisinopril	•	• (post-MI)[a]		
Moexipril	•			
Perindopril	•			
Quinapril	•	•		
Ramipril	•	• (post-MI)		•
Trandolapril	•	• (post-MI)		

[a]Captopril and lisinopril are indicated for CHF treatment both post-MI and as adjunctive therapy in general heart failure therapy.

[b]Enalapril is indicated for asymptomatic left ventricular dysfunction.

CHF, congestive heart failure; HTN, hypertension; MI, myocardial infarction.

hour treatment period (62). Likewise, in the treatment of CHF, ACE inhibitors indicated for once-daily dosing can be split dosed if BP drops excessively with a single dose.

An often asked question is what to do if an ACE inhibitor fails to normalize BP. One approach is simply to raise the dose; however, the dose–response curve for ACE inhibitors, like many antihypertensive agents, is fairly steep at the beginning doses and thereafter becomes shallow to flat (63,64). Responders to ACE inhibition typically do so at doses well below those necessary for complete 24-hour suppression of ACE.

If a partial response has occurred with an ACE inhibitor, then therapy can be continued because an additional drop in BP usually follows over the next several weeks. This late-stage response may involve factors (e.g., vascular remodeling and improvement in endothelial function) above and beyond inhibition of ACE (51). Thus, only with complete failure to respond to an ACE inhibitor does an alternative drug class need to be considered. Alternatively, an additional compound, such as a diuretic, calcium channel blocker (CCB), or peripheral α-blocker can be combined with an ACE inhibitor to effect BP control (see the next section).

ACE INHIBITORS IN COMBINATION WITH OTHER AGENTS

The BP-lowering effect of an ACE inhibitor is enhanced with the concurrent administration of a diuretic, particularly in the salt-sensitive form of hypertension characteristic of the elderly, African-American, or diabetic hypertensive (65). This pattern of response has encouraged the development of several fixed-dose combination products comprised of an ACE inhibitor and varying doses (as low as 12.5 mg) of a thiazide-type diuretic (65). The rationale for combining these two drug classes arises from the observation that diuretic-related sodium depletion activates the RAA axis; therein, BP shifts to an Ang-II-dependent mode, which is the most favorable circumstance for an ACE inhibitor to reduce BP.

β-Blockers have been administered in conjunction with ACE inhibitors, an approach that was commonly used per protocol in the Antihypertensive and Lipid-Lowering Treatment to Prevent Heart Attack Trial (53). The physiological basis for this combination is that of β-blockade blunting the rise in plasma renin activity, which is a feature of ACE inhibitor therapy; however, in the elderly the reactive hyperreninemic response to ACE inhibitors is nominal (66). Thus, in principle this combination (if intended for BP control) would seem to offer little chance of additivity in elderly hypertensives.

When a meaningful drop in BP follows from the addition of a β-blocker to an ACE inhibitor, it often occurs in tandem with a reduction in pulse rate. Alternatively, adding a peripheral α-antagonist, such as doxazosin, to an ACE inhibitor can further reduce BP, albeit without a clear mechanistic basis (67).

Finally, the BP-lowering effect of an ACE inhibitor is reinforced with the addition of a CCB, whether a dihydropyridine or a nondihydropyridine, and this additivity has been the basis for several products combining both drug classes (68–70). Adding an ACE inhibitor to a CCB is also helpful in attenuating the peripheral edema commonly seen with CCB therapy. This is germane to the elderly because CCB-related edema is more frequent in the elderly (71). In addition, preliminary evidence exists in support of CCB therapy attenuating the drop in glomerular filtration rate (GFR) that can accompany ACE inhibitor therapy (72). This is of potential importance to the elderly because one reason for underuse of ACE inhibitors in older subjects is fear of a further decline in renal function when baseline function is already reduced. This CCB and ACE inhibitor hemodynamic interaction at a renal level may also occasionally result in false-positive captopril renography studies (73).

The efficacy of both ACE inhibitors and angiotensin-receptor blockers (ARBs) as antihypertensive agents is well established. This has fueled the belief that in combination these two drug classes may provide an incremental benefit in both BP reduction and end-organ protection. However, there is insufficient evidence to support a general recommendation for the combination of these two drug classes (74,75).

Finally, studies have established the utility of ACE inhibitors in the management of hypertensive patients otherwise unresponsive to multiple drug combinations, such as a diuretic together with minoxidil, a CCB and a peripheral α-blocker (76). In addition, if an acute reduction in BP is needed, oral or sublingual captopril—with an onset of action as soon as 15 minutes after administration—can be given. An additional option for the management of hypertensive emergencies is that of intravenous enalaprilat (77). ACE inhibitors should be administered cautiously in patients suspected of a marked activation of the RAA axis (e.g., prior treatment with diuretics). In such subjects, sudden and extreme drops in BP—so-called first-dose hypotension—have been observed (78).

ACE INHIBITORS IN HYPERTENSION ASSOCIATED WITH OTHER DISORDERS

ACE inhibitors effectively regress left ventricular hypertrophy (79). This is an important characteristic of ACE inhibitors in that the presence of left ventricular hypertrophy portends a significant future risk of sudden death or MI (80). ACE inhibitors can be safely utilized in patients with coronary artery disease and are indicated for secondary prevention in coronary heart disease after acute MI. Also, the ACE inhibitor perindopril has been shown to reduce cardiovascular risk in a low-risk population with stable coronary artery disease and no apparent heart failure (81). Although they are not coronary vasodilators, they do improve hemodynamic factors that influence myocardial oxygen consumption and thereby have a favorable impact on ischemia development (Table 2). For example, ACE inhibitors do not reflexly increase myocardial sympathetic tone in hypertensive patients with angina, as can take place with other antihypertensives (82). These issues are only as relevant as the use of ACE inhibitors and to that end a prescribing inertia often surrounds the use of ACE inhibitors after MI, particularly in the elderly (83).

ACE inhibitors are also useful in the treatment of either isolated systolic hypertension or systolic-predominant forms of hypertension, which partly relates to their ability to improve artery compliance (51,84). In addition, ACE inhibitors are of value in the treatment of patients with cerebrovascular disease because they preserve cerebral autoregulatory ability despite their reducing BP *(85)*. This is particularly noteworthy in the treatment of the elderly hypertensive *(85)*. ACE inhibitors dilate both small and large arteries and can be used safely in patients with peripheral arterial disease (PAD) disease and on occasion favorably modify the pattern and/or the course of intermittent claudication *(86)*. For example, 4051 of the 9297 patients in the HOPE study had PAD—defined by a history of PAD, claudication, or an ankle–brachial index less than 0.90. These patients had a similar reduction in the primary end point when compared with those without PAD, thus demonstrating that an ACE inhibitor, in this case ramipril, lowered the risk of fatal and nonfatal ischemic events in patients with PAD *(19)*.

ACE inhibitors are also viewed as preferred agents—but not exclusively so—in the hypertensive diabetic patient *(87,88)*. ACE inhibitors are used in the hypertensive diabetic patient for two purposes: (a) organ protection, an occurrence presumably independent of BP; and (b) for BP reduction. In the instance of the latter, diuretic coadministration is often required because the BP-lowering effects of an ACE inhibitor are modest in the typically low-renin, volume-expanded hypertensive diabetic. A final consideration with ACE inhibitors in the hypertensive diabetic relates to their effect on hyperlipidemia and insulin resistance. In this regard, ACE inhibitors have yet to demonstrate an unambiguous effect on serum lipids or insulin resistance *(89)*. However, in both the CAPtopril Prevention Project (CAPPP) and the HOPE studies, the ACE inhibitors captopril and ramipril, respectively, decreased the incidence of new-onset type 2 diabetes mellitus *(90,91)*.

END-ORGAN EFFECTS

Renal

JNC 7 advises the use of ACE inhibitors in patients with hypertension and chronic renal disease both to control hypertension and to slow the rate of progression of CKD *(59)*. Irrespective of the renoprotective effects of ACE inhibitors, the most important element in the management of the patient with hypertension and CKD remains tight BP control. JNC 7 recommendations advise a goal BP of 130/80 mmHg in albuminuric patients (>300 mg/day) with or without CKD *(59)*. In CKD, ACE inhibitor monotherapy is seldom able to achieve goal BP, partly because of the volume dependency of this form of hypertension. For example, in the African-American Study of Kidney Disease, the ACE inhibitor ramipril was used, and the average number of medications required to achieve BP control was approximately three *(92)*.

Proteinuria has emerged as a strong marker for the rate of CKD progression as well as an independent risk factor for CVD *(93)*. Microalbuminuria typically foreshadows the progression of diabetic nephropathy and is now routinely measured in all diabetics *(94)*. Screening for microalbuminuria is recommended in diabetes and increasingly in others perceived to be at high risk for renal or CVD *(95)*. Most guidelines now advise efforts be undertaken to reduce proteinuria in both diabetic and nondiabetic renal disease *(96)*. In this regard, ACE inhibitors and more recently ARBs have been shown to reduce protein excretion and are important treatment components in the patient (with or without hypertension) with micro- or macroalbuminuria.

ACE inhibitors have proved useful in the setting of established type 1 insulin-dependent diabetic nephropathy *(24)*, type 2 non-insulin-dependent diabetic nephropathy *(97)*, normotensive type 1 patients with microalbuminuria *(98)*, and a variety of nondiabetic renal diseases *(99–101)*. However, renal outcomes with ACE inhibitors have occasionally been negative. The Ramipril Efficacy in Nephropathy study did not identify a renoprotective effect with ramipril in type 2 diabetic nephropathy patients. Of note, in the Ramipril Efficacy in Nephropathy study ramipril-treated patients lost renal function at a significantly faster rate than did patients treated with a conventional non-ACE inhibitor antihypertensive regimen *(102)*. Conversely, ramipril prevented or delayed the progression of albuminuria in the HOPE trial *(103)*. ACE inhibitor regimens shown to slow the rate of CKD progression include 25 mg of captopril three times a day, 5 to 10 mg per day of enalapril, 10 mg per day of benazepril, and 2.5 to 5 mg of ramipril per day *(3)*. These compounds are all renally cleared; thus, it can be presumed that reduced renal clearance under these circumstances enhances the pharmacological effect of each of these compounds *(104)*. The beneficial effect of ACE inhibitors is typically greatest when preexisting high rates of urinary protein excretion (>3 g/24 hours) can be substantially reduced because, if left untreated, these patients generally progress quite rapidly *(105)*.

Therapies directed at reducing the production or effects of Ang II provide a mixture of potentially beneficial renal, hemodynamic, cellular, and possibly lipid-related effects. For example, in chronic nephropathies, ACE inhibitor uptitration to maximum tolerated doses improves hypertriglyceridemia by a direct, dose-dependent effect and hypercholesterolemia through amelioration of the nephrotic syndrome *(106)*. ACE inhibitors also transiently reduce GFR in parallel with reduction of glomerular capillary pressures *(107)*. Such decrements are typically modest and on the order of a 10 to 15% drop in GFR; moreover, these changes are reversible and actually predictive of long-term renal protection *(108)*.

The elderly are prone to greater reductions in GFR with ACE inhibitors at least partly because of their frequent micro- and macrovascular renal disease (*see* Side Effects of Angiotensin-Converting Enzyme Inhibitors). A question commonly posed with ACE inhibitors, particularly in the elderly, is whether there is a specific level of renal function at which an ACE inhibitor cannot be started. Current practice considerations suggest that there is not a specific level of renal function that precludes starting an ACE inhibitor unless significant hyperkalemia is expected to develop.

Three factors can be considered as potential modifiers of the renal response to ACE inhibition. First, a low sodium intake enhances the antiproteinuric and antihypertensive effects of ACE inhibition *(109)*. Second, short-term studies suggested that dietary protein restriction complements the ACE inhibitor effect on protein excretion in nephrotic patients. This would seem to imply that the combination of ACE inhibition and protein restriction could prove more effective than an ACE inhibition alone in slowing the progression of renal failure *(110)*. However, this approach may be ill advised in the elderly, for whom nutritional intake may already be suboptimal.

A third factor is that of inherited variation in the activity of ACE. Two common forms of the ACE gene I (insertion) and D (deletion) give rise to three potential genotypes: II, ID, and DD. The DD phenotype is associated with higher levels of circulating ACE and a heightened pressor response to infused Ang-I as compared to the Ang-II phenotype, with the ID phenotype exhibiting intermediate characteristics *(111)*. The finding that DD patients are at increased risk for MI and ischemic cardiomyopathy first established the clinical significance of inherited variation in ACE activity *(112)*. Studies suggested that the GFR declines more rapidly in DD than II nephropathic patients, and that such patients do not show significant reductions in proteinuria or slowing in the rate of CKD progression when given ACE inhibitors *(113)*. Although a promising concept, pharmacogenetic studies performed to date have not provided a definitive answer regarding whether the antiproteinuric effect of ACE inhibition is influenced by the ACE genotype *(114)*.

Cardiac

Data from both placebo-controlled and open-label trials suggested that ACE inhibitors substantially reduce the risk of death and hospitalization for CHF while improving its symptomatology, making ACE inhibitors first-line therapy for the treatment of CHF *(115)*. ACE inhibitors reduce Ang-II generation (at least in the short term) and thereby alter the pathophysiological consequences of neurohumoral change in CHF

(116,117). Even at low doses, ACE inhibitors improve exercise tolerance and symptomatology in CHF; however, successfully altering the status of these surrogates does not imply that similar success will be obtained relating to the mortality of CHF. Improvement in CHF mortality at least partly requires high-dose ACE inhibitor therapy. One aspect of ACE inhibitor dosing relative to the elderly relates to CHF-related weight loss or the cachexia of CHF. Weight loss is a common finding in the elderly CHF patient, and its presence often prompts a diagnostic workup to seek other causes of weight loss. In this regard, effective ACE inhibitor therapy will arrest the weight loss otherwise seen with progressive CHF *(118)*.

Several ACE inhibitors—including captopril, fosinopril, lisinopril, quinapril, ramipril, and trandolapril—now have favorable outcome data in various forms of CHF *(115,119)*. Although ACE inhibitors are almost universally recommended as a cost-effective strategy for the treatment of CHF, physician prescribing practice is such that only a modest number (50–70%) of those patients eligible for treatment with ACE inhibitors actually receive them *(120)*. Moreover, the dosages used in "real-world practice" are substantially lower than those proven effective in RCTs. For example, in a retrospective review of 554 elderly hospital-discharged CHF patients older than 65 years, target (dosage recommended in practice guidelines), subtarget (dosages used in clinical trials but lower than guideline recommendations), and low-dose ACE inhibitor doses were given in 19, 63, and 18% of the patients, respectively. Few demographic or clinical criteria were related to the use of lower dosages *(121)*.

On average, overall mean doses of ACE inhibitors are less than one-half the targeted dose. Factors forecasting either the use or optimal dose administration of ACE inhibitors include variables relating to the treatment setting (prior hospitalization and/or specialty clinic follow-up), the prescribing physician (cardiology specialty vs family practitioner/general internist), the patient status (increased severity of symptoms, male, younger), and the drug (lower frequency of administration) *(120)*.

Enalapril, captopril, lisinopril, and trandolapril have also been shown to significantly reduce morbidity and mortality rates in the post-MI patient with a wide range of ventricular function. In a hemodynamically stable patient after an MI, an oral ACE inhibitor should be initiated, generally within 24-hours of the event, particularly if the MI is anterior and accompanied by depressed left ventricular function. The hemodynamic effects and overall benefit of ACE inhibition are seen early with 40% of the increase in 30-day survival seen in the first day, 45% in days 2 through 7, and approximately 15% after day 7 *(122)*. Currently, only captopril, lisinopril, ramipril, and trandolapril are specifically approved in post-MI left ventricular dysfunction, although enalapril is approved in asymptomatic left ventricular dysfunction. Trends show an increase in ACE inhibitor prescriptions in patients discharged followed an acute MI *(123)*.

There are presently insufficient data to determine if clinically significant differences exist among the ACE inhibitors in the post-MI setting given the paucity of head-to-head trials among these agents and the fact that study-specific conditions for particular ACE inhibitors have been quite variable *(124,125)*. However, as in patients with CHF, numerous ACE inhibitors have established benefits in the post-MI patient, suggesting a class effect for this phenomenon *(125)*.

Several dosing strategies have been demonstrated as effective in reducing morbidity and mortality in patients with left ventricular systolic dysfunction. In this regard, a systematic effort must be made to reach target ACE inhibitor doses shown effective in the randomized therapeutic CHF trials. Emerging data would seem to suggest that the doses of ACE inhibitors used in clinical practice (range of 50 and 10 mg/day for captopril and enalapril, respectively) are less effective than the relatively high doses (captopril and enalapril doses approaching 150 and 40 mg, respectively) used in the RCTs *(28,31)*.

Until incontrovertible evidence otherwise becomes available, the treatment of CHF should include sequential dose titration to those ACE inhibitor doses shown successful in RCTs. The ability to reach these doses in the CHF patient can sometimes prove challenging because a major deterrent is the development of systemic hypotension and/or a decline in GFR *(126,127)*. Thus, reaching goal ACE inhibitor doses necessitates a keen understanding of the critical relationship among volume status, BP, and the final desired ACE inhibitor dose. Probably the single most important variable that allows effective dose titration is the understanding of the relationship between volume status and BP *(126–128)*.

Stroke

Given the significant public health impact of stroke and the identification of both nonmodifiable (age, gender, race/ethnicity) and modifiable (BP, diabetes, lipid profile, and lifestyle) risk factors, early prevention strategies are increasingly implemented. When an elderly or diabetic patient suffers a stroke, the focus of care becomes the prevention of secondary events. This can be accomplished with antiplatelet and lipid-lowering as well as BP reduction strategies.

Despite the clear risk reduction with effective implementation of these preventative strategies, new approaches are needed. In particular, it is unclear whether the stroke benefit gained from BP reduction is unique to the agent employed (e.g., an ACE inhibitor or an ARB) or a simple consequence of upgrading the hemodynamic profile *(129–131)*.

The Perindopril Protection Against Recurrent Stroke Study (PROG-RESS) reported for the first time that antihypertensive therapy with a combination of the ACE inhibitor perindopril and the thiazide diuretic indapamide reduced the stroke recurrence rate even in patients with normal BP *(129)*. In this study, 6105 hypertensive and nonhypertensive patients who had sustained a stroke without a major disability within the past 5 years were randomly assigned to a 4-mg dose of perindopril with or without a 2.5-mg dose of indapamide (diuretic therapy was at the discretion of the treating physician). After 4 years of follow-up (40% received perindopril alone and 60% combination therapy) in the sub-group of patients receiving perindopril and indapamide, BP was reduced by 12/5 mmHg, and the risk of stroke fell by 43%, and those receiving perindopril monotherapy (BP reduced by 5/3 mmHg) had no significant reduction in the risk of stroke *(129)*. Based on the degree of BP reduction in the perindopril-only group, a 20% reduction in stroke risk would have been anticipated; thus, the absence of a positive stroke effect is puzzling. Of note, in the PROGRESS trial, treatment with perindopril and indapamide was associated with reduced risks of dementia and cognitive decline associated with recurrent stroke *(132)*.

A similar observation to that of the PROGRESS study was made in the CAPPP trial, for which—despite its design problems—fatal or non-fatal stroke was 1.25 times more common in patients randomly assigned to captopril than in those assigned to conventional therapy with diuretics and/or β-blockers *(133)*. Nevertheless, the beneficial effect of combination therapy with perindopril and indapamide is consistent with prior studies showing a positive effect of diuretics on recurrent stroke rate.

In contradistinction to the PROGRESS and CAPPP studies, the HOPE study provided compelling evidence that treatment with the ACE inhibitor ramipril can further reduce the risk of stroke in high-risk patients without left ventricular dysfunction by mechanisms presumably above and beyond simple BP reduction *(19)*. Ramipril at a dose of 10 mg/day achieved a highly significant 32% reduction in total stroke rate, and recurrent strokes were reduced by 33%. In a subanalysis of this trial, nonfatal stroke was reduced by 24% and fatal stroke by 61%. Interest-ingly, in the HOPE study ramipril was given at night, and therefore its peak effect, whether hemodynamic or otherwise, occurred in the morn-ing hours, a time when strokes occur more frequently *(134)*.

Based on the HOPE study, the American Heart Association guide-lines for the primary prevention of stroke recommend ramipril to prevent stroke in high-risk patients and in patients with diabetes and hypertension *(135)*. Thus, it would appear that ACE inhibitor therapy is warranted if primary prevention is contemplated in a high-risk patient or secondary prevention is under consideration in a patient already having sustained a cerebrovascular event.

SIDE EFFECTS OF ACE INHIBITORS

Soon after their release, a syndrome of functional renal insufficiency was observed as a class effect with ACE inhibitors *(136)*. This phenomenon was initially reported in patients with renal artery stenosis and a solitary kidney or in the presence of bilateral renal artery stenosis. Predisposing conditions to this process include dehydration, CHF, and either macro- or microvascular renal disease. All of these conditions are common occurrences in the elderly.

The mechanistic prompt in these conditions is a fall in afferent arteriolar flow. When this occurs, glomerular filtration temporarily declines. In response to this reduction in glomerular filtration, local production of Ang-II rises. In concert with this increase in Ang-II, the efferent or postglomerular arteriole constricts, restoring upstream hydrostatic pressures within the glomerular capillary bed.

The abrupt removal of Ang-II, as occurs with an ACE inhibitor (or an ARB), will suddenly dilate the efferent arteriole in tandem with a reduction in systemic BP. In combination, these hemodynamic changes drop glomerular hydrostatic pressure to do away with glomerular filtration. This type of functional renal insufficiency is best treated by discontinuation of the offending agent, careful volume expansion if intravascular volume contraction exists, and if suspected on clinical grounds, evaluation for the presence of renal artery stenosis *(126)*.

An additional ACE inhibitor-associated side effect relevant to the elderly is hyperkalemia *(137)*. ACE inhibitor-related hyperkalemia is uncommon unless a specific predisposition to hyperkalemia is present, such as in a diabetic or CHF patient with renal failure receiving potassium-sparing diuretics or potassium supplements *(138)*. Alternatively, ACE inhibitors will minimize the potassium loss accompanying diuretic therapy.

A dry, irritating, nonproductive cough is a common complication with ACE inhibitors, with its incidence estimated at between 0% and 44% *(139)*. Cough is a class phenomenon with ACE inhibitors and has ostensibly been attributed to an increase in bradykinin or other vasoactive peptides, such as substance P, which may play a second messenger role in triggering the cough reflex (343). Although numerous therapies have been tried, few have had any lasting success in eliminating ACE inhibitor-induced cough. The onset of cough with an ACE inhibitor is problematic in an elderly patient, particularly one with a past history of smoking, because it may instigate an unnecessary search for malignancy. The more prudent maneuver in such a case is to reassess the cough several weeks after discontinuing ACE inhibitor therapy.

ACE inhibitor-related nonspecific side effects are generally uncommon, with the exception of taste disturbances, leucopenia, skin rash, and dysgeusia, which are almost exclusively seen in captopril-treated patients *(140)*. The taste disturbance observed with captopril can be particularly troubling in the elderly, for whom taste abnormalities are already quite common *(141)*. Angioneurotic edema is a potentially life-threatening complication of ACE inhibitors that is more common in blacks *(142)*. ACE inhibitor-related angioedema is not more common in the elderly (defined as ≥65 years of age) *(143)*. ACE inhibitor-induced angioedema of the intestine can also occur. This typically presents with acute abdominal symptoms with or without facial or oropharyngeal swelling. Angioedema of the intestine is more common in females, and its occurrence is independent of age.

A final consideration with ACE inhibitors is that of anemia. ACE inhibitors suppress the production of erythropoietin in a dose-dependent manner, which is a particular problem when ACE inhibitors are administered in the presence of renal failure *(144)*.

CONCLUSIONS

ACE inhibitors are commonly used drugs in the elderly patient. These compounds are employed in their capacity either to reduce BP or to take advantage of their cardio- and/or renoprotective effects. ACE inhibitors can be expected to provide the greatest end-organ protection in the elderly with CHF or proteinuric renal disease or in the post-MI setting. Dosing guidelines exist for each of these scenarios, although such guidelines may not be followed as closely in clinical practice as is advised. ACE inhibitor-related side effects are for the most part easily recognized and, other than functional renal insufficiency, which is occasionally seen with their use, do not occur more commonly in the elderly.

REFERENCES

1. The Sixth Report of the Joint National Committee on Prevention, Detection, Evaluation, and Treatment of High Blood Pressure. *Arch Intern Med* 1997;157:2413–2446.
2. Strandberg TE, Pitkala K, Berglind S, et al. Possibilities of multifactorial cardiovascular disease prevention in patients aged 75 and older: a randomized controlled trial:

Drugs and Evidence Based Medicine in the Elderly (DEBATE) Study. E*ur Heart J* 2003;24:1216–1222.

3. Sica DA, Gehr TWB. Angiotensin converting enzyme inhibitors. In Oparil S, Weber M, eds. *Hypertension, a Companion to the Kidney.* Philadelphia: Saunders; 2000:599–608.

4. Strandberg T, Pitkala K, Tilvis R. Benefits of optimising drug treatment in home-dwelling elderly patients with coronary artery disease. *Drugs Aging* 2003;20:585–595.

5. White CM. Pharmacologic, pharmacokinetic, and therapeutic differences among ACE inhibitors. *Pharmacotherapy* 1998;18:588–599.

6. Cody R. Optimizing ACE inhibitor therapy of congestive heart failure: insights from pharmacodynamic studies. *Clin Pharmacokinet* 1993;24:59–70.

7. Sica DA. Angiotensin converting enzyme inhibitors: Fosinopril. In Messerli F, ed. *Cardiovascular Drug Therapy.* 2nd ed. Philadelphia: Saunders; 1996:801–809.

8. Chalmers D, Whitehead A, Lawson DH. Postmarketing surveillance of captopril for hypertension. *Br J Clin Pharmacol* 1992;34:215–223.

9. Brockmeier D. Tight binding influencing the future of pharmacokinetics. *Meth Find Exp Clin Pharmacol* 1998;20:505–516.

10. Reid JL. From kinetics to dynamics: are there differences between ACE inhibitors? *Eur Heart J* 1997;18(suppl E):E14–E18.

11. Hoyer J, Schulte K-L, Lenz T. Clinical pharmacokinetics of angiotensin converting enzyme inhibitors in renal failure. *Clin Pharmacokinet* 1993;24:230–254.

12. Dzau VJ, Bernstein K, Celermajer D, et al. The relevance of tissue angiotensin-converting enzyme: manifestations in mechanistic and endpoint data. *Am J Cardiol* 2001;88(suppl 9):1L–20L.

13. Ebihara A, Fujimura A. Metabolites of antihypertensive drugs. An updated review of their clinical pharmacokinetic and therapeutic implications. *Clin Pharmacokinet* 1991;21:331–343.

14. Hui KK, Duchin KL, Kripalani KJ, et al. Pharmacokinetics of fosinopril in patients with various degrees of renal function. *Clin Pharmacol Ther* 1991;49:457–467.

15. Danielson B, Querin S, LaRochelle P, et al. Pharmacokinetics and pharmacodynamics of trandolapril after repeated administration of 2 mg to patients with chronic renal failure and healthy control subjects. *J Cardiovasc Pharmacol* 1994;23(suppl 4):S50–S59.

16. Sica DA, Deedwania PC. Renal considerations in the use of angiotensin-converting enzyme inhibitors in the treatment of congestive heart failure. *Congest Heart Fail* 1997;3:54–59.

17. Brown NJ, Vaughn DE. Angiotensin-converting enzyme inhibitors. *Circulation* 1998;97:1411–1420.

18. Johnston CI, Fabris B, Yamada H, et al. Comparative studies of tissue inhibition by angiotensin converting enzyme inhibitors. *J Hypertens* 1989;7(suppl):S11–S16.

19. Yusuf S, Sleight P, Pogue J, et al. Effects of an angiotensin-converting enzyme inhibitor, ramipril, on cardiovascular events in high-risk patients. The Heart Outcomes Prevention Evaluation Study Investigators. *N Engl J Med* 2000;342:145–153.

20. Leonetti G, Cuspidi C. Choosing the right ACE inhibitor. A guide to selection. *Drugs* 1995;49:516–535.

21. Zeitz CJ, Campbell DJ, Horowitz JD. Myocardial uptake and biochemical and hemodynamic effects of ACE inhibitors in humans. *Hypertension* 2003;41:482–487.

22. Nordmann AJ, Krahn M, Logan AG, et al. The cost effectiveness of ACE inhibitors as first-line antihypertensive therapy. *Pharmacoeconomics* 2003;21:573–585.

23. The SOLVD investigators. Effect of enalapril on survival in patients with reduced left ventricular ejection fractions and congestive heart failure. *N Engl J Med* 1991;325:293–302.
24. Lewis EJ, Hunsicker LG, Bain RP, Rohde RD. The effect of angiotensin converting enzyme inhibition on diabetic nephropathy. The Collaborative Study Group. *N Engl J Med* 1993;329:1456–1462.
25. Sica DA. The HOPE Study: ACE inhibitors—are their benefits a class effect or do individual agents differ? *Curr Opin Nephrol Hypertens* 2001;10:597–601.
26. Jafar TH, Stark PC, Schmid CH, et al. Proteinuria as a modifiable risk factor for the progression of non-diabetic renal disease. *Kidney Int* 2001;60:1131–1140.
27. Wilson Tang WH, Vagelos RH, et al. Neurohormonal and clinical responses to high- vs low-dose enalapril therapy in chronic heart failure. *J Am Coll Cardiol* 2002;39:70–78.
28. Packer M, Poole-Wilson PA, Armstrong PW, et al. Comparative effects of low and high doses of the angiotensin-converting enzyme inhibitor, lisinopril, on morbidity and mortality in chronic heart failure. ATLAS Study Group. *Circulation* 1999;100: 2312–2318.
29. Massie B. Neurohormonal blockade in chronic heart failure; How much is enough? Can there be too much? *J Am Coll Cardiol* 2002;39:79–82.
30. Tang WH, Vagelos RH, Yee YG, et al. Impact of angiotensin-converting enzyme gene polymorphism on neurohormonal responses to high- versus low-dose enalapril in advanced heart failure. *Am Heart J* 2004;148:889–894.
31. Van Veldhuisen DJ, Genth-Zotz S, Brouwer J, et al. High vs low-dose ACE inhibition in chronic heart failure. A double-blind, placebo-controlled study of imidapril. *J Am Coll Cardiol* 1998;32:1811–1818.
32. Carretero OA, Scicli AG. The kallikrein-kinin system as a regulator of cardiovascular and renal function. In Brenner BM, Laragh JH, eds. Hypertension: *Pathophysiology, Diagnosis, and Management.* 2nd ed. New York: Raven Press; 1995:983–999.
33. Urata H. Nishimura H, Ganten D. Chymase-dependent angiotensin II forming system in humans. *Am J Hypertens* 1996;9:277–284.
34. Petrie MC, Padmanabhan N, McDonald JE, et al. Angiotensin converting enzyme and non-ACE dependent angiotensin II generation in resistance arteries from patients with heart failure and coronary heart disease. *J Am Coll Cardiol* 2001;37:1056–1061.
35. Ennezat PV, Berlowitz M, Sonnenblick EH, Le Jemtel TH. Therapeutic implications of escape from angiotensin-converting enzyme inhibition in patients with chronic heart failure. *Curr Cardiol Rep* 2000;2:258–262.
36. Mooser V, Nussberger J, Juillerat L, et al. Reactive hyperreninemia is a major determinant of plasma angiotensin II during ACE inhibition. *J Cardiovasc Pharmacol* 1990;15:276–282.
37. Swedberg K, Eneroth P, Kjekshus J, Wilhelmsen L. Hormones regulating cardiovascular function in patients with severe congestive heart failure and their relation to mortality. CONSENSUS Trial Study Group. *Circulation* 1990;82:1730–1736.
38. Gainer JV, Morrow JD, Loveland A, et al. Effect of bradykinin-receptor blockade on the response to angiotensin-converting enzyme inhibitor in normotensive and hypertensive subjects. *N Engl J Med* 1998;339:1285–1292.
39. Squire IB, O'Kane KP, Anderson N, Reid JL. Bradykinin B(2) receptor antagonism attenuates blood pressure response to acute angiotensin-converting enzyme inhibition in normal men. *Hypertension* 2000;36:132–136.
40. Rodriguez-Garcia JL, Villa E, Serrano M, Gallardo J, Garcia-Robles R. Prostacyclin: its pathogenic role in essential hypertension and the class effect of ACE inhibitors on prostaglandin metabolism. *Blood Press* 1999;8:279–284.

41. Johnson AG. NSAIDs and increased blood pressure. What is the clinical significance? *Drug Saf* 1997;17:277–289.
42. Morgan T, Anderson A. The effect of nonsteroidal anti-inflammatory drugs on blood pressure in patients treated with different antihypertensive drugs. *J Clin Hypertens (Greenwich)* 2003;5:53–57.
43. Nawarskas JJ, Townsend RR, Cirigliano MD, Spinler SA. Effect of aspirin on blood pressure in hypertensive patients taking enalapril or losartan. *Am J Hypertens* 1999;12:784–789.
44. Zanchetti A, Hansson L, Leonetti G, et al. Low-dose aspirin does not interfere with the blood pressure-lowering effects of antihypertensive therapy. *J Hypertens* 2002;20:1015–1022.
45. Nawarskas JJ, Spinler SA. Does aspirin interfere with the therapeutic efficacy of angiotensin-converting enzyme inhibitors in hypertension or congestive heart failure. *Pharmacotherapy* 1998;18:1041–1052.
46. Lang CC, Stein M, He HB, et al. Angiotensin converting enzyme inhibition and sympathetic activity in healthy subjects. *Clin Pharmacol Ther* 1996;59:668–674.
47. Ranadive SA, Chen AX, Serajuddin AT. Relative lipophilicities and structural-pharmacological considerations of various angiotensin-converting enzyme (ACE) inhibitors. *Pharm Res* 1992;9:1480–1486.
48. Fagard R, Amery A, Reybrouck T, et al. Acute and chronic systemic and hemodynamic effects of angiotensin converting enzyme inhibition with captopril in hypertensive patients. *Am J Cardiol* 1980;46:295–300.
49. Slavachevsky I, Rachmani R, Levi Z, et al. Effect of enalapril and nifedipine on orthostatic hypotension in older hypertensive patients. *J Am Geriatr Soc* 2000;48:807–810.
50. Vanhoutte PM. Endothelial dysfunction and inhibition of converting enzyme. Eur Heart J 1998;19(suppl J):J7–J15.
51. Schiffrin EL. Effects of antihypertensive drugs on vascular remodeling: do they predict outcome in response to antihypertensive therapy? *Curr Opin Nephrol Hypertens* 2001;10:617–624.
52. Wing LM, Reid CM, Ryan P, et al. A comparison of outcomes with angiotensin-converting enzyme inhibitors and diuretics for hypertension in the elderly. *N Engl J Med* 2002;348:583–592.
53. The ALLHAT Officers and Co-ordinators for the ALLHAT Collaborative Group. Major outcomes in high-risk hypertensive patients randomized to angiotensin converting enzyme inhibitor or calcium channel blocker vs diuretic. The Antihypertensive and Lipid-Lowering Treatment to Prevent Heart Attack Trial (ALLHAT). *JAMA* 2002;288:1981–1997.
54. Materson BJ, Reda DJ, Cushman WC, et al. Single-drug therapy for hypertension in men. A comparison of six antihypertensive agents with placebo. *N Engl J Med* 1993;328:914–921.
55. Smith RD, Franklin SS. Comparison of effects of enalapril plus hydrochlorothiazide vs standard triple therapy on renal function in renovascular hypertension. *Am J Med* 1985;79(suppl 3C):14–23.
56. Cheng A, Frishman WH. Use of angiotensin-converting enzyme inhibitors as monotherapy and in combination with diuretics and calcium channel blockers. *J Clin Pharmacol* 1998;38:477–491.
57. Weidmann P, De Myttenaere-Bursztein S, Maxwell MH. Effect of aging on plasma renin and aldosterone in normal man. *Kidney Int* 1975;8:325–333.
58. Israili ZH, Hall WD. ACE inhibitors: differential use in elderly patients with hypertension. *Drugs Aging* 1995;7:355–371.
59. Chobanian AV, Bakris GL, Black HR, et al. The Seventh Report of the Joint National Committee on Prevention, Detection, Evaluation, and Treatment of High Blood Pressure: the JNC 7 report. *JAMA* 2003;289:2560–2572.

60. Guidelines Committee. 2003 European Society of Hypertension-European Society of Cardiology guidelines for the management of arterial hypertension. *J Hypertens* 2003;21:1011–1053.

61. Omboni S, Fogari R, Palatini P, et al. Reproducibility and clinical value of the trough-to-peak ratio of the antihypertensive effect. Evidence from the Sample Study. *Hypertension* 1998;32:424–429.

62. Morgan TO, Morgan O, Anderson A. Effect of dose on trough peak ratio of antihypertensive drugs in elderly hypertensive males. *Clin Exp Pharmacol Physiol* 1995;22:778–780.

63. Sica DA, Gehr TWB. Dose-response relationship and dose adjustments. In: Izzo JL, Black HR, eds. *Hypertension Primer*. 2nd ed. Baltimore, MD: Lippincott, Williams, and Wilkins; 1999:342–344.

64. Elung-Jensen T, Heisterberg J, Kamper AL, et al. Blood pressure response to conventional and low-dose enalapril in chronic renal failure. *Br J Clin Pharmacol* 2003;55:139–146.

65. Sica DA. Rationale for fixed-dose combinations in the treatment of hypertension: the cycle repeats. *Drugs* 2002;62:443–462.

66. Belz GG, Essig J, Erb K, et al. Pharmacokinetic and pharmacodynamic interactions between the ACE inhibitor cilazapril and beta-adrenoreceptor antagonist propranolol in healthy subjects and in hypertensive patients. *Brit J Clin Pharmacol* 1989;27(suppl 2):317S–322S.

67. Black HR, Sollins JS, Garofalo JL. The addition of doxazosin to the therapeutic regimen of hypertensive patients inadequately controlled with other antihypertensive medications: a randomized, placebo-controlled study. *Am J Hypertens* 2000;13:468–474.

68. Gradman AH, Cutler NR, Davis PJ, et al. Combined enalapril and felodipine extended release for systemic hypertension. Enalapril-Felodipine ER Factorial Study Group. *Am J Cardiol* 1997;79:431–435.

69. DeQuattro V, Lee D. Fixed-dose combination therapy with trandolapril and verapamil SR is effective in primary hypertension. *Am J Hypertens* 1997;10(suppl 2):138S–145S.

70. Pool J, Kaihlanen P, Lewis G, et al. Once-daily treatment of patients with hypertension: a placebo-controlled study of amlodipine and benazepril vs amlodipine or benazepril alone. *J Hum Hypertens* 2001;15:495–498.

71. Sica DA. Calcium-channel blocker edema: can it be resolved? *J Clin Hypertens (Greenwich)* 2003;5:291–294.

72. Zuccala G, Onder G, Pedone C, et al. Use of calcium antagonists and worsening renal function in patients receiving angiotensin-converting-enzyme inhibitors. *Eur J Clin Pharmacol* 2003;58:695–699.

73. Ludwig V, Martin WH, Delbeke D. Calcium channel blockers: a potential cause of false-positive captopril renography. *Clin Nucl Med* 2003;28:108–112.

74. Sica DA. The practical aspects of combination therapy with angiotensin-receptor blockers and angiotensin-converting enzyme inhibitors. *J Renin Angiotensin Aldosterone Syst* 2002;3:66–71.

75. Taylor AA. Is there a place for combining angiotensin-converting enzyme inhibitors and angiotensin-receptor antagonists in the treatment of hypertension, renal disease or congestive heart failure? *Curr Opin Nephrol Hypertens* 2001;10:643–648.

76. Dufloux JJ, Prasquier R, Chatellier G, et al. Effects of captopril and minoxidil on left ventricular hypertrophy in resistant hypertensive patients: a 6-month double-blind comparison. *J Am Coll Cardiol* 1990;16:137–142.

77. Hirschl MM, Binder M, Bur A, et al. Impact of the renin-angiotensin-aldosterone system on blood pressure response to intravenous enalaprilat in patients with hypertensive crises. *J Hum Hypertens* 1997;11:177–183.
78. Sica DA. Dosage considerations with perindopril for hypertension. *Am J Cardiol* 2001;88(suppl 1):13–18.
79. Gottdiener JS, Reda DJ, Massie BM, et al. for the VA Cooperative Study Group on Antihypertensive Agents. Effect of single-drug therapy on reduction of left ventricular mass in mild to moderate hypertension. Comparison of six antihypertensive agents. *Circulation* 1997;95:2007–2014.
80. Koren MJ, Devereux RB, Casale PN, et al. Relation of left ventricular mass and geometry to morbidity and mortality in uncomplicated essential hypertension. *Ann Intern Med* 1991;114:345–352.
81. The European Trial on Reduction of Cardiac Events With Perindopril in Stable Coronary Artery Disease investigators. Efficacy of perindopril in reduction of cardiovascular events among patients with stable coronary artery disease: randomised, double-blind, placebo-controlled, multicentre trial (the EUROPA study). *Lancet* 2003;362:782–788.
82. Daly P, Mettauer B, Rouleau JL, et al. Lack of reflex increase in myocardial sympathetic tone after captopril: potential antianginal mechanism. *Circulation* 1985;71:317–325.
83. Strandberg T, Pitkala K, Tilvis R. Benefits of optimising drug treatment in home-dwelling elderly patients with coronary artery disease. *Drugs Aging* 2003;20:585–595.
84. Chrysant SG. Vascular remodeling: the role of angiotensin converting enzyme inhibitors. *Am Heart J* 1998;135:S21–S30.
85. Waldemar G, Ibsen H, Strandgaard S, et al. The effect of fosinopril sodium on cerebral blood flow in moderate essential hypertension. *Am J Hypertens* 1990;3:464–470.
86. Regensteiner JG, Hiatt WR. Current medical therapies for patients with peripheral arterial disease: a critical review. *Am J Med* 2002;112:49–57.
87. American Diabetes Association. Treatment of hypertension in adults with diabetes. *Diabetes Care* 2003;26:S80–S82.
88. Kirpichnikov D, Sowers JR. Role of ACE inhibitors in treating hypertensive diabetic patients. *Curr Diab Rep* 2002;2:251–257.
89. Lithell HO, Pollare T, Berne C. Insulin sensitivity in newly detected hypertensive patients: influence of captopril and other antihypertensive agents on insulin sensitivity and related biological parameters. *J Cardiovasc Pharmacol* 1990;15(suppl 5):S46–S52.
90. Yusuf S, Gerstein H, Hoogwerf B, et al. Ramipril and the development of diabetes. *JAMA* 2001;286:1882–1885.
91. Hansson L, Lindholm L, Niskanen L, et al. Effect of angiotensin-converting-enzyme inhibition compared with conventional therapy on cardiovascular morbidity and mortality in hypertension: the Captopril Prevention Project (CAPPP) randomised trial. *Lancet* 1999;353:611–616.
92. Wright JT Jr, Agodoa L, Contreras G, et al. Successful blood pressure control in the African American Study of Kidney Disease and Hypertension. *Arch Intern Med* 2002;162:1636–1643.
93. Yu HT. Progression of chronic renal failure. *Arch Intern Med* 2003;163:1417–1429.
94. Donnelly R, Yeung JM, Manning G. Microalbuminuria: a common, independent cardiovascular risk factor, especially but not exclusively in type 2 diabetes. *J Hypertens* 2003;21(suppl 1):S7–S12.

95. Brown WW, Peters RM, Ohmit SE, et al. Early detection of kidney disease in community settings: the Kidney Early Evaluation Program (KEEP). *Am J Kidney Dis* 2003;42:22–35.

96. Jafar TH, Schmid CH, Landa M, et al. Angiotensin-converting enzyme inhibitors and progression of nondiabetic renal disease. A meta-analysis of patient-level data. *Ann Intern Med* 2001;135:73–87.

97. Ravid M, Lang R, Rachmani R, et al. Long-term renoprotective effect of angiotensin converting enzyme inhibition in non-insulin dependent diabetes mellitus. A 7-year follow-up study. *Arch Int Med* 1996;156:286–289.

98. Viberti G, Mogensen CE, Groop LC, Pauls JF. Effect of captopril on progression to clinical proteinuria in patients with insulin-dependent diabetes mellitus and microalbuminuria: European Microalbuminuria Captopril Study Group. *JAMA* 1994;271:275–279.

99. Uhle BU, Whitworth JA, Shahinfar S, et al. Angiotensin-converting enzyme inhibition in nondiabetic progressive renal insufficiency: a controlled double-blind trial. *Am J Kidney Dis* 1996;27:489–495.

100. Giatras I, Lau J, Levey AS, et al. for the Angiotensin-Converting Enzyme Inhibition and Progressive Renal Disease Study Group. Effect of angiotensin-converting enzyme inhibitors on the progression of nondiabetic renal disease: a meta-analysis of randomized trials. *Ann Intern Med* 1997;127:337–347.

101. Jafar TH, Stark PC, Schmid CH, et al. Progression of chronic kidney disease: the role of blood pressure control, proteinuria, and angiotensin converting enzyme inhibition. A patient level meta-analysis. *Ann Intern Med* 2003;39:244–252.

102. Ruggenenti P, Perna A, Gherardi G, et al. Chronic proteinuric nephropathies: outcomes and response to treatment in a prospective cohort of 352 patients with different patterns of renal injury. *Am J Kidney Dis* 2000;35:1155–1165.

103. Mann JF, Gerstein HC, Yi QL, et al. Development of renal disease in people at high cardiovascular risk: results of the HOPE randomized study. *J Am Soc Nephrol* 2003;14:641–647.

104. Sica DA. Kinetics of angiotensin converting enzyme inhibitors in renal failure. *J Cardiovasc Pharmacol* 1992;20(suppl 10):S13–S20.

105. Jafar TH, Stark PC, Schmid CH, et al. Angiotensin-converting enzyme inhibition and progression of renal disease. Proteinuria as a modifiable risk factor for the progression of non-diabetic renal disease. *Kidney Int* 2001;60:1131–1140.

106. Ruggenenti P, Mise N, Pisoni R, et al. Diverse effects of increasing lisinopril doses on lipid abnormalities in chronic nephropathies. *Circulation* 2003;107:586–592.

107. Bakris GL, Weir MR. Angiotensin-converting enzyme inhibitor-associated elevations in serum creatinine: is this a cause for concern? *Arch Intern Med* 2000;160:685–693.

108. Apperloo AJ, de Zeeuw D, de Jong PE. A short-term antihypertensive-treatment induced drop in glomerular filtration rate predicts long-term stability of renal function. *Kidney Int* 1997;51:793–797.

109. Heeg JE, de Jong PE, van der Hem GK, et al. Efficacy and variability of the antiproteinuric effect of ACE inhibition by lisinopril *Kidney Int* 1989;36:272–279.

110. Gansevoort RT, de Zeeuw D, de Jong PE. Additive antiproteinuric effect of ACE inhibition and a low protein diet in human renal disease. *Nephrol Dial Transplant* 1995;10:497–504.

111. Ueda S, Elliott, Morton JJ, et al. Enhanced pressor response to angiotensin I in normotensive men with the deletion genotype (DD) for angiotensin-converting enzyme. *Hypertension* 1995;25:1266–1269.

112. Cambien F, Poirier O, Lecerf L, et al. Deletion polymorphism in the gene for angiotensin-converting enzyme is a potent risk factor for myocardial infarction. *Nature* 1992;359:641–644.

113. Parving HH, Jacobsen P, Tarnow L, et al. Effect of deletion polymorphism of angiotensin converting enzyme gene on progression of diabetic nephropathy during inhibition of angiotensin converting enzyme. Observational follow-up study. *BMJ* 1996;313:591–594.

114. Rudnicki M, Mayer G. Pharmacogenomics of angiotensin converting enzyme inhibitors in renal disease—pathophysiological considerations. *Pharmacogenomics* 2003;4:153–162.

115. Garg R, Yusuf S, for the Collaborative Group on ACE Inhibitor Trials. Overview of randomized trials of angiotensin-converting enzyme inhibitors on mortality and morbidity in patients with heart failure. *JAMA* 1995;273:1450–1456.

116. Massie B. Neurohormonal blockade in chronic heart failure; How much is enough? Can there be too much? *J Am Coll Cardiol* 2002;39:79–82.

117. Remme WJ. Effect of ACE inhibition on neurohormones. *Eur Heart J* 1998; 19(suppl J):J16–J23.

118. Anker SD, Negassa A, Coats AJ, et al. Prognostic importance of weight loss in chronic heart failure and the effect of treatment with angiotensin-converting-enzyme inhibitors: an observational study. *Lancet* 2003;361:1077–1083.

119. Flather MD, Yusuf S, Kober L, et al. Long-term ACE-inhibitor therapy in patients with heart failure or left-ventricular dysfunction: a systematic overview of data from individual patients. ACE-Inhibitor Myocardial Infarction Collaborative Group. *Lancet* 2000;355:1575–1581.

120. Bungard TJ, McAlister FA, Johnson JA, Tsuyuki RT. Underutilization of ACE inhibitors in patients with congestive heart failure. *Drugs* 2001;61:2021–2033.

121. Chen YT, Wang Y, Radford MJ, Krumholz HM. Angiotensin-converting enzyme inhibitor dosages in elderly patients with heart failure. *Am Heart J* 2001;141:410–417.

122. Naccarella F, Naccarelli GV, Maranga SS, et al. Do ACE inhibitors or angiotensin II antagonists reduce total mortality and arrhythmic mortality? A critical review of controlled clinical trials. *Curr Opin Cardiol* 2002;17:6–18.

123. Burwen DR, Galusha DH, Lewis JM, et al. National and state trends in quality of care for acute myocardial infarction between 1994–1995 and 1998–1999: the Medicare health care quality improvement program. *Arch Intern Med* 2003;163:1430–1439.

124. Megarry M, Sapsford R, Hall AS, et al. Do ACE inhibitors provide protection for the heart in the clinical setting of acute myocardial infarction? *Drugs* 1997;54(suppl 5):48–58.

125. Indications for ACE inhibitors in the early treatment of acute myocardial infarction: systematic review of individual data from 100,000 patients in randomised trials. *Circulation* 1998;97:2202–2212.

126. Schoolwerth AC, Sica DA, Ballermann BJ, Wilcox CS. Renal considerations in angiotensin converting enzyme inhibitor therapy: a statement for healthcare professionals from the Council on the Kidney in Cardiovascular Disease and the Council for High Blood Pressure Research of the American Heart Association. *Circulation* 2001;104:1985–1991.

127. Kittleson M, Hurwitz S, Shah MR, et al. Development of circulatory-renal limitations to angiotensin-converting enzyme inhibitors identifies patients with severe heart failure and early mortality. *J Am Coll Cardiol* 2003;41:2029–2035.

128. Ahmed A, Kiefe CI, Allman RM, et al. Survival benefits of angiotensin-converting enzyme inhibitors in older heart failure patients with perceived contraindications. *J Am Geriatr Soc* 2002;50:1659–1666.

129. Randomised trial of a perindopril-based blood-pressure-lowering regimen among 6105 individuals with previous stroke or transient ischaemic attack. *Lancet* 2001;358:1033–1041.

130. Anderson C. Blood pressure-lowering for secondary prevention of stroke: ACE inhibition is the key. *Stroke* 2003;34:1333–1334.

131. Bath P. Blood pressure-lowering for secondary prevention of stroke: ACE inhibition is not the key. *Stroke* 2003;34:1334–1335.

132. Tzourio C, Anderson C, Chapman N, et al. Effects of blood pressure lowering with perindopril and indapamide therapy on dementia and cognitive decline in patients with cerebrovascular disease. *Arch Intern Med* 2003;163:1069–1075.

133. Hansson L, Lindholm L, Niskanen L, et al. Effect of angiotensin-converting-enzyme inhibition compared with conventional therapy on cardiovascular morbidity and mortality in hypertension: the Captopril Prevention Project (CAPPP) randomised trial. *Lancet* 1999;353:611–616.

134. Svensson P, de Faire U, Sleight P, et al. Comparative effects of ramipril on ambulatory and office blood pressures: a HOPE Substudy. *Hypertension* 2001;38:E28–E32.

135. Goldstein LB, Adams R, Becker K, et al. Primary prevention of ischemic stroke: a statement for healthcare professionals from the Stroke Council of the American Heart Association. *Stroke* 2001;32:280–299.

136. Textor SC. Renal failure related to angiotensin-converting enzyme inhibitors. *Semin Nephrol* 1997;17:67–76.

137. Textor SC, Bravo EL, Fouad FM, Tarazi RC. Hyperkalemia in azotemic patients during angiotensin-converting enzyme inhibition and aldosterone reduction with captopril. *Am J Med* 1982;73:719–725.

138. Juurlink DN, Mamdani M, Kopp A, et al. Drug-drug interactions among elderly patients hospitalized for drug toxicity. *JAMA* 2003;289:1652–1658.

139. Israili ZH, Hall WD. Cough and angioneurotic associated with angiotensin-converting enzyme inhibitor therapy: a review of the literature and pathophysiology. *Ann Intern Med* 1992;117:234–242.

140. Chalmers D, Dombey SL, Lawson DH. Post-marketing surveillance of captopril (for hypertension): a preliminary report. *Br J Clin Pharmacol* 1987;24:343–349.

141. Morley JE. Decreased food intake with aging. *J Gerontol A Biol Sci Med Sci* 2001;56:81–88.

142. Gibbs CR, Lip GYH, Beevers DG. Angioedema due to ACE inhibitors: increased risk in patients of African origin. *Br J Clin Pharmacol* 1999;48:861–865.

143. Available at: http://www.fda.gov/ohrms/dockets/ac/02/briefing/3877B2_01_BristolMeyersSquibb.pdf. Accessed August 10th, 2003.

144. Sica DA, Gehr TWB. The pharmacokinetics and pharmacodynamics of angiotensin receptor blockers in end-stage renal disease. *J Renin Angiotensin Aldosterone Syst* 2002;3:247–254.

17 Use of Angiotensin Receptor Blockers in the Elderly

L. Michael Prisant, MD, FACC, FACP

CONTENTS

INTRODUCTION

No class of drugs has been more popular than the angiotensin-receptor blockers (ARBs). Their side-effect profile has resulted in increasing prescriptions because they are better tolerated than any other class of antihypertensive drugs. The outcome trials (Table 1) with these drugs are now being reported and are showing benefits for target organ protection (1–15). ARBs are proven to be effective in reducing the rate of renal insufficiency among diabetic hypertensives (3,5), reducing strokes for elderly patients (10) and hypertensive patients with left ventricular hypertrophy (7), and reducing cardiovascular mortality and total mortality compared to atenolol in diabetic hypertensive patients (9). Valsartan is as effective as captopril in patients sustaining a myocardial infarction complicated by heart failure, left ventricular dysfunction, or both (15).

From: *Clinical Hypertension and Vascular Diseases: Hypertension in the Elderly*
Edited by: L. M. Prisant © Humana Press Inc., Totowa, NJ

Table 1
Outcome Trials With Angiotensin Receptor Blockers

Trial	Drug	Comparison	Number	Mean age	Population	End point	Outcome
ELITE II	Losartan 50 mg qd	Captopril 50 mg tid	3152	71.5	Heart failure	All-cause mortality	No difference in outcome
RENAAL	Losartan 100 mg qd	Placebo	1513	60.0	Diabetic nephropathy	ESRD, 2X SCr, an total mortality	Decreased ESRD and 2X SCr, but not total mortality
LIFE	Losartan 100 mg qd	Atenolol 100 mg qd	9193	66.9	Electrocardiographic left ventricular hypertrophy	Cardiovascular mortality, MI, and stroke	Decreased strokes, but not MI or mortality; however, diabetics had a reduction in total and cardiovascular mortality
OPTIMAAL	Losartan 50 mg qd	Captopril 50 tid	5477	67.4	Acute MI with heart failure or new Q-wave anterior infarction or reinfarction	All-cause mortality	No difference in outcome
Val-HEFT	Valsartan 160 mg bid	Placebo	5010	62.7	Heart failure	All-cause mortality or mortality and morbidity	No difference in overall mortality; fewer heart failure hospitalizations; benefit not seen in patients not receiving an ACE inhibitor
VALIANT	Valsartan 160 bid alone or with captopril 50 tid	Placebo or captopril 50 tid	14,703	64.8	Acute MI and heart failure or left ventricular systolic dysfunction	All-cause mortality	Valsartan not inferior to captopril; valsartan and captopril not additive
VALUE	Valsartan 80–160 mg qd	Amlodipine 5–10 mg qd	14,400		Hypertension	Cardiovascular morbidity and mortality	No difference in primary endpoint or total mortality. Few MIs with amlodipine. Less new-onset diabetes with valsartan.

						All-cause mortality	
CHARM	Candesartan 32 mg qd	Placebo	7599	66.0	Heart failure		Total and cardiovascular mortality reduced; heart failure admissions decreased
SCOPE	Candesartan 16 mg ± HCTZ 12.5 mg	Placebo ± HCTZ 12.5 mg	4964	76.4	Elderly hypertensives	Cardiovascular death, MI, and CVA	Nonfatal CVA reduction, but fatal CVA, cardiovascular death, or MI
IDNT	Irbesartan 300 mg qd	Placebo or amlodipine 10 mg qd	1715	58.9	Diabetic nephropathy	ESRD, 2X SCr or mortality	Reduction in 2X SCr, but not ESRD or death
I-PRESERVE	Irbesartan	Placebo	3600		Heart failure with preserved systolic function	All-cause mortality and cardiovascular hospitalization	Pending
ONTARGET	Telmisartan alone or with captopril	Placebo or captopril	23,400		High-risk vascular disease	MI, CVA, CV death, heart failure	Pending
TRANSCEND	Telmisartan	Placebo	5000		ACE inhibitor intolerant and high-risk vascular disease	MI, CVA, CV death, heart failure	Pending

ACE, angiotensin-converting enzyme; CV, cardiovascular; CVA, cerebrovascular accident; ESRD, end-stage renal disease; HCTZ, hydrochlorothiazide; MI, myocardial infarction; SCr, serum creatinine. CHARM, Candesartan in Heart Failure—Assessment of Reduction in Mortality and Morbidity; ELITE, Evaluation of Losartan in the Elderly; IDNT, Irbesartan Diabetic Nephropathy Trial; I-PRESERVE, Irbesartan in Heart Failure With Preserved Systolic Function; LIFE, Losartan Intervention for Endpoint reduction in hypertension; ONTARGET, Ongoing Telmisartan Alone or in Combination With Ramipril Global Endpoint Trial; OPTIMAAL, Optimal Trial in Myocardial Infarction With Angiotensin II Antagonist Losartan; RENAAL, Reduction of Endpoints in NIDDM With Angiotensin II Antagonist Losartan; SCOPE, Study on Cognition and Prognosis in the Elderly; TRANSCEND, Telmisartan Randomized Assessment Study of ACE-I Intolerant Patients With Cardiovascular Disease; Val-HEFT, Valsartan Heart Failure Trial; Valiant, Valsartan in Acute Myocardial Infarction; VALUE, Valsartan Antihypertensive Long-Term Use Evaluation.

A large amount of data is available concerning heart failure. Valsartan and candesartan reduced cardiovascular morbidity and mortality in heart failure patients intolerant to converting enzyme inhibitors *(4,13)*. Also, candesartan reduced total mortality and cardiovascular mortality and heart failure hospitalizations in patients with chronic heart failure *(11)*. Furthermore, cardiovascular mortality and hospitalizations for heart failure were significantly reduced in patients receiving candesartan and a β-blocker or an angiotensin-converting enzyme (ACE) inhibitor *(12)*. Heart failure hospitalizations were reduced in patients treated with candesartan who had a preserved ejection fraction *(14)*.

There are pharmacological differences among the seven ARBs currently marketed (Table 2). Losartan and its active metabolite E3174 reduce blood pressure (BP). Candesartan cilexetil and olmesartan medoxomil are prodrugs that form an active metabolite. Losartan has a uricosuric effect. Telmisartan has the longest terminal half-life. In addition, there are differences in type I angiotensin II (AT_1) receptor binding affinity. Olmesartan, valsartan, candesartan, irbesartan, and telmisartan are insurmountable antagonists of angiotensin (Ang)-II. Eprosartan acts at vascular AT_1 receptors postsynaptically and at presynaptic AT_1 receptors, where it inhibits sympathetically stimulated noradrenaline release.

The ARBs do not cause a cough like ACE inhibitors do. In addition, these drugs are less likely to cause angioneurotic edema *(16)*. Care is required in dosing these drugs in patients with renal insufficiency. Close monitoring of potassium is required when used with potassium-sparing diuretics and exogenous potassium intake. Losartan and irbesartan have a greater affinity for cytochrome P450 isoenzymes, but this theoretical possibility has not been a problem to date. Candesartan, valsartan and eprosartan have modest affinity and telmisartan has no affinity for any of the cytochrome P450 isoenzymes.

It might be predicted that the response rate of ARBs for elderly patients might be less than for younger patients because there is reduced activity of the renin–angiotensin system in older persons. However, age does not seem to be a factor in reducing the overall response rate of ARBs. This is supported in the analysis of the studies with individual ARBs.

CANDESARTAN CILEXETIL

Pharmacokinetics parameters were measured in 33 elderly and 51 younger subjects after a single dose and after 7 days of once-daily administration of candesartan dosed between 2 and 16 mg *(17)*. The maximum concentration and the area under the curve (AUC) were 50% higher in the elderly subjects compared to the younger subjects. Also, the half-life

Table 2
Characteristics of Angiotensin Receptor Blockers

	Candesartan	Eprosartan	Irbesartan	Losartan	Olmesartan	Valsartan	Telmisartan
Brand	Atacand	Teveten	Avapro	Cozaar	Benicar	Diovan	Micardis
Dosing, mg	8–32	400–800	75–300	25–100	20–40	80–320	40–80
Terminal half-life, hours	5–9	5–9	11–15	6–9	13	6–9	24
Bioavailability, %	40	13	60–80	~30	26	25	30–60
Protein binding, %	>99	98	90–92	99.8	99	94–97	>98
Renal elimination, %	26	7	25	4	13	13	<1
Active metabolite	Yes			Yes	Yes		
Food effect						Yes	

was slightly longer among elderly participants. There was no accumulation of candesartan or its metabolite. No alteration in dosing is required for elderly patients.

The efficacy and tolerability of candesartan were evaluated in a prospective, randomized, double-blind, multicenter, parallel design trial *(18)*. After a 4- to 8-week placebo run-in period, 193 hypertensive subjects between 65 and 87 years were treated with 8–16 mg candesartan or placebo for 12 weeks. The mean reduction in supine BP was −13.6/−7.5 mmHg with candesartan compared with placebo therapy ($p < 0.001$ for systolic and diastolic). The proportion of patients achieving a supine diastolic blood pressure (DBP) of 90 mmHg or less was 41.7% with candesartan vs 16.8% with placebo ($p < 0.001$). There was no evidence of orthostatic hypotension, and active therapy with candesartan was well tolerated.

A multicenter, randomized, double-blind, parallel-group design trial studied 185 patients 75 years or older with a mean sitting DBP 95–114 mmHg after a placebo run-in period of 4–8 weeks *(19)*. Once-daily candesartan (8–16 mg) or hydrochlorothiazide (12.5–25 mg) was given for 24 weeks. The mean reduction in BP was not significantly different between treatments (Fig. 1). Similar numbers of adverse events were reported with each drug, although hypokalemia and hyperuricemia were more common with the diuretic.

A double-blind, randomized, crossover, placebo-controlled study using a factorial design compared once-daily placebo, 16 mg candesartan, 5 mg of felodipine, or the combination of each drug *(20)*. There were 31 subjects older than 65 years with a systolic blood pressure (SBP) 160 mmHg or higher treated for 1 month for four periods after an initial washout run-in phase. Ambulatory BP reading was performed after each treatment period. The average declines in 24-hour SBP were −12.2, −11.9, and −21.0 mmHg for candesartan, felodipine, and the combination, respectively. Thus, the combination of an ARB and dihydropyridine calcium antagonist improves overall response rate and is additive.

The Study on Cognition and Prognosis in the Elderly trial of candesartan in 4964 patients aged 70 to 89 years with SBP 160–179 mmHg and/or DBP 90–99 mmHg observed a reduction in nonfatal strokes *(10)*. This study is discussed in more detail in Chapter 7. Also, the Acute Candesartan Cilexetil Therapy in Stroke Survivors study evaluated the effect of BP reduction in the early treatment of stroke in a prospective, double-blind, placebo-controlled study of 342 patients *(21)*. After 12 months, there were fewer vascular events with candesartan compared with placebo (9.8% vs 18.7%, $p = 0.026$). There may be a special benefit of candesartan for modifying cerebrovascular events.

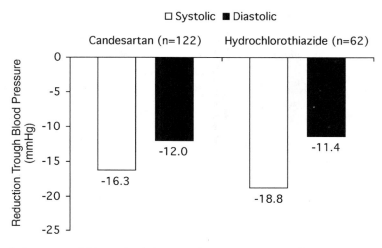

Fig. 1. Outcome of 12-week trial comparing candesartan and hydrochlorothiazide in older hypertensive patients. Each drug was equally effective in reducing systolic and diastolic blood pressure. (Data from ref. *19*.)

EPROSARTAN

In comparing eight young and eight elderly males after a single 200-mg dose of oral eprosartan, the AUC and the maximum concentration were twice as high among elderly subjects *(22)*. The time to maximal concentration was delayed by 3.4 hours. These differences may be related to increased bioavailability as a result of prolonged absorption. The elimination half-life was greater, possibly owing to decreased elimination rate in the elderly.

A 12-week, double-blind trial was conducted comparing eprosartan ($n = 264$) dosed 200–300 mg twice daily with enalapril ($n = 264$) dosed 5–20 mg once daily in 528 patients with a sitting DBP between 95 and 114 mmHg *(23)*. After 12 weeks, 12.5 to 25 mg hydrochlorothiazide dosed once daily could be added if the DBP was 90 mmHg or higher. Approximately 24% of the study participants were 65 years or older. The change in BP from baseline is displayed in Fig. 2. There was no difference between elderly and younger patients. Elderly patients did not require more or less medication than younger patients. Cough was more common with enalapril treatment; however, there was no difference by age group.

Another study enrolled 334 elderly patients with a sitting SBP 160 mmHg or higher in a 12-week multicenter, double-blind study with a single-blind placebo lead-in phase of 3 to 4 weeks *(24)*. Patients were

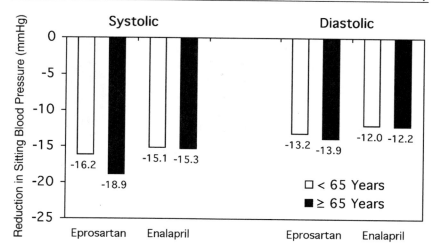

Fig. 2. Outcome of 12-week trial comparing eprosartan and enalapril in older and younger hypertensive patients. There was no difference in the response of either drug or the effectiveness based on age. (Data from ref. *23*.)

randomly assigned to 600 mg of eprosartan once daily or 5 mg of enalapril once daily. To achieve an SBP less than 140 mmHg during follow-up every 3 weeks, the dose of eprosartan could be titrated to 800 mg and enalapril to 20 mg once daily. After 12 weeks, the average reduction in BP was not significantly different: −18.0/−9.4 mmHg for eprosartan and −17.4/−9.6 mmHg for enalapril. Normalization of sitting SBP occurred in less than 25% for both drugs. More adverse events were observed with enalapril (50.9%) than with eprosartan (35.7%).

IRBESARTAN

In an open-label, single-dose, parallel group design that dosed 50 mg of irbesartan after a 10-hour overnight fast, the geometric mean AUC was 43% higher in elderly subjects than in younger subjects *(25)*. The maximum concentration was increased by 49%, and the time to peak concentration was shorter. Renal clearance was reduced by 56% in elderly females but not males. These differences in pharmacokinetics were thought unimportant because less than 3% of irbesartan is excreted in the urine *(26)*. In a 12-month open-label study of 32 elderly hypertensive subjects with creatinine clearance less than 45 mL/minute per 1.73 m², 150 mg of irbesartan alone or in combination with other drugs reduced BP and decreased proteinuria without worsening renal function *(27)*.

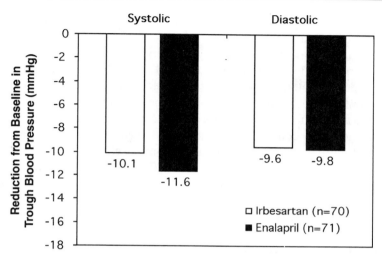

Fig. 3. Outcome of 8-week study comparing irbesartan and enalapril in older hypertensive volunteers. There was no difference in the change in blood pressure. (Data from ref. *28*.)

There does not appear to be any difference in the response rate of irbesartan on the basis of age *(28)*. Irbesartan in doses of 37.5–300 mg alone or in combination with 6.25–25 mg hydrochlorothiazide dosed once daily reduced trough seated SBP and DBP similarly in younger ($n = 520$) and older ($n = 110$) patients *(29)*. One randomized double-blind study of patients 65 years or older compared 150–300 mg irbesartan with 10–20 mg enalapril over an 8-week period *(30)*. There was no difference in the change in BP (Fig. 3). The diastolic control rate was similar for irbesartan (52.9%) and enalapril (54.9%, $p = 0.81$). Cough was less frequent with irbesartan than enalapril (15.5% vs 4.3%, $p = 0.046$).

LOSARTAN POTASSIUM

No significant difference in the plasma concentration of losartan or EXP3174 was observed between elderly or younger patients *(31)*.

The Evaluation of Losartan in the Elderly (ELITE) Studies I ($n = 722$) and II ($n = 3152$) were conducted in patients with heart failure *(1,2)*. Each double-blind trial compared 50 mg of losartan dosed once daily with 50 mg of captopril dosed three times daily in subjects with class II–IV heart failure and an ejection fraction of 40% or less. There was an unexpected reduction in total mortality in ELITE I, a safety-and-efficacy trial *(1)*. There was no superiority of losartan in reduction in mortality in ELITE II, an outcomes trial *(2)*. The results were attributed to the dosing of losartan. However, both trials consistently documented enhanced tolerability of losartan.

Several studies with isolated systolic hypertension have been completed. In a double-blind, randomized trial, 273 subjects (mean age 66.3 years) received 50 mg of losartan or atenolol once daily for 16 weeks of treatment after a 4-week single-blind placebo run-in period *(32)*. For subjects not controlled on monotherapy, 12.5 mg of hydrochlorothiazide dosed once daily could be added at week 8 to achieve a sitting SBP less than 160 mmHg. The average change from baseline of seated SBP for subjects *not* receiving a diuretic was –25.0 mmHg for losartan (n = 89) and –25.4 mmHg for atenolol (n = 88). At week 16, the average change from baseline was –24.7/–3.3 for losartan and –25.3/–4.3 for atenolol. More clinical adverse events necessitating withdrawal occurred with atenolol than with losartan (7.2% vs 1.5%, p = 0.035).

In a 16-week prospective study of 504 Spanish hypertensive patients 60 years or older, 50 mg losartan was given *(33)*. If BP exceeded 159/89 mmHg after 6 weeks, then 50 mg losartan with 12.5 mg hydrochlorothiazide was given. If BP was still elevated after 6 weeks, then 100 mg losartan with 25 mg hydrochlorothiazide was given. After 16 weeks, 77.8% of subjects had BPs less than 160/90 mmHg.

After a 4-week placebo run-in period, 50–100 mg losartan (n = 89) or 5–10 mg felodipine extended release (n = 43) was titrated to a sitting DBP less than 90 mmHg over 12 weeks in a double-blind study of older patients *(34)*. The trough BP reduction at week 12 was similar with losartan (–17.2/–13.2 mmHg) and felodipine extended release (–19.0/–14.0 mmHg). Although each drug was effective in reducing BP, there were more treatment withdrawals as the result of edema with the calcium antagonist.

There were 140 hypertensive patients 65 years or older randomly assigned in a double-blind study to losartan or nifedipine GITS (gastrointestinal therapeutic system) after a 4-week placebo lead-in period *(35)*. Every 4 weeks, treatment could be titrated to achieve a DBP less than 90 mmHg. Nifedipine GITS could be titrated from 30 to 90 mg daily. Losartan was dosed initially at 50 mg daily, but 12.5–25 mg of hydrochlorothiazide could be added. All medications were administered with a matching placebo. The change from baseline after 12 weeks was not significantly different between the drugs (Fig. 4). More patients achieved a DBP less than 90 mmHg with nifedipine (82%) than with losartan (68%).

A multicenter, double-blind, randomized study enrolled younger and older hypertensive subjects with mild-to-moderate hypertension *(36)*. After a 4-week placebo lead-in period, participants received a fixed dose

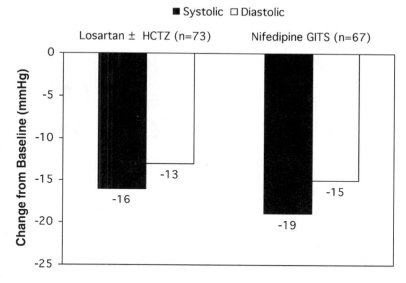

Fig. 4. Outcome of 12-week trial comparing losartan with or without a diuretic vs nifedipine gastrointestinal therapeutic system (GITS) in elderly hypertensive patients. There was no difference between the treatment groups. ±HCTZ, with or without hydrochlorothiazide. (Data from ref. *35*.)

of 50 mg of losartan with 12.5 mg of hydrochlorothiazide (*n* = 216) or 50 mg of captopril with 25 mg of hydrochlorothiazide (*n* = 109) once daily for 12 weeks. The change in trough BP is shown in Fig. 5. There was no difference in efficacy by age group or treatment. Cough and headache occurred more commonly in elderly patients receiving captopril than in those receiving losartan. Serum creatinine and uric acid increased, and serum potassium decreased from baseline more with captopril than with losartan.

OLMESARTAN MEDOXOMIL

Olmesartan medoxomil is absorbed and converted to olmesartan rapidly in elderly hypertensive patients *(37)*. After olmesartan dosed at 80 mg once daily, elderly patients had a higher steady-state maximum concentration and AUC and a longer elimination half-life compared with younger patients. Dosing adjustment in the elderly is not considered necessary except with severe renal impairment.

An integrated analysis of seven randomized, double-blind, placebo-controlled studies with an entry DBP between 100 and 115 mmHg was performed *(38)*. Of 2693 patients, approximately 20% were 65 years or

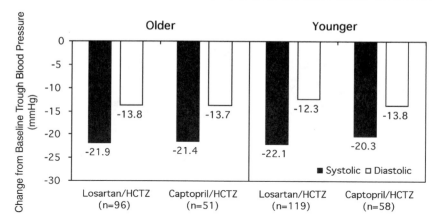

Fig. 5. Outcome of 12-week study in older and younger hypertensive patients of fixed-dose combination of hydrochlorothiazide (HCTZ) with either captopril or losartan. There was no difference in the response of either drug or the effectiveness based on age. (Data from ref. *36*.)

older. The duration of treatment was 6 to 12 weeks. Placebo and olmesartan at 2.5, 5, 10, 20, 40, and 80 mg were compared. The average decline in trough BP was −14.7/−11.3 mmHg in younger patients and −12.5/−11.8 mmHg in older patients.

TELMISARTAN

The pharmacokinetics of telmisartan in 12 elderly normotensive volunteers was studied *(39)*. Telmisartan (20 and 120 mg) was given orally in an open-label crossover study with a 14-day washout between doses. At steady state, the time to maximum concentration was 30 to 60 minutes, and the geometric mean half-life was 36 to 37 hours. There was no appreciable accumulation of telmisartan in elderly patients. However, the maximum concentration of telmisartan and AUC were higher in women than in men.

Telmisartan is effective in reducing BP in both younger and older patients (Fig. 6) *(40)*. The addition of hydrochlorothiazide enhances the BP response *(40)*. A 26-week, double-blind parallel study compared telmisartan and enalapril in 278 hypertensive patients 65 years and older after a 3- to 5-week placebo run-in phase *(41)*. Titration of 20 to 80 mg of telmisartan or 5 to 20 mg of enalapril was done to achieve a DBP less than 90 mmHg. If BP was controlled, then 12.5 to 25 mg of hydrochlorothiazide could be added after 12 weeks of monotherapy. Then, the titrated medications were maintained for the final 10 weeks of the study.

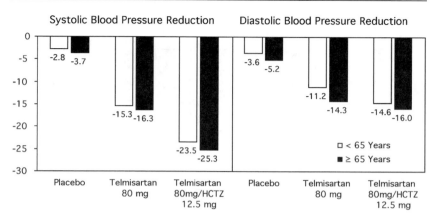

Fig. 6. Comparison of the change in baseline blood pressure in older and younger hypertensive patients with placebo, telmisartan, and telmisartan with hydrochlorothiazide (HCTZ). The combination of a diuretic with telmisartan significantly improved overall blood pressure reduction. (Data from ref. *40*.)

There was no significant difference in the reduction in trough BP between the treatment groups (Fig. 7). DBP was reduced to less than 90 mmHg in 63% of telmisartan-treated subjects and 62% of enalapril-treated subjects. SBP was reduced 10 mmHg or more in 70% of the telmisartan group and 67% of the enalapril group. There were fewer treatment-related adverse events with telmisartan (25.2%) compared with enalapril (37.4%) because of the higher rate of coughing with enalapril.

VALSARTAN

The pharmacokinetics of a single dose of 80 mg of valsartan was studied in 12 young and 12 elderly volunteers after a 12-hour fast *(42)*. The maximum concentration was 24% higher, and the AUC was 52% higher in elderly subjects compared to younger subjects. Also, the median terminal elimination half-life was 7.4 hours in elderly participants compared to 5.1 hours in younger participants. These differences may be caused by decreased renal elimination in the older subjects.

The efficacy of valsartan was studied in 146 older patients with SBP 160 mmHg or greater *(43)*. After a placebo run-in period, patients received 80 mg of valsartan dosed once daily or placebo in a randomized, double-blind, placebo-controlled trial. After 4 weeks, the placebo or valsartan dose was doubled for an additional 4 weeks. The placebo-correct decline in BP with valsartan was −10.4/−4.0 mmHg (Fig. 8). There was no symptomatic orthostatic hypotension, and treatment-related adverse events were similar between valsartan and placebo.

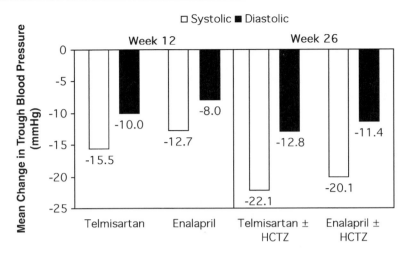

Fig. 7. Results of a trial in older hypertensive patients comparing blood pressure reduction with telmisartan or enalapril alone or with hydrochlorothiazide (HCTZ). There was no difference between the drugs. (Data from ref. *41.*)

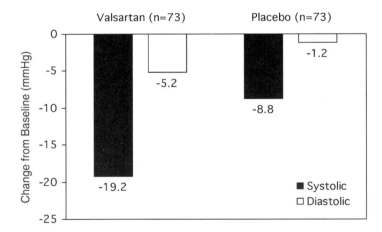

Fig. 8. Results of a study of systolic hypertension in older subjects with valsartan or placebo after 8 weeks. Blood pressure was significantly reduced with valsartan. (Data from ref. *43.*)

An analysis of nine randomized, placebo-controlled trials of valsartan or placebo was performed *(44)*. There were 4067 patients, including 998 patients who were 65 years or older. Figure 9 displays the results of this analysis, showing significant reductions in both SBP and DBP. The

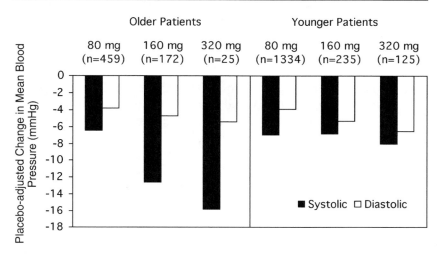

Fig. 9. Results of an integrated analysis of nine randomized, placebo-controlled trials comparing various doses of valsartan on blood pressure reduction in younger and older hypertensive subjects. There was a dose-dependent antihypertensive response for both older and younger patients. Systolic blood pressure reductions were greater in older than in younger patients. (Data from ref. *44*.)

results indicate an increasing antihypertensive response with escalating doses of valsartan. The SBP response was greater in elderly patients compared with younger patients.

A multicenter, double-blind, parallel group trial was conducted in 501 elderly hypertensive patients *(45,46)*. The volunteers were randomly assigned to receive 40 mg of valsartan (*n* = 334) or 2.5 mg of lisinopril (*n* = 167) daily with subsequent titration up to 80 mg of valsartan or 20 mg of lisinopril over 4 weeks if the DBP was 90 mmHg or greater. At weeks 8 and 12, the addition of 12.5 to 25 mg of hydrochlorothiazide could be made to achieve BP control. A DBP response, a sitting DBP less than 90 mmHg or 10 mmHg or greater decline from baseline, was 80% in both valsartan and lisinopril groups at 12 weeks. At 12 weeks, the mean BP was decreased by –19.7/–14.6 mmHg in the valsartan group and -21.0/ –15.1 mmHg in the lisinopril group. This benefit continued to be observed at 52 weeks. At 52 weeks, there was a similar nonsignificant decrease of –20.3/–14.4 mmHg in the valsartan group and –20.2/–15.4 mmHg in the lisinopril group. The overall incidence of drug-related adverse events was slightly higher in lisinopril-treated patients (35.3%) compared to valsartan-treated patients (29.3%). This difference was caused by the higher frequency (17.4%) of cough for the lisinopril-treated patients compared to patients treated with valsartan (7.5%). An extension of the trial with 69 patients continued to observe a similar BP response with each drug *(45)*. However, valsartan was better tolerated.

A 24-week, randomized, double-blind trial compared valsartan and amlodipine in older Italian patients with isolated systolic hypertension *(47)*. After a 2-week placebo lead-in period, patients with an SBP of 160–220 mmHg and a DBP less than 90 mmHg were given 5 mg of amlodipine or 80 mg of valsartan once daily. The dose of each drug was doubled after 8 weeks if the SBP was 140 mmHg or higher. After an additional 8 weeks, if the SBP goal was not achieved, then 12.5 mg of hydrochlorothiazide daily could be added. Baseline BP was 170/84 mmHg among 410 patients. The mean decline in BP at the end of the study was −30.7/−5.6 mmHg for valsartan and −32.2/−6.6 mmHg for amlodipine. The target SBP was achieved in 74.7% of patients treated with valsartan and 73% of patients treated with amlodipine. However, there was more peripheral edema with amlodipine compared to valsartan (26.8% vs 4.8%, $p < 0.001$).

SUMMARY

BP reduction is effectively achieved with ARBs. Some studies suggested a dose-dependent reduction in BP. Equivalent reduction in BP was observed when directly comparing ARBs with ACE inhibitors, β-blockers, or calcium antagonists. ARBs, when combined with a diuretic or a calcium antagonist, resulted in greater declines in BP than monotherapy. Combinations of drugs increased the likelihood of reaching SBP goals. These drugs are well tolerated compared with older antihypertensive agents.

REFERENCES

1. Pitt B, Segal R, Martinez FA, et al. Randomised trial of losartan vs captopril in patients over 65 with heart failure (Evaluation of Losartan in the Elderly Study, ELITE). *Lancet* 1997;349:747–752.
2. Pitt B, Poole-Wilson PA, Segal R, et al. Effect of losartan compared with captopril on mortality in patients with symptomatic heart failure: randomised trial—the Losartan Heart Failure Survival Study ELITE II. *Lancet* 2000;355:1582–1587.
3. Brenner BM, Cooper ME, de Zeeuw D, et al. Effects of losartan on renal and cardiovascular outcomes in patients with type 2 diabetes and nephropathy. *N Engl J Med* 2001;345:861–869.
4. Cohn JN, Tognoni G. A randomized trial of the angiotensin-receptor blocker valsartan in chronic heart failure. *N Engl J Med* 2001;345:1667–1675.
5. Lewis EJ, Hunsicker LG, Clarke WR, et al. Renoprotective effect of the angiotensin-receptor antagonist irbesartan in patients with nephropathy due to type 2 diabetes. *N Engl J Med* 2001;345:851–860.

6. Parving HH, Lehnert H, Brochner-Mortensen J, Gomis R, Andersen S, Arner P. The effect of irbesartan on the development of diabetic nephropathy in patients with type 2 diabetes. *N Engl J Med* 2001;345:870–878.

7. Dahlof B, Devereux RB, Kjeldsen SE, et al. Cardiovascular morbidity and mortality in the Losartan Intervention for Endpoint reduction in hypertension study (LIFE): a randomised trial against atenolol. *Lancet* 2002;359:995–1003.

8. Dickstein K, Kjekshus J. Effects of losartan and captopril on mortality and morbidity in high-risk patients after acute myocardial infarction: the OPTIMAAL randomised trial. Optimal Trial in Myocardial Infarction With Angiotensin II Antagonist Losartan. *Lancet* 2002;360:752–760.

9. Lindholm LH, Ibsen H, Dahlof B, et al. Cardiovascular morbidity and mortality in patients with diabetes in the Losartan Intervention for Endpoint reduction in hypertension study (LIFE): a randomised trial against atenolol. *Lancet* 2002;359:1004–1010.

10. Lithell H, Hansson L, Skoog I, et al. The Study on Cognition and Prognosis in the Elderly (SCOPE): principal results of a randomized double-blind intervention trial. *J Hypertens* 2003;21:875–886.

11. Pfeffer MA, Swedberg K, Granger CB, et al. Effects of candesartan on mortality and morbidity in patients with chronic heart failure: the CHARM-Overall programme. *Lancet* 2003;362:759–766.

12. McMurray JJ, Ostergren J, Swedberg K, et al. Effects of candesartan in patients with chronic heart failure and reduced left-ventricular systolic function taking angiotensin-converting-enzyme inhibitors: the CHARM-Added trial. *Lancet* 2003;362:767–771.

13. Granger CB, McMurray JJ, Yusuf S, et al. Effects of candesartan in patients with chronic heart failure and reduced left-ventricular systolic function intolerant to angiotensin-converting-enzyme inhibitors: the CHARM-Alternative trial. *Lancet* 2003;362:772–776.

14. Yusuf S, Pfeffer MA, Swedberg K, et al. Effects of candesartan in patients with chronic heart failure and preserved left-ventricular ejection fraction: the CHARM-Preserved Trial. *Lancet* 2003;362:777–781.

15. Pfeffer MA, McMurray JJ, Velazquez EJ, et al. Valsartan, captopril, or both in myocardial infarction complicated by heart failure, left ventricular dysfunction, or both. *N Engl J Med* 2003;349:1893–1906.

16. Prisant LM. Angioneurotic edema. *J Clin Hypertens (Greenwich)* 2001;3:262–263.

17. Hübner R, Högemann AM, Sunzel M, Riddell JG. Pharmacokinetics of candesartan after single and repeated doses of candesartan cilexetil in young and elderly healthy volunteers. *J Hum Hypertens* 1997;11(suppl 2):S19–S25.

18. McInnes GT, O'Kane KP, Jonker J, Roth J. The efficacy and tolerability of candesartan cilexetil in an elderly hypertensive population. *J Hum Hypertens* 1997;11(suppl 2):S75–S80.

19. Neldam S, Forsen B. Antihypertensive treatment in elderly patients aged 75 years or over: a 24-week study of the tolerability of candesartan cilexetil in relation to hydrochlorothiazide. *Drugs Aging* 2001;18:225–232.

20. Morgan T, Anderson A. A comparison of candesartan, felodipine, and their combination in the treatment of elderly patients with systolic hypertension. *Am J Hypertens* 2002;15:544–549.

21. Schrader J, Luders S, Kulschewski A, et al. The ACCESS Study: evaluation of Acute Candesartan Cilexetil Therapy in Stroke Survivors. *Stroke* 2003;34:1699–1703.

22. Tenero DM, Martin DE, Miller AK, et al. Effect of age and gender on the pharmacokinetics of eprosartan. *Br J Clin Pharmacol* 1998;46:267–270.

23. Argenziano L, Trimarco B. Effect of eprosartan and enalapril in the treatment of elderly hypertensive patients: subgroup analysis of a 26-week, double-blind, multicentre study. Eprosartan Multinational Study Group. *Curr Med Res Opin* 1999;15:9–14.

24. Ruilope L, Jager B, Prichard B. Eprosartan vs enalapril in elderly patients with hypertension: a double-blind, randomized trial. *Blood Press* 2001;10:223–229.

25. Vachharajani NN, Shyu WC, Smith RA, Greene DS. The effects of age and gender on the pharmacokinetics of irbesartan. *Br J Clin Pharmacol* 1998;46:611–613.

26. Gillis JC, Markham A. Irbesartan. A review of its pharmacodynamic and pharmacokinetic properties and therapeutic use in the management of hypertension. *Drugs* 1997;54:885–902.

27. De Rosa ML, Cardace P, Rossi M, Baiano A, de Cristofaro A. Evaluation of long-term efficacy and tolerability of irbesartan in elderly hypertensive patients with renal impairment in an open-label study. *Curr Ther Res* 2002;63:201–215.

28. Pool JL, Guthrie RM, Littlejohn TW 3rd, et al. Dose-related antihypertensive effects of irbesartan in patients with mild-to-moderate hypertension. *Am J Hypertens* 1998;11(4 pt 1):462–470.

29. Kochar M, Guthrie R, Triscari J, Kassler-Taub K, Reeves RA. Matrix study of irbesartan with hydrochlorothiazide in mild-to-moderate hypertension. *Am J Hypertens* 1999;12(8 pt 1):797–805.

30. Lacourciere Y. A multicenter, randomized, double-blind study of the antihypertensive efficacy and tolerability of irbesartan in patients aged > or = 65 years with mild to moderate hypertension. *Clin Ther* 2000;22:1213–1224.

31. Schaefer KL, Porter JA. Angiotensin II receptor antagonists: the prototype losartan. *Ann Pharmacother* 1996;30:625–636.

32. Farsang C, Garcia-Puig J, Niegowska J, Baiz AQ, Vrijens F, Bortman G. The efficacy and tolerability of losartan vs atenolol in patients with isolated systolic hypertension. Losartan ISH Investigators Group. *J Hypertens* 2000;18:795–801.

33. Fernández-Vega F, Abellan J, Sanz de Castro S, Cucalón JM, Maceira B, Gomez de la Cámara A. A study on the efficacy and safety of losartan in elderly patients with mild to moderate essential hypertension. *Int Urol Nephrol* 2001;32:519–523.

34. Chan JC, Critchley JA, Lappe JT, et al. Randomised, double-blind, parallel study of the anti-hypertensive efficacy and safety of losartan potassium compared with felodipine ER in elderly patients with mild to moderate hypertension. *J Hum Hypertens* 1995;9:765–771.

35. Conlin PR, Elkins M, Liss C, Vrecenak AJ, Barr E, Edelman JM. A study of losartan, alone or with hydrochlorothiazide vs nifedipine GITS in elderly patients with diastolic hypertension. *J Hum Hypertens* 1998;12:693–699.

36. Critchley JAJH, Gilchrist N, Ikeda L, et al. A randomized, double-masked comparison of the antihypertensive efficacy and safety of combination therapy with losartan and hydrochlorothiazide vs captopril and hydrochlorothiazide in elderly and younger patients. *Curr Ther Res* 1996;57:392–407.

37. von Bergmann K, Laeis P, Puchler K, Sudhop T, Schwocho LR, Gonzalez L. Olmesartan medoxomil: influence of age, renal and hepatic function on the pharmacokinetics of olmesartan medoxomil. *J Hypertens Suppl* 2001;19(suppl 1):S33–S40.

38. Neutel JM. Clinical studies of CS-866, the newest angiotensin II receptor antagonist. *Am J Cardiol* 2001;87:37C–43C.

39. Stangier J, Su CA, Roth W. Pharmacokinetics of orally and intravenously administered telmisartan in healthy young and elderly volunteers and in hypertensive patients. *J Int Med Res* 2000;28:149–167.

40. McGill JB, Reilly PA. Telmisartan plus hydrochlorothiazide vs telmisartan or hydrochlorothiazide monotherapy in patients with mild to moderate hypertension: a multicenter, randomized, double-blind, placebo-controlled, parallel-group trial. *Clin Ther* 2001;23:833–850.
41. Karlberg BE, Lins LE, Hermansson K. Efficacy and safety of telmisartan, a selective AT1 receptor antagonist, compared with enalapril in elderly patients with primary hypertension. TEES Study Group. *J Hypertens* 1999;17:293–302.
42. Sioufi A, Marfil F, Jaouen A, et al. The effect of age on the pharmacokinetics of valsartan. *Biopharm Drug Dispos* 1998;19:237–244.
43. Neutel JM, Bedigian MP. Efficacy of valsartan in patients aged > or = 65 years with systolic hypertension. *Clin Ther* 2000;22:961–969.
44. Hedner T, Pool JL, Oparil S, Glazer R, Chiang Y. Valsartan provides effective antihypertensive response in older patients: an integrated analysis. *J Hypertens* 2000;18(suppl 2):S42.
45. Bremner AD, Mehring GH, Meilenbrock S. Long-term systemic tolerability of valsartan compared with lisinopril in elderly hypertensive patients. *Adv Ther* 1997;14:245–253.
46. Bremner AD, Baur M, Oddou-Stock P, Bodin F. Valsartan: long-term efficacy and tolerability compared to lisinopril in elderly patients with essential hypertension. *Clin Exp Hypertens* 1997;19:1263–1285.
47. Malacco E, Vari N, Capuano V, Spagnuolo V, Borgnino C, Palatini P. A randomized, double-blind, active-controlled, parallel-group comparison of valsartan and amlodipine in the treatment of isolated systolic hypertension in elderly patients: the Val-Syst study. *Clin Ther* 2003;25:2765–2780.

18 Clinical Trials With Calcium Antagonists in Older Patients With Hypertension

William B. White, MD *and Sumeska Thavarajah, MD*

CONTENTS

INTRODUCTION

Although certain classes of medications provide additional benefits beyond blood pressure (BP) reduction in older patients with comorbid conditions, the greatest factor in reduction of cardiovascular and cerebrovascular events and preservation of renal function is BP reduction. The Hypertension Detection and Follow-up Program demonstrated that

From: Clinical Hypertension and Vascular Diseases: Hypertension in the Elderly
Edited by: L. M. Prisant © Humana Press Inc., Totowa, NJ

a reduction in systolic blood pressure (SBP) of 1 mmHg correlated with a 1% decline in mortality *(1)*. However, to achieve newly targeted BP levels based on the Seventh Report of the Joint National Committee on the Prevention, Detection, Evaluation, and Treatment of High Blood Pressure, the majority of individuals will require two to four agents *(2,3)*.

Calcium antagonists have long been utilized for the treatment of hypertension in older patients. Although guidelines support the use of calcium antagonists primarily in elderly individuals with isolated systolic hypertension, angina, or contraindications to use of β-blockers and diuretics *(4,5)*, these drugs have clearly been used far more widely in clinical practice. Marred by controversy during the course of the 1990s, there have been mixed reviews on the benefits and risks of this important class of antihypertensive therapy. The purpose of this chapter is to review the clinical trials that in fact do support the use of the calcium antagonists in elderly patients with hypertension and certain related complications.

THE CALCIUM ANTAGONIST CONTROVERSY IN THE TREATMENT OF HYPERTENSION

In the mid-1990s, clinicians avoided the use of the calcium antagonists in response to a series of retrospective analyses and reports of increased cancer incidence rates *(6)*, gastrointestinal bleeding episodes, and cardiovascular events *(7)*. These observational studies and pooled analyses along with widely publicized concerns of these adverse events in the lay press nearly immediately led to alterations in prescribing patterns for the calcium antagonists. For example, in British Columbia, Canada, calcium antagonist use fell from a 22% share of the antihypertensive prescriptions in 1994 to 15% of all the antihypertensive agents prescribed in 1996 *(8)*. A review of the prescription database in Ontario, Canada, demonstrated a similar decline in calcium antagonist use, falling from 22% to 14 % between 1993 and 1998 *(9)*. Although a number of placebo-controlled randomized trials with long-term follow-up have been published *(3,10–13)* to challenge earlier reports of adverse cardiovascular events, it is useful to review the studies that led to controversy and concern regarding calcium antagonist safety.

The observational studies, case reports, and meta-analyses increased concerns that cancer and cardiovascular events were higher on calcium antagonists compared to diuretics, β-blockers, and other commonly used antihypertensive therapies. For example, Pahor et al. reported a twofold greater incidence of cancer in elderly patients taking short-acting calcium antagonists in comparison to those prescribed β-adrenergic blockers *(6)*. However, there was no account of duration of exposure in relation to discovery of malignancy. Subsequent studies with calcium antagonists have failed to demonstrate an increased cancer incidence *(3)*.

Another meta-analysis *(7)* and a cohort study *(14)* reported an increased number of coronary events and gastrointestinal bleeds with the use of the immediate-release formulations of verapamil, diltiazem, and nifedipine. In a retrospective case–control study from the physician staff model Group Health Cooperative in Seattle, Washington, a dose-related 60% increase in acute myocardial infarction (MI) incidence was reported with the use of nifedipine compared to patients treated with diuretic therapy *(7)*. A meta-analysis by Stason and colleagues noted an increased incidence of angina with use of short-acting nifedipine in patients with coronary artery disease *(15)*.

It is important to note that subsequent placebo-controlled studies with long-acting calcium antagonists contradicted the majority of these retrospective studies that suggested greater cardiovascular risk for the calcium antagonists. For example, one of the first studies to demonstrate a reduction of cardiovascular events relative to placebo was the Shanghai Trial of Nifedipine in the Elderly *(16)*. This nonrandomized placebo-controlled trial involved 1632 subjects between the ages of 60 and 79 years with elevated BP (>160/90 mmHg). There was 40% risk reduction in stroke and arrhythmia incidence but an equivalent risk of myocardial events in the group treated with nifedipine. Shortly thereafter, the Systolic Hypertension in Europe (Syst-Eur) trial showed that, in isolated systolic hypertension in the elderly, the dihydropyridine calcium antagonist nitrendipine induced a significant reduction in cardiovascular morbidity and mortality compared to the placebo group *(12,17)*.

OVERVIEW OF THE CALCIUM ANTAGONIST CLINICAL TRIALS (1997–2003)

During the last decade, a number of controlled clinical trials with intermediate and long-term follow-up have shown the benefit of BP reduction and prevention of cardiovascular and cerebrovascular events using calcium antagonists (Fig. 1). It is clear from these trials that the reduction in morbidity and mortality is related to the amount of BP reduction, especially in the higher risk patient subgroups *(18,19)*.

For example, in the Hypertension Optimal Treatment study, which used the dihydropyridine calcium antagonist felodipine, there was a 2.5-fold increase for stroke incidence in the diabetic hypertensive group compared to the nondiabetic group *(20)*. Aggressive treatment of BP is the main means of slowing the progression of renal disease and preventing vascular events in both diabetic and nondiabetic individuals. The

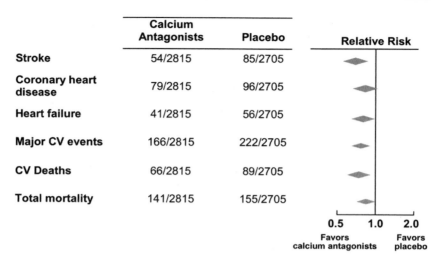

	Calcium Antagonists	Placebo
Stroke	54/2815	85/2705
Coronary heart disease	79/2815	96/2705
Heart failure	41/2815	56/2705
Major CV events	166/2815	222/2705
CV Deaths	66/2815	89/2705
Total mortality	141/2815	155/2705

Fig. 1. The relative risk of cardiovascular (CV) events on calcium antagonists vs placebo in pooled clinical trials. (Modified with permission from ref. 27.)

cohort of subjects in the Hypertension Optimal Treatment trial randomly assigned to a target diastolic blood pressure (DBP) of less than 80 mmHg had a 51% reduction in vascular events in comparison to the group with a target DBP below 90 mmHg (20). The tight control (average BP 144/82 mmHg) group in the United Kingdom Prospective Diabetes Study had a 44% risk reduction in stroke incidence compared to the less tightly controlled group using a variety of drugs, including calcium antagonists (average BP 154/87mmHg) (21). As described in the next sections, there have been several trials that have demonstrated the value of calcium channel blockers in cardiovascular risk modification, including the Nordic Diltiazem (NORDIL) trial (11), Syst-Eur trial (12), Systolic Hypertension in China (Syst-China) (22), Antihypertensive, Lipid-Lowering Treatment to Prevent Heart Attack Trial (ALLHAT) (3), and the Controlled-Onset Verapamil Investigation for Cardiovascular End-points (CONVINCE) (13).

PLACEBO-CONTROLLED TRIALS: SYST-EUR AND SYST-CHINA

The Syst-Eur trial followed 4695 elderly (>60 years old) individuals with systolic hypertension (defined as an SBP > 160 mmHg and DBP < 90 mmHg) for at least 2 years after randomization to nitrendipine or placebo dosed once or twice daily (12). The investigators were given the

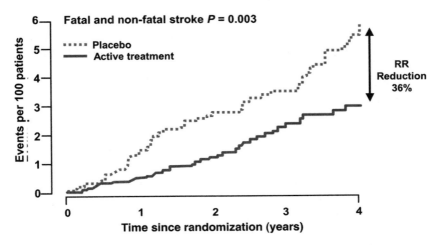

Fig. 2. Primary end point in the Syst-Eur Trial: nitrendipine, a dihydropyridine calcium antagonist, reduces the relative risk of stroke by 36%. (Modified with permission from ref. *12*.)

option of adding an angiotensin-converting enzyme (ACE) inhibitor (enalapril) or a diuretic (hydrochlorothiazide) to achieve target BP. Compared to placebo, treatment with nitrendipine was associated with a 42% reduction in stroke incidence (Fig. 2) ($p = 0.003$), 27% reduction in cardiovascular mortality ($p = 0.007$), 56% reduction in fatal MI ($p = 0.08$), 26% reduction in nonfatal MI ($p = 0.03$), and 31% reduction in combined cardiovascular morbidity and mortality ($p < 0.001$). In those subjects who remained on nitrendipine monotherapy, a 45% reduction in cardiovascular mortality was noted *(23,24)*. The reduction in cardiovascular end points in the diabetic subgroup ($n = 492$) was much higher (–69%) than in the nondiabetic ($n = 4203$) patients in Syst-Eur (–26%) *(24)*.

The Syst-China trial was similar to Syst-Eur in that it compared the same calcium antagonist, nitrendipine, to placebo in a cohort of 2394 patients with isolated systolic hypertension. There was also the potential to add captopril or hydrochlorothiazide to achieve targeted BP goals below 160 mmHg systolic. A similar reduction in stroke incidence (38% in Syst-China vs 42% in Syst-Eur) was achieved *(12,22)*. There were no differences in cardiovascular morbidity and mortality with nitrendipine monotherapy vs combination therapy if similar BP levels were achieved. These studies were among the very first to demonstrate the ability of a dihydropyridine calcium antagonist to significantly reduce cardiovascular morbidity and mortality in older patients with hypertension.

Based on data from these placebo-controlled studies, the relative benefits of the calcium antagonists compared to other antihypertensive therapeutic strategies can be derived from the analysis of two trials from the late 1990s: the Systolic Hypertension in the Elderly Program (SHEP) and the Swedish Trial in Old Patients With Hypertension 2 (STOP-Hypertension 2) (25,26). The SHEP trial followed 4736 elderly (>60 years old) subjects over 5 years treated with the diuretic chlorthalidone for SBP control. Among the nondiabetic individuals, there were similar reductions in mortality (15% in SHEP vs 18% in Syst-Eur), stroke incidence (38% in SHEP vs 39% in Syst-Eur), and cardiovascular end points (34% in SHEP vs 30% in Syst-Eur) (12,25). Within the diabetic subgroup of the Syst-Eur trial, a reduction of 73% in stroke incidence and 69% in all cardiovascular end points was achieved. The results emphasize the importance of BP reduction regardless of the agent used and the fact that BP reduction plays a greater role than blood glucose control in reduction of macrovascular events. The STOP-Hypertension 2 trial was a PROBE (prospective, randomized, open-label, blinded end point design) study of 6000 elderly patients (aged 70–84 years) randomly assigned to treatment with β-adrenergic blockers, thiazide diuretics, or calcium antagonists (26). Across the different treatment arms, there were similar numbers of cardiovascular end points.

ACTIVE CONTROL COMPARATOR TRIALS: NORDIL AND INSIGHT

Following the placebo-controlled studies of the dihydropyridines in the older patient population with systolic hypertension, it became obvious that it would be unethical to use a placebo in patients whose SBP was above 160 mmHg regardless of age. The next focus was on establishing equivalency of calcium antagonists with other classes of antihypertensive agents in prospective, randomized, double-blind trials.

The NORDIL trial and International Nifedipine GITS Study: Intervention as a Goal in Hypertension Treatment (INSIGHT) were the first two randomized clinical trials that compared the effects of calcium antagonists with diuretics and β-blockers on major cardiovascular end points, including fatal and nonfatal MI, fatal and nonfatal stroke, and other cardiovascular deaths (10,11). NORDIL followed for a mean of 4.5 years 10,881 patients, aged 50–74 years, with DBPs above 100 mmHg (11). Compared to the control regimen of diuretics and β-blockers, the diltiazem patient group achieved smaller SBP reduction and equivalent reduction in DBP (20/19 mmHg in diltiazem group vs 23/19 mmHg in diuretic/β-blocker group, $p < 0.001$ for SBP). The treatment groups did not differ in combined primary end points ($p = 0.97$), cardiovascular death ($p = 0.41$), all-cause mortality ($p = 0.99$), all cardiac events, and the development of diabetes mellitus. There was a numerical increase in MIs (7.4 in the diltiazem group vs 6.3 events per 1000 patient-years in the diuretic/β-blocker group), but this failed to reach clinical significance. In addition, a nonsignificant trend toward fewer strokes was noted in the diltiazem group compared to the control regimen (6.4 vs 7.9 events per 1000 patient-years).

INSIGHT involved 6321 subjects aged 55 to 88 years old with SBP above 160 mmHg or BP of more than 150/95 mmHg and one additional cardiovascular risk factor *(10)*. The inclusion criteria of an additional cardiovascular risk factor was designed to look at the equivalence of the effect of calcium antagonists on individuals at high risk for cardiovascular events. Subjects were randomly assigned to treatment with nifedipine and co-amilozide (hydrochlorothiazide plus amiloride) and were followed for at least 3 years for the end points of cardiovascular death, MI, heart failure, and stroke. There was no difference between treatments in BP reduction, the composite end point, all-cause or cause-specific mortality, sudden death, stroke, nonfatal cardiovascular events, and fatal heart failure (Fig. 3). The incidence of withdrawal because of adverse effects ($p < 0.001$), fatal MI ($p < 0.017$), and nonfatal heart failure ($p = 0.028$) was more common in the nifedipine group. The principal findings of NORDIL and INSIGHT demonstrated that calcium antagonists were similar to diuretics and β-adrenergic blocking agents in preventing cardiovascular and cerebrovascular events in older patients with hypertension.

ALLHAT

ALLHAT was designed to examine the effects of a calcium antagonist (amlodipine), ACE inhibitor (lisinopril), and α_1-adrenergic blocker (doxazosin) on the incidence of fatal and nonfatal coronary heart disease (CHD) events in comparison to treatment with a long-acting thiazidelike diuretic (chlorthalidone) *(3)*. In 2000, the doxazosin arm was discontinued because of a large excess in the number of treatment-emergent cases of congestive heart failure. Thus, the study was completed by examining the 33,357 patients, aged 55 years and older, with stage I–II hypertension and an additional CHD risk factor randomly assigned to chlorthalidone, amlodipine, and lisinopril.

The primary outcome end point of ALLHAT was combined fatal CHD or nonfatal MI. Secondary outcome measures included all-cause mortality, combined cardiovascular disease (stroke, heart failure, periph-

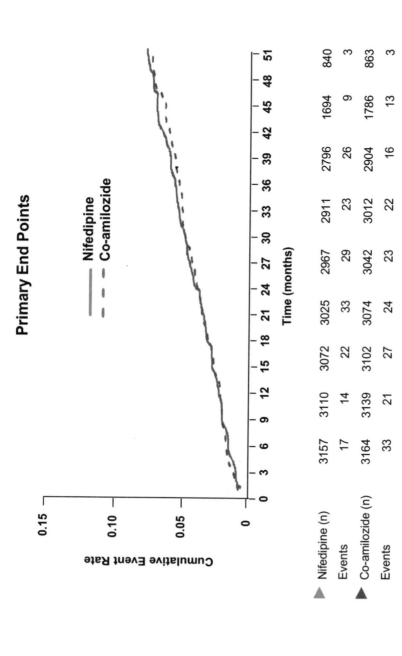

Fig. 3. Cumulative primary end points in the INSIGHT trial. BP control was similar in the two treatment groups during the 4 years of therapy. (Modified with permission from ref. *10*.)

eral arterial disease, and CHD), stroke, combined CHD (angina, revascularization, and all MIs), cancer, and end-stage renal disease.

Compared to the control group, the amlodipine treatment group showed no differences in the primary outcome of combined CHD incidence or in the secondary outcomes of cancer, end-stage renal disease, stroke, composite CHD, and composite cardiovascular disease. Although not specified as a discrete end point, there was a higher risk of developing edema and congestive heart failure in the calcium antagonist treatment group compared to the chlorthalidone group. In addition, chlorthalidone was found to be superior to lisinopril in the prevention of stroke in the African-American patient subgroup, a finding that most likely is associated with discrepancies in BP control for the two treatment groups as the SBP reductions in the lisinopril treated group were on average 4 mmHg lower than the chlorthalidone group.

CONVINCE

In 2003, the results of the CONVINCE trial were published despite an early termination of the trial by the study sponsor Pharmacia prior to achieving the required number of cardiovascular end points *(13)*. CONVINCE enrolled nearly 17,000 patients at least 55 years of age with hypertension and another established cardiovascular risk factor, such as smoking or diabetes, obesity, or prior vascular events. Patients were randomly assigned to treatment with the calcium antagonist, controlled-onset extended-release (COER) verapamil dosed at bedtime, or a standard-of-care (SOC) arm, which could have included the β-adrenergic blocker atenolol or the thiazide diuretic hydrochlorothiazide. The diuretic could also be added to COER verapamil as a second agent for BP control, and ACE inhibitors were recommended as the third level of treatment.

The COER verapamil group had similar reductions in BP as in the SOC group, 13.6/7.8 and 13.5/7.1 mmHg, respectively. The trial was terminated by the sponsor after only 3 of the 5 anticipated years of follow-up, so only about one-third of the number of events required in the original statistical power calculations had occurred. Despite this, there was reasonable confidence that the two regimens were similar in their ability to prevent cardiovascular end points. For example, there was a hazard ratio of 1.02 ($p = 0.77$) in the COER verapamil group for the primary composite end point of MI, stroke, and cardiovascular disease-related death compared to the SOC group.

Examining each component of the composite end points, there were nonsignificant increased hazard ratios for stroke of 1.15 ($p = 0.26$) and cardiovascular death of 1.09 ($p = 0.47$) in the calcium antagonist treatment group. In contrast, there was a decreased hazard ratio of 0.82 ($p =$ 0.09) for the incidence of fatal/nonfatal MI in the COER verapamil group. Secondary outcomes within this trial included an expanded cardiovascular end point encompassing hospitalizations for angina, accelerated hypertension, transient ischemic attacks, heart failure, revascularization, all-cause mortality, cancer, hospitalization for bleeding, and morning (6 AM to noon) incidence of primary end points. Among the secondary end points, hospitalizations for heart failure ($p =$ 0.051) and bleeding unrelated to stroke ($p = 0.003$) had significantly higher hazard ratios in the COER verapamil treatment arm. For the other end points, the hazard ratios were close to 1, and the differences between the treatment groups were not clinically significant.

The increased risk of bleeding and stroke and lower incidence of MI were postulated as secondary to platelet inhibition on verapamil relative to the control drugs. The increased risk of heart failure in the COER verapamil group was attributed to the fact that both diuretics and β-blockers are agents that improve congestive symptoms and signs of heart failure. In any event, conclusions from CONVINCE are limited because of the shortened follow-up period and the smaller-than-expected number of clinical events.

CONCLUSIONS

The use of calcium antagonists as initial therapy or as part of combination therapy for the control of hypertension in older patients has been a subject of debate over the years. As a result of observational data, case-controlled studies, and meta-analyses, increased incidence of cancer, bleeding, and cardiovascular events were attributed to the entire class of calcium antagonists, leading to a documented decline in usage of these agents by clinicians. However, there have been several well-conducted randomized clinical trials that have demonstrated the reduction of cardiovascular events with calcium antagonists in the elderly hypertensive population.

Similar levels of benefit for preventing cardiovascular end points for calcium antagonists with β-blockers and diuretics have been demonstrated in older patients in the INSIGHT and NORDIL trials. The large randomized trials of ALLHAT, CONVINCE, and INSIGHT established that both dihydropyridine and nondihydropyridine calcium antagonists are similar to other antihypertensive agents for reductions in cardiovascular events in high-risk hypertensive patients. One exception is that, in some comparisons, patients treated with calcium antagonists did have significantly higher incidences of heart failure because of the known benefits of downregulation of the sympathetic nervous system by β-blockers and removal of volume and improvement in pulmonary vascular congestion with diuretics, agents that are both recommended for the treatment of heart failure.

Earlier reports of increased cancer incidence and bleeding risks for the calcium antagonists have not proven to be significant in most of these trials. Thus, the effectiveness and safety of the calcium antagonist class of antihypertensives in older patients has been proven in comparison to placebo and several other types of antihypertensive agents. The findings from the large clinical trials of the 1990s that studied calcium antagonists stress the fact that to achieve reduction in cardiovascular events in older patients, reduction in SBP is paramount regardless of the pharmacological properties of any particular agent.

REFERENCES:

1. Hypertension Detection and Follow-up Program Cooperative Group. Five-year findings of the Hypertension Detection and Follow-up Program I: Reduction in the mortality of persons with high blood pressure, including mild hypertension. *JAMA* 1979;242:2562–2571.
2. Elliot WJ, Montoro R, Smith D, et al. Comparison of two strategies for intensifying antihypertensive treatment: low-dose combination (enalapril and felodipine ER) vs increased dose of monotherapy (enalapril). LEVEL (Lexxel vs Enalapril) Study Group. *Am J Hypertens* 1999;12:691–696.
3. The ALLHAT Officers and Coordinators for the ALLHAT Collaborative Research Group. Major outcomes in high-risk hypertensive patients randomized to angiotensin-converting enzyme inhibitor or calcium channel blocker vs. diuretic. The Antihypertensive and Lipid-Lowering Treatment to Prevent Heart Attack Trial (ALLHAT). *JAMA* 2002;288:2981–2997.
4. The Seventh Report of the Joint National Committee of Prevention, Detection, Evaluation, and Treatment of High Blood Pressure. *JAMA* 2003;289:2560–2572.
5. Chalmers J. 1999 World Health Organization-International Society of Hypertension guidelines for management of hypertension: Guidelines Subcommittee. *J Hypertens* 1999;17:151–183.
6. Pahor M, Guralnick JM, Ferrucci L, et al. Calcium-channel blockade and incidence of cancer in aged populations. *Lancet* 1996;348:493–497.
7. Psaty PM, Heckbert SR, Koepsell TD, et al. The risk of myocardial infarction associated with antihypertensive drug therapies. *JAMA* 1995;92:1326–1331.
8. Maclure M, Dormuth C, Naumann T, et al. Influence of educational interventions and adverse news about calcium-channel blockers on first-line prescribing of antihypertensive drugs to elderly people in British Columbia. *Lancet* 1998;352:943–948.
9. Tu K, Mamdani MM, Tu J. Hypertension guidelines in elderly patients. Is anybody listening? Am J Med 2002;113:52–58.
10. Brown MJ, Palmer CR, Castaigne A, et al. Morbidity and mortality in patients randomized to double-blind treatment with a long-acting calcium-channel blocker or diuretic in the International Nifedipine GITS Study Intervention as a Goal in Hypertension Treatment (INSIGHT). *Lancet* 2000;356:366–372.

11. Hansson L, Hedner T, Lund-Johansen P, et al. Randomised trial of effects of calcium antagonists compared with diuretics and beta-blockers on cardiovascular morbidity and mortality in hypertension: the Nordic Diltiazem (NORDIL) Study. *Lancet* 2000;356:359–365.
12. Staessen JA, Fagard R, Thijs L, et al. Randomised double-blind comparison of placebo and active treatment for older patients with isolated systolic hypertension. The Systolic Hypertension in Europe (Syst-Eur) Trial Investigators. *Lancet* 1997;350:757–764.
13. Black HR, Elliott WJ, Grandits G, et al. Principal results of the Controlled Onset Verapamil Investigation of Cardiovascular Endpoints (CONVINCE) trial. *JAMA* 2003;289:2073–2087.
14. Pahor M, Guralnick JM, Corti MC, et al. Long-term survival and use of antihypertensive medications in older persons. *J Am Geriatr Soc* 1995;43:1191–1197.
15. Stason WB, Schmid CH, Niedzwiecki D, et al. Safety of nifedipine in angina pectoris: a meta-analysis. *Hypertension* 1999;33:24–31.
16. Gong L, Zhang W, Zhu Y, et al. Shanghai Trial of Nifedipine in the Elderly (STONE). *Hypertension* 1996;14:1237–1245.
17. Staessen JA, Thijs L, Fagard RH, et al. Calcium channel blockade and cardiovascular prognosis in the European trial on isolated systolic hypertension. *Hypertension* 1998;32:410–416.
18. Laing C, Unwin RJ. Are calcium antagonists effective in preventing complications of hypertension and progression of renal disease? *Curr Opin Nephrol Hypertens* 2000;9:489–495.
19. Grossman E, Messerli FH, Goldburt U. High blood pressure and diabetes mellitus: are all antihypertensive drugs created equal? *Arch Intern Med* 2000;160:2447–2452.
20. Hansson L, Zanchetti A, Carruthers SG, et al. for the HOT Study Group. Effects of intensive blood-pressure lowering and low-dose aspirin in patients with hypertension: principal results of the Hypertension Optimal Treatment (HOT) randomized trial. *Lancet* 1998;351:1755–1762.
21. UK Prospective Diabetes Study Group. Tight blood pressure control and risk of macrovascular and microvascular complications in type 2 diabetes: UKPDS. *BMJ* 1998;317:703–713.
22. Liu L, Wang JG, Gong L, et al. Comparison of active treatment and placebo in older Chinese patients with isolated systolic hypertension. Systolic Hypertension in China (Syst-China) Collaborative Group. *J Hypertens* 1998;16:1823–1829.
23. White WB. Clinical trial experience around the globe: focus on calcium-channel blockers. *Clin Cardiol* 2003;26(suppl 2):1–5.
24. Tuomilehto J, Rastenyte D, Birkenhager WH, et al. for Systolic Hypertension in Europe Trial Investigators. Effects of calcium-channel blockade in older patients with diabetes and systolic hypertension. *N Engl J Med* 1999;340:677–684.
25. SHEP Cooperative Research Group. Prevention of stroke by antihypertensive drug treatment in older persons with isolated systolic hypertension. Final results of the Systolic Hypertension in the Elderly Program (SHEP). *JAMA* 1991;265:3255–3264.
26. Hansson L, Lindholm LH, Ekbom T, et al. Randomised trial of old and new antihypertensive drugs in elderly patients: cardiovascular mortality and morbidity the Swedish Trial in Old Patients With Hypertension-2 Study. *Lancet* 1999;354:1751–1756.
27. Neal B, MacMahon S, Chapman N, Blood Pressure Lowering Treatment Trialists' Collaboration. Effects of ACE inhibitors, calcium antagonists, and other blood-pressure-lowering drugs: results of prospectively designed overviews of randomised trials. Blood Pressure Lowering Treatment Trialists' Collaboration. *Lancet* 2000;356:1955–1964.

19 α-Adrenoceptor Blockers for Management of Hypertension in the Elderly

James L. Pool, MD

CONTENTS

From: *Clinical Hypertension and Vascular Diseases: Hypertension in the Elderly*
Edited by: L. M. Prisant © Humana Press Inc., Totowa, NJ

INTRODUCTION TO THE SYMPATHETIC
NERVOUS SYSTEM IN HYPERTENSION

The arterial pressure is regulated by changes in cardiac output and/or systemic vascular resistance. Effective perfusion of body organs requires appropriate resistance to blood flow to maintain arterial pressure. In the systemic vasculature, the major factor of vascular resistance is smooth muscle tone, which helps regulate the most important determinant of resistance to flow, the cross-sectional area of a vessel. There are two major neurohormonal systems that regulate cardiovascular function, including smooth muscle tone: the autonomic nervous system and the renin–angiotensin system. The peripheral autonomic nervous system has three main components: (a) the sympathetic nervous system (SNS), which comprises the autonomic outflow from the thoracic and high lumbar segments of the spinal cord; (b) the parasympathetic nervous system, which includes the outflow from the cranial nerves and the low lumbar and sacral spinal cord; and (c) the enteric nervous system, which is intrinsic neurons in the wall of the gut. In addition to the blood vessels, the urinary bladder, penis, and prostate also have smooth muscle cells (SMCs) innervated by SNS and parasympathetic nervous system neurons to help regulate micturition, erection, and ejaculation (1).

In the elderly with elevated systemic arterial blood pressure (BP), increased sympathetic activity has been reflected in a marked increase in arterial norepinephrine (NE), SNS predominance in regulating cardiac rate, and increased microneurographic signal in peripheral sympathetic neurons (2,3). In general, blood vessels are innervated by the SNS, which plays an important role in the regulation of BP. A number of sympathetic abnormalities have been identified in high BP, most notably increased SNS activity, which contributes to an increase in vasoconstriction and total peripheral vascular resistance. Studies have demonstrated an increased cardiac β-adrenergic drive and an increased vascular α-adrenergic drive in both borderline and mild hypertension (4). Almost all vasomotor nerves are adrenergic, with the transmitter NE producing vasoconstriction by acting on a specific type of transmembrane structure of the vascular smooth muscle, the α-adrenergic receptor (α-adrenoceptor). This knowledge contributed to the development of drugs that inhibit α- and β-adrenoceptors.

α-ADRENOCEPTORS IN THE VASCULATURE

In the human vasculature, there are two types of adrenoceptors (α and β), which are transmembrane receptors that initiate biological signals via these cell membrane receptors (5). Within these two types of α- and

Table 1
α_1-Adrenoceptor Subtypes

1995 Classification			
Native receptors	Cloned receptors	Cloned receptors (historical)	Human chromosome location
α_{1A}	α_{1a}	α_{1a}	C8
α_{1B}	α_{1b}	α_{1b}	C5
α_{1D}	α_{1d}	$\alpha_{1a/d}$, α_{1a}	C20

β-adrenoceptors, there are now identified nine subtypes (designated α_{1A}, α_{1B}, α_{1D}, α_{2A}, α_{2B}, α_{2C}, β_1, β_2, and β_3) and two other candidates (α_{1L} and β_4), which may be conformational states of α_{1A} and β_1 adrenoceptors, respectively *(6,7)*. Table 1 lists further details about the six α-adrenoceptor subtypes.

Furthermore, the vascular endothelium is now known to be more than a passive anatomic barrier that contacts the blood. Instead, the endothelium is an important organ possessing at least five different adrenoceptor subtypes (α_{2A}, α_{2C}, β_1, β_2, and β_3), which either directly or through the release of nitric oxide actively participate in the regulation of the vascular tone. The precise roles for each of these multiple subtypes of adrenoceptors in the regulation of BP are not completely defined.

STRUCTURE AND ACTIVATION
OF α_1-ADRENOCEPTORS

The innervation of smooth muscle by sympathetic nerve terminals involves a tight junction or "synapse" so there is proximity of neural membranes to SMCs *(8)*. The synaptic gap (or "cleft") between the neural endings and the SMCs is visible only with an electron microscope. The neural components of these synapses are described as *presynaptic*; the smooth muscle components, including the α_1-adrenoceptors, are *postsynaptic*. Sympathetic nerve impulses travel down the nerve, depolarize the nerve terminal, and stimulate the release of NE into the synaptic cleft by exocytosis. Exocytosis occurs when NE-containing vesicles in the nerve terminals bind to presynaptic neural membranes; the fused vesicles then open and empty their neurotransmitter NE into the synaptic cleft, where it is available to bind to postsynaptic adrenoceptors.

The postsynaptic α_1-adrenoceptor is a complex structure that spans the width of the SMC membrane, with specific topographical features on its outer surface that "recognize" and bind the newly released NE (Fig. 1). This α_1-adrenoceptor complex includes (a) the α_1-adrenoceptor; (b) a transducer subunit, the guanine nucleotide-releasing protein; (c) a catalytic subunit, phospholipase C (PLC); and (d) the dual second messengers inositol 1,4,5-trisphosphate (IP$_3$) and diacylglyerol (DAG). When circulating NE binds to the transmembrane α_1-adrenoceptor, this "activates" the receptor and initiates a cascade of events that modulates ionized calcium (Ca^{2+}) channels through a distinct, dual-action transduction pathway that acts via the second messengers IP$_3$ and DAG to initiate a sharp, transient rise in cytoplasmic calcium. This in turn initiates the vascular smooth muscle contraction that is the ultimate result of the physiological binding of NE to the adrenoceptors.

Stimulation of the α-adrenergic receptor complex begins when circulating NE binds to the postsynaptic α_1-adrenoceptor, thus activating the receptor. The activated α_1-adrenoceptor couples with a guanine nucleotide-releasing protein to activate PLC, which hydrolyses phosphatidylinositol 4,5-bisphosphate to generate IP$_3$ and DAG. Release of the newly synthesized IP$_3$ initiates a sharp rise in the cytoplasmic Ca^{2+} by releasing intracellular stored Ca^{2+}. The large and transient increase in Ca^{2+} activates chloride channels, leading to a membrane depolarization, which opens voltage-gated Ca^{2+} channels, releasing Ca^{2+} into the cytoplasm, resulting in contraction of the SMC. In addition, the other second messenger, DAG, transiently activates protein kinase C, which increases the opening probability of Ca^{2+} channels through a phosphorylation-dependent process, thus increasing cytoplasmic Ca^{2+}.

Many signals from the extracellular milieu, from adjacent cells, or from a distant part of the cell itself can cause a sharp rise in the cytoplasmic Ca^{2+} concentration (the so-called calcium transient). Calcium transients can occur via Ca^{2+} release through channels in the plasma membrane or those in the endoplasmic reticulum (ER), which functions as an intracellular Ca^{2+} store. In the case of Ca^{2+} release from the ER, IP$_3$, generated through the hydrolysis of phosphatidylinositol 4,5-bisphosphate by PLC, is critical because it opens a specific calcium channel in the ER called the IP$_3$ receptor. The IP$_3$ receptor is also regulated by other molecules, including calmodulin and Ca^{2+} itself.

In general, it is the α_1-subtype that is located postsynaptically in smooth muscle and that, when stimulated, produces vasoconstriction of the blood vessel. Sympathetic overactivity in hypertension results in excess stimulation of postsynaptic α_1-adrenoceptors.

Consequently, there has been a sound physiological rationale for the use of selective α_1-adrenoceptor inhibitors in the treatment of hypertension. By selectively inhibiting the vascular α_1-adrenoceptors and thereby

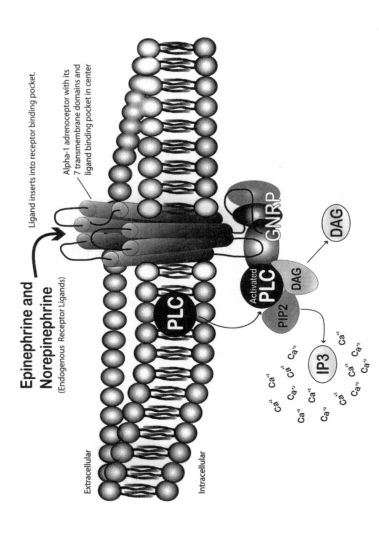

Fig. 1. The α_1-adrenoceptor receptor is a member of the G protein-coupled receptor superfamily of membrane proteins that mediate the actions of the endogenous catecholamines norepinephrine and epinephrine. As shown, these proteins traverse the membrane in seven transmembrane-spanning α–helical domains linked by three intracellular and three extracellular loops. Ca^{2+}, cytoplasmic calcium; DAG, diacylglyerol; GNRP, guanine nucleotide-releasing protein; IP3, inositol 1,4,5-trisphosphate; PIP2, phosphatidylinositol 4,5-bisphosphate; PLC, phospholipase C.

inhibiting the receptor-mediated response to NE, these agents reduce BP via a decrease in peripheral vascular resistance. The reduction in BP is achieved with little or no change in central hemodynamic parameters, such as heart rate or cardiac output. The favorable hemodynamic effects of selective α_1-inhibitors are evident during exercise, when cardiac performance is better preserved with α_1-blockers than β-blockers.

α-ADRENOCEPTORS IN THE URINARY BLADDER AND LUMBOSACRAL SPINAL CORD

The exact role of the SNS in the regulation of micturition remains uncertain *(9,10)*. Early findings suggested that two types of spinal α_1-adrenoceptor mechanisms are involved in reflex bladder activity. There are facilitatory α_1-adrenoceptors in bulbospinal pathways from the brain stem to the lumbosacral spinal cord, and these contribute to neural control of the lower urinary tract. In the urinary outflow tract, α_1-adrenoceptors are located in SMCs of the neck of the urinary bladder, capsule of the prostate, and fibromuscular stroma of the prostate. Stimulation of α_1-adrenoceptors in the bladder outflow tract increases resistance to urine flow. The frequency of the reflex to urinate is inhibited by afferent α_1-adrenoceptors in the spinal cord. The descending limb of the micturition reflex pathway may be facilitated by α_1-adrenoceptors.

For control of the micturition reflex, selective α_1-adrenoceptor antagonists may be used, and it is thought that these have dual sites of action: the central nervous system and the smooth muscle of the lower urinary tract. During the development of benign prostatic hyperplasia (BPH) and lower urinary tract symptoms (LUTS) in males, obstruction to urine flow is primarily attributed to a static or anatomic component (enlarged prostate gland) and a dynamic or functional component (smooth muscle tone in bladder neck and the surgical capsule and fibromuscular stroma of the prostate gland) *(11,12)*.

Up to 40% of total urethral pressure is caused by α-adrenergic tone, and the rest is caused by static pressure from the enlarged prostate. Relaxation of this muscle tone by α_1-adrenoceptor blockade increases urinary flow and improves LUTS in patients with BPH. Consequently, α-adrenoceptor blockers emerged as treatment for symptomatic BPH *(13)*.

AN OVERVIEW OF α-ADRENOCEPTOR ANTAGONISTS

α-Adrenoceptor antagonists (or *blockers*) are categorized by the type (or subtype) of adrenoceptor(s) each drug inhibits (Table 2). Several types of α-adrenoceptor blockers have been introduced, including nonselective (α_1 and α_2), presynaptic α_2, and postsynaptic α_1-adrenoceptor

Table 2
α-Adrenoceptor Antagonists

Antagonist compound	Selective α_1	Nonselective α_1 and α_2	Selective α_1 and nonselective $\beta_1 + \beta_2$
Alfuzosin[a]	✓		
BMY-7378	✓		
Bunazosin	✓		
Carvedilol[a]			✓
Chloroethylclonidine	✓		
Cyclazosin	✓		
Doxazosin[a]	✓		
Labetolol[a]			✓
Phenoxybenzamine[a]		✓	
Phentolamine[a]		✓	
Prazosin[a]	✓		
RS 17053	✓		
SK&F 105854	✓		
SNAP 5150	✓		
(+)Niguldipine	✓		
Tamsulosin[a]	✓		
Terazosin[a]	✓		
5-Methyl-urapidil	✓		
WB-4101	✓		

[a]Approved by US Food and Drug Administration.

antagonists *(14)*. Selective α_1-adrenoceptor blockers lower BP primarily by blocking postsynaptic α_1-adrenoceptors. In this respect, selective α_1-receptor antagonists differ from nonselective α-blockers like the competitive inhibitor phentolamine and the noncompetitive inhibitor phenoxybenzamine. Importantly, the presynaptic α_2-adrenoceptors inhibit NE release.

Nonspecific α-blockade causes these α_2-receptors to increase NE release with β-adrenoceptor-mediated tachycardia, enhanced renin secretion, and attenuation of postsynaptic α_1-inhibition. Selective blockade of these presynaptic α_2-adrenoceptors with a drug such as yohimbine can lead to a rise in BP. In contrast, the selective α_1-antagonists may reduce vascular tone in capacitance vessels as well as resistance vessels to provide a balance of preload and afterload reduction, thus avoiding vasodilation (afterload reduction) without venodilation (preload reduction), which would promote an increase in cardiac output and heart rate.

As a result of these pharmacological differences between nonselective and selective agents, nonselective α-blockers were unsuccessful in attempts to treat essential hypertension and symptomatic BPH. Phentolamine, a parenteral drug, is used almost exclusively for emergent and urgent severe hypertension with excess catecholamine release. The oral, nonselective, and noncompetitive α-inhibitor phenoxybenzamine remains an important agent in the preoperative management of pheochromocytomas and cases of inoperable, metastatic pheochromocytoma.

Another unique feature of two of the selective α_1-adrenoceptor blockers is blockade of β_1- and β_2-adrenoceptors. The combination α plus β agent, labetalol, is predominately a selective α_1-adrenoceptor antagonist during acute intravenous or chronic oral administration. Labetolol is a nonselective β-blocker and a selective α_1-blocker that is equal to about 10% of α-blockade with phentolamine. In contrast, carvedilol is predominantly a nonselective β-blocker with less-selective α_1-blockade, which is indicated for the treatment of heart failure or hypertension.

SELECTIVE α_1-ADRENOCEPTOR ANTAGONISTS FOR TREATMENT OF HYPERTENSION AND BENIGN PROSTATIC HYPERPLASIA

In 1976, prazosin was the first of three (prazosin, terazosin, and doxazosin) quinazoline compounds (Table 3), which are selective postsynaptic α_1-adrenoceptor antagonists, to be approved in the United States for the treatment of hypertension (15). These drugs are highly selective for α_1-adrenoceptor subtypes (α_{1A}, α_{1B}, α_{1D}). When given in large doses, they do not inhibit the α_2-adrenoceptors (α_{2A}, α_{2B}, α_{2C}), the β-adrenoceptors (β_1, β_2, β_3), or other receptors, such as acetylcholine (muscarinic), dopamine, and 5-hydroxytryptamine receptors.

These selective α_1-blockers are used mainly in the management of hypertension and relief of urinary obstruction in BPH. Because of limited treatment options in mild BPH, selective α_1-blockers have been widely used to treat LUTS, and 50% of men have histological evidence of BPH by 60 years of age (16). BPH frequently causes prostatic obstruction and LUTS, which are predominantly caused by bladder outlet obstruction. In the Sixth Report of the Joint National Committee on Prevention, Detection, Evaluation, and Treatment of High Blood Pressure, selective α_1-blockers are recommended not only as second-line antihypertensive therapy after low-dose diuretics and β-blockers, but also for specific indications such as therapy in men with hypertension and LUTS (17). The National Ambulatory Medical Care Survey reported that the number of people on any type of selective α_1-blockers in 1995 was

Table 3

Selective α-1 Adrenoceptor Antagonists Marketed in the United States for Hypertension

Generic Name (Brand Name)	Chemical Structure	Plasma Half-Life (hrs)	Frequency of Dose Per Day
Prazosin (Minipress®)	•HCl	2-4	2-3
Terazosin (Hytrin®)	•HCl • 2H$_2$O	12	1
Doxazosin (Cardura®)	•CH$_3$SO$_3$H	22	1

Terazosin: The saturated furan configuration provides the molecule with one optically active chemical center(*) so terazosin has 2 enantiomeric forms.

Doxazosin: The 6- and 7-hydroxy metabolites of doxazosin have demonstrated in vitro antioxidant properties.

389

approximately 6 to 7% of those with hypertension *(18)*. About 80% of surveyed physicians would choose these drugs as a first-line BP agent for patients with hypertension and symptoms of BPH.

SELECTIVE α_1-ANTAGONISTS IN HYPERTENSION TREATMENT

Selective α_1-blockers (prazosin, terazosin, and doxazosin) have been shown to be effective antihypertensive agents whether used as monotherapy or as part of a regimen of multiple antihypertensive drugs. The longer acting drugs (doxazosin and terazosin), which can be prescribed once per day, have generally replaced prazosin, which requires multiple doses (i.e., two to three times per day) for control of high BP. In large, placebo-controlled studies of mild-to-moderate essential hypertension, doxazosin or terazosin given once daily lowered BP at 24 hours by about 9/5 mmHg in the supine position compared to placebo and about 10/8 mmHg in the standing position. Their effects are additive to those of angiotensin-converting enzyme (ACE) inhibitors, angiotensin receptor antagonists, β-blockers, calcium channel blockers, diuretics, and direct-acting vasodilators *(19)*.

About 50% of mild-to-moderate essential hypertensives treated with α_1-blocker monotherapy achieve diastolic BPs below 90 mmHg, but only 30% achieve combined reductions of systolic and diastolic BPs below 140/90 mmHg. Age, race, and gender do not influence BP response with selective α_1-blocker treatment.

Although less pronounced than with potent vasodilators, monotherapy with α_1-blockers promotes sodium and water retention. Use of a diuretic prevents fluid retention and can markedly enhance the antihypertensive effect of the drugs. In clinical practice, α_1-blockers have their widest application as one component of multiple drug regimens for the treatment of mild-to-severe hypertension.

SIDE EFFECTS OF SELECTIVE α_1-ANTAGONISTS

Selective α_1-antagonists are generally well tolerated with a short list of potential adverse effects. In controlled trials, the symptoms that most commonly caused discontinuation of α_1-antagonist therapy were asthenia (2%), nasal congestion (2%), and dizziness (1%). Generally, there is no drug dose relationship for clinical adverse effects. The dizziness with α_1-blockers is not entirely understood because many patients experience this sensation without postural hypotension. In males, priapism is rare. But, individuals with alterations of urinary bladder function can develop incontinence with α_1-blocker-mediated relaxation of the bladder outlet.

Syncope

The *first-dose phenomenon*, with severe hypotension after the first dose of α_1-antagonist, is well known, but syncope is uncommon, occurring in less than 1% of patients when an initial, small dose (1 mg or less) was taken at bedtime as monotherapy. If the patient had prior treatment with one or more agents (especially a diuretic, β-blocker, sildenafil, or verapamil), additional caution with the first dose is advisable. In one study of unblinded, long-term treatment, 364 patients who received terazosin monotherapy or combination therapy with diuretic and/or β-blocker for up to 4.7 years, 262 patients were treated for at least 1 year and 139 for 2 years or more *(20)*. Only 1 patient discontinued the study because of syncope.

Laboratory Test Changes

There are no clinically important adverse effects on laboratory tests. Serum electrolytes, serum urea nitrogen, creatinine, glucose, and uric acid are not altered. There are no significant effects on renal function in hypertensive patients with normal, moderate, or severe renal impairment. In placebo-controlled trials, a greater percentage of α_1-blocker patients have small decreases in hematocrit, hemoglobin, white blood cell count, total protein, and albumin levels from baseline values. Except for the white blood cell count, these changes have been attributed to hemodilution secondary to hemodynamic changes and/or mild fluid retention. The reduction of white blood cell counts remains unexplained, but individual reductions have been small, and prolonged drug treatment has not been associated with progressive white blood cell count reductions.

Fluid Retention and Weight

The Veterans Administration Cooperative Study on Antihypertensive agents was a double-blind, randomized controlled trial comparing atenolol, captopril, clonidine, diltiazem, hydrochlorothiazide, prazosin, and placebo for differences in antihypertensive efficacy in 1105 men who had mild diastolic hypertension *(21)*. At 8 weeks, a highly significant weight gain of 1 kg was observed with prazosin compared to baseline ($p < 0.001$). In all other treatment groups, there was either weight loss or no mean weight change. However, the average weight gain of 0.5 kg from baseline was no longer statistically significant at 1 year of therapy when compared to the original baseline weight or the other therapies.

In 1984, Bauer et al. showed increases in plasma volume, interstitial fluid volume, and extracellular fluid volume following both short- and long-term prazosin therapy *(22)*. Within 3 to 6 weeks of initiation of this study of 14 hypertensive men, there was a significant 1.4 L average increase in extracellular fluid volume and a 200 mL average increase in plasma volume without weight gain that lasted during 5 to 6 months of chronic therapy. In these subjects, the authors postulated a net increase in total body sodium from an acute renal effect of prazosin, followed by chronic sodium homeostasis and maintenance of the increased total body sodium. Other studies demonstrated both an increase in weight and laboratory changes consistent with volume expansion with prazosin.

BENEFICIAL METABOLIC EFFECTS OF SELECTIVE α_1-ANTAGONISTS

Selective α_1-adrenoceptor antagonists have proven beneficial effects on the serum lipid profile of hypertensive patients (23,24). A large number of controlled studies have demonstrated that they lower the levels of total cholesterol, low-density lipoprotein cholesterol (LDL-C), and triglycerides and increase the levels of high-density lipoprotein (HDL) cholesterol and the ratio of HDL cholesterol to total cholesterol. In predominantly normocholesterolemic patients, doxazosin produced small reductions in total serum cholesterol (2–3%) and LDL cholesterol (4%) and a similarly small increase in HDL/total cholesterol ratio (4%).

These modifications of the serum lipid profile are the result of several different mechanisms. These include an increase in LDL-C receptor number, a decrease in LDL-C synthesis, stimulation of lipoprotein lipase activity, reduction of very-low-density lipoprotein cholesterol synthesis and secretion, and reduction in the absorption of dietary cholesterol. In addition, one of the unique features of doxazosin, or rather the 6-hydroxy and 7-hydroxy metabolites of doxazosin, is the ability to inhibit the oxidation of LDL-C (25). Oxidized LDL plays an important role in the initiation and progression of atherosclerosis.

Treatment with selective α_1-inhibitors in hypertensive patients with and without non-insulin-dependent diabetes mellitus has shown not only reductions in BP and improvement in the lipid profile, but also improvements in insulin sensitivity, reductions in elevated serum insulin levels, and trends toward reducing fasting glucose (26,27).

SELECTIVE α_1-ANTAGONISTS DO NOT IMPROVE HEART FAILURE

Sympathetic stimulation of the cardiac α_1-adrenoceptor has marked trophic effects. As expected, regression of left ventricular hypertrophy can be achieved with selective α_1-adrenoceptor inhibitors. But, α-blockers have not shown sustained benefits in chronic congestive heart failure. Mortality from this left ventricular dysfunction is not improved by selective α_1-adrenoceptor inhibitors. In the 1986 Veterans Administration Cooperative Study of the effect of vasodilator therapy in chronic congestive heart failure, mortality in the prazosin treatment group was similar to that in the placebo group *(21)*. Furthermore, chronic therapy with α_1-blocker (doxazosin) plus β-blocker (metoprolol) in heart failure produces identical effects as those seen in patients receiving β-blocker alone *(28)*.

MAJOR CLINICAL TRIALS
WITH SELECTIVE α_1-ANTAGONISTS

The prevention of coronary heart disease (CHD) remains one of the greatest challenges for antihypertensive therapy. Previous trials have identified a shortfall in the protection of hypertensive patients against CHD compared with that predicted from observational studies. The question has been whether newer classes of drugs can rectify the shortfall compared with older agents (i.e., diuretics).

The Antihypertensive and Lipid-Lowering Treatment to Prevent Heart Attack Trial (ALLHAT) is the largest double-blind, antihypertensive trial designed to determine whether three newer agents—amlodipine (calcium channel blocker), doxazosin (α_1-blocker), or lisinopril (ACE inhibitor)—are superior to standard diuretic therapy (chlorthalidone) in reducing coronary events *(29)*. Because of the favorable effects of α_1-blockers on several surrogate end points (e.g., cholesterol and glucose), doxazosin was selected as one of the three agents for comparison with chlorthalidone. The total of 42,418 participants were men and women aged 55 years and older with hypertension plus an additional risk factor for CHD.

In February 2000, the doxazosin component of the study was terminated because of a 25% greater incidence of combined cardiovascular disease (CVD) events compared with the chlorthalidone arm. About half of the 25% was accounted for by the increased risk of heart failure, but there was no significant difference between the chlorthalidone and doxazosin groups for the primary CHD end point of combined nonfatal myocardial infarction and CHD death, all-cause mortality, or combined CHD. Premature termination of the doxazosin arm for a secondary end point was justified also because doxazosin was highly unlikely to achieve superiority if this arm was continued. Since publication of these preliminary ALLHAT results, the role of α_1-blocker in the treatment of hypertension has become controversial.

Table 4
ALLHAT Final Outcomes of Chlorthalidone vs Doxazosin

Outcomes	Relative risk	Δ 4-Year rate per 100 patients[a]	p[b]
Primary end point			
• CHD (Fatal CHD + Nonfatal MI)	1.02	0.2	NS
Secondary end points			
• All-cause mortality	1.03	0.5	NS
• Combined CHD	1.07	1.1	NS
• Hospitalized or treated angina	1.13	1.0	0.01
• Stroke	1.26	1.4	0.001
• Combined CVD	1.20	3.5	<0.001
• HF (fatal, hospitalized)	1.66	2.2	<0.001
• HF (fatal, hospitalized, treated)	1.80	3.5	<0.001

[a]Difference between doxazosin minus chlorthalidone 4-year event rates per 100 patients.
[b]To adjust for multiple comparisons, compare p value to 0.018 rather than 0.05; NS, not significant.
CHD, coronary heart disease; CVD, cardiovascular disease; HF, heart failure; MI, myocardial infarction. Combined CHD = CHD death, nonfatal MI, coronary revascularization procedures and hospitalized angina. Combined CVD = CHD death, nonfatal MI, stroke, coronary revascularization procedures, hospitalized or treated angina, treated or hospitalized heart failure, and peripheral vascular disease (hospitalized or outpatient revascularization).

As shown in Table 4, significant ($p < 0.001$) increases in combined CVD, heart failure, and stroke events were experienced by participants randomly assigned to doxazosin compared with the chlorthalidone group. Specifically, participants randomly assigned to doxazosin experienced a 26% higher risk of stroke, a 66% to 80% higher risk of heart failure, a 12% higher risk of coronary revascularization, and a 13% higher risk of hospitalized or treated angina. Thus, the combined CVD risk was 20% higher among participants randomly assigned to doxazosin compared with chlorthalidone. About half of the 20% was accounted for by the increased risk of heart failure. When the outcome measure for heart failure was restricted to only hospitalized or fatal cases, the heart failure risk was 66% higher for doxazosin compared with chlorthalidone. The observed clinical events for these significant outcomes included 1 to 3.5 more events per 100 patients over 4 years in participants randomized to doxazosin.

In the final analysis, there were noteworthy differences in treatment effects between the doxazosin and chlorthalidone groups. Mean BP at randomization was 146/84 mmHg for both groups, and after the first year, it was 137/79 mmHg for the chlorthalidone group and 140/80 mmHg for the doxazosin group, which were 3 and 1 mmHg higher systolic and diastolic BPs, respectively, than the control group. Starting at 24 months, the systolic difference narrowed to 2.3 mmHg and diastolic to 0.1 mmHg, but the systolic difference remained 2.1 mmHg throughout the final 24 months of the trial. At their 4-year follow-up visit, more chlorthalidone than doxazosin subjects (63 vs 58%) were at goal pressure below 140/90 mmHg.

Of the 24,316 participants in the doxazosin and chlorthalidone comparison, nearly 90% of the study participants had received antihypertensive therapy before randomization. At the end of 4 years of follow-up, there were differences in treatment. There were 481 (3.2%) lost to follow-up in the chlorthalidone group and 447 (4.9%) in the doxazosin group, but person-years of observation were 95% of those expected and were similar in both arms of the trial. At 4 years of follow-up, 78% of the chlorthalidone group and 71% of the doxazosin group had remained on their assigned treatment, which occurred mostly by the end of the first year. Exclusive use of assigned medication was 34% for chlorthalidone and 23% for doxazosin. Conversely, 23% of the doxazosin participants were prescribed a diuretic, and 4% of chlorthalidone participants were prescribed an α-blocker. Two-medication use was 35% for chlorthalidone and 37% for doxazosin (~18% of the chlorthalidone group and 18% of the doxazosin group were on atenolol). About 19% of those in the chlorthalidone group were prescribed three or more medications to lower their BP, compared with 27% of participants in the doxazosin group.

As anticipated from earlier clinical trials, favorable metabolic effects were demonstrated with doxazosin compared to chlorthalidone. Serum cholesterol, initially 216 mg/dL for the chlorthalidone group and 215 mg/dL for the doxazosin group, fell to 197 and 187 mg/dL, respectively, at 4 years ($p < 0.001$). About 25% of each group had participated in the lipid-lowering arm of the ALLHAT trial. Fasting serum glucose, initially 123 mg/dL in the chlorthalidone group and 122 mg/dL in the doxazosin group, was 125 and 117 mg/dL, respectively, at the 4-year visit ($p < 0.001$).

From the final data for the chlorthalidone vs doxazosin arm of ALLHAT, the Steering Committee concluded that chlorthalidone compared with doxazosin provided superior BP control, enhanced tolerability, and reduced cardiovascular morbidity. Furthermore, because the α_1-blocker class lacks clinical trial evidence for cardioprotection superior to placebo, they recommended the α_1-blockers no longer be considered appropriate initial therapy for hypertension.

SUMMARY

Recent clinical trials combined with four decades of additional α_1-blocker research have clarified their role in treatment of hypertension, especially in the elderly, who often fit the ALLHAT cardiovascular risk profile. Thiazide-type diuretics have emerged as preferred initial therapy for moderate-to-high-risk hypertensives. In this new treatment paradigm for the elderly, the α_1-blockers are added to the treatment regimen along with ACE inhibitors, angiotensin-receptor blockers, and calcium channel blockers to achieve goal BPs. In the elderly male, treatment for BPH with LUTS will often require α_1-blocker to reduce symptoms and the risk of acute urinary retention. But, the majority of males with BPH will also develop hypertension and need management of their high BP, which will require adherence to low-dose thiazide diuretic treatment. Because hypertension and BPH occur commonly together in elderly males, this drug combination will continue to exploit these dual therapeutic roles of α_1-blockers.

REFERENCES

1. Andersson KE. Pharmacology of penile erection. *Pharmacol Rev* 2001;53:417–450.
2. Anderson EA, Sinkey CA, Lawton WJ, Mark AL. Elevated sympathetic nerve activity in borderline hypertensive humans. Evidence from direct intraneural recordings. *Hypertension* 1989;14:177–183.
3. Somers VK, Anderson EA, Mark AL. Sympathetic neural mechanisms in human hypertension. *Curr Opin Nephrol Hypertens* 1993;2:96–105.
4. Julius S. Autonomic nervous system dysregulation in human hypertension. *Am J Cardiol* 1991;67:3B–7B.
5. Guimaraes S, Moura D. Vascular adrenoceptors: an update. *Pharmacol Rev* 2001;53:319–356.
6. Bylund DB, Eikenberg DC, Hieble JP, et al. International Union of Pharmacology nomenclature of adrenoceptors. *Pharmacol Rev* 1994;46:121–136.
7. Civantos Calzada B, Aleixandre de Artinano A. α-Adrenoceptor subtypes. *Pharmacol Res* 2001;44:195–208.
8. Varma DR, Deng XF. Cardiovascular α_1-adrenoceptor subtypes: functions and signaling. *Can J Physiol Pharmacol* 2000;78:267–292.
9. Andersson KE. Bladder activation: afferent mechanisms. *Urology* 2002;59(5 suppl 1):43–50.
10. Andersson KE. Treatment of the overactive bladder: possible central nervous system drug targets. *Urology* 2002;59(5 suppl 1):18–24.
11. Denis L, McConnell J, Yoshida O, et al. Recommendations of the International Scientific Committee: the evaluation and treatment of lower urinary tract symptoms (LUTS) suggestive of benign prostatic obstruction. In: Denis L, Griffiths K, Khoury S, Cockett ATK, et al., eds. *Fourth International Consultation on Benign Prostatic Hyperplasia*. Plymouth, UK: Plymbridge Distributors; 1998:669–684.
12. Roehrborn CG, Bartsch G, Kirby R, et al. Guidelines for the diagnosis and treatment of benign prostatic hyperplasia: a comparative, international overview. *Urology* 2001;58:642–650.

13. Kirby RS, Pool JL. α-Adrenoceptor blockade in the treatment of benign prostatic hyperplasia: past, present and future. *Br J Urol* 1997;80:521–532.
14. Frishman WH, Kotob F. α-Adrenergic blocking drugs in clinical medicine. *J Clin Pharmacol* 1999;39:7–16.
15. Stanaszek WF, Kellerman D, Brogden RN, Romankiewicz JA. Prazosin update. A review of its pharmacological properties and therapeutic use in hypertension and congestive heart failure. *Drugs* 1983;25:339–384.
16. Berry SJ, Coffey DS, Walsh PC, Ewing LL. The development of human benign prostatic hyperplasia with age. *J Urol* 1984;132:474–479.
17. The sixth report of the Joint National Committee on Prevention, Detection, Evaluation, and Treatment of High Blood Pressure. *Arch Intern Med* 1997;157:2413–2446.
18. Mehta SS, Wilcox CS, Schulman KA. Treatment of hypertension in patients with comorbidities: results from the study of hypertensive prescribing practices (SHyPP). *Am J Hypertens* 1999;12(4 pt 1):333–340.
19. Pool JL. Combination antihypertensive therapy with terazosin and other antihypertensive agents: results of clinical trials. *Am Heart J* 1991;122(3 pt 2):926–931.
20. Luther RR, Glassman HN, Estep CB, Schmitz PJ, Horton JK, Jordan DC. Terazosin, a new selective α₁-adrenergic blocking agent. Results of long-term treatment in patients with essential hypertension. *Am J Hypertens* 1988;1(3 pt 3):237S–240S.
21. Cohn JN, Archibald DG, Ziesche S, et al. Effect of vasodilator therapy on mortality in chronic congestive heart failure. Results of a Veterans Administration Cooperative Study. *N Engl J Med* 1986;314:1547–1552.
22. Bauer JH, Jones LB, Gaddy P. Effects of prazosin therapy on BP, renal function, and body fluid composition. *Arch Intern Med* 1984;144:1196–1200.
23. Cubeddu LX, Pool JL, Bloomfield R, et al. Effect of doxazosin monotherapy on blood pressure and plasma lipids in patients with essential hypertension. *Am J Hypertens* 1988;1:158–167.
24. Pool JL. Effects of doxazosin on serum lipids: a review of the clinical data and molecular basis for altered lipid metabolism. *Am Heart J* 1991;121(1 pt 2):251–259.
25. Chait A, Gilmore M, Kawamura M. Inhibition of low density lipoprotein oxidation in vitro by the 6- and 7-hydroxy-metabolites of doxazosin, an α₁-adrenergic antihypertensive agent. *Am J Hypertens* 1994;7:159–167.
26. Andersson PE, Johansson J, Berne C, Lithell H. Effects of selective α₁- and β₁-adrenoreceptor blockade on lipoprotein and carbohydrate metabolism in hypertensive subjects, with special emphasis on insulin sensitivity. *J Hum Hypertens* 1994;8:219–226.
27. Reaven GM, Lithell H, Landsberg L. Hypertension and associated metabolic abnormalities—the role of insulin resistance and the sympathoadrenal system. *N Engl J Med* 1996;334:374–381.
28. Kukin ML, Kalman J, Mannino M, Freudenberger R, Buchholz C, Ocampo O. Combined α-β blockade (doxazosin plus metoprolol) compared with β-blockade alone in chronic congestive heart failure. Am J Cardiol 1996;77:486–491.
29. Diuretic vs α-blocker as first-step antihypertensive therapy: final results from the Antihypertensive and Lipid-Lowering Treatment to Prevent Heart Attack Trial (ALLHAT). Hypertension 2003;42:239–246.

20 Combination Drug Therapy in the Elderly

L. Michael Prisant, MD, FACC, FACP and Laura Lyngby Mulloy, DO, FACP

INTRODUCTION

Awareness, treatment, and control of hypertension in the United States have been improving for geriatric patients *(1)*. However, awareness, treatment, and control remain the lowest among the oldest age group *(2)*.

From: *Clinical Hypertension and Vascular Diseases: Hypertension in the Elderly*
Edited by: L. M. Prisant © Humana Press Inc., Totowa, NJ

This is ironic given the fact that the largest body of outcomes trials documents the reduction of morbidity and mortality in the elderly population. These trials are reviewed in detail in Chapter 7.

After the diagnosis of systemic hypertension is confirmed, nonpharmacological treatment with weight reduction, sodium restriction, alcohol intake reduction, and aerobic exercise is recommended initially *(3,4)*.The studies of nonpharmacological therapy in the elderly are reviewed in Chapter 6. If there is an inadequate blood pressure (BP) response to nutritional and hygienic therapy, then pharmacological therapy is initiated *(see* Fig. 1). Although diuretics, β-blockers, angiotensin converting enzyme (ACE) inhibitors, calcium channel blockers (CCBs), and angiotensin II receptor blockers (ARBs) are possible choices for the initial treatment of hypertension, diuretics are endorsed as initial therapy because of trials supporting a reduction in both morbidity and mortality *(3)*.

THERAPEUTIC APPROACHES TO BLOOD PRESSURE CONTROL

There are three options for the treatment of hypertension if the initial drug choice fails to achieve the target of BP control: (a) drug titration, (b) drug substitution, and (c) drug combination *(5)*. Drug titration is potentially beneficial because monotherapy is maintained for the treatment of hypertension, drug therapy costs are contained, and compliance is increased compared to the use of multiple drugs. However, there are disadvantages of progressive drug titrations: (a) diminishing increments of BP reduction and (b) increasing side effects (Fig. 2) *(6)*. Most important, monotherapy achieves BP control in fewer than 50% of patients (Fig. 3) *(7–9)*.

Sequential monotherapy or substitution therapy attempts to select an agent that is synchronized with the underlying pathophysiology of the patient's hypertension *(10)*. Thus, if a patient fails a diuretic or a CCB as initial therapy because of lack of BP control, then a β-blocker, ACE inhibitors, or an ARB would be tried next. The disadvantage of such a lengthy testing of each drug and switching to another agent is the patient's loss of confidence in the physician and decreased adherence *(11)*. Substitution of an alternative drug is sensible if adverse effects limit the use of the chosen initial therapy.

RATIONALE FOR COMBINATION DRUG THERAPY

Combination drug therapy achieves a higher control rate, especially when an algorithm approach is used *(12–16)*. The diastolic and systolic BP control rates that can be achieved are respectively about 90 and 70%

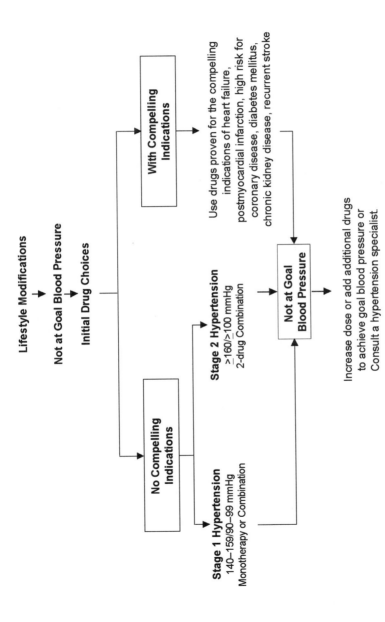

Fig. 1. Algorithm for hypertension treatment. The current algorithm of the Joint National Committee emphasizes the use of combination drug therapy for the treatment of hypertension. (Modified from ref. 3.)

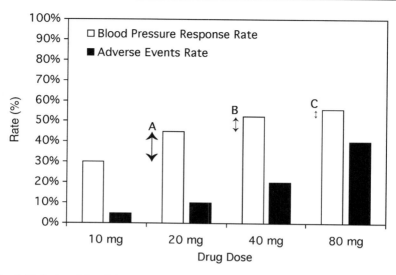

Fig. 2. Relationship of drug dose–response rate and side effects. As the dose of a drug is increased, there is a diminishing increment in blood pressure reduction (C < B < A) and an increase in adverse events.

in patients without chronic kidney disease and diabetes mellitus (DM). However, combinations of multiple drugs increase the exposure of dose-independent side effects, drug–drug interactions, higher drug costs, and nonadherence, especially when the dosing intervals are not synchronized.

Fixed-dose combinations (Table 1) are usually less expensive than the purchase of each drug separately *(17)*. The fixed-dose combination products include a thiazide diuretic with a potassium-sparing diuretic, a β-blocker, an ACE inhibitor, or an ARB. The combination of a CCB and an ACE inhibitor is also obtainable. The combination of a dihydropyridine CCB and β-blocker is accessible outside the United States. There have been six fixed-dose combinations that are approved for the *initial* treatment of hypertension: Capozide, Ziac, Moduretic, Dyazide, Maxzide, and Aldactazide *(20)*. The major disadvantages of fixed-dose combination therapy are potential loss of dosing flexibility and difficulty in determining which agent in the combination is causing the side effect.

The Seventh Report from the Joint National Committee on the Prevention, Detection, Evaluation, and Treatment of High Blood Pressure emphasizes the use of combination drug therapy to achieve BP control (Fig. 1) *(4)*. Two drugs or more are usually required to reach a target BP below 140/90 mmHg *(3)*. The percentage of patients requiring two or more drugs to achieve the BP goals was 63% in the Antihypertensive and

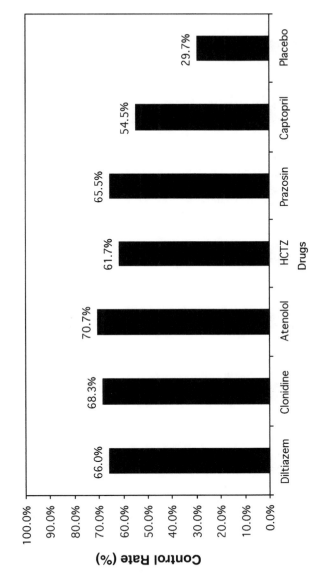

Fig. 3. Control rate of diastolic blood pressure (<90 mmHg) among older white males after 1 year of treatment. The placebo-corrected control rate is less than 45% for elderly white males. HCTZ, hydrochlorothiazide. (Data from ref. 8.)

Table 1
Currently Marketed Fixed-Dose Combination Drugs in the United States

Angiotensin-converting enzyme inhibitors and calcium antagonists
- Lexxel: Enalapril-felodipine (5/5)
- Lotrel: Amlodipine-benazepril hydrochloride (2.5/10, 5/10, 5/20, 10/20)
- Tarka: Trandolapril-verapamil (2/180, 1/240, 2/240, 4/240)

Angiotensin-converting enzyme inhibitors and diuretics
- Accuretic: Quinapril-hydrochlorothiazide (10/12.5, 20/12.5, 20/25)
- Capozide: Captopril-hydrochlorothiazide (25/15, 25/25, 50/15, 50/25)
- Lotensin HCT: Benazepril-hydrochlorothiazide (5/6.25, 10/12.5, 20/12.5, 20/25)
- Monopril/HCT: Fosinopril-hydrochlorothiazide (10/12.5, 20/12.5)
- Prinzide: Lisinopril-hydrochlorothiazide (10/12.5, 20/12.5, 20/25)
- Uniretic: Moexipril-hydrochlorothiazide (7.5/12.5, 15/25)
- Vaseretic: Enalapril-hydrochlorothiazide (5/12.5, 10/25)
- Zestoretic: Lisinopril-hydrochlorothiazide (10/12.5, 20/12.5, 20/25)

Angiotensin receptor blockers and diuretics
- Atacand HCT: Candesartan-hydrochlorothiazide (16/12.5, 32/12.5)
- Avalide: Irbesartan-hydrochlorothiazide (150/12.5, 300/12.5)
- Benicar HCT: Olmesartan medoxomil-hydrochlorothiazide (20/12.5, 40/12.5, 40/25)
- Diovan-HCT: Valsartan-hydrochlorothiazide (80/12.5, 160/12.5, 160/25)
- Hyzaar: Losartan-hydrochlorothiazide (50/12.5, 100/25)
- Micardis-HCT: Telmisartan-hydrochlorothiazide (40/12.5, 80/12.5)
- Teveten-HCT: Eprosartan-hydrochlorothiazide (600/12.5, 600/25)

β-Blockers and diuretics
- Corzide: Nadolol-bendroflumethiazide (40/5, 80/5)
- Inderide LA: Propranolol LA-hydrochlorothiazide (40/25, 80/25)
- Lopressor HCT: Metoprolol-hydrochlorothiazide (50/25, 100/25)
- Tenoretic: Atenolol-chlorthalidone (50/25, 100/25)
- Timolide: Timolol-hydrochlorothiazide (10/25)
- Ziac: Bisoprolol-hydrochlorothiazide (2.5/6.25, 5/6.25, 10/6.25)

Centrally acting drug and diuretics
- Aldoril methyldopa-hydrochlorothiazide (250/15, 250/25, 500/30, 500/50)
- Demi-Regroton, Regroton: Reserpine-chlorthalidone (0.125/25, 0.25/50)
- Diupres reserpine-chlorothiazide (0.125/250, 0.25/500)
- Hydropres reserpine-hydrochlorothiazide (0.125/25, 0.125/50)

Diuretic and potassium-sparing diuretic
- Aldactazide: Spironolactone-hydrochlorothiazide (25/25, 50/50)
- Dyazide: Triamterene-hydrochlorothiazide (37.5/25, 75/50)
- Maxzide: Triamterene-hydrochlorothiazide (37.5/25, 75/50)
- Moduretic: Amiloride-hydrochlorothiazide (5/50)

Lipid-Lowering Treatment to Prevent Heart Attack Trial, 73% in the Controlled Onset Verapamil Investigation of Cardiovascular End Points trial, and 49% in the International Verapamil-Trandolapril Study *(12,14,16)*. To achieve a target diastolic blood pressure (DBP) less than 90 mmHg, 63% of participants in the Hypertension Optimal Treatment Study required two or more drugs *(21)*. The percentage was 74% if the target was less than 80 mmHg.

The target BP for DM and chronic kidney disease is less than 130/80 mmHg. Thus, the presence of DM and chronic kidney disease as well as systolic hypertension and African-American ethnicity increases the probability of the requirement of two or more drugs. The benefits of lower BP treatment goals translated into a reduction of cardiovascular events among the diabetic subjects in Hypertension Optimal Treatment Study *(21)* and the United Kingdom Prospective Diabetes Study 38 *(22)*. Among patients with a previous stroke in the Perindopril Protection Against Recurrent Stroke Study, the combination of perindopril and indapamide decreased recurrent strokes by 43% *(23)*.

The rationale for using combination drug therapy (Fig. 4) obviously is to maximize BP control *(24)*. The efficacy is achieved by combining drugs, which act by dissimilar mechanisms and thereby produce additive or perhaps synergistic effects on BP reduction (Fig. 4) *(25,26)*. Because diuretics activate renin release by volume contraction and β-blockers reduce renin, their mechanisms are complementary by blocking opposing homeostatic mechanisms. This reduces the potassium wasting of the diuretic. If small doses of two drugs with different modes of action are used, dose-dependent adverse events are diminished *(30)*.

There are other benefits of combining antihypertensive medications. The combination of a dihydropyridine CCB and an ACE inhibitor reduces the peripheral edema associated with dihydropyridine CCB monotherapy *(31)*. The combination of sustained-release (SR) verapamil and trandolapril is additive for lowering BP and reducing proteinuria *(32)*. African Americans have a diminished BP response to ACE inhibitors, ARBs, and β-blockers compared to diuretics or CCBs *(33–35)*. However, the addition of a diuretic to those drugs results in equal efficacy in both blacks and whites *(36,37)*.

If the goal of combining two antihypertensive drug is to lower BP, then it should be noted that the combination of ACE inhibitors and β-blockers (Fig. 4) *(38,39)*, α_2-stimulants and β-blockers, α_1-blockers and α_2-stimulants, and possibly ACE inhibitors and ARBs are not fully additive when *appropriate* doses of each drug are used *(40,41)*. However, for target organ protection, the combination of ACE inhibitors and β-blockers is protective for both ischemic heart disease *(42–48)* and

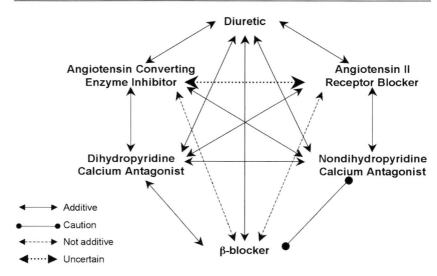

Fig. 4. Potential combinations for treating hypertension. Most drugs are additive with each other, but there appears to be a less-than-additive effect of the combination of β-blockers and angiotensin-converting enzyme inhibitor or angiotensin receptor blockers.

heart failure *(49–51)*. Similar observations have been made for the combination of ACE inhibitors and ARBs for renal protection *(52)*.

Care must be taken in combining α_1-blockers with CCBs because they may have a synergistic effect *(26,53,54)*. Also, the combination of the nondihydropyridine CCBs diltiazem and verapamil with a β-blocker potentially could cause severe myocardial depression, extreme bradycardia, or advanced heart block. Alternatively, it could be cautiously used in patients with a preserved ejection fraction and hyperkinetic heart syndrome, hypertrophic cardiomyopathy, and diastolic heart failure.

There are several additional combinations that are controversial (Fig. 4). Dihydropyridine and nondihydropyridine CCBs appear to be additive *(55,56)*. This is caused by a pharmacokinetic interaction owing to diltiazem and verapamil increasing plasma concentrations of nifedipine *(56)*. The combination of CCBs and diuretics is controversial *(57–59)*. The sequence of which drug is added to the opposite drug may be important. For instance, the addition of isradipine or propranolol to hydrochlorothiazide-treated patients is equally efficacious *(60)*. Factorial design trials combining a diuretic with verapamil or diltiazem showed an additive antihypertensive effect *(61,62)*. However, not all studies documented additivity *(63)*. Currently, there are no fixed-dose combinations of a diuretic and calcium antagonist marketed.

POTASSIUM-SPARING DIURETICS
WITH HYDROCHLOROTHIAZIDE

Diuretic-induced hypokalemia and hypomagnesemia occur with diuretic use in the elderly *(64, 65)*. Hypokalemia associated with diuretic use in the Systolic Hypertension in the Elderly Program was associated with a higher stroke rate than in the placebo group *(66)*. The combination of hydrochlorothiazide with potassium-sparing diuretics decreases the need to supplement potassium *(24,67)*. In a randomized, double-blind, placebo-controlled study of 130 elderly patients, 25 mg of hydrochlorothiazide or 25/2.5 mg of hydrochlorothiazide/amiloride were given after a 4-week placebo run-in period *(67)*. Drug doses were doubled at weeks 8 and 12 to achieve a DBP less than 90 mmHg. At week 16, the reduction from baseline was similar for each drug. Hypokalemia occurred in 15% of the hydrochlorothiazide-treated patients and 3% of the study participants receiving hydrochlorothiazide/amiloride ($p < 0.02$). The amiloride did not add to the antihypertensive effect.

Care must be taken in using potassium-sparing diuretics in the elderly. A serum creatinine greater than 1.3 mg/dL should be viewed as abnormal because older patients have less muscle mass. Serious hyperkalemia may occur in older patients with type IV renal tubular acidosis, DM, renal insufficiency, or treatment with nonsteroidal anti-inflammatory drugs, ACE inhibitors, ARBs, or oral potassium supplements and potassium-sparing diuretics *(68,69)*.

β-BLOCKER AND DIURETIC COMBINATION

β-Blockers are effective therapy in elderly patients *(70)*. The combination of β-blockers and diuretics reduced cardiovascular morbidity and mortality and total mortality in the Swedish Trial of Older Persons *(71)*.Elderly hypertensive patients may benefit from the use of β-blockers, especially if there is concomitant ischemic heart disease, atrial arrhythmias, or systolic heart failure. Alterations of lipids, glucose, and potassium are not seen when low-dose diuretics (e.g., 6.25 and 12.5 mg of hydrochlorothiazide) are combined with β-blockers *(30,72,73)*. Figure 5 compares the antihypertensive effect of placebo, 25 mg of hydrochlorothiazide, 5 mg of bisoprolol, and the combination of 5/6.25 mg of bisoprolol/hydrochlorothiazide each dosed once daily in a randomized, double-blind trial in older patients *(28)*. The low-dose combination was more effective than diuretic or β-blocker monotherapy. The incidence of hypokalemia was 6.5% for the diuretic monotherapy and 0.7% for the low-dose diuretic and β-blocker combination.

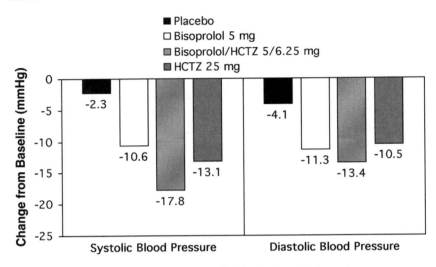

Fig. 5. Combination of a diuretic and a β-blocker in elderly patients. The combination of bisoprolol with an ultra low dose of hydrochlorothiazide (HCTZ) is significantly more effective than hydrochlorothiazide. (Data from ref. *28*.)

An open-labeled study randomly assigned 308 older persons (65 years and older) with isolated systolic hypertension to no treatment or one of four drug regimens: (a) 25/2.5 mg of hydrochlorothiazide/amiloride, one tablet once daily; (b) 50 mg of atenolol dosed once daily; (c) 10 mg of nifedipine slow release dosed twice daily; and (d) 25/6.25 mg of atenolol/chlorthalidone, one tablet dosed once daily *(74,75)*. After 90 days, the drug dose could be doubled if the systolic blood pressure (SBP) was 160 mmHg or higher. Each group significantly attained a greater reduction of SBP compared with the control group at 3 months. However, at 6 months, this was no longer true for the atenolol group. The mean change in BP at 6 months was control,–8.1/–0.7 mmHg; hydrochlorothiazide and amiloride, –21.8/–3.7 mmHg; nifedipine, –22.7/–4.8 mmHg; atenolol, –26.4/–3.6 mmHg; and atenolol/chlorthalidone, –26.4/ –5.4 mmHg. Postural hypotension did not occur more than in the control group.

In a randomized, double-blind trial of isolated SBP, 164 patients older than 60 years were allocated to 2.5/6.25 mg of bisoprolol/hydrochlorothiazide or 5 mg of amlodipine dosed once daily for 12 weeks *(76)*. Figure 6 shows that there was no difference between the combination and amlodipine in the change from the baseline for SBP and DBPs. Heart rate was lowered more with combination. Quality of life improved similarly with each treatment.

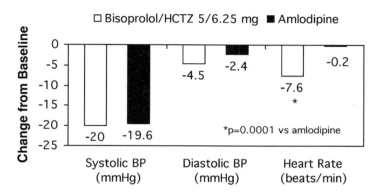

Fig. 6. Comparison of low-dose combination and amlodipine in isolated systolic hypertension. The combination of bisoprolol with an ultra low dose of hydrochlorothiazide (HCTZ) was as effective as amlodipine in reducing systolic blood pressure (BP). (Data from ref. *76*.)

β-BLOCKER AND CALCIUM ANTAGONIST COMBINATION

Calcium antagonists combined with β-blockers are useful for patients who have hypertension and stable angina *(58)*. The mechanism of action is considered complementary, reducing cardiac output and dilating peripheral blood vessels *(77)*. Dihydropyridines (amlodipine, felodipine, isradipine, nicardipine, nifedipine, or nisoldipine) are preferred calcium antagonists in these combinations. It is unfortunate that there are no such fixed combinations available in the United States.

Twenty-one elderly study participants with isolated systolic hypertension completed a double-blind, four-period, crossover design after an initial 4-week single-blind placebo run-in period *(78)*. Each treatment period lasted 6 weeks. Patients were randomly assigned to placebo, 50–200 mg of metoprolol, 5–20 mg of felodipine, or the combination of metoprolol and felodipine. Medication during the first 3 weeks of each period was titrated to achieve a supine SBP goal less than 140 mmHg. The average placebo-corrected decline in supine BP at the end of treatment was –17/–5 mmHg for felodipine, –6/–5 mmHg for metoprolol, –19/–9 mmHg for the combination. The percentage of patients who achieved a SBP less than 140 mmHg 2 hours postdose at the end of each treatment period was 0% for placebo, 45% for felodipine, 24% for metoprolol, and 70% for the combination. The benefits diminished when measured 12 hours postdose.

Using 50 mg controlled-release metoprolol and 5 mg extended-release felodipine given as a fixed combination or individual drug combination, 23 elderly (60–77 years old) subjects were studied in a randomized, double-blind, placebo-controlled, three-way crossover design *(77)*. Each treatment period lasted 4 weeks. Using ambulatory BP monitoring, compared to placebo treatment the average 24-hour decline in BP was –15/–11 mmHg when dispensed individually and –18/–11 when dispensed as a fixed combination.

ANGIOTENSIN-CONVERTING ENZYME INHIBITOR AND DIURETIC COMBINATIONS

Diuretics potentiate ACE inhibitors by stimulating the release of renin. Combining an ACE inhibitor with a diuretic results in similar efficacy for blacks vs whites and younger vs elderly *(39,79)*. The combination should be advantageous for elderly hypertensive individuals with systolic heart failure, DM, renal insufficiency, and a previous stroke. However, care is necessary, especially in the elderly, to avoid an excessive, prolonged decline in BP *(39,80)*. Attention to overall volume status and the use of low doses of medications are prudent to initiate treatment to avoid a disproportionate and extended decline in BP. Thereafter, the combination should be gradually titrated to achieve the therapeutic effect *(39)*.

Low-dose diuretics combined with an ACE inhibitor are effective. In an open-label study after a 2-week placebo lead-in period, 99 subjects 60 years or older with a DBP of 92–110 mmHg were treated with 25 mg of captopril twice daily *(81)*. After 2 weeks, if the DBP was 90 mmHg or higher, then patients were randomly assigned to 25/15 mg of captopril/hydrochlorothiazide or 50 mg of captopril twice daily.

A randomized, double-blind, placebo-controlled study was conducted in patients with stage I and II hypertension *(79)*. Figure 7 shows the change in seated DBP after 12 weeks with active therapy in the 69 elderly patients treated with placebo, 10 mg of lisinopril, 12.5 mg of hydrochlorothiazide, 25 mg of hydrochlorothiazide, 10/12.5 mg of lisinopril/hydrochlorothiazide, and 10/25 mg of lisinopril/hydrochlorothiazide dosed once daily *(79)*. The overall treatment response of the older cohort was 1 to 3 mmHg higher for each treatment category compared with the total group of 467 subjects.

A double-blind, randomized, parallel group study enrolled 278 subjects aged 65 to 80 years *(82)*. After a 2-week, single-blind, placebo run-in period, patients received once-daily dosed 20 mg of lisinopril, 12.5 mg of hydrochlorothiazide, or a fixed-dose combination 20/12.5 mg of lisinopril/hydrochlorothiazide. There were 153 patients who completed

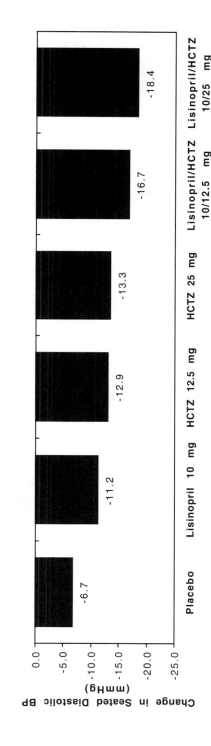

Fig. 7. Change in seated diastolic blood pressure from baseline treated with a diuretic, converting enzyme inhibitor, or combination. The antihypertensive effect of the combination of hydrochlorothiazide (HCTZ) and lisinopril was superior to monotherapy. (Data from ref. 79.)

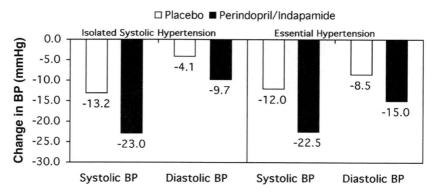

Fig. 8. Mean change in supine blood pressure from baseline at week 12 of fixed, low-dose combination therapy. Perindopril/indapamide 2/0.625 mg was significantly better than placebo. BP, blood pressure. (Data from ref. *83*.)

the protocol. The average decline in sitting BP at the end of 8 weeks was −16.2/−15.6, −16.6/−13.1, and −24.5/−17.6 mmHg for the ACE inhibitor, diuretic, and combination treatment, respectively. Only the change in DBP with lisinopril was not significantly different from the combination of lisinopril and hydrochlorothiazide.

A double-blind study randomly assigned 383 older patients to placebo or 2/0.625 mg of perindopril/indapamide dosed one to two tablets once daily to achieve a treatment goal of a SBP less than 160 mmHg or a DBP less than 90 mmHg *(83)*. After 12 weeks, the average decline in BP was −12.3/−7.3 for placebo-treated patients and −22.5/−13.2 for the indapamide/perindopril combination (Fig. 8) *(84)*. The response rate, defined as a DBP decline of 10 mmHg or a DBP of 90 mmHg or less, was 81.3% for the combination vs 48.9% for placebo. Normalization of SBP below 160 mmHg was less than DBP to 90 mmHg or less. The average change in potassium for placebo treatment was −0.01 mmol/L and for active therapy was −0.07 mmol/L for one tablet and 0.16 mmol/L for two tablets *(83)*.

ANGIOTENSIN-CONVERTING ENZYME INHIBITOR AND CALCIUM ANTAGONIST COMBINATIONS

Why an ACE inhibitor and a CCB are additive for the treatment of hypertension is less clear than other combinations. A modest stimulatory effect on renin by CCBs because of increased sympathetic activity has been suggested for the additivity with CCBs *(24,39)*. In addition, each drug class vasodilates and promotes salt and water excretion by different mechanisms *(9,24)*.

There have been several ACE inhibitor and CCB combinations that have been approved for the treatment of hypertension: (a) amlodipine and benazepril, Lotrel; (b) felodipine and enalapril, Lexxel; (c) verapamil and trandolapril, Tarka; and (d) diltiazem and enalapril, Teczem, which is no longer manufactured. These agents do not alter lipids; however, there is the risk of renal dysfunction and hyperkalemia caused by the ACE inhibitor in susceptible patients. In a 20-week, double-blind study of 463 hypertensive diabetics, a comparison of the combination of verapamil and trandolapril with atenolol and chlorthalidone found that hemoglobin A1c increased with β-blocker–diuretic combination, but not with the CCB–ACE inhibitor (85).

Figure 9 shows the change in systolic and DBPs in 36 elderly men and women with a supine DBP 95–115 mmHg in a double-blind, three-way, crossover design 18 weeks long with a 4-week, single-blind run in period (31). The BP at the end of the placebo period was designated as the baseline BP, which was used for the comparison of 5–10 mg extended-release felodipine, 5–10 mg of enalapril, and 5/5 mg of felodipine/enalapril dosed once daily. Each treatment period lasted 6 weeks. The study showed the superiority of the combination of felodipine and enalapril compared to the baseline BPs or monotherapy. The combination of felodipine and enalapril was tolerated better and associated with less ankle edema than felodipine alone.

Another factorial design trial compared placebo, 5–20 mg extended-release felodipine, 5–20 mg of enalapril, and their combination in 6-week periods (86). Twenty older patients with a supine SBP 160 mmHg or greater and DBP less than 95 mmHg were randomly assigned in this double-blind, crossover study. The drugs could be titrated every 2 weeks to achieve a SBP less than 140 mmHg. The placebo-corrected change in BP was –13/–5, –5/–3, –18/–7 mmHg for felodipine, enalapril, and the combination. The combination was additive.

A 3×2 factorial design trial studied 120 and 240 mg SR diltiazem alone or with 10 mg lisinopril dosed once daily, 10 mg lisinopril once daily, and placebo (87). The study population was 156 Chinese persons 65 years and older with a DBP of 95–114 mmHg after a 4-week placebo lead-in period. The active treatment phase of this double-blind, randomized study lasted 12 weeks. Figure 10 displays the mean seated change in trough SBP (Panel A) and DBP (Panel B). Active treatment reduced BP significantly compared with placebo. The combination of diltiazem and lisinopril at each dose lowered BP more than the same dose of diltiazem alone. However, the effect was less than additive. Peripheral edema occurred with the same frequency in each treated group, but cough was the most common adverse event among the patients treated with lisinopril monotherapy or combination therapy.

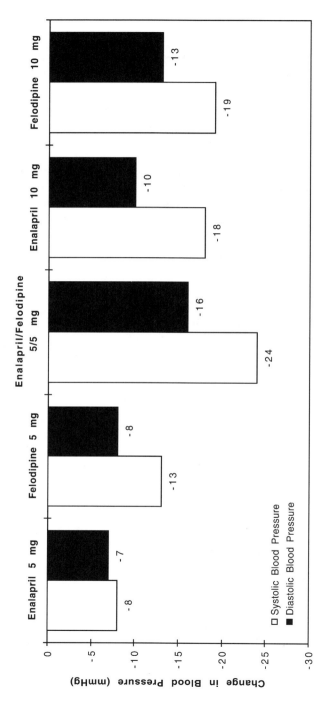

Fig. 9. Double-blind three-way crossover design study of 36 elderly hypertensive subjects. Low doses of an angiotensin-converting enzyme inhibitor and a dihydropyridine calcium channel blocker lowered blood pressure more than what was achieved by the titration of individual drugs. (Data from ref. *31*.)

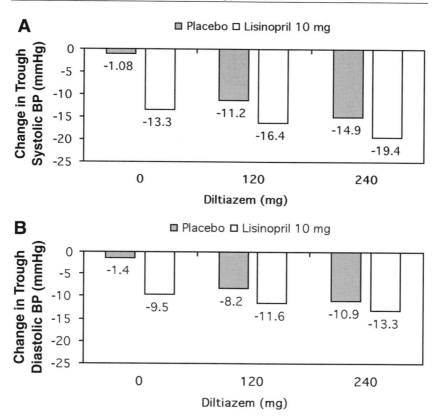

Fig. 10. Factorial design trial in elderly Chinese subjects. The combination of each drug lowered systolic (Panel A) and diastolic (Panel B) blood pressure (BP) more than diltiazem monotherapy ($p < 0.05$ for systolic and diastolic). However, the combination was less than additive. (Data from ref. *87*.)

A multicenter, double-blind, parallel-group trial randomized 308 patients after a 2- to 4-week placebo run-in period *(88)*. Entry DBP was required to be between 100 and 120 mmHg. Subjects were allocated to one of four groups: (a) placebo; (b) 20 mg of benazepril; (c) 5 mg of amlodipine; or (d) 5/20 mg of amlodipine/benazepril. Medication was dosed once daily and continued for 8 weeks. The combination was statistically superior in each comparison. Furthermore, it was similarly effective in younger and older patients (Fig. 11).

After a 4-week, single-blind placebo run-in period, 254 elderly hypertensive patients with a DBP of 95–115 mmHg were treated with the fixed

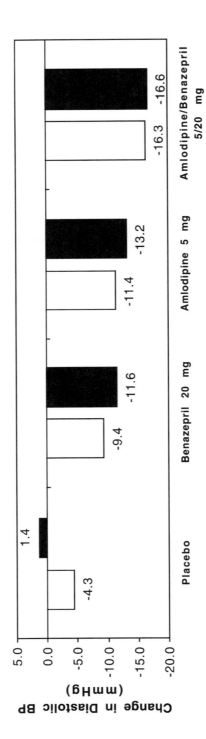

Fig. 11. Mean change from baseline in mean sitting diastolic blood pressure (BP) by age and treatment. The combination of benazepril and amlodipine lowered blood pressure more than the individual drugs. There was no difference in effectiveness of the combination by age group. (Data from ref. 88.)

combination of verapamil SR/trandolapril (89). Treatment was initiated with 120/0.5 mg of verapamil SR/trandolapril dosed once daily and titrated to 180/2 mg of verapamil SR/trandolapril at 4-week intervals until the DBP was less 90 mmHg during the first 12 weeks. After 3 months of treatment, patients who did not achieve the target BP were excluded from additional 3-month follow-up. Verapamil SR/trandolapril was highly effective in reducing BP. The mean reduction in BP was –21.9/ –17.1 mm Hg for responders and nonresponders. The combination was tolerated well.

ANGIOTENSIN RECEPTOR BLOCKER AND DIURETIC COMBINATION

The mechanism of combining an ARB and a diuretic is similar to the combination with an ACE inhibitor. This combination should be particularly useful for patients with left ventricular hypertrophy (LVH[90]), DM with renal insufficiency (91,92) or LVH (93), heart failure (94–97), and myocardial infarction (98).

A multicenter, double-blind, randomized study enrolled younger and older hypertensive subjects with mild-to-moderate hypertension (99). After a 4-week placebo lead-in period, participants received a fixed dose of 50 mg of losartan with 12.5 mg of hydrochlorothiazide (n = 216) or 50 mg of captopril with 25 mg of hydrochlorothiazide (n = 109) once daily for 12 weeks. There was no difference in efficacy by age group or treatment. Cough and headache occurred more commonly in elderly patients receiving captopril than those receiving losartan. Serum creatinine and uric acid increased and serum potassium decreased from baseline more with captopril than with losartan.

A randomized, double-blind, parallel-group trial of 2002 hypertensive subjects compared 160/12.5 mg of valsartan/hydrochlorothiazide, 160/25 mg of valsartan/hydrochlorothiazide, and 160 mg of valsartan dosed once daily for 8 weeks in patients who were inadequately controlled on 160 mg of valsartan after 4 weeks (100). Approximately 21% were 65 years or older. The response rate (sitting DBP less than 90 mmHg and/or a 10 mmHg decline in DBP) was 59.1, 66.7, and 70.7% for 160 mg of valsartan, 160/12.5 mg of valsartan/hydrochlorothiazide, and 160/25 mg of valsartan/hydrochlorothiazide, respectively. The response rate for younger patients was less. The mean change in BP was –15.4/–12.5, –18.7/–13.7, and –20.4/–14.3 mmHg for 160 mg of valsartan, 160/12.5 mg of valsartan/hydrochlorothiazide, and 160/25 mg of valsartan/hydrochlorothiazide, respectively.

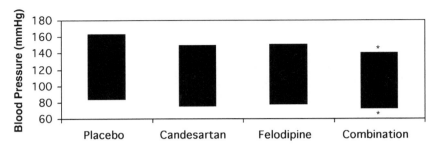

Fig. 12. A 24-hour ambulatory blood pressure comparison of placebo, candesartan, felodipine, and combination. The combination of candesartan and felodipine was additive. *$p < 0.005$ vs candesartan and felodipine. (Data from ref. *101*.)

CALCIUM ANTAGONIST AND ANGIOTENSIN RECEPTOR BLOCKER COMBINATION

Few studies assessed the combination of an ARB with a CCB. One study examined 31 subjects older than 65 years who had a SBP of 160 mmHg or higher after their medications were stopped 3 to 7 days prior to randomization *(101)*. Subjects were randomly assigned in a double-blind, crossover design to each of the following 4-week treatments: (a) placebo, (b) 16 mg of candesartan, (c) 5 mg of felodipine, and (d) 16/5 mg of candesartan/felodipine, each dosed once daily. Ambulatory BP reading was performed after each treatment period. The average decline in 24-hour SBP was −12.2, −11.9, and −21.0 mmHg for candesartan, felodipine, and the combination, respectively (Fig. 12). The combination of an ARB and dihydropyridine calcium antagonist was additive.

CALCIUM ANTAGONIST AND DIURETIC COMBINATION

Two outcomes trials documented the benefit of a diuretic chlorthalidone or the calcium antagonist nitrendipine for reducing cardiovascular events in older patients with isolated systolic hypertension *(102,103)*. It is logical to ask whether the combination of these drugs might be beneficial. A randomized, double-blind, crossover trial of 19 elderly patients with isolated systolic hypertension compared placebo, 2 to 4 mg of lacidipine, 25 to 50 mg of hydrochlorothiazide, or their combination dosed once daily during 4-week treatment cycles *(104)*. Each treatment could be titrated from a low dose to a higher dose after 2 weeks to achieve the goal

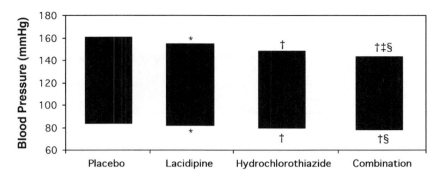

Fig. 13. Factorial design trial in elderly patients with isolated systolic hypertension: results of 24-hour ambulatory blood pressure. Lacidipine and hydrochlorothiazide were fully additive. $*p < 0.001$; $\dagger p < 0.001$ vs placebo; $\ddagger p < 0.01$ vs hydrochlorothiazide; $\S p < 0.001$ vs lacidipine. (Data from ref. *104*.)

SBP, which was 160 mmHg or lower for a SBP greater than 180 mmHg or a reduction of 20 mmHg or greater for a SBP between 160 and 180 mmHg. In addition to clinic BP measurements, ambulatory BP monitoring was performed. Factorial analysis documented that hydrochlorothiazide was more effective than lacidipine, and the combination was additive (Fig. 13).

SUMMARY

BP control remains the lowest among the oldest age group, despite the documented reduction in morbidity and mortality in randomized controlled trials. Combination drug therapy achieves a higher control rate and is endorsed by the most recent report of the Joint National Committee on the Prevention, Detection, Evaluation, and Treatment of High Blood Pressure. The rational combination of drugs should be used to treat underlying coexisting illnesses that are more common in older patients. Fixed-dose combinations may be dispensed, when appropriate, to achieve BP treatment goals and to treat coexisting illnesses.

REFERENCES

1. Hajjar I, Kotchen TA. Trends in prevalence, awareness, treatment, and control of hypertension in the United States, 1988–2000. *JAMA 2003;290:199–206.*
2. Hyman DJ, Pavlik VN. Characteristics of patients with uncontrolled hypertension in the United States. *N Engl J Med* 2001;345:479–486.
3. Chobanian AV, Bakris GL, Black HR, et al. Seventh report of the Joint National Committee on Prevention, Detection, Evaluation, and Treatment of High Blood Pressure. *Hypertension* 2003;42:1206–1252.

4. Chobanian AV, Bakris GL, Black HR, et al. The seventh report of the Joint National Committee on Prevention, Detection, Evaluation, and Treatment of High Blood Pressure: the JNC 7 report. *JAMA* 2003;289:2560–2572.

5. Prisant LM. Fixed low-dose combination therapy: current recommendations. *Manag Care* 2003;12(8 suppl Hypertension):45–50.

6. Fagan TC. Remembering the lessons of basic pharmacology. *Arch Intern Med* 1994;154:1430–1431.

7. Materson BJ, Reda DJ, Cushman WC, et al. Single-drug therapy for hypertension in men. A comparison of six antihypertensive agents with placebo. The Department of Veterans Affairs Cooperative Study Group on Antihypertensive Agents. *N Engl J Med* 1993;328:914–921.

8. Materson BJ, Reda DJ, Cushman WC. Department of Veterans Affairs single-drug therapy of hypertension study. Revised figures and new data. Department of Veterans Affairs Cooperative Study Group on Antihypertensive Agents. *Am J Hypertens* 1995;8:189–192.

9. Ruzicka M, Leenen FH. Monotherapy vs combination therapy as first line treatment of uncomplicated arterial hypertension. *Drugs* 2001;61:943–954.

10. Brunner HR, Ménard J, Waeber B, et al. Treating the individual patient: considerations on dose, sequential monotherapy and drug combinations. *J Hypertens* 1990;8:3–11.

11. Mancia G, Failla M, Grappiolo A, Giannattasio C. Present and future role of combination treatment in hypertension. *J Cardiovasc Pharmacol* 1998;31(suppl 2):S41–S44.

12. Black HR, Elliott WJ, Neaton JD, et al. Baseline characteristics and early blood pressure control in the CONVINCE Trial. *Hypertension* 2001;37:12–18.

13. Black HR, Elliott WJ, Grandits G, et al. Principal results of the Controlled Onset Verapamil Investigation of Cardiovascular End Points (CONVINCE) trial. *JAMA* 2003;289:2073–2082.

14. Cushman WC, Ford CE, Cutler JA, et al. Success and predictors of blood pressure control in diverse North American settings: the antihypertensive and lipid-lowering treatment to prevent heart attack trial (ALLHAT). *J Clin Hypertens (Greenwich)* 2002;4:393–404.

15. Major outcomes in high-risk hypertensive patients randomized to angiotensin-converting enzyme inhibitor or calcium channel blocker vs diuretic: the Antihypertensive and Lipid-Lowering Treatment to Prevent Heart Attack Trial (ALLHAT). *JAMA* 2002;288:2981–2997.

16. Pepine CJ, Handberg EM, Cooper-DeHoff RM, et al. A calcium antagonist vs a non-calcium antagonist hypertension treatment strategy for patients with coronary artery disease. The International Verapamil-Trandolapril Study (INVEST): a randomized controlled trial. *JAMA* 2003;290:2805–2816.

17. Kaplan NM. Implications for cost-effectiveness. Combination therapy for systemic hypertension. *Am J Cardiol* 1995;76:595–597.

18. Fenichel RR, Lipicky RJ. Combination products as first-line pharmacotherapy. *Arch Intern Med* 1994;154:1429–1430.

19. Fenichel RR, Lipicky RJ. Combination products as first-line pharmacotherapy. *Arch Intern Med* 1995;155:117.

20. Prisant LM, Doll NC. Hypertension: the rediscovery of combination therapy. *Geriatrics* 1997;52:28–30, 33–38.

21. Hansson L, Zanchetti A, Carruthers SG, et al. Effects of intensive blood-pressure lowering and low-dose aspirin in patients with hypertension: principal results of the Hypertension Optimal Treatment (HOT) randomised trial. HOT Study Group. *Lancet* 1998;351:1755–1762.

22. UK Prospective Diabetes Study Group. Tight blood pressure control and risk of macrovascular and microvascular complications in type 2 diabetes: UKPDS 38. *BMJ* 1998;317:703–713.
23. Randomised trial of a perindopril-based blood-pressure-lowering regimen among 6105 individuals with previous stroke or transient ischaemic attack. *Lancet* 2001;358:1033–1041.
24. Sica DA. Rationale for fixed-dose combinations in the treatment of hypertension: the cycle repeats. *Drugs* 2002;62:443–462.
25. Oster JR, Epstein M. Fixed-dose combination medications for the treatment of hypertension: a critical review. *J Clin Hypertens* 1987;3:278–293.
26. Elliott HL, Meredith PA, Reid JL. Verapamil and prazosin in essential hypertension: evidence of a synergistic combination? *J Cardiovasc Pharmacol* 1987; 10(suppl 10):S108–S110.
27. Frishman WH, Bryzinski BS, Coulson LR, et al. A multifactorial trial design to assess combination therapy in hypertension. Treatment with bisoprolol and hydrochlorothiazide. *Arch Intern Med* 1994;154:1461–1468.
28. Frishman WH, Burris JF, Mroczek WJ, et al. First-line therapy option with low-dose bisoprolol fumarate and low-dose hydrochlorothiazide in patients with stage I and stage II systemic hypertension. *J Clin Pharmacol* 1995;35:182–188.
29. Prisant LM, Weir MR, Papademetriou V, et al. Low-dose drug combination therapy: an alternative first-line approach to hypertension treatment. *Am Heart J* 1995;130: 359–366.
30. Neutel JM, Rolf CN, Valentine SN, Li J, Lucas C, Marmorstein BL. Low-dose combination therapy as first line treatment of mild-to-moderate hypertension: the efficacy and safety of bisoprolol/HCTZ vs amlodipine, enalapril, and placebo. *Cardiovasc Rev Rep* 1996;17:33–45.
31. Morgan TO, Anderson A, Jones E. Comparison and interaction of low dose felodipine and enalapril in the treatment of essential hypertension in elderly subjects. *Am J Hypertens* 1992;5:238–243.
32. Bakris GL, Weir MR, DeQuattro V, McMahon FG. Effects of an ACE inhibitor/calcium antagonist combination on proteinuria in diabetic nephropathy. *Kidney Int* 1998;54:1283–1289.
33. Saunders E, Weir MR, Kong BW, et al. A comparison of the efficacy and safety of a beta-blocker, a calcium channel blocker, and a converting enzyme inhibitor in hypertensive blacks. *Arch Intern Med* 1990;150:1707–1713.
34. Prisant LM, Mensah GA. Use of β-adrenergic receptor blockers in blacks. *J Clin Pharmacol* 1996;36:867–873.
35. Prisant LM. Meet the experts: effective use of combination drug therapy in the treatment of minority hypertensive populations. Combination Therapy: Rediscovered. *Ethn Dis* 1997;7:165–168.
36. Prisant LM, Neutel JM, Ferdinand K, et al. Low-dose combination therapy as first-line hypertension treatment for blacks and nonblacks. *J Natl Med Assoc* 1999;91:40–48.
37. Vidt DG. A controlled multiclinic study to compare the antihypertensive effects of MK-421, hydrochlorothiazide, and MK-421 combined with hydrochlorothiazide in patients with mild to moderate essential hypertension. *J Hypertens Suppl* 1984;2:S81–S88.
38. MacGregor GA, Markandu ND, Smith SJ, Sagnella GA. Captopril: contrasting effects of adding hydrochlorothiazide, propranolol, or nifedipine. *J Cardiovasc Pharmacol* 1985;7(suppl 1):S82–S87.
39. Cheng A, Frishman WH. Use of angiotensin-converting enzyme inhibitors as monotherapy and in combination with diuretics and calcium channel blockers. *J Clin Pharmacol* 1998;38:477–491.

40. Sutton JM, Bagby SP. Nontraditional combination pharmacotherapy of hypertension. *Cleve Clin J Med* 1992;59:459–468.
41. Sica DA, Elliott WJ. Angiotensin-converting enzyme inhibitors and angiotensin receptor blockers in combination: theory and practice. *J Clin Hypertens (Greenwich)* 2001;3:383–387.
42. Pfeffer MA, Braunwald E, Moye LA, et al. Effect of captopril on mortality and morbidity in patients with left ventricular dysfunction after myocardial infarction. Results of the survival and ventricular enlargement trial. The SAVE Investigators. *N Engl J Med* 1992;327:669–677.
43. Effect of ramipril on mortality and morbidity of survivors of acute myocardial infarction with clinical evidence of heart failure. The Acute Infarction Ramipril Efficacy (AIRE) Study Investigators. *Lancet* 1993;342:821–828.
44. GISSI-3: effects of lisinopril and transdermal glyceryl trinitrate singly and together on 6-week mortality and ventricular function after acute myocardial infarction. Gruppo Italiano per lo Studio della Sopravvivenza nell'infarto Miocardico. *Lancet* 1994;343:1115–1122.
45. ISIS-4: a randomised factorial trial assessing early oral captopril, oral mononitrate, and intravenous magnesium sulphate in 58,050 patients with suspected acute myocardial infarction. ISIS-4 (Fourth International Study of Infarct Survival) Collaborative Group. *Lancet* 1995;345:669–685.
46. Ambrosioni E, Borghi C, Magnani B. The effect of the angiotensin-converting-enzyme inhibitor zofenopril on mortality and morbidity after anterior myocardial infarction. The Survival of Myocardial Infarction Long-Term Evaluation (SMILE) Study Investigators. *N Engl J Med* 1995;332:80–85.
47. Kober L, Torp-Pedersen C, Carlsen JE, et al. A clinical trial of the angiotensin-converting-enzyme inhibitor trandolapril in patients with left ventricular dysfunction after myocardial infarction. Trandolapril Cardiac Evaluation (TRACE) Study Group. *N Engl J Med* 1995;333:1670–1676.
48. Fox KM. Efficacy of perindopril in reduction of cardiovascular events among patients with stable coronary artery disease: randomised, double-blind, placebo-controlled, multicentre trial (the EUROPA study). *Lancet* 2003;362:782–788.
49. Effect of metoprolol CR/XL in chronic heart failure: Metoprolol CR/XL Randomised Intervention Trial in Congestive Heart Failure (MERIT-HF). *Lancet* 1999;353:2001–2007.
50. The Cardiac Insufficiency Bisoprolol Study II (CIBIS-II): a randomised trial. *Lancet* 1999;353:9–13.
51. Packer M, Coats AJ, Fowler MB, et al. Effect of carvedilol on survival in severe chronic heart failure. *N Engl J Med* 2001;344:1651–1658.
52. Nakao N, Yoshimura A, Morita H, Takada M, Kayano T, Ideura T. Combination treatment of angiotensin-II receptor blocker and angiotensin-converting-enzyme inhibitor in non-diabetic renal disease (COOPERATE): a randomised controlled trial. *Lancet* 2003;361:117–124.
53. Lenz ML, Pool JL, Laddu AR, Varghese A, Johnston W, Taylor AA. Combined terazosin and verapamil therapy in essential hypertension. Hemodynamic and pharmacokinetic interactions. *Am J Hypertens* 1995;8:133–145.
54. Nalbantgil S, Nalbantgil I, Onder R. Clinically additive effect between doxazosin and amlodipine in the treatment of essential hypertension. *Am J Hypertens* 2000;13:921–926.
55. Kaesemeyer WH, Carr AA, Bottini PB, Prisant LM. Verapamil and nifedipine in combination for the treatment of hypertension. *J Clin Pharmacol* 1994;34:48–51.

56. Saseen JJ, Carter BL, Brown TE, Elliott WJ, Black HR. Comparison of nifedipine alone and with diltiazem or verapamil in hypertension. *Hypertension* 1996;28: 109–114.
57. Severs PS, Poulter NR. Calcium antagonists and diuretics as combined therapy. *J Hypertens* 1987;5(suppl 4):S123–S126.
58. Frishman WH, Landau A, Cretkovic A. Combination drug therapy with calcium-channel blockers in the treatment of systemic hypertension. *J Clin Pharmacol* 1993;33:752–755.
59. Nicholson JP, Resnick LM, Laragh JH. Hydrochlorothiazide is not additive to verapamil in treating essential hypertension. *Arch Intern Med* 1989;149:125–128.
60. Prisant LM, Carr AA, Nelson EB, Winer N, Velasquez MT, Gonasun LM. Isradipine vs propranolol in hydrochlorothiazide-treated hypertensives. A multicenter evaluation. *Arch Intern Med* 1989;149:2453–2457.
61. Letzel H, Bluemner E. Dose–response curves in antihypertensive combination therapy: results of a controlled clinical trial. *J Hypertens Suppl* 1990;8:S83–S86.
62. Burris JF, Weir MR, Oparil S, Weber M, Cady WJ, Stewart WH. An assessment of diltiazem and hydrochlorothiazide in hypertension. Application of factorial trial design to a multicenter clinical trial of combination therapy. *JAMA* 1990;263: 1507–1512.
63. Prisant LM. Ambulatory blood pressure profiles in patients treated with once-daily diltiazem extended-release or indapamide alone or in combination. *Am J Ther* 2000;7:177–184.
64. Martin BJ, Milligan K. Diuretic-associated hypomagnesemia in the elderly. *Arch Intern Med* 1987;147:1768–1771.
65. Petri M, Cumber P, Grimes L, et al. The metabolic effects of thiazide therapy in the elderly: a population study. *Age Ageing* 1986;15:151–155.
66. Franse LV, Pahor M, Di Bari M, Somes GW, Cushman WC, Applegate WB. Hypokalemia associated with diuretic use and cardiovascular events in the Systolic Hypertension in the Elderly Program. *Hypertension* 2000;35:1025–1030.
67. Myers MG. Hydrochlorothiazide with or without amiloride for hypertension in the elderly. A dose-titration study. *Arch Intern Med* 1987;147:1026–1030.
68. Vanpee D, Swine CH. Elderly heart failure patients with drug-induced serious hyperkalemia. *Aging (Milano)* 2000;12:315–319.
69. Schepkens H, Vanholder R, Billiouw JM, Lameire N. Life-threatening hyperkalemia during combined therapy with angiotensin-converting enzyme inhibitors and spironolactone: an analysis of 25 cases. *Am J Med* 2001;110:438–441.
70. Prisant LM. Should β-blockers be used in the treatment of hypertension in the elderly? *J Clin Hypertens (Greenwich)* 2002;4:286–294.
71. Dahlöf B, Lindholm LH, Hansson L, Scherstén B, Ekbom T, Wester PO. Morbidity and mortality in the Swedish Trial in Old Patients with Hypertension (STOP-Hypertension). *Lancet* 1991;338:1281–1285.
72. Neutel JM. Metabolic manifestations of low-dose diuretics. *Am J Med* 1996;101: 71S–82S.
73. Neutel JM, Black HR, Weber MA. Combination therapy with diuretics: an evolution of understanding. *Am J Med* 1996;101:61S–70S.
74. Avanzini F, Alli C, Bettelli G, et al. Antihypertensive efficacy and tolerability of different drug regimens in isolated systolic hypertension in the elderly. *Eur Heart J* 1994;15:206–212.
75. Tognoni G, Alli C, Avanzini F, et al. Randomised clinical trials in general practice: lessons from a failure. *BMJ* 1991;303:969–971.

76. Benetos A, Consoli S, Safavian A, Dubanchet A, Safar M. Efficacy, safety, and effects on quality of life of bisoprolol/hydrochlorothiazide vs amlodipine in elderly patients with systolic hypertension. *Am Heart J* 2000;140:E11.

77. McLay JS, MacDonald TM, Hosie J, Elliott HL. The pharmacodynamic and pharmacokinetic profiles of controlled-release formulations of felodipine and metoprolol in free and fixed combinations in elderly hypertensive patients. *Eur J Clin Pharmacol* 2000;56:529–535.

78. Wing LM, Russell AE, Tonkin AL, Bune AJ, West MJ, Chalmers JP. Felodipine, metoprolol and their combination compared with placebo in isolated systolic hypertension in the elderly. *Blood Press* 1994;3:82–89.

79. Chrysant SG. Antihypertensive effectiveness of low-dose lisinopril-hydrochlorothiazide combination. A large multicenter study. Lisinopril-Hydrochlorothiazide Group. *Arch Intern Med* 1994;154:737–743.

80. Israili ZH, Hall WD. ACE inhibitors. Differential use in elderly patients with hypertension. *Drugs Aging* 1995;7:355–371.

81. Tuck ML, Katz LA, Kirkendall WM, Koeppe PR, Ruoff GE, Sapir DG. Low-dose captopril in mild to moderate geriatric hypertension. *J Am Geriatr Soc* 1986;34: 693–696.

82. Hart W. Lisinopril-hydrochlorothiazide combination compared with the monocomponents in elderly hypertensive patients. *J Hum Hypertens* 1991;5(suppl 2):85–89.

83. Chalmers J, Castaigne A, Morgan T, Chastang C. Long-term efficacy of a new, fixed, very-low-dose angiotensin-converting enzyme-inhibitor/diuretic combination as first-line therapy in elderly hypertensive patients. *J Hypertens* 2000;18:327–337.

84. Castaigne A, Chalmers J, Morgan T, Chastang C, Feldmann L, Guez D. Efficacy and safety of an oral fixed low-dose perindopril 2 mg/indapamide 0.625 mg combination: a randomized, double-blind, placebo-controlled study in elderly patients with mild to moderate hypertension. *Clin Exp Hypertens* 1999;21:1097–1110.

85. Holzgreve H, Nakov R, Beck K, Janka HU. Antihypertensive therapy with verapamil SR plus trandolapril vs atenolol plus chlorthalidone on glycemic control. *Am J Hypertens* 2003;16(5 pt 1):381–386.

86. Wing LM, Russell AE, Tonkin AL, et al. Mono- and combination therapy with felodipine or enalapril in elderly patients with systolic hypertension. *Blood Press* 1994;3:90–96.

87. Chan P, Lin CN, Tomlinson B, Lin TH, Lee YS. Additive effects of diltiazem and lisinopril in the treatment of elderly patients with mild-to-moderate hypertension. *Am J Hypertens* 1997;10(7 pt 1):743–749.

88. Kuschnir E, Acuna E, Sevilla D, et al. Treatment of patients with essential hypertension: amlodipine 5 mg/benazepril 20 mg compared with amlodipine 5 mg, benazepril 20 mg, and placebo. *Clin Ther* 1996;18:1213–1224.

89. Holzgreve H, Compagnone D, Zilles P. Verapamil SR/trandolapril combination therapy for the elderly hypertensive patient. German VeraTran Hypertension Study Group. *J Hum Hypertens* 1999;13:61–67.

90. Dahlof B, Devereux RB, Kjeldsen SE, et al. Cardiovascular morbidity and mortality in the Losartan Intervention For Endpoint reduction in hypertension study (LIFE): a randomised trial against atenolol. *Lancet* 2002;359:995–1003.

91. Lewis EJ, Hunsicker LG, Clarke WR, et al. Renoprotective effect of the angiotensin-receptor antagonist irbesartan in patients with nephropathy due to type 2 diabetes. *N Engl J Med* 2001;345:851–860.

92. Brenner BM, Cooper ME, de Zeeuw D, et al. Effects of losartan on renal and cardiovascular outcomes in patients with type 2 diabetes and nephropathy. *N Engl J Med* 2001;345:861–869.

93. Lindholm LH, Ibsen H, Dahlof B, et al. Cardiovascular morbidity and mortality in patients with diabetes in the Losartan Intervention for Endpoint reduction in hypertension study (LIFE): a randomised trial against atenolol. *Lancet* 2002;359:1004–1010.

94. Yusuf S, Pfeffer MA, Swedberg K, et al. Effects of candesartan in patients with chronic heart failure and preserved left-ventricular ejection fraction: the CHARM-Preserved Trial. *Lancet* 2003;362:777–781.

95. Granger CB, McMurray JJ, Yusuf S, et al. Effects of candesartan in patients with chronic heart failure and reduced left-ventricular systolic function intolerant to angiotensin-converting-enzyme inhibitors: the CHARM-Alternative trial. *Lancet* 2003;362:772–776.

96. McMurray JJ, Ostergren J, Swedberg K, et al. Effects of candesartan in patients with chronic heart failure and reduced left-ventricular systolic function taking angiotensin-converting-enzyme inhibitors: the CHARM-Added trial. *Lancet* 2003;362: 767–771.

97. Pfeffer MA, Swedberg K, Granger CB, et al. Effects of candesartan on mortality and morbidity in patients with chronic heart failure: the CHARM-Overall programme. *Lancet* 2003;362:759–766.

98. Pfeffer MA, McMurray JJ, Velazquez EJ, et al. Valsartan, captopril, or both in myocardial infarction complicated by heart failure, left ventricular dysfunction, or both. *N Engl J Med* 2003;349:1893–1906.

99. Critchley JAJH, Gilchrist N, Ikeda L, et al. A randomized, double-masked comparison of the antihypertensive efficacy and safety of combination therapy with losartan and hydrochlorothiazide vs captopril and hydrochlorothiazide in elderly and younger patients. *Curr Ther Res* 1996;57:392–407.

100. Mallion JM, Carretta R, Trenkwalder P, et al. Valsartan/hydrochlorothiazide is effective in hypertensive patients inadequately controlled by valsartan monotherapy. *Blood Press Suppl* 2003;suppl 1:36–43.

101. Morgan T, Anderson A. A comparison of candesartan, felodipine, and their combination in the treatment of elderly patients with systolic hypertension. *Am J Hypertens* 2002;15:544–549.

102. Prevention of stroke by antihypertensive drug treatment in older persons with isolated systolic hypertension. Final results of the Systolic Hypertension in the Elderly Program (SHEP). SHEP Cooperative Research Group. *JAMA* 1991;265: 3255–3264.

103. Staessen JA, Fagard R, Thijs L, et al. Randomised double-blind comparison of placebo and active treatment for older patients with isolated systolic hypertension. The Systolic Hypertension in Europe (Syst-Eur) Trial Investigators. *Lancet* 1997;350:757–764.

104. Wing LM, Arnolda LF, Harvey PJ, et al. Lacidipine, hydrochlorothiazide and their combination in systolic hypertension in the elderly. *J Hypertens* 1997;15(12 pt 1):1503–1510.

V SPECIAL POPULATIONS

21 Attitudes Regarding Hypertension Among Older African-American Adults

Wallace R. Johnson, Jr., MD
and Elijah Saunders, MD

CONTENTS

MAJOR BARRIERS TO EFFECTIVE ANTIHYPERTENSIVE THERAPY

Before hypertension can be effectively treated in older African-American patients, the clinician must become familiar with the attitudes of this population regarding this disease. One of the major barriers to effective antihypertensive therapy is having a clinician who is not aware of potential impact that patient attitudes have on compliance with office visits and pharmacological therapy. One group of investigators did a survey of African Americans, Hispanic Americans, and non-Hispanic white adults over the age of 75 years that assessed ethnic differences in perceptions regarding the cause, prevention, and treatment of hyperten-

From: *Clinical Hypertension and Vascular Diseases: Hypertension in the Elderly*
Edited by: L. M. Prisant © Humana Press Inc., Totowa, NJ

sion as well as associations between perceptions and the use of preventive health services (1). The survey found that African Americans felt that hypertension resulted from poor health behaviors and stress, but that it was both preventable and treatable. In contrast, non-Hispanic whites felt that hypertension is a result of various mechanistic causes and heredity; also, they felt hypertension was treatable but not preventable. Finally, Hispanic Americans were more likely to state that hypertension was the result of aging and poor health behaviors and was not susceptible to treatment.

How do the above findings potentially affect the use of health services? First, participants in all three ethnic groups who identified hypertension as their major health problem were much more likely to have had a physical, to have their blood pressure (BP) checked, and to have a primary care physician than normotensives. However, African Americans were less likely to have received a BP check or have a primary care physician but more likely to have had a physical and to have visited an emergency room. These differences were noted despite the fact that all the participants in the study were eligible for Medicare and within easy driving distance of a major medical center. In addition, these differences persisted even when controlling for other factors such as age, gender, education, and living arrangements (1). African Americans, who attributed hypertension to poor health behaviors and stress, were most likely to believe that high BP could be prevented and did show a slightly lower utilization of preventive services than non-Hispanic whites.

These findings may have an impact on the treatment of hypertension in several ways, such as (a) patient-specific lifestyle modifications are imperative for all African-American hypertensives because many perceive hypertension as preventable; (b) BP checks should be incorporated into the office visit of any elderly African-American patient; (c) community health fairs are still necessary because many elderly have difficulty getting to a physician's office and/or do not have a regular primary care physician; (d) mechanisms must be put into place to facilitate the process of assigning a patient to a primary care provider; (e) emergency room providers must be included in any hypertension education initiatives because African Americans get a disproportionate amount of their care in the emergency room; and (f) stress and other psychosocial factors must be addressed by clinicians during an office visit or by specialty referrals. Once clinicians understand the perceptions and attitudes of older adults regarding hypertension, they can begin behavioral modification and pharmacological therapy programs specifically tailored to the needs of elderly African-American patients.

PHARMACOLOGICAL THERAPY

Diuretics

The Antihypertensive Lipid-Lowering Treatment to Prevent Heart Attack Trial (ALLHAT) and Systolic Hypertension in the Elderly Program (SHEP) study have given strong support to the use of diuretics in elderly African Americans *(2,3)*. Both clinical trials used the thiazide diuretic chlorthalidone either alone or in combination with other antihypertensive therapy. ALLHAT was the largest BP study ever completed, and the participants had a mean age of 67 years, with about 6000 people in the trial older than 85 years. ALLHAT consisted of a population that was approximately 35% African American; thus, it has particular relevance to the treatment of elderly African-American hypertensives. The ALLHAT study authors concluded that (a) thiazide-type diuretics are the preferred first step in the treatment of most hypertensive patients, (b) combination therapy that includes a diuretic will be required in most patients, and (c) goal BPs are achievable in most hypertensive patients.

A review by Moser *(4)* of the ALLHAT findings in the elderly subgroup was even more revealing. ALLHAT included 13,000 patients over the age of 65 years who were followed over 5 years. Over that 5-year period, mean BP was reduced from 147/81 to 135/77 mmHg with minimal clinically significant differences in the achieved BP in the group older than 65 years among the calcium antagonist and diuretic subgroups. Although the overall difference between the achieved BP in the calcium antagonist (amlodipine) and diuretic (chlorthalidone) groups was less than 1 mmHg, the large number of patients resulted in a difference that achieved statistical significance.

The morbidity/mortality data in the group 75 years and older was analyzed and used to compare the amlodipine, chlorthalidone, and angiotensin-converting enzyme (ACE) inhibitor (lisinopril) groups. When comparing chlorthalidone with amlodipine, there were no statistically significant differences between the two drugs in myocardial infarctions (MIs), strokes, all-cause mortality, and coronary heart disease, but there was a statistically significant difference in the occurrence of heart failure. The chlorthalidone-based treatment group had a 22% lower occurrence of heart failure compared with the amlodipine-based treatment program. In the lisinopril-based group, there were more episodes of heart failure, with a statistically significant 20% increase in the lisinopril group vs the diuretic group. The African-American cohort contributed disproportionately to the increased rate of cardiovascular events noted in the lisinopril-treated group.

However, several factors should be kept in mind before deciding on diuretic therapy based on the ALLHAT results. First, after 5 years of study, the African-American participants taking diuretic-based therapy had a systolic blood pressure (SBP) that was 4 mmHg lower than that of the lisinopril group. Second, the BP difference may explain why the diuretic group had fewer adverse outcomes. Third, the ACE inhibitor reduced the incidence of new-onset diabetes compared with the other agents (lisinopril 8%, amlodipine 10%, and chlorthalidone 12%). Last, it is important to remember that ALLHAT was a trial in which there was no statistically significant difference in the primary outcome (fatal and nonfatal MI) despite the superior efficacy noted in the diuretic group.

The SHEP trial included 4736 participants aged 60 years and older with an SBP between 160 and 219 mmHg and a diastolic blood pressure (DBP) less than 90 mmHg. African Americans accounted for 14% of the subjects in this trial (3). The trial was primarily designed to determine whether treatment with chlorthalidone and atenolol or reserpine, if needed, could reduce the risk of fatal and nonfatal stroke in elderly patients with isolated systolic hypertension. Participants were randomly assigned to a placebo vs stepped care regimen. All the subjects in the active treatment were initially started on 12.5 mg chlorthalidone, which could be titrated up to 25 mg if they were not at goal BP. Participants who were still not at goal on chlorthalidone could have 25–50 mg atenolol added to their regimen. Reserpine could be used if atenolol was contraindicated.

The active treatment group was noted to have mean reductions in SBP and DBP of 26 mmHg and 9 mmHg, respectively, when compared with baseline (3). The average follow-up was 4.5 years, and the active treatment group had a significant reduction in several clinical outcomes. Active treatment was associated with a 36% reduction in fatal and nonfatal strokes, a 27% reduction in MIs and coronary death, a 32% reduction in major cardiovascular events, and a 13% reduction in all-cause mortality compared with placebo. Interestingly, African-American women, white women, and white men benefited from active treatment, but this was not evident in African-American men (5). However, the lack of a significant benefit in African-American men may have partly been caused by the small number of stroke events in this cohort.

The excess risk associated with hypertension in African Americans compels clinicians to strive to reach goal BP in this group. In general, when treating hypertensive elderly African Americans with diuretics, clinicians can certainly expect significant efficacy in most patients. However, the real clinical question is whether diuretics confer any special advantage over other antihypertensives in reducing the cardiovascular outcomes that disproportionately affect African Americans. An article by Messerli et al. suggested that thiazide diuretics confer a particular benefit in reducing the risk of stroke and stated that this benefit may be independent of the BP-lowering effect *(6)*. The authors recommended that low-dose diuretics should be used alone or in combination for all hypertensive patients at risk for cerebrovascular disease. African Americans with hypertension have a higher overall risk of stroke in comparison to their hypertensive white counterparts; however, more data are needed before making the recommendation to use diuretics in all African Americans with hypertension.

In summary, thiazide diuretics are an attractive choice for elderly African-American hypertensives for several reasons, including (a) good efficacy and cardiovascular benefit were noted in both the ALLHAT and SHEP trials; (b) the low cost of diuretics will allow many senior citizens on fixed incomes to afford them; (c) thiazide diuretics have good synergy when combined with most other antihypertensives; and (d) thiazide diuretics seem to have particularly significant effects in those cardiovascular outcomes that disproportionately affect the elderly, such as congestive heart failure (CHF) and stroke. There will probably always be a debate regarding whether thiazide diuretics should be first-line therapy in most hypertensives, but it can certainly be argued that they certainly have a place in the management of elderly African-American patients with high BP.

Non-Thiazide Diuretics

The loop diuretics can also be very useful in reducing the BP of selected patients, but the available data are minimal compared with that for the thiazide diuretics. At present, the main indication for loop diuretics in hypertension has been in patients with abnormal kidney function because thiazide diuretics often become ineffective as the serum creatinine rises above 2 mg/dL. The disadvantage of loop diuretics is that they often must be dosed two to three times a day and therefore reduce compliance. Also, the significant increase in diuretic potency compared with thiazide diuretics can make this class of drugs an unattractive alternative for incontinent patients and those elderly hypertensives who have poor mobility.

The potassium-sparing diuretics, which are also called the aldosterone antagonists, have recently generated a lot of interest because a new agent, eplerenone, has been approved for the treatment of hypertension. The old standard aldosterone antagonist spironolactone has generated renewed interest because of its clinical efficacy in patients with CHF *(7)*. These drugs have two unique advantages over other diuretics: (a) a different mode of action (i.e., aldosterone antagonism) and (b) the potassium-sparing property, making patients less prone to hypokalemia. Hypokalemia has been found to induce arrhythmias in selected groups of patients, and in the SHEP trial, the subset of patients with hypokalemia did not have the same benefit from diuretic therapy as those with normal electrolytes. This class of drugs has also been recommended by the Seventh Report of the Joint National Committee on the Prevention, Detection, Evaluation, and Treatment of High Blood Pressure (JNC 7) as a therapy in post-MI and CHF patients with hypertension *(7–9)*.

Eplerenone was evaluated in a clinical trial consisting of 348 African-American and 203 white patients with mild-to-moderate hypertension *(10)*. Patients were randomly assigned to double-blind treatment with 50 mg of eplerenone, the 50 mg of angiotensin II receptor antagonist losartan, or placebo once daily. For reduction of SBP, eplerenone was superior to placebo and losartan in black patients. Eplerenone was as effective as losartan in reducing SBP and DBP in the high-renin patient, but more effective than losartan in the low-renin patient. This last finding has particular significance for elderly African-American hypertensives, who are often low renin and salt sensitive.

In clinical practice, this class of drugs will probably be used in the following groups of patients: (a) those with refractory hypertension because aldosterone-antagonists have a unique mechanism of action; (b) post-MI and CHF patients already on conventional therapy with β-blockers and ACE inhibitors; (c) those with aldosterone excess; and (d) patients prone to hypokalemia secondary to pharmacological therapy.

An important message for treating the elderly with diuretics is to do frequent monitoring of the electrolytes because these patients are especially prone to hypokalemia, dehydration, and renal insufficiency. Unfortunately, eplerenone is not recommended in diabetes because the Food and Drug Administration was concerned about the risk of hyperkalemia in diabetic nephropathy. It is hoped that postmarketing surveillance and more clinical trials will result in approval for use in diabetics.

Angiotensin-Converting Enzyme Inhibitors

Treating elderly African-American hypertensives with the ACE inhibitor class of drugs has particular appeal because this group of patients is especially prone to renal insufficiency, CHF, and stroke. The African American Study of Kidney Disease (AASK) evaluated 1094 African-American patients with hypertension and renal disease, defined as having a glomerular filtration rate (GFR) between 20 and 65 mL/minute/ 1.73 m^2 *(11)*. The study was designed to evaluate the impact of three different treatment regimens (ramipril, amlodipine, and metoprolol) and two different BP goals (low and usual) on the progression of hypertensive renal disease. The patients were assigned to receive ramipril (2.5– 10 mg/day), amlodipine (5–10 mg/day), or metoprolol (50–200 mg/ day). They were further randomly assigned into a usual BP goal group (mean arterial pressure [MAP] of 102–107 mmHg) and low BP goal group (MAP <92 mmHg).

This trial was not specifically aimed at the elderly, but the results are worthy of closer attention. AASK found that a ramipril-based treatment regimen slowed the progression of renal disease to a significantly greater extent than amlodipine and metoprolol when renal disease was looked at as a composite of a 50% decline in GFR, deaths, and end-stage renal disease (ESRD). Of note, a significant proportion of patients were able to achieve target BP levels irrespective of age, sex, body mass index, education level, insurance, or employment status. The majority of patients needed multiple drugs to reach their target BP; however, the ACE inhibitor-based therapy produced the above findings despite a similar reduction in BP when compared to the other two agents. Therefore, elderly African-American hypertensives with renal insufficiency should be considered for ACE inhibitor therapy in view of the AASK study and the lack of other significant data on therapy for this population.

The Heart Outcomes Prevention Evaluation trial evaluated high-risk patients who were treated with the ACE inhibitor ramipril *(12)*. Although the study did not include a significant number of African Americans, it is worth mentioning because the results suggest that the treatment drug has some benefit that extends beyond BP lowering. Also, the target population was composed of older patients with multiple comorbid conditions.

Significant controversy still exists concerning whether the Heart Outcomes Prevention Evaluation trial results are truly independent of a BP difference between the study populations *(13)*. A subsequent substudy found that when 24-hour BP monitoring was performed, the BP reduction in the ACE inhibitor group was greater than that of the placebo group *(14)*. This was largely because office BP taken during the day did not reveal the large BP reductions at night that were captured by 24-hour BP monitoring. This nocturnal drop in BP in the ramipril group was caused by evening dosing of the study medication.

Many clinicians rarely prescribe ACE inhibitors as monotherapy because of the belief that they will not be effective in African-American patients. This belief that ACE inhibitors have poor efficacy in this population is based on the fact that ACE inhibitors have been found in some cases to lower BP less in African Americans vs white hypertensives *(13,15)*. Also, because African-American and elderly populations tend to have low circulating levels of renin vs other groups, some clinicians and researchers feel drugs that inhibit the renin–angiotensin system will theoretically have less effectiveness in low-renin patients. This low-renin hypothesis is supported by clinical trials, which have found that both diuretics and calcium antagonists have better BP-lowering efficacy than ACE inhibitors in African Americans *(16,17)*.

The Hypertension in African-Americans Working Group of the International Society on Hypertension in Blacks published a consensus statement that revealed some of the limitations in the prior data, suggesting that ACE inhibitors may be less-effective agents: (a) prior studies generally did not report SBP responses; (b) response rates are generally reported as a reduction of 10 mmHg or more from baseline rather than achievement of target BP; (c) individual hypertensive agents cannot be used as a proxy for class effect; (d) conclusions cannot be drawn regarding the best course of treatment in patients who did not have an effective BP-lowering response to antihypertensive treatment; and (e) the high doses of thiazide diuretics (50–100 mg) used in prior studies are rarely used in current clinical practice *(18)*. Physicians are also concerned about literature indicating that African-Americans have a higher incidence of ACE inhibitor-induced angioedema and cough than whites *(19,20)*.

Stroke prevention is an important issue in the elderly African-American population, and thus the Perindopril Protection Against Recurrent Stroke study is worthy of review *(21)*. This study was a double-blind, placebo-controlled, randomized trial that evaluated 6105 individuals (mean age 64 years; range 26–91 years) with a prior history of stroke or transient ischemic attack from 172 centers in Europe, Asia, and Australasia. The active treatment group received a flexible regimen of the ACE inhibitor perindopril (4 mg daily) with the addition of the diuretic indapamide if deemed necessary by the treating physicians. The primary outcome was both fatal and nonfatal stroke. Combination therapy with perindopril plus indapamide reduced BP by 12/5 mmHg and stroke risk by 43%; perindopril alone reduced BP by 5/3 mmHg but did not result in a statistically significant reduction in stroke. Also, both hypertensives and nonhypertensives were included, and both groups had similar reductions in strokes. The JNC 7 subsequently recommended diuretics plus ACE inhibitors as a treatment for recurrent stroke prevention *(8)*. The lack of participation by the United States and the absence of any reference to persons of African descent by the investigators will increase concern that this trial may not be applicable to African Americans.

Overall, we feel that the use of a diuretic with the ACE inhibitor and the use of a higher dose of the perindopril (8 mg or more) should give the clinician some reassurance that these findings will be applicable to their African-American patient population.

Should ACE inhibitors be used in elderly African-American hypertensives? Overall, the evidence suggests that this class of agents should provide significant protection from target end-organ damage. Therefore, these drugs seem to have a special indication in the so-called complicated hypertensive patient, defined as a person with diabetes, evidence of target end-organ damage, or a history of a cardiovascular event *(22)*. It is also important to remember that in the AASK trial the ACE inhibitor group had a 46% reduction in ESRD or death compared with the amlodipine group. When the AASK study findings are coupled with the fact that African Americans are six times more likely to develop ESRD than whites, it is difficult to exclude ACE inhibitors or other renin–angiotensin blocking agents unless they are specifically contraindicated *(23)*.

Angiotensin II Receptor Blockers

According to the JNC 7, angiotensin II receptor blockers (ARBs) are indicated for hypertensive patients with high coronary disease risk, diabetes, and heart failure *(8)*. The elderly African-American hypertensive population may potentially benefit from this hypertensive drug class if these drugs can be proven to have all the clinical benefits of an ACE inhibitor without the adverse effects. Unfortunately, the number of African Americans in clinical trials evaluating the effectiveness of ARBs is small.

The Losartan Intervention for Endpoint reduction in hypertension trial is a double-blind, randomized, parallel-group study designed to test the effectiveness of the ARB losartan vs the β-blocker atenolol in reducing cardiovascular morbidity, MI, and stroke in 9193 patients with hypertension and left ventricular hypertrophy *(24)*. In the subgroup of 533 African Americans, the atenolol-treated group had a lower risk of the primary end point vs losartan-treated African Americans (6% atenolol vs 11% losartan). In contrast, losartan reduced the primary end point more than atenolol in the general study population. Overall, the take-home message is probably to be careful when interpreting trial results, which come from small subgroups; thus, we await larger clinical trials.

Diabetics have a special need for ARBs, as seen in clinical trials *(25,26)*. The Irbesartan Diabetic Nephropathy Trial was designed to determine whether the use of an ARB or calcium channel blocker would provide protection against the progression of nephropathy caused by type 2 diabetes beyond that attributable to BP lowering. The participants (mean age 59 years) had to have type 2 diabetes, hypertension, and proteinuria, with protein excretion of at least 900 mg per 24 hours, to be eligible *(25)*. There were 228 African-American participants out of a total study population of 1715 hypertensive patients, with all enrollees followed for a mean duration of 2.6 years. Treatment with irbesartan was associated with a relative risk of ESRD that was 23% lower than in both the placebo and amlodipine groups. The irbesartan group also had a 37% lower risk of doubling the serum creatinine than the amlodipine-treated patients. These findings were independent of BP.

The Reduction in Renal Endpoints in Type 2 Diabetes with Angiotensin II Antagonist Losartan trial was also performed on type 2 diabetics with hypertension and proteinuria *(26)*. There were 1513 patients (15.2% African-American) enrolled in this randomized, double-blind study comparing losartan (50–100mg once daily) with placebo, both taken in addition to conventional antihypertensive treatment (calcium antagonist, diuretics, α-blockers, β-blockers, and centrally acting agents) for a mean follow-up of 3.4 years. The primary outcome was the composite of a doubling of the baseline serum creatinine concentration, ESRD, or death. Losartan reduced the incidence of a doubling of serum creatinine (25% risk reduction) and ESRD (28% risk reduction) but had no effect on the rate of death. The level of proteinuria declined by 35% in the losartan group compared to the placebo group. The benefit was found to exceed that purely attributable to BP, and losartan was well tolerated. Overall, both irbesartan and losartan were found to be beneficial in type 2 diabetics with nephropathy.

African Americans represent 12% of the US population but still account for 30% of the new cases entering dialysis programs and have the highest incidence (1996–1999) of hypertension-related ESRD *(27)*. Unfortunately, the proportions of African-American patients in the above trials involving ARBs is not representative of the proportion of black patients among those with ESRD in the United States. In addition, the reports of the Irbesartan Diabetic Nephropathy Trial and Reduction in Renal Endpoints in Type 2 Diabetes with Angiotensin II Antagonist Losartan studies do not include subgroup analysis of the treatment response according to race *(28)*. However, the higher incidence of ESRD in African Americans and the low adverse event rate of ARBs will continue to make this class of agents a frequent first-line or adjunct therapy for clinicians.

We also suggest that clinicians treating elderly African Americans with ARBs should remember to give relatively high doses as is recommended with ACE inhibitors and to do cost comparisons among the various agents because many senior citizens do not have adequate drug benefits. Last, it is important to expect a rise in serum creatinine levels during initial therapy with either ARBs or ACE-inhibitors, but the drugs should not be discontinued unless there is at least a 30% rise in creatinine or significant hyperkalemia. Given the very high incidence of ESRD in blacks, it is advisable to seek specialty consultation before trying to manage African-American patients without renin–angiotensin antagonists.

Calcium Antagonists

As a class, calcium antagonists appear to make good physiological sense as a treatment modality for elderly, hypertensive African Americans. Prior investigations have found that, compared with whites, African Americans appear to have lower plasma renin levels, a potentially larger plasma volume, more peripheral and renal vascular resistance, and greater sensitivity to sodium *(29–31)*. Also, the fact that one group of investigators found that calcium sensitivity in African Americans appears to contribute to more arteriolar vasoconstriction (peripheral resistance) suggests that calcium antagonists should be considered for therapy in this population *(29,32)*. Furthermore, calcium antagonists appear to have a mild diuretic effect during the initial stages of therapy *(32)*.

African Americans, especially those residing in the southeastern United States, are exposed to various high-sodium and high-fat foods known as "soul food" as well as a large variety of "fast foods" that are often similar to soul food in terms of their fat and sodium contents. Fortunately, calcium antagonists have been found to retain their antihypertensive efficacy in the setting of high dietary sodium intake *(33)*. In addition, elderly populations can benefit from the fact that at least one clinical study has noted that calcium antagonists appear to maintain good antihypertensive efficacy in patients taking concomitant nonsteroidal anti-inflammatory drugs *(34)*. The above findings may be related to the natriuretic and diuretic activity of calcium antagonists, which in itself results from augmentation of renal blood flow and GFR seen with these agents *(29,35)*

A number of clinical trials have found that calcium channel antagonists are beneficial in African-American hypertensives. The clinical trials did not specifically focus on the elderly, but older patients were included, and it would reasonable to do some extrapolation of the data when treating elderly African-American hypertensives. One early trial demonstrated the superior efficacy of verapamil over atenolol and captopril in more than 300 African-American hypertensives *(16,29)*. The Veterans Administration Cooperative Study found that African-

American males responded better to diltiazem and hydrochlorothiazide than their white counterparts (15). All calcium channel antagonists are not created equal, and thus they are classified as dihydropyridines (nifedipine, felodipine, isradipine, nicardipine, nisoldipine, and amlodipine) and non-dihydropyridines (verapamil and diltiazem). The differences between these two subgroups may have potential clinical implications, and thus large outcome-based studies are needed to evaluate the impact these differences have on clinical outcomes.

There are two large recent clinical trials that involved calcium antagonists: ALLHAT and the International Verapamil-Trandolapril Study. ALLHAT included more than 15,000 African Americans with hypertension who were at least 55 years old and had at least one risk factor for cardiovascular disease (2). The subjects were randomly assigned to receive amlodipine (2.5–10 mg), chlorthalidone (12.5–25 mg), or lisinopril (10–40 mg). The α-blocker (doxazosin) was prematurely discontinued from the study because of an excess incidence of heart failure. The amlodipine arm was not different from the diuretic or ACE inhibitor group in the rate of nonfatal myocardial infarctions and fatal coronary disease (the primary end point) or in mortality (2,5). There also was no statistically significant difference found between amlodipine-treated and chlorthalidone-treated participants in terms of cerebrovascular events. The main difference in outcome was seen in heart failure, with the amlodipine group having a 1.47 relative risk of heart failure vs the chlorthalidone group. Given these findings, it is important to remember that the SBP was 1 mmHg lower in the diuretic-treated cohort vs the amlodipine cohort as a whole, and more than 60% of the participants needed two or more drugs to reach target BP. The difference in BP between the chlorthalidone group and the other treated groups was even more pronounced in the African-American ALLHAT cohort, which is likely to account partly for the outcome advantage noted in the chlorthalidone arm. However, the ALLHAT investigators stated that although the differences in outcome between the diuretic group and the lisinopril and amlodipine groups were not statistically reduced by statistically adjusting for the BP difference, one cannot exclude an effect of the BP difference on the treatment outcomes noted in this trial (5).

The International Verapamil-Trandolapril Study was a large, randomized, open-label, blinded end-point trial with 22,576 hypertensive coronary artery disease patients, including 3029 African Americans and 7523 patients over 70 years old from the entire cohort (36). Participants were randomly assigned to either a calcium antagonist strategy (CAS) or a non-calcium antagonist strategy (NCAS). If the participants did not achieve their target BP on CAS (verapamil sustained release) or NCAS (atenolol), trandolapril and/or hydrochlorothiazide was administered to get the BP to the goal BP as determined by the Sixth Report of the Joint National Committee on Prevention, Detection, Evaluation, and Treatment of High Blood Pressure *(37)*. The primary outcome was the first occurrence of death (all cause), nonfatal MI, or nonfatal stroke. Secondary outcomes included new-onset diabetes, time to most serious event, cardiovascular death, angina, cardiovascular hospitalizations, BP control, cancer, Alzheimer's disease, Parkinson's disease, and gastrointestinal tract bleeding at 24 months. After 2 years of follow-up, 2269 patients had a primary outcome event with no statistically significant difference between the verapamil-based treatment group and the atenolol-based treatment strategies (9.93% vs 10.17%, relative risk 0.98, 95% confidence interval 0.90–1.06). The BP control at 2 years was similar for both groups, with 72% of the CAS group and 71% of the NCAS group achieving a BP less than 140/90 mmHg. Overall, the conclusion was that the verapamil-based strategy was as clinically effective as the β-blocker-based strategy in hypertensive coronary artery disease patients *(36)*. As far as secondary outcomes, the main difference was seen in the development of new-onset diabetes. Of the 8098 CAS patients without diabetes at entry, 569 (7%) were diagnosed as having diabetes after 2 years of follow-up; 665 (8.2%) of the 8078 NCAS patients without diabetes at entry developed diabetes during the follow-up. Otherwise, no statistically significant difference in the incidence of the previously named secondary outcomes was found between the two groups.

In summary, elderly hypertensive African Americans would appear based on the literature presented here to be good candidates for treatment with calcium antagonists. The elderly are often low-renin hypertensives, and many are on nonsteroidal therapy. The question of whether calcium antagonists should be preferred initial therapy in this population will continue to be debated; however, the continued need for combination therapy to reach goal BP will certainly lead to fewer patients who will be seen as candidates for monotherapy.

Because there are two types of calcium antagonists, the second unresolved question is whether dihydropyridines or non-dihydropyridines should be the preferred choice from this drug class. The high incidence of hypertension-related renal disease in African Americans coupled with data indicating there may be differences in the degree of renal protection achieved by the two types of calcium antagonists illustrate the need for a carefully designed clinical trial in this area *(40)*. In summary, calcium antagonists should be used to achieve goal BP, especially if there are compelling indications, with the main caveat that African Americans with renal disease probably should not receive dihydropyridine calcium antagonists as monotherapy *(23)*.

β-*Blockers*

The use of β-blockers in the elderly and in special populations like African Americans has not been without considerable controversy. There have been claims of less antihypertensive efficacy in the elderly and African Americans, which may be partly or fully because these special populations also tend to have lower renin levels *(41)*. Saunders and colleagues published data that provide strong evidence that African Americans seem to have less BP response with β-blockers, but the literature concerning the elderly is less uniform *(15,16)*. The higher prevalence of stage 2 hypertension in the African-American population vs their white counterparts has also been a likely contributor to the reluctance in using a β-blocker when significant BP reduction is often needed. Furthermore, the response in African Americans with heart failure to β-blockers parallels that seen in hypertension; namely, the benefit is not as significant as that of non-black populations. The β-Blocker Evaluation of Survival Trial found that African Americans did not respond as effectively as non-blacks when using the β-blocker bucindolol to treat heart failure *(42)*.

The above findings have resulted in more attention focused on carvedilol because it is unique in its antioxidant properties and ability to inhibit both α_1-adrenergic and β_2-adrenergic receptors *(43)*. As far as heart failure, the US Carvedilol Heart Failure Trials Program found that, in contrast to the β-Blocker Evaluation of Survival Trial, the benefit of the β-blocker (carvedilol) was of a similar magnitude in both black and non-black patients with heart failure *(44)*. The antihypertensive response to this subclass of β-blockers is also very promising because the resistance to β-blockers in African Americans can be overcome by the use of a β-blocker with α-blocking properties *(45)*.

The elderly African-American population may also benefit from the finding that combined α- and β-blockade may diminish the adverse effects of β-blockade alone on blood lipids and insulin sensitivity *(46,47)*. Also, prior studies have found that African Americans have greater responses to cardiac β_2-adrenergic stimuli and peripheral α_1-stimuli than whites, particularly during states of potassium depletion *(48)*. Hypertensive African Americans often have potassium-deficient diets and frequently require diuretic therapy to reach goal blood pressure; thus. an agent that is able to maintain its efficacy during potassium depletion would be especially appealing.

In summary, elderly African Americans with hypertension can derive significant benefit from β-blockers beyond their ability to lower BP especially because the elderly have a greater prevalence of heart failure and MIs than younger populations. In sharp contrast to prior conventional wisdom, the JNC 7 now lists diabetes as a compelling indication for β-blocker therapy based largely on the results in the UK Prospective Diabetes Study *(39,49)*. Therefore, clinicians should always consider use of β-blockers in patients with hypertension plus heart failure, post-MI status, high coronary disease risk, or diabetes unless contraindicated. β-Blockers also have additive BP-lowering effects in hypertensive patients with baseline pulse rates greater than 84 beats per minute *(38)*. Patients who are taking first-generation β-blockers, like propanolol or atenolol, but need both aggressive BP reduction and β-blockade, may benefit from agents with combined α- and β-blocking properties like labetalol and carvedilol. However, more head-to-head comparisons will be needed before investigators can make strong conclusions about the superiority or inferiority of one β-blocker vs another in elderly African-American hypertensives.

Combination Therapy

The consensus statements of the Hypertension in African-Americans Working (HAAW) Group and the JNC 7 have both endorsed the use of combination therapy in many, if not the majority, of hypertensive patients *(18,39)*. In addition to the clinical data, there is reason to believe that combination therapy may also be cost-effective and improve compliance in African Americans *(50)*. An analysis was done to assess the potential financial impact of substituting a combination ACE inhibitor and calcium channel blocker (CCB) therapy (benazepril-amlodipine) for the two-drug treatment using benazepril and amlodipine as two separate prescriptions. In this cost analysis, they found that using a fixed-dose combination resulted in a savings of $1080 per patient per year vs the treatment plan using two separate drugs. This has particular significance for senior citizens, who are usually on a fixed income and often do not have pharmacy benefits.

Combination therapy in African Americans is often required if you are going to use β-blockers, ACE inhibitors, or ARBs. Also, not all combinations make good physiological sense or are equally efficacious in treating hypertension. A review of the available clinical data from randomized controlled clinical trials revealed that the following two-drug combinations may be considered effective: ACE inhibitor/diuretic, ARB/diuretic, β-blocker/diuretic, and ACE inhibitor/CCB *(18)*. Although some clinical trials have not had large numbers of African Americans, race should not be used as a rationale for avoiding certain classes of antihypertensives. In fact, some of the racial differences with monotherapy can be overcome by combining two drugs, a diuretic with a renin-angiotensin system-blocking agent *(51)*. The additional reduction in BP achieved by combining low doses of two antihypertensive drugs can be substantial, with an additional 4 to 6 mmHg reduction in diastolic pressure and 8–11 mmHg additional reduction in systolic pressure compared to monotherapy *(51)*.

Are there some combinations of antihypertensive drugs that will provide better efficacy and a larger reduction in cardiovascular outcomes? Unfortunately, there is scarce clinical trial outcome evidence to support the recommendation of an optimal combination therapy for African Americans or any other subpopulation. At present, we would agree with the recommendations by the HAWW Group, which is not to assume that individual African-American patients will not respond to available therapy. Combining two drugs may also reduce the potential adverse effects of one of the drugs, for example, the reduced incidence of peripheral edema in patients on both an ACE inhibitor and CCB vs CCB monotherapy. A new clinical trial, Avoiding Cardiovascular Events Through Combination therapy in Patients Living With Systolic Hypertension (ACCOMPLISH), will directly compare cardiovascular mortality and morbidity rates for two fixed-dose combination therapies *(53,54)*. While clinicians await the completion of this trial, elderly African-American hypertensives should be treated with combination therapy according to the HAAW Group guidelines (Fig. 1). Also, because cost and compliance are often correlated, clinicians should get pharmacy prices for fixed-dose combinations whenever two-drug therapy is used to see if the fixed-dose preparations are more cost-effective.

ADDITIONAL CONSIDERATIONS IN TREATING ELDERLY AFRICAN AMERICANS

There are two well-known guidelines on hypertension treatment that have been discussed: those of the JNC 7 and of the HAAW Group *(8,18)*. The guidelines have very similar recommendations; however, the differences should be understood to avoid confusion when treating patients. The main differences are the recommendation by the HAAW Group that combination therapy be instituted for a BP 155/100 mmHg or greater; the JNC 7 recommends the same therapy if the BP is 160/100 mmHg or greater in uncomplicated hypertensives with a goal BP less than 140/90 mmHg. Patients with diabetes and/or chronic kidney disease are recommended for combination therapy if the BP is 15/10 mmHg or greater above goal BP of 130/80 mmHg in the HAAW Group guidelines, and the JNC 7 consensus panel recommended the same treatment if the BP is 20/10 mmHg or greater above goal BP (Fig. 1).

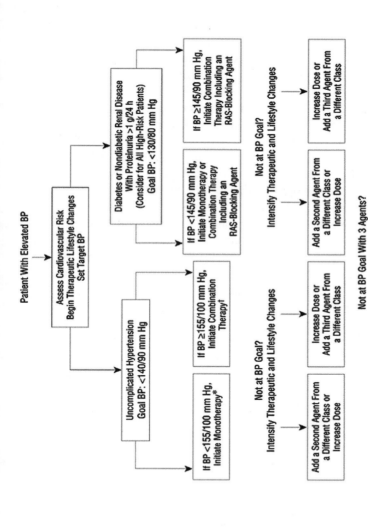

Fig. 1. Clinical algorithm for achieving target blood pressure (BP) in African-American patients with high BP. Asterisk (*)Initiate monotherapy at the recommended starting dose with an agent from any of the following classes: diuretics, β-blockers, calcium channel blockers (CCBs), angiotensin-converting enzyme (ACE) inhibitors, or angiotensin II receptor blockers (ARBs). †Initiate low-dose combination therapy with any of the following combinations: β-blocker/diuretic, ACE inhibitor/diuretic, ACE inhibitor/CCB, or ARB/diuretic. RAS, renin–angiotensin system. (Reproduced with permission from ref. 18.)

The other difference is that the JNC 7 panel gives a stronger endorsement than the HAAW group for the use of thiazide diuretics as initial therapy in both diabetic and nondiabetic patients who are eligible for monotherapy. Fortunately, it is not difficult to decide how to treat most African-American patients because the majority will usually benefit from combination therapy. Because so many patients require combination therapy, issues related to initial monotherapy will not have as much importance in the treatment of elderly African Americans.

As far as the difference in the levels of BP recommended to initiate treatment, namely, 160/100 mmHg or greater in the JNC 7 vs 155/100 mmHg or greater in the HAAW guidelines, the difference is small enough such that clinicians can use their own judgment to treat hypertensive patients as long as goal BP is reached. In summary, both guidelines recommend diuretics, ACE inhibitors, ARBs, calcium antagonists, β-blockers, or a combination of these to treat most patients *(8,18)*.

Last, the role of religion in the health care of elderly hypertensive African Americans should not be ignored. The belief in the power of religion has been a guiding force in African-American health care since slavery *(55)*. Research has shown that individuals who believe in the therapeutic power of faith find that regular church attendance, Bible study, and prayer lower BP, prevent depression, and promote healthy lifestyles and a longer life. Furthermore, patients who find comfort in prayer and their religious faith are three times more likely to survive than their nonreligious counterparts *(56)*.

In all, over 350 studies have examined the effects of religious involvement on health *(57)*. Results of these studies essentially showed that people who were considered religious had healthy lifestyles and required fewer health services. As clinicians struggle to increase compliance with a healthy lifestyle, understanding the role of religion in the African-American community will certainly have a positive impact on the health of their patients.

How should clinicians improve their understanding of the African-American church? First, we would encourage visiting churches in communities during worship services as opposed to just coming for health fairs. Second, consider setting up a special time to meet with some members of clergy; this will allow you to find out different health concerns in the community. Last, do not forget to inquire about whether a patient attends church; this is important because some elderly patients may have few living relatives, and thus church members may be your only source of information in an emergency situation.

REFERENCES

1. Ontiveras JA, Black SA, Jakobi PL, Goodwin JS. Ethnic variation in attitudes toward hypertension in adults ages 75 and older. *Prev Med* 1999;29:443–449.
2. The ALLHAT Collaborative Research Group. Major outcomes in high-risk hypertensive patients randomized to angiotensin-converting enzyme inhibitor or calcium channel blocker vs diuretic: the Antihypertensive and Lipid-Lowering Treatment to Prevent Heart Attack Trial (ALLHAT). *JAMA* 2002;288:2981–2997.
3. SHEP Cooperative Research Group. Prevention of stroke by antihypertensive drug treatment in older persons with isolated systolic hypertension. *JAMA* 1991;265: 3255–3264.
4. Moser M. Treatment of hypertension in the very elderly: a clinician's point of view. *J Clin Hypertens (Greenwich)* 2003;5:310–312.
5. Wright JT, Douglas J. Optimal treatment of hypertension and cardiovascular risk reduction in African-Americans: treatment approaches for outpatients. *J Clin Hypertens (Greenwich)* 2003;5(1 suppl 1):18–25.
6. Messerli FH, Grossman E, Lever AF. Do thiazide diuretics confer specific protection against strokes? *Arch Intern Med* 2003;163:2557–2560.
7. Pitt B, Zannad F, Remme WJ, et al. for Randomized Aldactone Evaluation Study Investigators. The effect of spironolactone on morbidity and mortality in patients with severe heart failure. *N Engl J Med* 1999;341:709–717.
8. Chobanian AV, Bakris GL, Black HR, et al. The seventh report of the Joint National Committee on Prevention, Detection, Evaluation, and Treatment of High Blood Pressure: the JNC 7 report. *JAMA* 2003;289:2560–2571.
9. Pitt B, Remme W, Zannad F, et al. Eplerenone, a selective aldosterone blocker, in patients with left ventricular dysfunction after myocardial infarction. *N Engl J Med* 2003;348:1309–1321.
10. Flack JM, Oparil S, Pratt JH, Roniker B, et al. Efficacy and tolerability of eplerenone and losartan in hypertensive black and white patients. *J Am Coll Cardiol* 2003;41:1148–1155.
11. Agodoa LY, Appel L, Bakris GL, et al. Effect of ramipril vs amlodipine on renal outcomes in hypertensive nephrosclerosis. A randomized controlled trial. *JAMA* 2001;285:2719–2728.
12. The Heart Outcomes Prevention Evaluation Study Investigators. Effects of an angiotensin-converting enzyme inhibitor, ramipril, on cardiovascular events in high-risk patients. *N Engl J Med* 2000;342:145–153.
13. Saunders E, Gavin JR 3rd. Blockade of the renin-angiotensin System in African-Americans with hypertension and cardiovascular disease. *J Clin Hypertens (Greenwich)* 2003;5:12–17.
14. Svensson P, de Faire U, Sleight P, et al. Comparative effects of ramipril on ambulatory and office blood pressures. A HOPE substudy. *Hypertension* 2001;38:e28–e32.
15. Materson BJ, Reda DJ, Cushman WC, et al. Single-drug therapy for hypertension in men. A comparison of six antihypertensive agents with placebo. *N Engl J Med* 1993:328:914–921.
16. Saunders E, Weir M, Kong BW, et al. A comparison of the efficacy and safety of a β-blocker, a calcium channel blocker, and a converting enzyme inhibitor in hypertensive blacks. *Arch Intern Med* 1990;150:1707–1713.
17. Materson BJ, Reda DJ, Williams D, for the Department of Veterans Affairs Cooperative Study Group on Antihypertensive Agents. Lessons from combination therapy in Veterans Affairs Studies. *Am J Hypertens* 1996;9:187S–191S.

18. Douglas JG, Bakris GL, Epstein M, et al. Management of high blood pressure in African-Americans. Consensus statement of the Hypertension in African-Americans Working Group of the International Society on Hypertension in Blacks. *Arch Intern Med* 2003;163:525–541.

19. Brown NJ, Ray WA, Snowden M, Griffin MR. Black Americans have an increased rate of angiotensin converting enzyme inhibitor-associated angioedema. *Clin Pharmacol Ther* 1996;60:8–13.

20. Elliott WJ. Higher incidence of discontinuation of angiotensin enzyme inhibitors due to cough in black subjects. *Clin Pharmacol Ther* 1996;60:582–588.

21. PROGRESS Collaborative Group. Randomized trial of a perindopril-based blood-pressure-lowering regimen among 6105 individuals with previous stroke or transient ischemic attack. *Lancet* 2001;358:1033–1041.

22. Johnson WR, Saunders E, Jones-Burton C: Hypertension in African-Americans. In Egan BM, Basile JN, Lackland DT, eds. *Hot Topics in Hypertension*. Philadelphia: Hanley and Belfus; 2004: 406–407.

23. Wright JT Jr, Bakris G, Greene T, et al. Effect of blood pressure lowering and antihypertensive drug class on progression of hypertensive kidney disease: results from the AASK trial. *JAMA* 2002;288:2421–2431.

24. Dahlof B, Devereux RB, Kjeldsen SE, et al. Cardiovascular morbidity and mortality in the Losartan Intervention For Endpoint reduction in hypertension study (LIFE): a randomized trial against atenolol. *Lancet* 2002;359:995–1003.

25. Lewis EJ, Hunsicker LG, Clarke WR, et al. Renoprotective effect of the angiotensin-receptor antagonist irbesartan in patients with nephropathy due to type 2 diabetes. *N Engl J Med* 2001;345:851–860.

26. Brenner BM, Cooper ME, De Zeeuw D, et al. Effects of losartan on renal and cardiovascular outcomes in patients with type 2 diabetes and nephropathy. *N Engl J Med* 2001;345:861–869.

27. Kaperonis N, Bakris G. Blood pressure, antihypertensive therapy and risk for renal injury in African-Americans. *Curr Opin Nephrol Hypertens* 2003;12:79–84.

28. Hostetter TH. Editorial. *N Engl J Med* 2001;345:910–912.

29. Saunders E. Benefits of calcium channel antagonists in controlling hypertension in African-American patients: factors in drug selection. *ABC Digest Urban Cardiol* 1999;6:11–15.

30. Weir MR. Population characteristics and the modulation of the renin-angiotensin system in the treatment of hypertension. *J Hum Hypertens* 1997;11:17–21.

31. Krieger N, et al. Discrimination in African-Americans: the effect on the incidence of hypertension. *Am J Pub Health* 1996;86:1370–1378.

32. Leonetti G. The effects of calcium antagonists on electrolytes and water balance in hypertensive patients. *J Cardiovasc Pharmacol* 1994;24(suppl A):S25–S29.

33. Redon J, Lozano JV, de la Figuera M, et al. Do changes in dietary influence blood pressure of hypertensive patients pharmacologically controlled with verapamil? The Salt-Switching-Study (SSS). *J Hum Hypertens* 1995;9:143–147.

34. Houston MC, Weir MR, Gray J, et al. The effects of nonsteroidal anti-inflammatory drugs on blood pressures of patients with hypertension controlled by verapamil. *Arch Intern Med* 1995;155:1049–1054.

35. Krishna GC, Riley LJ, Deuter G, et al. Natriuretic effect of calcium-channel blockers in hypertensives. *Am J Kidney Dis* 1991;18:566–572.

36. Pepine CJ, Handberg EM, Cooper-Dehoff RM, et al. A calcium antagonist vs a non-calcium antagonist hypertension treatment strategy for patients with coronary artery disease. The International Verapamil-Trandolapril Study (INVEST): a randomized controlled trial. *JAMA* 2003;290:2805–2816.

37. The Sixth Report of the Joint National Committee on Prevention, Detection, Evaluation, and Treatment of High Blood pressure. National Institutes of Health; National Heart, Lung, and Blood Institute; National High Blood Pressure Education Program. November 1997. NIH Publication No. 98-4080.

38. Bakris GL, Dworkin WH, Elliott WJ, et al. Preserving renal function in adults with hypertension and diabetes; a consensus approach. National Kidney Foundation Hypertension and Diabetes Executive Committee Working Group. *Am J Kidney Dis* 2000;36:646–661.

39. Chobanian AV, Bakris GL, Black HR, et al. Joint National Committee on Prevention, Detection, Evaluation, and Treatment of high Blood Pressure. Seventh report of the Joint National Committee on Prevention, Detection, Evaluation, and treatment of High Blood Pressure. *Hypertension* 2003;42:1206–1252.

40. Bakris GL, Williams M, Dworkin L, et al. Preserving renal function in adults with hypertension and diabetes: a consensus approach. *Am J Kidney Dis* 2000;36:646–661.

41. Kaplan NM. Clinical Hypertension. 7th ed. Baltimore, MD: Williams and Wilkins; 1998:210–211.

42. A trial of the β-blocker bucindolol in patients with advanced chronic heart failure. *N Engl J Med* 2001;344:1659–1667.

43. Feuerstein G, Yue TL, Ma X, Ruffolo RR. Novel mechanisms in the treatment of heart failure: inhibition of oxygen radicals and apoptosis by carvedilol. *Prog Cardiovasc Dis* 1998;41(1 suppl 1):17–24.

44. Yancy CW, Fowler MB, Colucci WS, et al. Race and the response to adrenergic blockade with carvedilol in patients with chronic heart failure. *N Engl J Med* 2001;344:1358–1365.

45. Flamenbaum W, Weber MA, McMahon FG, et al. Monotherapy with labetalol compared with propanolol: differential effects by race. *J Clin Hypertens* 1985;1:56–69.

46. Jacob S, Rett K, Wicklmayr M, et al. Differential effect of chronic treatment with two beta-blocking agents on insulin sensitivity: the carvedilol-metoprolol study. *J Hypertens* 1996;14:489–494.

47. Giugliano MD, Acampora R, Marfella R, et al. Metabolic and cardiovascular effects of carvedilol and atenolol in non-insulin-dependent diabetes mellitus and hypertension: a randomized, controlled trial. *Ann Intern Med* 1997;126:955–959.

48. Sudhir K, Forman A, Yi SL, et al. Reduced dietary potassium reversibly enhances vasopressor response to stress in African-Americans. *Hypertension* 1997;29: 1083–1090.

49. UK Prospective Diabetes Study Group. Efficacy of atenolol and captopril in reducing risk of macrovascular and microvascular complications in type 2 diabetes: UKPDS 39. *BMJ* 1998;317:713–720.

50. Kountz DS. Cost containment for treating hypertension in African-Americans: impact of a combined ACE-inhibitor-calcium channel blocker. *J Natl Med Assoc* 1997;89:457–460.

51. Ferdinand KC. Recommendations for the management of special populations: racial and ethnic populations. *Am J Hypertens* 2003;16(11 pt 2):50S–54S.

52. Messerili FH, Oparil S, Feng Z. Comparison of efficacy and side effects of combination therapy of angiotensin-converting enzyme inhibitor (benazepril) with calcium antagonist (either nifedipine or amlodipine) vs high-dose calcium antagonist monotherapy for systemic hypertension. *Am J Cardiol* 2000;86:1182–1187.

53. Jamerson KA, Bakris GL, Douglas JG, et al. Design of the ACCOMPLISH (Avoiding Cardiovascular Events Through Combination Therapy in Patients Living With Systolic Hypertension) trial [abstract P-431]. *Am J Hypertens* 2003;16:193A.

54. Jamerson KA. The first hypertension trial comparing the effects of two fixed-dose combination therapy regimens on cardiovascular events: Avoiding Cardiovascular Events Through Combination Therapy in Patients Living With Systolic Hypertension (ACCOMPLISH). *J Clin Hypertens* 2003;5(4 suppl 3):29–35.
55. Lincoln C. Race, *religion, and the Continuing American Dilemma*. New York: Hill and Wang; 1984.
56. Koenig H. *The Healing Power of Faith*. New York: Simon and Schuster; 1999.
57. Walker CC, Kong BW, Benjamin TG, Ofili EO. *The Healing Power of Faith*. ABC Digest Urban Cardiol 2002;9:8–16.

22 Treatment of Hypertension in the Elderly Patient With Diabetes

James R. Sowers, MD, FACE, FACP, FAHA and L. Michael Prisant, MD, FACC, FACP

CONTENTS

OVERVIEW

More than 16 million people in the United States have diabetes mellitus (DM), and another 40 million have hypertension. These chronic diseases often coexist in our aging population. Both diseases are important predisposing factors for the development of cardiovascular and renal disease, and the coexistence of these risk factors is a very powerful pro-

From: *Clinical Hypertension and Vascular Diseases: Hypertension in the Elderly*
Edited by: L. M. Prisant © Humana Press Inc., Totowa, NJ

moter of both cardiovascular and renal disease. There is accumulating evidence that the rigorous treatment of hypertension and other risk factors such as dyslipidemia and hyperglycemia lessen the burden of cardiovascular disease (CVD), stroke, and renal disease in patients with DM.

Optimal therapy in these patients includes treatment with an aspirin, statins, aggressive control of hyperglycemia, and lowering of blood pressure (BP) to less than 130/80 mmHg *(1)*. There is also considerable data to suggest that the treatment strategies that interrupt the renin–angiotensin system have special benefits in diabetic patients and may prevent the development of clinical diabetes in hypertensive patients with impaired glucose tolerance. Reports indicated that angiotensin receptor blockers (ARBs) decrease the rate of development of proteinuria and diabetic renal disease. These observations will likely have a significant impact on new guidelines for treatment of hypertension in patients with type 2 DM.

DIABETES AND CARDIOVASCULAR DISEASE

Because the populations of many societies are getting older, more obese, and sedentary, the prevalence of diabetes, especially type 2 diabetes, is rapidly increasing throughout the world *(2–4)*. The disease will soon involve more than 20 million people in the United States and 300 million persons worldwide. Diabetes is now the leading cause in the United States of new blindness, end-stage renal disease (ESRD), and nontraumatic amputations *(2,3,5)*. Because diabetes is currently the leading cause of end-stage renal disease in the United States *(6)*, this increase in ESRD, necessitating dialysis and transplantation, is a tremendous burden on our health care resources as well as on families and individuals affected by this medical problem. CVD is the major cause of mortality in aging patients with type 2 diabetes *(7–11)* (Fig. 1), and hypertension is a major contributor to development of both CVD and renal disease in this population *(12)*. Accordingly, the pathophysiology of and therapeutic approaches to hypertension in the aging diabetic patient are discussed in this chapter.

HYPERTENSION IN THE AGING PATIENT
WITH TYPE 2 DIABETES

The prevalence of hypertension in patients with type 2 diabetes is up to three times greater than in age- and gender-matched non-diabetic patients *(6,12,13)*. Increasing age, obesity, and the onset of renal disease are all factors that increase the prevalence of hypertension in the diabetic

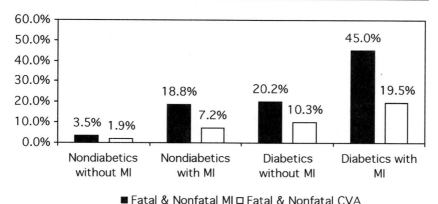

Fig. 1. Seven-year incidence of cardiovascular risk in type 2 diabetes mellitus. CVA, cerebrovascular accident; MI, myocardial infarction. (From ref. 7.)

patient *(6,12,13)*. Obesity, especially central/visceral obesity, is increasingly an important factor predisposing to the development of both diabetes and hypertension *(6,12,14)*. An increased prevalence of obesity in minority populations contributes to the greater incidence of both diabetes and hypertension in these populations *(6,14,15)*. As our population ages, an increasingly sedentary lifestyle also contributes to a high prevalence of diabetes and hypertension.

Persons with hypertension have a high prevalence of insulin resistance *(15)* and have a substantially increased risk of developing type 2 DM *(16,17)*. Further, as patients age they are more likely to have changes in skeletal muscle tissue that predispose to diabetes *(8)*. These changes include altered composition of skeletal muscle tissue (less slow-twitch insulin-sensitive muscle fibers and increased fat interspersed between skeletal muscle fibers) (Table 1). A sedentary lifestyle accentuates these changes with aging.

HYPERTENSION AND CARDIOVASCULAR DISEASE IN AGING PATIENTS WITH TYPE 2 DIABETES

Hypertension increases the risk for CVD *(12)* and stroke *(18–21)* in patients with type 2 diabetes. Within the Multiple Risk Factor Intervention Trial *(10)*, more than 5000 diabetic patients were followed for 12 years and compared to more than 350,000 persons without diabetes. The Multiple Risk Factor Intervention Trial confirmed that hypertension, elevated cholesterol, and cigarette use were independent CVD risk fac-

Table 1
Mechanism of Insulin Resistance in Hypertension

Decreased nonoxidative glucose metabolism by skeletal muscle

Postreceptor defect

*   Decreased insulin-mediated glucose transport
*   Decreased glycogen synthase activity

Altered skeletal muscle fiber type

*   Decreased insulin-sensitive slow-twitch fibers

Decreased delivery of insulin and glucose to skeletal muscle

*   Vascular rarefaction
*   Vascular hypertrophy
*   Increased vasoconstriction

tors in men with diabetes, and their presence had a greater impact on CVD risk in men with diabetes compared to those without diabetes *(10)*. In the United Kingdom Prospective Diabetes Study (UKPDS), a major risk factor for CVD in type 2 diabetes included systolic blood pressure (SBP) *(22)*. BP was also observed to be a strong CVD risk factor in type 2 diabetic patients in the Prospective Cardiovascular Münster study *(23)*.

There is considerable evidence from controlled clinical trials indicating that rigorous control of BP to levels below the conventional control levels of 140/90 mmHg markedly reduces CVD and stroke morbidity/ mortality as well as development of ESRD in persons with type 2 DM *(23–27)*. For example, in the UKPDS in patients assigned to "tight" BP control (144/82 mmHg), there was a 24% reduction in diabetes-related end points, 32% reduction in death-related end points caused by diabetes, 44% reduction in strokes, and 37% reduction in microvascular end points, especially diabetic retinopathy (Fig. 2) *(27)*. The relative benefit on CVD risk reduction was more powerful for intensive BP reduction than tight glucose control.

The Hypertension Optimal Treatment study reported that, in a diabetic subgroup ($n = 1501$), major CVD events were reduced by 51% in those randomly assigned to a diastolic blood pressure (DBP) goal below 80 mmHg compared to a goal of below 90 mmHg (Fig. 3) *(26)*. In a placebo-controlled trial of treatment of isolated SBP, the Systolic Hypertension in Europe (Syst-Eur) trial, the 492 older patients with diabetes were reported in a *post hoc* analysis to have significant reductions in CVD mortality, all CVD events, and stroke, with a reduction in mean SBPs from 175 to 153 mmHg *(28)*. These data from the Syst-Eur trial are similar to those of the Systolic Hypertension in the Elderly Program

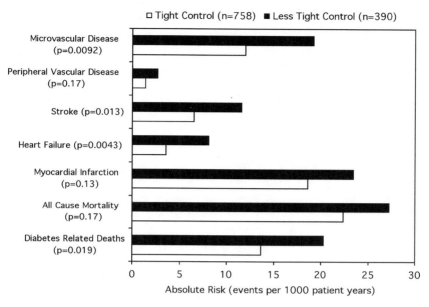

Fig. 2. United Kingdom Prospective Diabetes Study 38: tight vs less-tight blood pressure control. (Data from ref. *27.*)

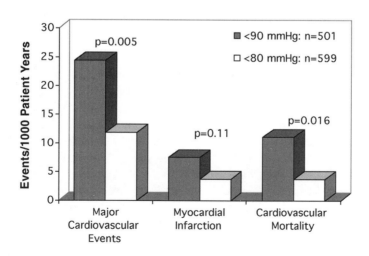

Fig. 3. Events in patients with diabetes mellitus at baseline in relation lower blood pressure levels (Hypertension Optimal Treatment trial). (Data from ref. *26.*)

study, for which elderly persons with type 2 diabetes derived more CVD reduction than those without diabetes *(29)*. In general, diabetic patients in these clinical trials required more antihypertensive agents (two or more drugs) to achieve these more aggressive goals *(6,30)*. The difficulty in achieving the goal BPs primarily relates to achieving an SBP of 130 mmHg *(31)*. Both aging and diabetes result in disproportionate elevations in SBPs *(12)*.

The Antihypertensive and Lipid-Lowering Treatment to Prevent Heart Attack Trial enrolled 15,297 diabetic hypertensive participants 55 years or older *(32)*. Thus, 36% of the entire cohort reported a history of diabetes *(33)*. To compare treatment with chlorthalidone, doxazosin, lisinopril, and amlodipine, the rates of fatal coronary heart disease and nonfatal myocardial infarction (MI) were measured as the primary end point *(33)*. Figure 4 shows what can be achieved by titrating therapy and combining additional drugs (β-blocker or reserpine and hydralazine). Many diabetic hypertensive patients will require three or more drugs to achieve a lower target BP *(34)*. For the primary end point or all-cause mortality among hypertensive diabetics, there were no differences among chlorthalidone, lisinopril, amlodipine, and doxazosin *(35,36)*. Only doxazosin was inferior to chlorthalidone for strokes ($p = 0.04$) *(35)*. All drugs were inferior to chlorthalidone for heart failure *(35–37)*.

STROKE IN THE AGING PATIENT WITH TYPE 2 DIABETES AND HYPERTENSION

Stroke is the third leading cause of death in the United States *(18–21)*. Age is one of the stronger predictors for an increase. There are more than 700,000 strokes annually, and currently there are over 4.5 million stroke survivors *(38,39)*. Diabetes and aging are well-documented independent modifiable stroke risk factors of increasing importance as the prevalence of diabetes and the numbers of elderly citizens increase *(2,18–21)*. Indeed, the incidence of stroke among diabetic patients is up to three times that in the general population *(18–21)* with an especially high-risk rates in the southeastern United States *(20,21)*. There is an increase in both short- and long-term mortality in diabetic patients following stroke *(18–21)*. High admission glucoses are one predictor of poor outcomes in these patients *(18–21)*, especially in the older patient with diabetes.

As the incidence of strokes is higher and the clinical outcome poorer in diabetic patients, prevention of stroke is very important *(18)*. Hypertension, heart failure, and cigarette and alcohol use are modifiable risk factors for stroke in patients with and without diabetes *(5,18,21)*. In the 8 years of observation in the UKPDS group, an increased risk of stroke

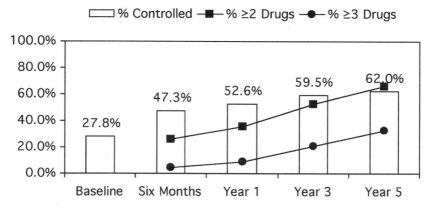

Fig. 4. Blood pressure control (<140/90 mmHg) and number of antihypertensive drugs in North American Diabetic ALLHAT Participants. (Data from ref. *34*.)

was strongly associated with systolic hypertension as well as atrial fibrillation *(38)*. Both of these risk factors are more common in the elderly patient with diabetes *(39)*.

Intervention trials have provided support for rigorous BP control in prevention of stroke in patients with diabetes. In the UKPDS trial for combined fatal and nonfatal stroke, tight BP control (mean BP achieved 144/82 mmHg) resulted in a striking 44% relative risk reduction compared with less-aggressive control (mean BP of 154/87 mmHg) *(38)*. This 44% risk reduction in stroke was even greater than the 22% reduction with antihypertensive treatment found in the diabetic cohort in the Systolic Hypertension Elderly Program *(29)*. Data from Syst-Eur for those treated with nitrendipine-based antihypertensive therapy showed that the excess risk of stroke associated with diabetes was abolished by antihypertensive treatment of older patients with type 2 diabetes and isolated systolic hypertension *(28)*.

In the Microalbuminuria, Cardiovascular, and Renal Outcomes-HOPE subset analysis of the Heart Outcomes Prevention Evaluation (HOPE) study, 3577 diabetic patients treated with ramipril showed a reduction of primary combined end points of MI, stroke, and CVD death by 25% and stroke reduction by 33% *(30)*. Studies have shown the beneficial effects of an ARB *(25,40)* and an angiotensin-converting enzyme (ACE)/diuretic combination *(41)* in reduction of primary and secondary strokes in high-risk patients, including diabetics.

These data support the guidelines of a BP of less than 130/80 mmHg that is recommended in patients with diabetes and hypertension (Fig. 5)

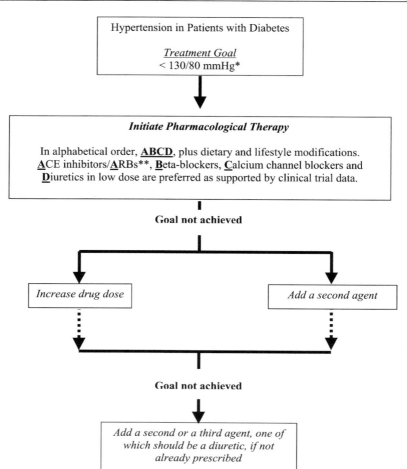

Fig. 5. Management of hypertension in diabetic patients. *In patients with more than 1 g proteinuria and renal insufficiency, the treatment goal is blood pressure less than 125/75 mmHg. **ARBs, angiotensin receptor blockers.

(6,42). Although this goal is more difficult to accomplish in the elderly, it can be achieved using combinations of antihypertensive medications that include a low-dose diuretic as part of the regimen *(39)*.

TREATMENT OF HYPERTENSION IN CASES OF DIABETIC NEPHROPATHY

Diabetic nephropathy has become the leading etiological cause of ESRD in the United States *(6,43,44)*. Approximately 35% of persons with diabetes will develop diabetic nephropathy characterized by proteinuria, decreased glomerular filtration rate, and increased BP *(6,43,44)*. In type 2 diabetic patients, the incidence of diabetic nephropathy is approximately 20% *(6,43–45)*. Because 95% of diabetic patients are type 2, more than half of ESRD in diabetes occurs in type 2 patients *(6,44)*.

Both the prevalence and incidence of ESRD are approximately twice what they were 10 years ago *(43)*. If the trends of the past two decades persist, approximately 175,000 new cases of ESRD will be diagnosed in 2010 *(44)*. This is partly because type 2 diabetes is expected to double within the next 10 to 15 years, and diabetic patients are living longer and thus are more likely to develop chronic problems, including ESRD. The cost associated with the management of ESRD is expected to exceed $28 billion by 2010 *(43)*. Elderly patients with ESRD will constitute an increasingly large proportion of this population.

A routine urinalysis should be performed in all newly diagnosed type 2 diabetes. If the urinalysis is negative for protein, the albumin to creatinine ratio (ACR) in a spot urine collection should be performed *(44)*. Microalbuminuria is present if urine albumin excretion is 30 mg/24 hours or greater (equivalent to 20 µg/minute on a timed specimen or 20 mg/g creatinine on a random collection) *(44)*. A number of factors can artificially increase urinary albumin excretion, including urinary tract infections, exercise, fever, poor glycemic control, and congestive heart failure *(44)*. The current recommendation by the American Diabetes Association *(44)*, as well as the National Kidney Foundation (6), is to have at least two elevated ACRs to affirm microalbuminuria. An adequate collection of urine, either spot or 24 hour, may be especially problematic in elderly patients, who are more prone to have urinary tract infections and heart failure *(39)*.

Microalbuminuria has been observed to predict the development of CVD and stroke as well as progression of diabetic nephropathy *(6,12,15,44–52)*. Microalbuminuria has also been associated with insulin resistance or hyperinsulinemia *(49)*, atherogenic dyslipidemia (12,52), and the absence of a nocturnal drop in both SBP and DBP *(12)* and is a part of the cardiometabolic syndrome (Table 2) *(12,15)*. Because microalbuminuria is part of the cardiometabolic syndrome and is related to endothelial dysfunction and increased oxidative stress *(6,12,53)*, it is not suprising that diabetic glomerulosclerosis parallels the process of diabetic atherosclerosis *(12)* and is a powerful risk factor for CVD and stroke *(12,54)*. Thus, even after adjustment for renal function, microalbuminuria remained a strong risk factor for CVD in the subset analysis of HOPE *(54)*.

In the HOPE trial, the presence of albuminuria doubled the risk for the composite end point of MI, stroke, or CVD death and all-cause mortality.

Table 2
Cardiovascular Disease Risk Factors Associated
With Cardiometabolic Syndrome

1. Systolic hypertension
2. Central obesity
3. Hyperinsulinemia/insulin resistance
4. Endothelial dysfunction
5. Microalbuminuria
6. Low high-density lipoprotein cholesterol levels
7. High triglyceride levels
8. Small, dense low-density lipoprotein cholesterol particles
9. Increased apolipoprotein B levels
10. Increased fibrinogen levels
11. Increased plasminogen activator inhibitor-1 and decreased plasminogen
    activator levels
12. Increased C-reactive protein and other inflammatory markers
13. Absent nocturnal dipping of blood pressure and heart rate
14. Salt sensitivity
15. Left ventricular hypertrophy
16. Premature/excess coronary artery disease, stroke, and peripheral vascular
    disease

The risk of heart failure was 3.7 times greater in type 2 diabetic patients with microalbuminuria compared to those without albuminuria *(50)*. The risks of the composite end points, all-cause mortality, and heart failure hospitalizations in diabetic patients with microalbuminuria were significantly reduced with treatment with the ACE inhibitor ramipril *(50)*. These data suggest that interruption of the renin–angiotensin–aldosterone system (RAAS) is important in preventing CVD, even in elderly patients with diabetes and hypertension *(12)*.

Several studies have provided evidence for unique benefits of anti-hypertensive agents that interrupt the RAAS in diabetic patients with hypertension *(30,40,55,56)*. In addition to their impact on CVD *(12,30, 40,55)*, ACE inhibitors in six small trials involving 352 type 2 diabetic patients with diabetic nephropathy were more effective in reducing pro-teinuria than other antihypertensive agents (ARBs were not included) *(57,58)*.

Studies have addressed renal protection from ARBs in type 2 DM. The Irbesartan Diabetic Nephropathy Trial (IDNT) evaluated the effects of irbesartan in 1715 patients with hypertension, type 2 diabetes, and proteinuria equal to or greater than 900 mg per day *(59)*. These patients were randomly assigned to the ARB irbesartan, a placebo-control group, or amlodipine and had an average follow-up of 2.6 years. The time to the event for the composite end point of doubled serum creatinine, ESRD, or death was 28% in the control group vs 19.8% in the irbesartan group. Amlodipine treatment was associated with a 25.2% reduction in composite end points, which was not different from the control group but less than the irbesartan group. In that study, the amlodipine treatment group had a higher rate of heart failure than in the placebo or irbesartan groups. This is of potential importance, particularly in elderly patients with type 2 DM.

In another trial, the Reduction of Endpoints in NIDDM With Angiotensin II Antagonist Losartan (RENAAL) study, the ARB losartan at 50 to 100 mg plus conventional hypertensive therapy was compared to placebo plus conventional hypertensive therapy in 1513 patients *(60)*. Creatinine was required to be between 1.3 and 3 mg/dL, and urine ACR had to be greater than 300 mg/g or 25 mg/mmol. The goal BP was less than 140/90 mmHg, and the patients were followed for 3.4 years. Losartan therapy was associated with a 28% reduction in the risk of ESRD and a 25% reduction in doubling of serum creatinine. Furthermore, there was a 32% reduction in the first hospitalization for congestive heart failure. There was a nonsignificant trend for a reduction in MI in the losartan group. Again, these observations are of relevance to an older population of type 2 diabetic patients.

The Irbesartan in Patients With Type 2 Diabetes and Microalbuminuria (IRMA2) study examined the possibility that the ARB irbesartan could delay or prevent the development of clinical proteinuria in patients with type 2 diabetes, microalbuminuria, and a normal serum creatinine level (1.3 mg/dL for men and 1.1 mg/dL for women) *(61)*. Type 2 diabetic patients whose overnight albumin excretion rates (UAER) were 20 to 200 µg/minute on two of three consecutive samples were randomly assigned to receive placebo or 150–300 mg irbesartan once daily. Goal BP was less than 135/85 mmHg 3 months after randomization; additional antihypertensive agents, except ACE inhibitors and dihydropyridine calcium channel blockers, were added to achieve that goal. The primary end point of the trial was defined as the occurrence of UAER of greater than 200 µg/minute and/or a UAER at least 30% higher than baseline on at least two consecutive measurements.

In the IRMA2 study, average BP values were slightly lower in the two groups treated with irbesartan than in the placebo group during the first 6 months of the study, but this small difference disappeared during the last 12 months of the study. Patients were followed for an average of 2 years. In the 150 mg irbesartan vs placebo group, there was a 39% reduction in the development rate of clinical proteinuria; however, in the

300 mg irbesartan treatment group, there was a 70% reduction in the primary end point. Return to a normal UAER, defined as a UAER of less than 20 µg/minute, was 34% more frequent among patients treated with 300 mg irbesartan than among patients in the placebo group. The results of this study demonstrate that the ARB irbesartan at a dose of 300 mg daily can delay progression of microalbuminuria to clinical proteinuria in patients with type 2 diabetes.

In all three of these trials using ARBs, there was a little problem with hyperkalemia, which is a key issue in elderly type 2 diabetic patients *(39)*.

There have also been trials examining the impact of combination of an ACE inhibitor and an ARB on diabetic nephropathy *(62–64)*. For instance the Candesartan and Lisinopril Microalbuminuria trial was a randomized study of the effect of combining the ARB candesartan and the ACE inhibitor lisinopril on microalbuminuria in 199 type 2 diabetic patients *(63)*. This was a 12-week combination therapy trial, with 12 weeks of prior monotherapy with either candesartan or lisinopril. In this study, the reduction in the urinary ACR in those receiving candesartan (16 mg/day) and lisinopril (20 mg/day) was significantly greater (50% reduction) than that observed with either agent alone (24% for candesartan and 39% for lisinopril). As is often the case with combination therapy, BP values were lower than with the individual agent, which makes interpretation of the findings difficult. After 24 weeks of therapy, DBP was reduced to a greater degree with combination therapy (−16.3 mmHg) than with either candesartan (−10.4 mmHg) or lisinopril (−10.7 mmHg) alone.

Thus, in conclusion, diabetic nephropathy is an increasingly common problem in our aging diabetic population *(39)*. To date, there is no established means to predictably reduce the primary rate of development of diabetic nephropathy. Instead, current practice typically addresses diabetic nephropathy when it is already present, either in the form of microalbuminuria or as the more advanced disease state characterized by macroproteinuria and declining renal function. Important elements of the treatment plan for diabetic nephropathy include meticulous BP control and reduction in urine protein excretion to below 1 g/day. In this regard, ACE inhibitors and/or ARBs are of considerable importance. In type 2 diabetic nephropathy, the available evidence supports the preferential use of ARBs or ACE inhibitors.

SUMMARY

There are limited data evaluating various interventions in the elderly diabetic with hypertension *(65)*. Most guidelines *(6,42,66)*, but not all

Table 3
Dietary and Lifestyle Modifications Recommended
for Management of Hypertension

1. Weight loss
2. Exercise (aerobic physical activity) 30–45 minutes at least three times a week
3. Reduced sodium intake to 100 mmol (2.4 g) per day
4. Smoking cessation
5. Adequate intake of dietary potassium, calcium, and magnesium
6. Reduced alcohol intake to less than 1 oz of ethanol (24 oz of beer) per day
7. Diet rich in fruits and vegetables but low in fat

guidelines *(65,67)*, favor a target BP of 130/80 mmHg. Thus, elderly patients with diabetes often require three or more medications to control their BP *(6,12,31)*. BP should be reduced gradually to avoid complications *(65)*. As noted in the treatment algorithm (Fig. 5), pharmacological therapy should be initialized in conjunction with hygienic measures (Table 3) *(6,12,31)*. Based on the results of the Dietary Approaches to Stop Hypertension intervention, the reduction of sodium intake to levels below 100 mmol per day along with a diet that is enriched in potassium and other minerals (i.e., magnesium, calcium) is beneficial *(68,69)*. Because many elderly persons are on a limited fixed income, this is often difficult to achieve *(39)*. In the absence of anginal symptoms and lower extremity problems (i.e., foot abnormalities, claudication), the elderly diabetic patient should be encouraged to participate in aerobic exercise, even if that means only walking on a safe surface (i.e., in shopping malls) *(39)*.

As stated, the consensus BP goal in diabetic patients is less than 130/80 mmHg *(6,42,66)*. Initial therapy is an ACE inhibitor or an ARB. Renal function and potassium levels should be checked within 1 or 2 weeks of initiation, with each titration, and yearly *(65)*. Current recommendations include the use of β-blockers, calcium antagonists, or low-dose diuretics in conjunction with an ACE inhibitor or an ARB *(6,12,31)*. Because of the results of the UKPDS *(27)* and other studies *(70)*, β-blockers are now considered important antihypertensive agents in elderly patients with diabetes, especially those who have angina. Low-dose diuretics and dihydropyridine calcium antagonists are often required to accomplish adequate BP control, especially systolic control in elderly patients with type 2 diabetes *(6,12)*.

In addition to BP control, these patients should receive aspirin in a dose of 81 mg to an adult aspirin dose *(12)*. A large study has demon-

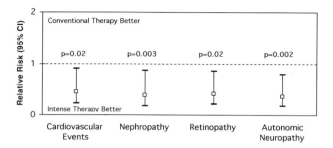

Fig. 6. Effectiveness of intense multifactorial intervention in type 2 diabetes: the Steno-2 Study. CI, confidence interval. (Data modified from ref. *72*.)

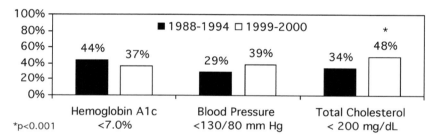

Fig. 7. Risk factor control of diabetes in the United Sates. Third National Health and Nutrition Examination Survey (NHANES III): 1988–1994 vs 1999–2000. (Data from ref. *75*.)

strated the benefits of statin therapy in elderly patients as well as those with diabetes *(71)*. Therefore, it is recommended that all elderly diabetic patients have their low-density lipoprotein cholesterol lowered to less than 100 mg/dL with statin therapy. The elderly diabetic patient also should have blood glucoses well controlled *(12)*, with glycated hemoglobins less than 7%. An intense, multiple risk-factor intervention in type 2 diabetes reduces the risk of CVD, nephropathy, retinopathy, and autonomic neuropathy (Fig. 6) compared to conventional treatment *(72)*. However, data indicated that hormone replacement therapy is generally not indicated in the elderly diabetic female *(73,74)*. Despite these data, little progress is being made in risk-factor control in diabetes (Fig. 7) *(75)*.

ACKNOWLEDGMENT

We wish to thank Paddy McGowan for her usual excellent work in preparing this chapter.

REFERENCES

1. Prisant LM. Diabetes mellitus and hypertension: a mandate for intense treatment according to new guidelines. *Am J Ther* 2003;10:363–369.
2. Amos AF, McCarty DJ, Zimmet P. The rising global burden of diabetes and its complications: estimates and projections to the year 2010. *Diabet Med* 1997; 14(suppl 5):S1–S85.
3. King H, Aubert RE, Herman WH. Global burden of diabetes, 1995–2025: prevalence, numerical estimates, and projections. *Diabetes Care* 1998;21:1414–1431.
4. Mokdad AH, Ford ES, Bowman BA, et al. Diabetes trends in the U.S.: 1990–1998. *Diabetes Care* 2000;23:1278–1283.
5. Fagan TC, Sowers J. Type 2 diabetes mellitus: greater cardiovascular risks and greater benefits of therapy. *Arch Intern Med* 1999;159:1033–1034.
6. Bakris GL, Williams M, Dworkin L, et al. Preserving renal function in adults with hypertension and diabetes: a consensus approach. National Kidney Foundation Hypertension and Diabetes Executive Committees Working Group. *Am J Kidney Dis* 2000;36:646–661.
7. Haffner SM, Lehto S, Ronnemaa T, Pyorala K, Laakso M. Mortality from coronary heart disease in subjects with type 2 diabetes and in nondiabetic subjects with and without prior myocardial infarction. *N Engl J Med* 1998;339:229–234.
8. Sowers JR, Lester MA. Diabetes and cardiovascular disease. *Diabetes Care* 1999;22(suppl 3):C14–C20.
9. Grundy SM, Benjamin IJ, Burke GL, et al. Diabetes and cardiovascular disease: a statement for healthcare professionals from the American Heart Association. *Circulation* 1999;100:1134–1146.
10. Stamler J, Vaccaro O, Neaton JD, Wentworth D. Diabetes, other risk factors, and 12-year cardiovascular mortality for men screened in the Multiple Risk Factor Intervention Trial. *Diabetes Care* 1993;16:434–444.
11. Sowers JR. Diabetes mellitus and cardiovascular disease in women. *Arch Intern Med* 1998;158:617–621.
12. Sowers JR, Epstein M, Frohlich ED. Diabetes, hypertension, and cardiovascular disease: an update. *Hypertension* 2001;37:1053–1059.
13. Sowers JR, Williams M, Epstein M, Bakris G. Hypertension in patients with diabetes. Strategies for drug therapy to reduce complications. *Postgrad Med* 2000;107:47–54,60.
14. Sowers JR. Obesity and cardiovascular disease. *Clin Chem* 1998;44(8 pt 2):1821–1825.
15. McFarlane SI, Banerji M, Sowers JR. Insulin resistance and cardiovascular disease. *J Clin Endocrinol Metab* 2001;86:713–718.
16. Gress TW, Nieto FJ, Shahar E, Wofford MR, Brancati FL. Hypertension and antihypertensive therapy as risk factors for type 2 diabetes mellitus. Atherosclerosis Risk in Communities Study. *N Engl J Med* 2000;342:905–912.
17. Sowers JR, Bakris GL. Antihypertensive therapy and the risk of type 2 diabetes mellitus. *N Engl J Med* 2000;342:969–970.
18. Goldstein LB, Adams R, Becker K, et al. Primary prevention of ischemic stroke: a statement for healthcare professionals from the Stroke Council of the American Heart Association. *Circulation* 2001;103:163–182.
19. Tuomilehto J, Rastenyte D. Diabetes and glucose intolerance as risk factors for stroke. *J Cardiovasc Risk* 1999;6:241–249.
20. Bell DS. Stroke in the diabetic patient. *Diabetes Care* 1994;17:213–219.
21. Sacco RL. Reducing the risk of stroke in diabetes: what have we learned that is new? *Diabetes Obes Metab* 2002;4(suppl 1):S27–S34.

22. Turner RC, Millns H, Neil HA, et al. Risk factors for coronary artery disease in non-insulin dependent diabetes mellitus: United Kingdom Prospective Diabetes Study (UKPDS: 23). *BMJ* 1998;316:823–828.

23. Assmann G, Cullen P, Schulte H. Simple scoring scheme for calculating the risk of acute coronary events based on the 10-year follow-up of the Prospective Cardiovascular Munster (PROCAM) study. *Circulation* 2002;105:310–315.

24. Yusuf S, Sleight P, Pogue J, Bosch J, Davies R, Dagenais G. Effects of an angiotensin-converting-enzyme inhibitor, ramipril, on cardiovascular events in high-risk patients. The Heart Outcomes Prevention Evaluation Study Investigators. *N Engl J Med* 2000;342:145–153.

25. Dahlof B, Devereux RB, Kjeldsen SE, et al. Cardiovascular morbidity and mortality in the Losartan Intervention for Endpoint reduction in hypertension study (LIFE): a randomised trial against atenolol. *Lancet* 2002;359:995–1003.

26. Hansson L, Zanchetti A, Carruthers SG, et al. Effects of intensive blood-pressure lowering and low-dose aspirin in patients with hypertension: principal results of the Hypertension Optimal Treatment (HOT) randomised trial. HOT Study Group. *Lancet* 1998;351:1755–1762.

27. Tight blood pressure control and risk of macrovascular and microvascular complications in type 2 diabetes: UKPDS 38. UK Prospective Diabetes Study Group. *BMJ* 1998;317:703–713.

28. Tuomilehto J, Rastenyte D, Birkenhager WH, et al. Effects of calcium-channel blockade in older patients with diabetes and systolic hypertension. Systolic Hypertension in Europe Trial Investigators. *N Engl J Med* 1999;340:677–684.

29. Curb JD, Pressel SL, Cutler JA, et al. Effect of diuretic-based antihypertensive treatment on cardiovascular disease risk in older diabetic patients with isolated systolic hypertension. Systolic Hypertension in the Elderly Program Cooperative Research Group. *JAMA* 1996;276:1886–1892.

30. Effects of ramipril on cardiovascular and microvascular outcomes in people with diabetes mellitus: results of the HOPE study and MICRO-HOPE substudy. Heart Outcomes Prevention Evaluation Study Investigators. *Lancet* 2000;355:253–259.

31. McFarlane SI, Jacober SJ, Winer N, et al. Control of cardiovascular risk factors in patients with diabetes and hypertension at urban academic medical centers. *Diabetes Care* 2002;25:718–723.

32. Barzilay JI, Jones CL, Davis BR, et al. Baseline characteristics of the diabetic participants in the Antihypertensive and Lipid-Lowering Treatment to Prevent Heart Attack Trial (ALLHAT). *Diabetes Care* 2001;24:654–658.

33. Grimm RH Jr, Margolis KL, Papademetriou VV, et al. Baseline characteristics of participants in the Antihypertensive and Lipid Lowering Treatment to Prevent Heart Attack Trial (ALLHAT). *Hypertension* 2001;37:19–27.

34. Cushman WC, Ford CE, Cutler JA, et al. Success and predictors of blood pressure control in diverse North American settings: the Antihypertensive and Lipid-Lowering Treatment to Prevent Heart Attack Trial (ALLHAT). *J Clin Hypertens (Greenwich)* 2002;4:393–404.

35. Major cardiovascular events in hypertensive patients randomized to doxazosin vs chlorthalidone: the antihypertensive and lipid-lowering treatment to prevent heart attack trial (ALLHAT). ALLHAT Collaborative Research Group. *JAMA* 2000;283:1967–1975.

36. Major outcomes in high-risk hypertensive patients randomized to angiotensin-converting enzyme inhibitor or calcium channel blocker vs diuretic: The Antihypertensive and Lipid-Lowering Treatment to Prevent Heart Attack Trial (ALLHAT). *JAMA* 2002;288:2981–2997.

37. Diuretic vs α-blocker as first-step antihypertensive therapy: final results from the Antihypertensive and Lipid-Lowering Treatment to Prevent Heart Attack Trial (ALLHAT). *Hypertension* 2003;42:239–246.
38. Davis TM, Millns H, Stratton IM, Holman RR, Turner RC. Risk factors for stroke in type 2 diabetes mellitus: United Kingdom Prospective Diabetes Study (UKPDS) 29. *Arch Intern Med* 1999;159:1097–1103.
39. Sowers JR, Farrow SL. Treatment of elderly hypertensive patients with diabetes, renal disease, and coronary heart disease. *Am J Geriatr Cardiol* 1996;5:57–70.
40. Lindholm LH, Ibsen H, Dahlof B, et al. Cardiovascular morbidity and mortality in patients with diabetes in the Losartan Intervention for Endpoint reduction in hypertension study (LIFE): a randomised trial against atenolol. *Lancet* 2002;359:1004–1010.
41. Randomised trial of a perindopril-based blood-pressure-lowering regimen among 6105 individuals with previous stroke or transient ischaemic attack. *Lancet* 2001;358:1033–1041.
42. Hypertension management in adults with diabetes. *Diabetes Care* 2004;27(suppl 1):S65–S67.
43. Excerpts from the United States Renal Data Systems 2002 annual report: atlas of end-stage renal disease in the United States. *Am J Kidney Dis* 2003;41(4 suppl 2):v–ix, S7–S254.
44. Molitch ME, DeFronzo RA, Franz MJ, et al. Nephropathy in diabetes. *Diabetes Care* 2004;27(suppl 1):S79–S83.
45. Ruddy MC. Angiotensin II receptor blockade in diabetic nephropathy. *Am J Hypertens* 2002;15:468–471.
46. Agewall S, Wikstrand J, Ljungman S, Fagerberg B. Usefulness of microalbuminuria in predicting cardiovascular mortality in treated hypertensive men with and without diabetes mellitus. Risk Factor Intervention Study Group. *Am J Cardiol* 1997;80:164–169.
47. Dinneen SF, Gerstein HC. The association of microalbuminuria and mortality in non-insulin-dependent diabetes mellitus. A systematic overview of the literature. *Arch Intern Med* 1997;157:1413–1418.
48. Bigazzi R, Bianchi S, Baldari D, Campese VM. Microalbuminuria predicts cardiovascular events and renal insufficiency in patients with essential hypertension. *J Hypertens* 1998;16:1325–1333.
49. Jager A, Kostense PJ, Ruhe HG, et al. Microalbuminuria and peripheral arterial disease are independent predictors of cardiovascular and all-cause mortality, especially among hypertensive subjects: five-year follow-up of the Hoorn Study. *Arterioscler Thromb Vasc Biol* 1999;19:617–624.
50. Gerstein HC, Mann JF, Pogue J, et al. Prevalence and determinants of microalbuminuria in high-risk diabetic and nondiabetic patients in the Heart Outcomes Prevention Evaluation Study. The HOPE Study Investigators. *Diabetes Care* 2000;23(suppl 2):B35–B39.
51. Jensen JS, Feldt-Rasmussen B, Strandgaard S, Schroll M, Borch-Johnsen K. Arterial hypertension, microalbuminuria, and risk of ischemic heart disease. *Hypertension* 2000;35:898–903.
52. Bianchi S, Bigazzi R, Quinones Galvan A, et al. Insulin resistance in microalbuminuric hypertension. Sites and mechanisms. *Hypertension* 1995;26:789–795.
53. Sowers JR. Hypertension, angiotensin II, and oxidative stress. *N Engl J Med* 2002;346:1999–2001.
54. Mann JF, Gerstein HC, Pogue J, Bosch J, Yusuf S. Renal insufficiency as a predictor of cardiovascular outcomes and the impact of ramipril: the HOPE randomized trial. *Ann Intern Med* 2001;134:629–636.

55. Hansson L, Lindholm LH, Niskanen L, et al. Effect of angiotensin-converting-enzyme inhibition compared with conventional therapy on cardiovascular morbidity and mortality in hypertension: the Captopril Prevention Project (CAPPP) randomised trial. *Lancet* 1999;353:611–616.

56. Lewis EJ, Hunsicker LG, Bain RP, Rohde RD. The effect of angiotensin-converting-enzyme inhibition on diabetic nephropathy. The Collaborative Study Group. *N Engl J Med* 1993;329:1456–1462.

57. Parving HH, Hovind P, Rossing K, Andersen S. Evolving strategies for renoprotection: diabetic nephropathy. *Curr Opin Nephrol Hypertens* 2001;10:515–522.

58. Remuzzi G, Schieppati A, Ruggenenti P. Clinical practice. Nephropathy in patients with type 2 diabetes. *N Engl J Med* 2002;346:1145–1151.

59. Lewis EJ, Hunsicker LG, Clarke WR, et al. Renoprotective effect of the angiotensin-receptor antagonist irbesartan in patients with nephropathy due to type 2 diabetes. *N Engl J Med* 2001;345:851–860.

60. Brenner BM, Cooper ME, de Zeeuw D, et al. Effects of losartan on renal and cardiovascular outcomes in patients with type 2 diabetes and nephropathy. *N Engl J Med* 2001;345:861–869.

61. Parving HH, Lehnert H, Brochner-Mortensen J, Gomis R, Andersen S, Arner P. The effect of irbesartan on the development of diabetic nephropathy in patients with type 2 diabetes. *N Engl J Med* 2001;345:870–878.

62. Agarwal R. Add-on angiotensin receptor blockade with maximized ACE inhibition. *Kidney Int* 2001;59:2282–2289.

63. Mogensen CE, Neldam S, Tikkanen I, et al. Randomised controlled trial of dual blockade of renin-angiotensin system in patients with hypertension, microalbuminuria, and non-insulin dependent diabetes: the candesartan and lisinopril microalbuminuria (CALM) study. *BMJ* 2000;321:1440–1444.

64. Sica DA, Elliott WJ. Angiotensin-converting enzyme inhibitors and angiotensin receptor blockers in combination: theory and practice. *J Clin Hypertens (Greenwich)* 2001;3:383–387.

65. Brown AF, Mangione CM, Saliba D, Sarkisian CA. Guidelines for improving the care of the older person with diabetes mellitus. *J Am Geriatr Soc* 2003;51(5 suppl guidelines):S265–S280.

66. Chobanian AV, Bakris GL, Black HR, et al. Seventh report of the Joint National Committee on Prevention, Detection, Evaluation, and Treatment of High Blood Pressure. *Hypertension* 2003;42:1206–1252.

67. Snow V, Weiss KB, Mottur-Pilson C. The evidence base for tight blood pressure control in the management of type 2 diabetes mellitus. *Ann Intern Med* 2003;138: 587–592.

68. Sacks FM, Svetkey LP, Vollmer WM, et al. Effects on blood pressure of reduced dietary sodium and the Dietary Approaches to Stop Hypertension (DASH) diet. DASH-Sodium Collaborative Research Group. *N Engl J Med* 2001;344:3–10.

69. Obarzanek E, Sacks FM, Vollmer WM, et al. Effects on blood lipids of a blood pressure-lowering diet: the Dietary Approaches to Stop Hypertension (DASH) Trial. *Am J Clin Nutr* 2001;74:80–89.

70. Prisant LM. Should β-blockers be used in the treatment of hypertension in the elderly? *J Clin Hypertens (Greenwich)* 2002;4:286–294.

71. Collins R, Armitage J, Parish S, Sleigh P, Peto R. MRC/BHF Heart Protection Study of cholesterol-lowering with simvastatin in 5963 people with diabetes: a randomised placebo-controlled trial. *Lancet* 2003;361:2005–2016.

72. Gæde P, Vedel P, Larsen N, Jensen GV, Parving HH, Pedersen O. Multifactorial intervention and cardiovascular disease in patients with type 2 diabetes. *N Engl J Med* 2003;348:383–393.
73. Humphrey LL, Chan BK, Sox HC. Postmenopausal hormone replacement therapy and the primary prevention of cardiovascular disease. *Ann Intern Med* 2002;137: 273–284.
74. Rossouw JE, Anderson GL, Prentice RL, et al. Risks and benefits of estrogen plus progestin in healthy postmenopausal women: principal results from the Women's Health Initiative randomized controlled trial. *JAMA* 2002;288:321–333.
75. Saydah SH, Fradkin J, Cowie CC. Poor control of risk factors for vascular disease among adults with previously diagnosed diabetes. *JAMA* 2004;291:335–342.

23 Management of Hypertension in Older Patients With Arthritis

Sumeska Thavarajah, MD and William B. White, MD

INTRODUCTION

Musculoskeletal disorders such as osteoarthritis, rheumatoid arthritis, and gouty arthritis are common problems among the elderly (over 65 years old) population and have an impact on functional status and disability. The National Health and Nutrition Examination Survey reported a greater than 80% incidence of osteoarthritis in people over the age of 55 years *(1–3)*. Far less common is rheumatoid arthritis, with an inci-

From: *Clinical Hypertension and Vascular Diseases: Hypertension in the Elderly*
Edited by: L. M. Prisant © Humana Press Inc., Totowa, NJ

dence of 30 per 100,000 persons; this disease has a peak onset between ages 30 and 55 years, with symptoms progressing later into life *(4)*.

The prevalence of arthritis among the elderly population has created a need for the use of nonsteroidal anti-inflammatory drugs (NSAIDs) and cyclooxygenase-2 (COX-2) inhibitors to provide analgesia and anti-inflammatory benefits *(5)*. Alternative agents such as acetaminophen or narcotic agents provide analgesia without relief from the inflammatory changes. Narcotic agents pose the risk of development of addiction and can be sedating. Therefore, NSAIDs have become the most commonly prescribed class of drugs, with estimates of 70 million prescriptions a year *(6,7)*. This is probably an underestimation of the utility of these agents, however, because the over-the-counter availability and usage is often not reported to the health care provider.

The heaviest users of NSAIDs are the elderly, with up to 10 to 15% of older adults using this class of medications on a regular basis *(8–11)*. NSAID and COX-2 inhibitor use may result in cardiovascular and renal complications in the elderly not only as a function of age but also owing to common comorbidities such as hypertension, congestive heart failure (CHF), concomitant drugs, and renal impairment *(12,13)*. The predisposition to a variety of clinical complications in individuals with hypertension has important implications for the use of NSAIDs and COX-2 inhibitors in elderly patients with arthritis.

IMPORTANCE OF PROSTAGLANDINS IN HYPERTENSION AND RENAL INSUFFICIENCY

Prostanoids, including prostaglandins, prostacyclin, and thromboxane, are the products of arachidonic acid metabolism, playing a key role in homeostasis (*see* Table 1).

Actions of the prostaglandins include maintenance of mucus secretion and mucosal circulation in the stomach, stimulation of platelet aggregation and vessel wall adhesion, modulation of renal blood flow, and activation of inflammatory mechanisms *(14)*. The key enzyme in the conversion of arachidonic acid is COX present in two isoforms, COX-1 and COX-2 (*see* Fig. 1).

COX-1 is expressed throughout the body and plays a key role in several constitutive functions. COX-2 is an inducible isoenzyme and plays a key role in inflammation. NSAIDs inhibit both isoforms of the COX enzyme, blocking inflammation and causing adverse effects by disruption of gastric protection and renal autoregulation. The COX-2 inhibitors were initially perceived to provide anti-inflammatory benefits in arthritis patients without untoward effects in the rest of the body.

Table 1
Homeostatic Role of Prostaglandins

Site of action	Physiological effects
Stomach	Mucous/bicarbonate secretion
	Mucosal circulation
Hemostasis	Platelet aggregation
	Vessel wall adhesion
Kidney	Modulate renin production
	Modulate renal plasma flow
	Sodium and water reabsorption
Inflammation	Vasodilation
	Generation of fever
	Vascular permeability

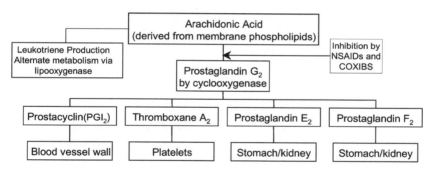

Fig. 1. Prostaglandin synthesis. NSAIDs, nonsteroidal anti-inflammatory drugs; COXIBS, COX-2 selective inhibitors.

Studies, including the Vioxx Gastrointestinal Outcomes Research (VIGOR) trial, have demonstrated that rofecoxib has a better gastrointestinal side-effect profile than nonselective NSAIDs, but they have similar or greater potential for blood pressure (BP) elevation, fluid retention, and nephrotoxicity *(14–16)*. Thus, the use of NSAIDs or COX-2 inhibitors can potentially disrupt renal and vascular mechanisms, resulting in BP elevation, fluid and electrolyte changes, and renal injury. Recognizing the development and the time course of the development of these adverse events along with patient risk factors will help in decision making for the appropriate use of these medications.

BLOOD PRESSURE EFFECTS OF NSAIDS
AND COX-2 INHIBITORS

Hypertension is a very common disease among the elderly, with a prevalence of 60 to 80% *(17)*. Given the widespread use of NSAIDs and COX-2 inhibitors, it is not surprising that a reported 12 to 15% or 12 to 20 million elderly patients use both antihypertensive agents and drugs for pain and arthritis *(18–20)*. The concomitant use of these agents makes it important to recognize the potential BP effects of these agents. Pooled analyses of numerous studies have shown an average increase in mean arterial pressure (MAP) of approx 5 mmHg associated with NSAID use in the elderly (Tables 2 and 3) *(11,21)*. In a meta-analysis by Johnson et al. of 50 studies (38 randomized, placebo-controlled, 12 randomized non-placebo-controlled), pooled data on multiple NSAIDs in 771 patients revealed an increase in supine MAP of 5 mmHg (1.2–8.7 mmHg) *(10)*. Another large meta-analysis by Pope et al. that included 1324 patients found an elevation of 1.1 mmHg in normotensive individuals and 3.3 mmHg in hypertensive individuals following NSAID administration *(22)*.

Studies have also evaluated the effect of the COX-2 inhibitors, including celecoxib and rofecoxib on BP in older patients with hypertension. A double-blind, randomized trial involving 1082 patients that evaluated celecoxib, rofecoxib, or placebo demonstrated an incidence of hypertension of 9.5% with active treatment vs 3.3% incidence in the placebo arm *(23)*. Another study involving 67 elderly (aged 60–80 years) subjects randomly assigned to celecoxib, rofecoxib, or placebo demonstrated similar increases of 3–4 mmHg in systolic BP in each treatment arm *(24)*.

Mechanisms of Blood Pressure Elevation

The elevation in BP associated with NSAIDs results from a combination of increased sodium and water reabsorption, expansion of intravascular volume, loss of vasodilatory signals, and increased peripheral vascular resistance. The administration of NSAIDs inhibits COX (isoforms 1 and 2), leading to diminished production of prostaglandin E2 (PGE_2) and prostacyclin (PGI_2), both of which have direct action in the kidney. PGE_2 inhibits the response of the thick ascending loop of Henle to antidiuretic hormone (vasopressin, antidiuretic hormone) and upregulates sodium reabsorption. The increased sodium and water retention manifests as a reported 2 to 5% incidence rate of edema *(25,26)*. Studies by Rossat et al. and Catella-Lawson et al. documented that, even with short-term use (7–14 days) of NSAIDs or COX-2 inhibitors, there was a decline in urinary sodium excretion in comparison to a placebo-treated group *(27,28)*. Even in the absence of intravascular volume expan-

Table 2
Blood Pressure Effects of Nonsteroidal Anti-Inflammatory Drugs

Author (reference)	Number	Agent	BP change	Duration of treatment
Johnson (29)	41	Indomethacin	↑ SBP 4.1 mmHg	4 weeks
Johnson (10)	771	Multiple	↑ MAP 5 mmHg	Meta-analysis
Gurwitz (35)	25	Ibuprofen	↑ Standing SBP 5.1 mmHg	4 weeks
Pope (22)	1324	Mixed, >50% indomethacin	↑ MAP 3.3 mmHg in hypertensives	Meta-analysis
Chrischilles (21)	2805	Mixed	↑ MAP 4.9 mmHg	>90 days

BP, blood pressure; MAP, mean arterial pressure; SBP, systolic blood pressure.

Table 3
Blood Pressure Effects of Cyclooxygenase-2 Inhibitors

Author (reference)	Number	Agent	BP change	Duration of treatment
Catella-Lawson (28)	36	Rofecoxib	No change	2 weeks
		Indomethacin	No change	
Whelton (52)	810	Rofecoxib	↑ SBP 2.6 mmHg	6 weeks
		Celecoxib	No change	
Whelton (60)	29	Celecoxib	No change	7 days
		Naproxen	No change	
Bombardier (15)	8000	Rofecoxib	↑ SBP 4.6 mmHg	9 months
		Naproxen	No change	

BP, blood pressure; SBP, systolic blood pressure.

sion, BP elevation can occur as a result of increases in vascular resistance (29).

There are three components that result in increased peripheral vascular resistance: inhibition of vasodilatory effect on arteriolar smooth muscle cells because of interference with PGI_2, alternative metabolism of arachidonic acid, and increased production of endothelin-1 (ET-1) (25,29). NSAIDs and COX-2 inhibitors block production of prostacyclin, an endothelial cell-derived vasodilator resulting in increased peripheral vascular resistance (7,30). Inhibition of prostaglandin synthesis shunts arachidonic acid metabolism into an alternative pathway involving cytochrome P450 enzymes. Epoxyeicosatrienoic acids and 20-hydroxyeicosatrienoic acids, metabolites of this alternative pathway, have vasoconstrictive effects that increase BP (31). The last component of increasing peripheral vascular resistance is through the production of ET-1. ET-1, a vasoactive peptide produced in the kidney, acts on peripheral arterial tone (32). Usually inhibited by prostaglandins, ET-1 production may be upregulated by NSAID or COX-2 inhibitor use.

Johnson and others demonstrated the role of ET-1 in BP elevation in a group of 41 elderly subjects treated with indomethacin. Increases in systolic blood pressure (SBP) of 4.1 mmHg and in diastolic blood pressure (DBP) of 2.7 mmHg with indomethacin administration occurred with unchanged cardiac output and an 83% increase in urinary ET-1 levels (20,29,33). Because COX-2, expressed in the vascular wall, plays a role in the peripheral production of vasodilator prostaglandins (34) and modulates sodium/water reabsorption in the kidneys, COX-2 inhibitors have the potential to have similar BP effects as NSAIDs.

Blood Pressure Dysregulation

Another mechanism by which NSAIDs or COX-2 inhibitors may affect BP is through attenuation of antihypertensive agents (*see* Table 4). The attenuation may occur via the enhancement of sodium and water reabsorption, which counteracts the action of diuretics. In a study of 25 elderly subjects (mean age 73 ± 7 years) treated with hydrochlorothiazide, patients receiving ibuprofen had higher supine SBPs (143.8 ± 21.0 vs 139.6 ± 15.9 mmHg for placebo, $p = 0.004$) *(35)*.

There has been a blunting of antihypertensive effects of those agents that act on the renin–angiotensin system. β-Blockers lower BP by decreasing renin synthesis and stimulate production of vasodilator prostaglandins *(10)*. Because NSAIDs decrease renin synthesis, the degree of reduction in BP achieved by β-blockers is attenuated. Similar blunting of effects is seen when NSAIDs are used with angiotensin-converting enzyme (ACE) inhibitors. In the case of ACE inhibitors, there is also a blunted production of bradykinin, thus removing some of its vasodilatory actions *(36)*. In the meta-analysis by Pope et al., there was a mean increase of 5.4 mmHg in those taking ACE inhibitors and β-blockers *(22)*. Minimal interactions have been noted with calcium channel blockers, presumably because their antihypertensive mechanism of action is not dependent on renal prostaglandin production *(19,37)*.

Angiotensin II receptor blockers (ARBs) have not been well studied in terms of interaction with NSAIDs. Although there is the theory that ARBs are not dependent on bradykinin production or blockade of renin production to lower BP, the interaction with NSAIDs is not necessarily less than that of ACE inhibitors.

The small increases in BP seen in clinical trials of pain and arthritis typically will not play a significant role in a normotensive individual. In contrast, within hypertensive subjects these small incremental differences seen in a population have implications toward cardiovascular and cerebrovascular event risk. For example, a difference of 3 to 4 mmHg between treatment arms in the Antihypertensive Lipid-Lowering Treatment to Prevent Heart Attack Trial was associated with a 15 to 19% reduction in stroke *(38)*. Other studies have demonstrated that a 5-mmHg reduction in MAP is associated with a decrease in stroke risk by 45% *(37,39)*.

In assessment of the development of hypertension in arthritis patients, both elevation in BP or uptitration of current antihypertensive therapy have been reported as a "diagnosis of hypertension." In a case–control study of 9411 elderly individuals, Gurwitz et al. found that recent NSAID users had an odds ratio of 2.10 (1.95–2.26) in comparison to non-NSAID

Table 4

Interaction Between Different Nonsteroidal Anti-Inflammatory Drugs (NSAIDs) and Antihypertensive Drugs

Author (reference)	Duration	NSAID	BP agent	BP change by NSAID
Johnson (10)	Variable	Mixed	β-Blockers	↑ SBP 6.2 mmHg
Klassen (61)	4 weeks	Naproxen	Nicardipine	<1 mmHg change
Klassen (62))	4 weeks	Naproxen Ibuprofen	Hydrochlorothiazide	↑ DBP 1.8–2.1 mmHg
Gurwitz (35)	4 weeks	Ibuprofen	Hydrochlorothiazide	↑ SBP 4.2 mmHg
Morgan (36)	3 weeks	Indomethacin	Enalapril	↑ SBP 10.1 mmHg
			Amlodipine	No change

BP, blood pressure; DBP, diastolic blood pressure; SBP, systolic blood pressure.

users for requiring initiation of a new antihypertensive agent *(7)*. Using an insurance claims database, Zhao et al. examined the incidence of BP destabilization and the associated cost of this problem in patients starting NSAIDs or COX-2 inhibitors *(40)*. The incidence of BP destabilization was 2.22 per 1000 days of celecoxib use compared to 2.66 per 1000 days of rofecoxib or 2.65 per 1000 days of nonspecific NSAID use ($p <$ 0.001). The average cost of a BP destabilization event for the first 90 days of the anti-inflammatory agent use was calculated at $459 (cost of office visit, lab work, new prescription).

Not all NSAIDs or COX-2 inhibitors result in the same degree of BP changes. The amount of BP elevation seems to be a function of the agent used, concomitant antihypertensive therapy, and duration of use of the anti-inflammatory medication. Piroxicam, indomethacin, and naproxen have been reported to interfere with BP control more than other agents, such as sulindac or diclofenac *(7,10,15,19,26,41)*. Based on a meta-analysis, piroxicam use was associated with the greatest BP elevation, 6.2 mmHg *(10,19)*. Certain COX-2 inhibitors may have smaller increases in BP than nonselective NSAIDs, depending on the dose. Among the COX-2 inhibitors, rofecoxib has a greater tendency to cause BP elevation, as seen in comparison to celecoxib and lower doses of valdecoxib *(40)*.

Other predictors of the degree of BP destabilization are the duration and extent of exposure. In Gurwitz's study of hypertension, after NSAID use there were higher rates of initiation of antihypertensive therapy in those receiving higher doses of NSAIDs (odds ratio = 1.83 in low-dose NSAID group vs 2.39 in high-dose NSAID group) *(7)*. In addition, it was demonstrated that the need for antihypertensive therapy started between 30 and 90 days after NSAID use *(7)*. In short-term studies of NSAIDs and COX-2 inhibitors, BP often changes very little compared to placebo *(27)*, and the clinical relevance of such studies should be questioned. In longer-term studies of 4 weeks or more, BP destabilization is predicted in part by the concomitant antihypertensive therapy. In analyses of both NSAIDs and COX-2 inhibitors *(22)*, patients treated with ACE inhibitors or β-blockers are more susceptible to BP destabilization than patients on nonspecific vasodilators or calcium channel blockers.

THE ROLE OF FLUID AND ELECTROLYTE BALANCE IN NSAID-INDUCED HYPERTENSION

Prostaglandin (especially renal PGE_2) inhibition leads to alterations in sodium and water balance, electrolyte levels, and renal blood flow *(42)*. These alterations can result in fluid retention and lead to weight gain, peripheral edema, hypertension, and rarely, pulmonary edema (43–45). In the euvolemic state, nonsteroidals and COX-2 inhibitors have little effect. Under conditions of renal insufficiency or reduced renal blood flow, maintaining renal function becomes more dependent on prostaglandin production. In the setting of hypertension and diminished circulating volume such as cirrhosis, CHF, volume depletion, or chronic diuretic use, there is more pronounced fluid retention with NSAID or COX-2 inhibitor administration.

Prostaglandins regulate renal sodium reabsorption by inhibiting active transport in the thick ascending limb of the loop of Henle and the collecting duct (35,46). Inhibition of COX-2 activity reduces renal medullary blood flow and downregulates sodium and water excretion. Because the COX-2 inhibition is the key component, similar fluid retention is seen with COX-2 inhibitors and NSAIDs. Mitigation of the diuretic and natriuretic effects of the prostaglandins leads to augmented renal sodium absorption and may manifest clinically as peripheral edema, hypertension, and in rare circumstances, pulmonary vascular congestion (47).

In a series of healthy older patients (ranging from 59 to 80 years of age) randomly assigned to receive 50 mg of rofecoxib once a day or 50 mg of indomethacin three times a day, a 20% decline in urinary sodium excretion occurred. There was no evidence of an increased incidence of edema or BP elevation in this setting (28,48). In a salt-restricted/depleted state, these same individuals developed a decline in renal function at lower doses of rofecoxib (28). Ferri et al. studied 35 salt-sensitive hospitalized patients with hypertension and demonstrated a significant decline in urinary sodium excretion with an associated 10 mmHg increase in DBP in 15 of those treated with a 5-day course of indomethacin (49). It was postulated that the variable BP effect was a reflection of the degree of renin dependence.

Two long-term studies, VIGOR (15) and the Celecoxib Long-Term Arthritis Safety Study (41), have helped us to understand the general effects of high-dose COX-2 inhibitor therapy on the incidence of hypertension. In the VIGOR trial, which compared 50 mg/day of rofecoxib to 1000 mg/dayof naproxen, the incidence rate of lower extremity edema was reported at 5.4% and 3.6%, respectively (15). The Celecoxib Long-Term Arthritis Safety Study reported data on the incidence of clinically significant upper and lower extremity edema as 3.7% with celecoxib, 3.5% with diclofenac, and 5.2% with ibuprofen (41). The degree and frequency of edema are a function of the total dose, length of exposure, and half-life of a particular NSAID or COX-2 inhibitor (50). The longer half-life and duration of action of rofecoxib may explain the higher incidence of edema and hypertension in comparison to celecoxib as shown in older subjects with osteoarthritis treated with either agent for 6 weeks *(51,52)*.

Although rare, salt and water retention can manifest as significant weight gain (>2 kg) or even CHF. In a retrospective analysis by Heerdink et al. of 10,519 patients chronically on diuretics, the incidence of hospitalizations for CHF was studied in relation to NSAID use *(53)*. Among the group using the combination of diuretics and NSAIDs, there were 228 hospitalizations, for a rate of 23.3 per 1000 person-years, in comparison to 161 hospitalizations or 9.3 per 1000 person-years in the group receiving diuretics alone (relative risk 2.5 [95% confidence interval 2.1–2.9]) *(53)*. Most (57%) of the hospitalizations occurred within the first month of NSAID initiation, with the greatest increase within the first 20 days (three times the incidence of heart failure within the diuretic-alone group).

In another analysis of 5000 participants of preregistration osteoarthritis trials, the incidence of cardiorenal adverse events in patients treated with rofecoxib, diclofenac, and nabumetone were not common—occurrences of significant weight gain or episodes of CHF in the general population were in fact rare *(54)*. This observation stresses the fact that the incidence of renal and cardiac events is greatest in the most susceptible, high-risk population, such as patients with underlying renal disease, CHF, or cirrhosis or on chronic diuretic therapy.

Another electrolyte derangement associated with NSAID or COX-2 inhibitor use is hyperkalemia *(55)*. Normal renal potassium excretion depends on the level of sodium delivery to the collecting duct and the presence of aldosterone. With NSAID and COX-2 inhibitor use, there is increased sodium reabsorption and decreased sodium delivery to the distal tubule, resulting in decreased renin levels *(46,56)*. In studies of both celecoxib and rofecoxib, those patients on a sodium-restricted diet had diminished urinary potassium excretion. Particularly susceptible to hyperkalemia are those individuals on potassium supplementation, ACE inhibitors or ARBs, or potassium-sparing diuretics and those with renal insufficiency *(44)*.

These changes in salt and water balance and electrolyte levels associated with NSAID or COX-2 inhibitor administration occur through disruption of renal function and are more prevalent in patients who have renal insufficiency and are more dependent on prostaglandins to maintain renal blood flow. Beyond fluid and electrolyte homeostasis, prostaglandin inhibition has more direct effects on the kidney, with the potential of irreversible, nephrotoxic effects.

RENAL EFFECTS OF THE NSAIDS
AND COX-2 INHIBITORS

As suggested, most of the adverse effects noted with NSAIDs and COX-2 inhibitors occur through disruption of renal hemodynamics and subsequent impairment of natriuresis and filtration. Although those individuals with preserved function in a euvolemic state typically can tolerate prostaglandin inhibition, in the setting of low-volume states and renal impairment, the impact of loss of prostaglandin stimulation is amplified. The development of edema, hypertension, and fluid/electrolyte changes are the result of alterations in sodium and water reabsorption, diminished renin/aldosterone release, and unopposed vasoconstriction signals. Beyond these adverse effects, NSAID and COX-2 inhibitor use can lead to the development of acute renal failure, nephrotic syndrome, interstitial nephritis, and papillary necrosis *(55,57)*. Unlike the fluid and electrolyte changes, if these adverse events are not recognized and interventions provided quickly, there is a potential for permanent parenchymal changes.

Prostaglandins act on several different pathways to maintain renal plasma flow. PGI_2 and PGE_2 cause arteriolar vasodilation to increase blood flow to the medulla and cortex. PGI_2, PGE_2, and thromboxane A_2 act on glomeruli to maintain autoregulation of the glomerular filtration rate (GFR). In the juxtaglomerular apparatus, there is an upregulation of renin release. Inhibition of these prostaglandins enhances renal vasoconstriction and exposure to the unopposed effects of catecholamines and angiotensin II *(44)*. The resultant reduction of renal plasma flow can proceed to oliguria or anuria and possibly acute renal failure. When unrecognized, there is potential for the development of acute tubular necrosis and irreversible parenchymal damage *(28,56,58,59)*. In a cohort of elderly (mean age 79 years) individuals followed over 6 years, it was demonstrated that NSAID users had an odds ratio of 1.9 for being in the highest quartile of serum urea nitrogen (BUN >23 mg/dL), 1.3 for the highest quartile of serum creatinine (Cr >1.4mg/dL), and 1.7 for the highest quartile of BUN/Cr ratio (>19.4) *(8)*. Gurwitz et al. studied renal function in 114 elderly subjects treated with either 600 mg/day of ibuprofen, 70 mg/day of indomethacin, 300 mg/day of sulindac, or 1000 mg/day of naproxen on a short-term basis and found significant increases in BUN levels without changes in the serum creatinine *(7)*.

Risk factors for deteriorations in renal function with NSAIDs or COX-2 inhibitors include prior renal insufficiency, cirrhosis, nephrotic syndrome, CHF, and diuretic use *(57)*. Renal function is known to decline with age independent of comorbid conditions, with an estimated 10% fall in creatinine clearance per decade after the age of 30 years. Despite this change, aging alone is not a risk factor for NSAID-induced renal failure.

The risk of acute renal failure is more dependent on the choice of medication, the dosage, the duration of therapy, and the baseline renal function. Those NSAIDs with short half-lives reach steady state in a shorter time frame and manifest nephrotoxic effects earlier. For example, ibuprofen can cause a decline in function within a few days of initiation, whereas sulindac (long half-life) takes about 11 days or more after initiation to induce renal dysfunction *(45,56,57)*. In patients with underlying renal insufficiency, treatment with short-acting agents such as ibuprofen may be less likely to significantly alter the GFR. Use of a longer acting agent such as piroxicam may result in significant reductions in GFR in those with renal insufficiency, especially when used long term *(50)*.

Direct Parenchymal Damage

There are three additional manifestations of NSAIDs on the kidneys that result in parenchymal damage and permanent reductions in renal function if prolonged exposure occurs. Administration of NSAIDs can lead to nephrotic syndrome with interstitial nephritis, acute papillary necrosis, or chronic papillary necrosis.

NSAID-induced interstitial nephritis differs from the classic presentation by the lack of fever, rash, eosinophilia, or eosinophiluria. Manifestations of the syndrome include edema, oliguria, foamy urine, nephrotic range proteinuria, and microscopic hematuria. The onset is typically about 5.5 months after initiation of therapy, but it can occur as early as within 2 weeks. The proposed mechanism for the development of the proteinuria and nephritis is through alternate metabolism of arachidonic acid via the lipo-oxygenase pathway *(56)*. This leads to increased leukotriene production, which potentially alters vascular permeability in the glomerular and peritubular capillaries. No risk factors have been identified for the development of this interstitial nephritis, although an increased association has been noted with autoimmune diseases. Treatment is somewhat controversial beyond discontinuation of the NSAID.

Two other nephrotoxic manifestations of NSAID use are acute and chronic papillary necrosis *(57)*. These syndromes can result in permanent parenchymal damage; the extent of renal failure is dependent on the degree of structural damage. The acute form of papillary necrosis is often the result of massive doses of NSAIDs in a volume-depleted individual. Because of the subtle presentation with flank pain and hematuria, it is often misdiagnosed as either nephrolithiasis or ureterolithiasis. The vascular supply within the renal papilla is highly prostaglandin dependent, and in the setting of volume depletion and vasoconstriction, ischemia and necrosis readily occur. The renal papillary lesion is a sharply demarcated lesion with a histological picture consistent with coagulative necrosis. As the papilla of the kidney is responsible for concentration of urine, the long-term consequences of papillary necrosis could include the inability to concentrate urine.

Chronic papillary necrosis tends to be a manifestation of long-standing NSAID use, usually about 5 to 20 years. There has been recognition of increased risk among those individuals on combination agents with NSAIDs, acetaminophen, and caffeine and those who take these agents on a daily basis. In fact, approx 2% of the dialysis population have end-stage renal disease as a result of analgesic abuse nephropathy *(43)*.

CONCLUSIONS

Arthritis is prevalent in the elderly population and has implications for functional status and disability. Especially with an expanding aging population, understanding how to best manage arthritis in patients with hypertension becomes more important. NSAIDs and COX-2 inhibitors still remain the optimal choice because of their analgesic and anti-inflammatory effects. As there is increased prevalence of renal impairment, diuretic use, hypertension, and CHF in older individuals, there is increased susceptibility to side effects from NSAID or COX-2 inhibitor use.

While inhibiting the prostaglandin synthesis associated with the inflammatory response, there is a disruption of fluid and electrolyte balance, BP control, and renal function, with the potential for permanent renal damage. The risk of these side effects does not prevent the use of these agents in an elderly patient but necessitates close monitoring for weight gain, fluid retention, BP changes, or renal dysfunction. NSAIDs and COX-2 inhibitors should be prescribed at the lowest dose possible and on a short-term basis if appropriate. Agents with shorter half-lives may minimize effects. Chronic requirements for these anti-inflammatory agents may necessitate a change in the class of antihypertensive agent or an uptitration of current antihypertensive agents to prevent clinically significant untoward effects.

ADDENDUM

Shortly, after this chapter went to press, several new findings that have created concerns were reported in the literature and media surrounding the COX-2 inhibitors and NSAIDs. We have listed these events and findings to be as comprehensive as possible regarding the use of these agents in older patients with hypertension and cardiovascular diseases.

Rofecoxib, a selective inhibitor of COX-2, was withdrawn voluntarily from the market in September 2004 amid growing data pointing to an increased risk of cardiovascular complications associated with its use. During the 9-month VIGOR trial *(15)*, serious thrombotic cardiovascular events occurred in 45 of 4047 patients (1.11%) taking 50 mg of rofecoxib one daily, compared to 19 of 4029 patients (0.47%) who were given 500 mg of naproxen, twice daily. A subsequent retrospective case–control study of 941 rofecoxib users concluded that the use of rofecoxib was associated with an elevated relative risk of acute myocardial infarciton (AMI) when compared to celecoxib use (odds ratio [OR] 1.24, $p = 0.11$) and a trend to an increased risk when compared to nonusers of NSAIDs (OR 1.14, $p = 0.054$) *(61)*. An unpublished study that led to the removal of rofecoxib from the market used 25-mg doses to study the prevention of adenomatous polyps of the colon—in this study there was a small but significant increased incidence of cardiovascular events on rofecoxib vs placebo (cumulative incidence of 3.5% vs 2.0%) after 18 months of taking the drug (APPROVe Trial).

Data on Celecoxib and Valdecoxib

In the Celecoxib Long-term Arthritis Safety Study (CLASS), no statistically significant increase in cardiovascular events was detected between high-dose celecoxib (400 mg twice daily) and comparator NSAIDs ibuprofen and diclofenac *(41,62)*. In a pooled analysis of nearly 32,000 patients in controlled clinical trials of celecoxib for arthritis, White et al. *(63)* showed no increase in AMI, stroke, or cardiovascular death on celecoxib relative to placebo or conventional NSAIDs. The maximal exposure to celecoxib in that study was 2 years. In the retrospective analysis by Solomon *(61)* comparing rofecoxib and celecoxib, celecoxib use in 1814 patients was also found not to increase the risk of MI and showed that the odds of having an MI was 1.7 fold higher on high doses of rofecoxib.

In one meta-analysis of almost 9000 patients in 10 randomized clinical trials (up to 1-year follow-up period), valdecoxib use was not found to increase the risk of thrombotic cardiovascular events when compared to traditional NSAIDs and placebo *(64)*. This was so across all dosages of valdecoxib, even those greater than recommended and included a subanalysis of approximately 1200 patients on low-dose aspirin who participated in the trials. However, this study has a relatively low number of cardiovascular events and the median exposure to valdecoxib was less than 6 months. Thus, longer term and large studies are still needed to evaluate the cardiovascular safety of valdecoxib.

Conclusions

In large database studies, rofecoxib does seem to increase the risk of AMI and stroke, but the effect was much more apparent at supra-therapeutic doses. Further study is needed to determine whether cardiovascular thrombotic disease is a class effect of all selective inhibitors of COX-2 or whether the development of hypertension on all NSAIDs could contribute to the development of myocardial infarction and stroke.

REFERENCES

1. Brandt K. Osteoarthritis: clinical patterns and pathology. In: Kelley WN, Harris ED Jr, Ruddy S, Sledge CE, eds. *Textbook of Rheumatology*. 5th ed. Philadelphia: Saunders; 1997:1383.
2. Hartz AJ, Fischer MG, Bril G, et al. The association of obesity with joint pain and osteoarthritis is the HANES data. *J Chronic Dis* 1986;39:311.
3. Lawrence JS, Bremner JM, Bier F. Osteoarthritis prevalence in the population and relationships between symptoms and X-ray changes. *Ann Rheum Dis* 1966;25:1.
4. Lawrence RC, Helmick CG, Arnett FC, et al. Estimates of the prevalence of arthritis and selected musculoskeletal disorders in the United States. *Arthritis Rheum* 1998;41:778–799.
5. Celis H, Thijs L, Staessen JA, et al. for Syst-Eur Investigators. Interaction between nonsteroidal antiinflammatory drug intake and calcium channel blocker- based antihypertensive treatment in the Syst-Eur Trial. *J Hum Hypertens* 2001;15:613–618.
6. Fierro-Carrion GA, Ram CVS. Nonsteroidal anti-inflammatory drugs (NSAIDs) and blood pressure. *Am J Cardiol* 1997;80:775–776.
7. Gurwitz JH, Avorn J, Bohn RL, et al. Initiation of antihypertensive treatment during nonsteroidal anti-inflammatory drug therapy. *JAMA* 1994;272:781–786.
8. Field TS, Gurwitz JH, Glynn RJ, et al. The renal effects of nonsteroidal anti-inflammatory drugs in older people: findings from the established populations for epidemiologic studies of the elderly. *J Am Geriatr Soc* 1999;47:507–511.
9. Ray WA, Griffin MR, Avorn J. Evaluating drugs after their approval for clinical use. *N Engl J Med* 1993;329:2029–2032.
10. Johnson AG, Nguyen TV, Day RO. Do nonsteroidal anti-inflammatory drugs affect blood pressure? *Ann Intern Med* 1994;121:289–300.
11. Johnson AG. NSAIDs and blood pressure. Clinical Importance for older patients. *Drugs Aging* 1998;12:17–27.
12. van den Ouweland FA, Gribnau FWJ, Meyboom RHB. Congestive heart failure due to nonsteroidal antiinflammatory drugs in the elderly. *Age Ageing* 1988;17:8–16.
13. Ailabouni W, Eknoyan G. Nonsteroidal anti-inflammatory drugs and acute renal failure in the elderly. A risk-benefit assessment. *Drugs Aging* 1996;9:341–351.
14. Bjorkman DJ. The effect of aspirin and nonsteroidal anti-inflammatory drugs on prostaglandins. *Am J Med* 1998;105:8S–12S.
15. Bombardier C, Laine L, Reicin A, et al. Comparison of upper gastrointestinal toxicity of rofecoxib and naproxen in patients with rheumatoid arthritis. *N Engl J Med* 2000;343:1520–1528.

16. Simon LS. Role and regulation of cyclooxygenase-2 during inflammation. *Am J Med* 1999;106:37S–42S.
17. Burt VL, Whelton P, Rocella EJ, et al. Prevalence of hypertension in the US adult population. Results from the Third National Health and Nutrition Examination Survey 1988–1991. *Hypertension* 1995;25:305–313.
18. Clyburn EB, DiPette DJ. Hypertension induced by drugs and other substances. *Semin Nephrol* 1995;15:72–86.
19. Kozuh JL. NSAIDs and antihypertensives: an unhappy union. *Am J Nurs* 2000;100:40–43.
20. Johnson AG. NSAIDs and increased blood pressure. What is the clinical significance? *Drug Safety* 1997;17:277–289.
21. Chrischilles EA, Wallace RB. Nonsteroidal anti-inflammatory drugs and blood pressure in an elderly population. *J Gerontol* 1993;48:M91–M96.
22. Pope JE, Anderson JJ, Felson DT. A meta-analysis of the effects nonsteroidal anti-inflammatory drugs on blood pressure. *Arch Intern Med* 1993;153:477–484.
23. Schitzer TJ, Kivitz AJ, Greenwald M, et al. Rofecoxib provides superior relief of symptoms of osteoarthritis (OA) compared to celecoxib. Presented at: EULAR; June 2001; Prague, Czech Republic. Abstract SAT0089.
24. Schwartz JI, Malice MP, Lasseter KC, et al. Effect of rofecoxib, celecoxib, and naproxen on blood pressure and urinary sodium excretion in elderly volunteers. Presented at: EULAR; June 2001; Prague Czech Republic. Abstract SAT0055.
25. Frishman WH. Effects of nonsteroidal anti-inflammatory drug therapy on blood pressure and peripheral edema. *Am J Cardiol* 2002;89(suppl):18D–25D.
26. Brook RD, Kramer MB, Blaxall BC, et al. Nonsteroidal anti-inflammatory drugs and hypertension. *J Clin Hypertens* 2000;2:319–325.
27. Rossat J, Maillard M, Nussberger J, et al. Renal effects of selective cyclooxygenase-2 inhibition in normotensive salt-depleted subjects. *Clin Pharmacol Ther* 1999;66:76–84.
28. Catella-Lawson F, McAdam B, Morrison BW, et al. Effects of specific inhibition of cyclooxygenase-2 on sodium balance, hemodynamics, and vasoactive eicosanoids. *J Pharmacol Exp Ther* 1999;289:735–741.
29. Johnson AG, Nguyen TV, Owe-Young R, et al. Potential mechanisms by which nonsteroidal anti-inflammatory drugs elevate blood pressure: the role of endothelin-1. *J Hum Hypertens* 1996;10:257–261.
30. Stoff JS. Prostaglandins and hypertension. *Am J Med* 1986;80(suppl):56–61.
31. Moreno C, Maier KG, Hoagland KM, et al. Abnormal pressure natriuresis in hypertension: role of cytochrome P450 metabolites of arachidonic acid. *Am J Hypertens* 2001;14:90S–97S.
32. Haynes WG, Webb DJ. Contribution of endogenous generation of endothelin-1 to basal vascular tone. *Lancet* 1994;344:852–854.
33. Firth JD, Ratcliffe PJ. Organ distribution of three rat endothelin messenger RNA's and the effects of ischemia in renal gene expression. *J Clin Invest* 1992;90:1023–1031.
34. McAdam BF, Catella-Lawson IA, Mardini S, et al. Systemic biosynthesis of prostacyclin by cyclooxygenase (COX)-2: the human pharmacology of a selective inhibitor of COX-2. *Proc Natl Acad Sci USA* 1999;96:272–277.
35. Gurwitz JH, Everett DE, Monane M, et al. The impact of ibuprofen on the efficacy of antihypertensive treatment with hydrochlorothiazide in elderly persons. *J Gerontol A Biol Sci Med Sci* 1996;51:M74–M79.
36. Morgan TO, Anderson A, Bertram D. Effect of indomethacin on blood pressure in elderly people with essential hypertension well controlled on amlodipine or enalapril. *Am J Hypertens* 2000;13:1161–1167.

37. Mene P, Pugliese F, Patrono C. The effects of nonsteroidal anti-inflammatory drugs on human hypertensive vascular disease. *Semin Nephrol* 1995;15:244–252.
38. ALLHAT Collaborative Research Group. Major cardiovascular events in hypertensive patients randomized to doxazosin vs chlorthalidone: the antihypertensive and lipid-lowering treatment to prevent heart attack trial (ALLHAT). *JAMA* 2000;283: 1967–1975.
39. DeLeeuw PW. Nonsteroidal anti-inflammatory drugs and hypertension. The risks in perspective. *Drugs* 1996;51:179–187.
40. Zhao SZ, Burke TA, Whelton A, et al. Blood pressure destabilization and related health care utilization among hypertensive patients using nonspecific NSAIDs and COX-2 inhibitors. *Am J Manag Care* 2002;8(15 suppl):S401–S413.
41. Silverstein FE, Faich G, Goldstein JL, et al. Gastrointestinal toxicity with celecoxib vs nonsteroidal anti-inflammatory drugs for osteoarthritis and rheumatoid arthritis: the CLASS study: a randomised controlled trial Celecoxib Long-Term Arthritis Safety Study. *JAMA* 2000;284:1247–1255.
42. Brater DC. Effect of indomethacin on salt and water homeostasis. *Clin Pharmacol Ther* 1979;25:322–330.
43. Brater DC. Effects of nonsteroidal anti-inflammatory drugs on renal function: focus on cyclooxygenase-2 selective inhibition. *Am J Med* 1999;107(suppl 6A):65S–71S.
44. Bell GM, Schnitzer TJ. COX-2 inhibitors and other nonsteroidal anti-inflammatory drugs in the treatment of pain in the elderly. *Clin Geriatr Med* 2001;17:489–502.
45. Breyer MD, Harris RC. Cyclooxygenase 2 and the kidney. *Curr Opin Nephrol Hypertens* 2001;10:89–98.
46. Traynor TR, Smart A, Briggs JP, et al. Inhibition of macula densa-stimulated renin secretion by pharmacological blockade of cyclooxygenase-2. *Am J Physiol* 1999;277:F706–F710.
47. Whelton A. Renal and related cardiovascular effects of conventional and COX-2 specific NSAIDs and non-NSAID analgesics. *Am J Ther* 2000;7:63–74.
48. Fitzgerald GA, Patrono C. The COXIBS, selective inhibitors of cyclooxygenase-2. *N Engl J Med* 2001;345:433–442.
49. Ferri C, Bellini C, Piccoli A, et al. Enhanced blood pressure response to cyclooxygenase inhibitor in SMT-sensitive human essential hypertension. *Hypertension* 1993;21:875–881.
50. Page J, Henry D. Consumption of NSAIDs and the development of congestive heart failure in elderly patients. An underrecognized public health problem. *Arch Intern Med* 2000;160:777–784.
51. Whelton A, Fort JG, Puma JG, et al. Cyclooxygenase-2 specific inhibitors and cardiorenal function: a randomized, controlled trial of celecoxib and rofecoxib in older hypertensive osteoarthritis patients. *Am J Ther* 2001;8:85–95.
52. Whelton A, White WB, Bello AE, et al. Effects of celecoxib and rofecoxib on blood pressure and edema in patients > or = 65 years of age with systemic hypertension and osteoarthritis. *Am J Cardiol* 2002;90:959–963.
53. Heerdink ER, Leufkens HG, Herings RM, et al. NSAIDs associated with risk of congestive heart failure in elderly patients taking diuretics. *Arch Intern Med* 1998;158:1108–1112.
54. Gertz BJ, Krupa D, Bolognese JA, et al. A comparison of adverse renovascular experiences among osteoarthritis patients treated with rofecoxib and comparator nonselective nonsteroidal anti-inflammatory agents. *Curr Med Res Opin* 2002;18: 82–91.
55. Breyer MD, Hao C, Qi Z. Cyclooxygenase-2 Selective inhibitors and the kidney. *Curr Opin Crit Care* 2001;7:393–400.

56. Tan SY, Shapiro R, Franco R, et al. Indomethacin induced prostaglandin inhibition with hyperkalemia. A reversible cause of hyporeninemic hypoaldosteronism. *Ann Intern Med* 1979;90:783–785.

57. Whelton A. Nephrotoxicity of nonsteroidal anti-inflammatory drugs: physiologic foundations and clinical implications. *Am J Med* 1999;106:13S–24S.

58. Ruoff G. Management of pain in patients with multiple health problems: a guide for the practicing physician. *Am J Med* 1998;105:53S–60S.

59. Atta MG, Whelton A. Acute papillary necrosis caused by ibuprofen. *Am J Ther* 1997;4:55–60.

60. Whelton A, Schulman G, Wallemark C. Effects of celecoxib and naproxen on renal function in the elderly. *Arch Intern Med* 2000;160:1465–1471.

61. Solomon DH, Schneeweiss S, Glynn RJ, et al. Relationship between selective cyclooxygenase-2 inhibitors and acute myocardial infarciton in older adults. *Circulation* 2004;109:2068.

62. White WB, Faich G, Whelton A, et al. Comparison of thromboembolic events in patients treated with celecoxib, a cyclooxygenase-2 specific inhibitor, versus ibuprofen or diclofenac. *Am J Cardiol* 2002;89:425–430.

63. White WB, Faich G, Borer J, Makuch R. Cardiovascular thrombotic events in arthritis trials of the cyclooxygenase inhibitor celecoxib. *Am J Cardiol* 2003;93:411–418.

64. White WB, Strand V, Whelton A, Roberts R. Effects of the cyclooxygenase-2 specific inhibitor valdecoxib versus nonsteroidal antiinflammatory agents and placebo on cardiovascular thrombotic events in patients with arthritis. *Am J Ther* 2004; 11:244.

VI ADHERENCE

24 The Clinician's Role in Improving Therapeutic Adherence and Blood Pressure Control in Older Hypertensive Patients

Brent M. Egan, MD
and Eni C. Okonofua, MD

CONTENTS

BACKGROUND

The prevalence of high blood pressure (BP), particularly isolated systolic hypertension, rises sharply with age along with the incidence of heart failure, stroke, and coronary heart disease (CHD) *(1–3)*. Antihypertensive treatment reduces these adverse outcomes, especially in older hypertensive patients. Unfortunately, hypertension control to less than 140/90 mmHg declines as a function of age and largely reflects inad-

From: *Clinical Hypertension and Vascular Diseases: Hypertension in the Elderly*
Edited by: L. M. Prisant © Humana Press Inc., Totowa, NJ

equate control of systolic blood pressure (SBP) and largely represents the challenges in controlling systolic hypertension (4,5). Systolic hypertension dominates diastolic as a cardiovascular risk factor in older patients (1,6). The progressive rise of SBP with aging coupled with the poorer control of systolic hypertension is a major contributor to preventable cardiovascular morbidity and mortality. More than 57% of uncontrolled hypertension in the United States is accounted for by hypertensive patients 65 years of age and older, who are seen an average of four times annually for health care (7). Thus, providers have multiple opportunities to improve BP control rates through prescribing affordable and effective medication regimens and by promoting adherence.

One important national health objective defined in the Healthy People 2010 Report was improving the percentage of all hypertensive patients with BP less than 140/90 mmHg to 50% from 31% in 1999–2000 (8). The goal is all the more challenging given the tremendous projected growth in Americans 60 years of age and older with hypertension control rates of only 27% in 1999–2000. There is also the projected addition of more than 30 million Americans 60 years and older in the next 20 years, more than 40% of whom will likely have the metabolic syndrome, which is associated with two- to fourfold higher rates of CHD and stroke (9,10).

Advanced calculus is not required to conclude that the health and economic toll from CHD, heart failure, and stroke will increase dramatically going forward unless effective strategies for controlling hypertension and related risk factors are implemented soon. This will require a concerted effort involving patients, payers, providers, and the public health sector. In this chapter, we focus on issues that can be efficiently implemented in the clinical setting to enhance hypertension awareness, treatment, and control in older hypertensive patients.

CLINICAL EPIDEMIOLOGY

The prevalence of hypertension among Americans 60 years and older has risen in the National Health and Nutrition Examination Surveys (NHANES), from approximately 58% in 1988–1991 to about 65% in 1999–2000 (Table 1) (4,5). Awareness of hypertension during this time period did not change significantly and remained in the 70% range. On a positive note, the proportion of older hypertensives on treatment increased from about 55% to 63%. Although the proportion of controlled-to-treated older hypertensive patients remained in the low 40% range, the proportion of older hypertensives with BP controlled to less than 140/90 mmHg rose from 22.5% in 1988–2001 to 27.4% in 1999–2000 or roughly one in four.

Table 1
Changes in Hypertension Prevalence, Awareness, Treatment,
and Control in Americans 60 Years and Older, 1988–2000

	1988–1991	1991–1994	1999–2000
Prevalence	58 ± 2	60 ± 1	65 ± 2*
Awareness	68 ± 1	69 ± 2	70 ± 2
Treatment	55 ± 1	57 ± 2	63 ± 2*
Control (Rx)	41 ± 3	35 ± 2	44 ± 3
Control (all)	23 ± 2	20 ± 2	27 ± 2*

*$p < 0.05$ for change over time.
Rx, medicated. (From ref. 5.)

More than half of patients with uncontrolled hypertension are 65 years and older (7). Most uncontrolled hypertensive patients have SBPs in the range of 140–159 mmHg. Unlike many younger hypertensive patients who are seen infrequently, these older Americans see their health care providers an average of four times annually. The clinician has multiple opportunities to diagnose hypertension and implement educational and therapeutic plans. As just one example of the potential benefits, heart failure is the most common diagnosis-related group in older Americans. heart failure accounts for approximately $60 billion in annual health care expenditures, and hospitalization makes up more than 50% of heart failure costs (11). Treatment of hypertension, including isolated systolic hypertension, reduces heart failure by approximately 50% (12).

TRANSLATING RESEARCH INTO PRACTICE: CLOSING THE GAP

Clinical trials demonstrated that BP can be controlled to less than 140/90 mmHg in approximately 62 to 70% of older hypertensive patients (13,14). The 1999–2000 NHANES found that hypertension was controlled to less than 140/90 mmHg in only 27.4% of hypertensive patients aged 60 years and 41.6% of hypertensives 40–59 years old (5). The NHANES 1999–2000 data indicated that constructive approaches to addressing the age-related disparity in BP control require attention to hypertension awareness, treatment, and control.

Awareness

For every 100 hypertensive patients 60 years or older, about 30 are unaware of the diagnosis, although most are receiving health care services. The majority of older Americans are focused on diastolic blood pressure (DBP). Of older Americans, 94% reported that their BP was measured in the past year, with more than 80% recalling a measurement in the past 4 months *(15)*. However, 30% of those who recalled that their SBP was more than 140 mmHg reported they had normal BP. Moreover, only one in seven older Americans reporting a normal BP believed they would develop high BP in their lifetime. Approximately 90% of normotensive 55- to 65-year-olds will develop hypertension, predominantly systolic, during their remaining lifetime *(16)*. Despite the current lack of knowledge, older Americans are interested in receiving information on the causes, consequences, prevention, and treatment of high BP.

Treatment

For every 100 hypertensives 60 years or older, about 37% or roughly 3 in 8 are not on treatment *(5)*. The good news is the majority (90%) of aware older hypertensives are treated.

Control

Control rates for all hypertensives 60 years and older compared to those 40 to 59 years old were noted. For every 100 older hypertensives in 1999–2000 on treatment, 43.7% had BP below 140/90 mmHg compared to 66.4% among patients 40 to 59 years old.

ATTAINABLE HYPERTENSION CONTROL RATES

Awareness

Because the majority of older Americans are receiving health care, BPs measured during outpatient visits are a major detection tool. Older individuals particularly require education that an SBP 140 mmHg or higher is elevated and associated with greater cardiovascular risk *(15)*. Older Americans should also receive more information from providers on the causes, consequences, prevention, and treatment of high BP. Information from providers should be reinforced by public health education. An increase of hypertension awareness from 70% to 85% of older Americans, which represents a 50% decrease in the unaware group, is a critical and realistic objective in achieving the Healthy People 2010 BP control goal *(17)*.

Treatment

Inertia on the part of providers and patients represents a barrier to BP control. Many patients, including the elderly, do not want to begin medication and, if on treatment, are reluctant to increase the number of medications. Of providers, 40% indicate they will not initiate or increase antihypertensive treatment when SBP values are 140–159 mmHg *(18)*. In actual practice, providers increase therapy on only about one in seven visits when the SBP is in the stage 1 range and about one in four visits when the SBP is stage 2 (>160 mmHg) *(19,20)*.

In defense of both patients and providers, there is not one randomized, double-blind, placebo-controlled trial that studied older patients with isolated, stage 1 systolic hypertension. Other evidence indirectly suggests benefits of treating BPs in this range. In the Systolic Hypertension in the Elderly Program, BP in the placebo group averaged 155/72 vs 143/68 mmHg in the group receiving chlorthalidone either with or without atenolol. Treatment was associated with a decrease of 27% in CHD, 36% in stroke, and 49% in heart failure *(12,21)*. And, in a cohort study of treated hypertensive men in France, those with SBP less than 140 mmHg had significantly fewer coronary and total cardiovascular events than men with readings of 140 mmHg to 159 mmHg after controlling for age and cigarette smoking *(22)*. To improve control rates, changes in both patient knowledge and provider behavior will be required.

Control

As noted, control rates of approximately 62 to 70% are attainable in clinical trials of older hypertensive patients *(13,14)*. Although clinical trials have some advantages with free medications and visits, structured return visit schedules, and medication titration schemes, the protocols often limit the classes of medications that can be used given the research question addressed. For example, in the Antihypertensive and Lipid-Lowering Treatment to Prevent Heart Attack Trial (ALLHAT), most patients in the angiotensin-converting enzyme arm did not receive diuretics or calcium channel blockers and vice versa *(23)*. Thus, many patients in a research project may not receive medication that could optimize their BP. That is a long way of saying that control rates in the range of about 62% to 70% of all older hypertensives on treatment are realistic in clinical practice.

Hypertension control rates could rise by about 12% of treated patients and approximately 6% overall if *measurement artifacts*, mainly office hypertension, are properly detected and documented *(24–26)*. The accuracy of some ambulatory BP monitors is sufficiently well established that these units could be used to verify the presence of office hypertension. Although the preponderance of outcome data are based on measurements in a clinical setting, a growing body of literature indicates that the ambulatory BP readings are more closely related to target organ damage and clinical outcomes, which includes elderly patients with systolic hypertension *(27–29)*.

Given the assumptions that the proportion of older hypertensives who are aware increases from 70% to 85% and treatment is maintained at the present level of 90% for aware patients, then approximately 77% of all older hypertensives will be treated. If BP control rates to less than 140/90 mmHg of in clinical trials of about 62% to 70% (approximately 66%) are attained, then about 51% of all older hypertensives would have a BP reading less than 140/90 mmHg. The 27% control rates among Americans 60 years and older in 1999–2000 will nearly double, and the Healthy People 2010 control goal will be achieved (Table 2). If office hypertension is documented, the goal will be more readily attained.

FACTORS CONTRIBUTING TO UNCONTROLLED SYSTOLIC HYPERTENSION

Factors contributing to low BP control rates, most often uncontrolled systolic hypertension, can be divided into four categories and include patient factors, physician or provider factors, treatment factors, and system factors. Examples of each include the following:

1. *Patient factors.* Some individuals do not obtain health insurance, even when they can afford it *(30)*. Even among individuals with insurance, preventive services are often not requested or received *(31)*. A high proportion of hypertensive patients does not take medications reliably or change their lifestyle when instructed to do so *(32)*.
2. *Provider factors.* Providers are often unaware of consensus guidelines *(18)*, fail to initiate and titrate medications when BP is not controlled *(19,20)*, and appear unaware of BP control rates in their patients *(33)*.
3. *Treatment factors.* Even when the patient and provider are motivated, access to care is ensured, and medication cost is not an issue, BPs are uncontrolled in approximately one-third or more *(13,14,34)*. These observations suggest that current medications, as utilized clinically, are not effective in controlling BP, especially the systolic value.
4. *Systems factors.* Limited access to regular primary care and medications *(35)*, inadequate public health information, lack of appointment reminders, and deficiencies in producing and disseminating guidelines *(36)* comprise some of the systems limitations to BP control.

Table 2
Attaining the Healthy People 2010 Blood Pressure Goal of 50% Control
in Patients 60 Years and Older, %

	Aware	Treated	Cont/Rx	Control
NHANES 1999–2000	70	63	44	27
NHANES 2010?	85	77	66	51

Cont, control; NHANES, National Health and Nutrition Examination Survey; Rx, on treatment. (Adapted from ref. *17*.)

Patient Factors

Focus on the Patient

In a survey, the majority (94%) of older individuals had their BP measured within the past year, and 81% had a measurement in the past 4 months. However, almost half did not know their BP value. Among older Americans reporting a systolic reading of 140 mmHg or higher, 30% stated that they did not currently have high BP. Thus, systolic hypertension is often not recognized by older Americans *(15)*.

Although the majority (approximately 80%) of older Americans acknowledging a diagnosis of hypertension report taking medications precisely as prescribed, 60% do not think that medications alone will control their BP. This attitude may partially reflect the fact that approximately 40% of providers would not initiate or increase treatment for an SBP of 140–159 mmHg *(18,36)*. Thus, a significant proportion of older Americans with systolic hypertension may not be receiving the medications required to attain BP control, although most have insurance and are seen in a medical care setting an average of four times annually *(7)*. Because many older Americans look to their physicians for information and guidance, the knowledge, attitudes, and practice patterns of providers about systolic hypertension probably contribute to the relatively low levels of patient awareness, treatment, and control *(7,18)*.

Knowledge

Many patients seem unaware of the importance of regular primary care in preventing disease *(35)*. Although this is a general problem, men, ethnic minorities, and individuals in the Southeast appear to make fewer primary health care visits each year than the US average *(35,37)*. The level of primary care utilization by men, especially from ethnic minorities, is very low and probably plays a major role in rates of uncontrolled hypertension, which tend to coincide with visit frequency *(4,5,38)*.

The vast majority of older Americans correctly identified stroke and heart disease as complications of hypertension *(15)*. Treatment of systolic hypertension in older Americans may be further enhanced by patient awareness that large absolute and relative reductions in risk for stroke, heart attack, and congestive heart failure are realized *(12,21–23)*. Renal disease is not as clearly linked with hypertension by older Americans. Awareness that hypertension contributes to cognitive decline with aging and that treatment is beneficial could enhance interest in BP treatment and control *(39)*. Similarly, osteoporosis is a concern for many older Americans, and several thiazide-type diuretics improve bone density and reduce fracture risk *(40)*. Of importance, older hypertensive patients tolerate treatment as well as younger individuals, and quality of life appears unchanged *(41)* or improved *(42)*.

Older Americans are seeking information on lifestyle change alternative approaches for treating and preventing hypertension *(15)*. Older Americans indicate that several lifestyle changes are effective in lowering BP. Consonant with the health belief model, 75% reported making a lifestyle change, with more than 60% of them indicating that change lowered their pressure. Thus, therapeutic strategies that encourage lifestyle change and incorporate effective alternative therapeutic approaches *(43)* as an adjunct to antihypertensive medications are likely to engender the most effective and enduring therapeutic alliance between the older patient and his or her health care provider.

HEALTH LITERACY

A rapidly growing body of literature indicates that low levels of health literacy are pervasive and affect nearly half of American adults *(44)*. Low levels of health literacy are associated with poorer outcomes for a variety of health conditions and may explain or contribute to a large portion of health disparities *(45)*. Risk factors for low levels of health literacy include older age, male sex, ethnic minority status, limited formal education, and low income. Low health literacy is rarely disclosed voluntarily by the patient and often goes undetected in the typical clinical setting *(46)*. Providers and support staff can address this limitation by asking patients in lay terms before they leave the office or clinic if they would like any additional explanation about diagnostic, therapeutic, or follow-up plans. Group visits, which include semiformal education sessions about chronic diseases, including hypertension, may improve health literacy and risk-factor control rates *(47)*.

HEALTH DISCOUNT RATES

Most of us discount the future. Resources (money and health) are worth more today than in the future. Knowledge of the risk factor and its consequences is not sufficient motivation to seek care, take medications, and change lifestyle if the perceived complications are estimated to be at a future time point that does not have sufficient value relative to other priorities today. The rates at which the future is discounted vary from person to person *(48–50)*. Individuals who discount future health at higher rates may be less likely to seek preventive services and obtain risk-factor control. Providers with higher discount rates for future health may be less likely to emphasize preventive services. Health discount rates of patients *and* providers may be a critical factor in treating and controlling risk factors such as hypertension.

LACK OF SELF-EFFICACY

Low levels of *self-efficacy*, defined as the capacity and/or confidence of an individual to effect change that benefits him or her, predict poorer outcomes. Self-efficacy has an impact on the likelihood that an individual will begin and maintain positive health change, such as physical activity and dietary patterns *(51)*. The link between self-efficacy and health behavior is present in both majority and minority populations *(52)*. Self-efficacy is associated with adherence patterns *(32,52)*.

SOCIAL SUPPORT AND ADHERENCE

A study of 50 African-American men hospitalized for severe hypertension, owing mainly to nonadherence, suggested that lack of social and community support were much more important barriers than either cost or side effects *(53)*. Appropriate feedback to patients from physicians, pharmacists, and other health professionals can convey a level of concern, potentially compensate for limited social support, and foster adherence.

LIMITED ACCESS TO CONTINUOUS PRIMARY CARE

Continuity of primary care is powerfully related to patient compliance and BP control. Patients with a regular source of primary care were eight times more likely to control their hypertension than patients who did not have a regular source of primary care *(54)*. Conversely, individuals receiving services for hypertension through the emergency room were one-eighth as likely as patients receiving care in a primary care setting to take antihypertensive mediations regularly *(55)*. Thus, efforts to ensure a regular source of primary care are a vital policy issue in the battle to achieve the Healthy People 2010 BP control rates. Improving access to primary health care will also contribute to the goals in reducing ethnic health disparities *(35,37)*.

LACK OF RESOURCES

Low income is associated with poorer health. Poverty is accompanied by barriers to medical care that include limited access to diagnostic and therapeutic health care services. However, differences in income and insurance do not appear to account for the majority of the health disparities associated with poverty and ethnicity *(35)*. The larger portion of the health disparity appears related to personal health habits and under-utilization of available preventive services. Evidence suggests a widening disparity in health knowledge for minorities and people living in poverty *(56)*.

Socioeconomic, educational, and ethnic factors have an impact on health knowledge, attitudes, and behaviors regarding dietary patterns *(57)*. African-Americans tend to consume more high-fat foods and fewer fresh fruits and vegetables, which in turn has an impact on the prevalence of heart disease, stroke, and cancer *(58,59)*. These dietary differences probably play an important role in racial variations in hypertension and cardiovascular outcomes such as stroke *(60,61)*. Moreover, the BP-lowering effects of a healthy diet are greater among African-Americans than Caucasians and are related in part to genetic polymorphisms involved in BP regulation *(8,62,63)*.

COMORBID DEPRESSION OR ALCOHOLISM

The management of long-term risk factors, including hypertension and diabetes, is poorer among patients with depression or alcohol use *(64,65)*.

PATIENT ADHERENCE

Approximately 70% of hypertensive patients are aware of the diagnosis, and the majority are receiving primary health care *(5,7)*. Most have received a prescription for antihypertensive medications. However, approximately 50% of individuals who begin antihypertensive therapy discontinue treatment within the first year *(66,67)*. Although some of them reenter therapy, even among those who remain in treatment approximately 50% take less than 80% of the medication prescribed *(68)*. Parenthetically, these data from previous studies on patient compliance are relatively consistent with more recent information on adherence patterns in a representative sample of hypertensive patients *(32)*. In this report, approximately 55% of hypertensive patients were identified as reliable in taking medications, and about 39% of all hypertensive patients were found to comply with both medication and lifestyle advice.

Approximately 45% of hypertensive patients had evidence of significant limitations to adherence with both medication and lifestyle measures required to control hypertension *(32)*. The "low" adherers were composed of two subgroups. One of the subgroups included more women than men, tended to be the most overweight, and was the most likely to forget medications. They also had lower levels of self-efficacy, which has an impact on adherence and outcomes *(51,52)*, and were not confident in their ability to sustain healthy lifestyle change. The other group was composed of more men than women and was generally disinterested in preventive care, unconvinced about the efficacy of pharmacotherapy, and disinclined to change lifestyle.

The self-reported rates of perfect medication adherence by 80% of hypertensive older Americans in a survey are remarkable *(15)*. Previous studies indicated that approximately 40% of hypertensive patients who report taking 100% of their antihypertensive medications are taking less than 75% by pill count *(68)*. Although the proportion of the sample overreporting medication adherence is unknown, noncompliance with medications probably exceeds the level reported.

COST OF MEDICATIONS

Adherence at 75% to 80% or greater with prescribed medication is regarded as the minimum level required to derive the desired pharmacological benefit. In a variety of medical settings with different cost structures, control rates of about 25% in hypertensive patients have been reported *(19,33,69,70)*. For the roughly 20% of older hypertensive Americans who reported not taking medications at all or as prescribed in a recent, cost was a significant issue for about 20% of them or approximately 4% of the entire sample *(15)*. Cost of medications lagged forgetfulness, BP under control, do not like taking medications, and side effects as a contributor to self-reported nonadherence. Although cost is clearly a critical issue that limits adherence for some patients, cost appears to trail efficacy and tolerability in importance among older patients *(15,71)*.

Focus on the Provider and Patient–Provider Interface

Providers encounter multiple barriers to controlling BP. One review identified almost 300 barriers in physician adherence to the treatment guidelines alone *(36)*. Another review classified barriers to reaching therapeutic goals into six categories: qualities of the guidelines, characteristics of the provider, characteristics of the practice setting, incentives, regulation, and patient factors *(72)*.

SUCCESS OF AUDIT AND FEEDBACK FOR IMPROVING BLOOD PRESSURE CONTROL

Hypertension control at the primary care level improved dramatically over 1 year with an intervention that included feedback on control rates to primary care providers *(33)*. The University of Pennsylvania conducted a chart review of 20,000 patients in their managed care program. Blood pressure was controlled to less than 140 mmHg systolic and less than 90 mmHg diastolic in only 19% of hypertensive patients at baseline. Charts were reviewed quarterly, and providers received feedback on hypertension control rates in their patients compared to their peers. Within 1 year, hypertension control rates nearly tripled from 19 to 53%. Chart audit and effective feedback to providers emerged as a major factor in the dramatic improvement in BP control. Of interest, the BP control rates among treated hypertensive patients in this managed care setting are identical to the 53% of treated hypertensive patients under control in the report from the NHANES 1999–2000 survey *(5)*. The fact that hypertension control rates, which have languished at 19% to 27% for many years *(9,33,69,70)*, can be dramatically improved with chart audit and feedback to providers raises the possibility that feedback enhances physicians' prescribing patterns and improves communication with patients, thus leading to greater therapeutic adherence.

IS INDIVIDUALIZED THERAPY PART OF THE PROBLEM?

Control of hypertension invariably improves when groups of patients are taken from their usual care settings with individualized therapy and placed in studies with relatively rigid treatment protocols *(13,14,34)*. ALLHAT is just one of many examples (Fig. 1) in which control rates improved dramatically, in this case from 27% at entry to 54% at 1 year and 66% at 5 years *(13)*.

Practical management algorithms "tailored" according to comorbidities with compelling treatment indications (e.g., systolic heart failure and prior myocardial infarction) together with monitoring and feedback might prove an especially useful tool for clinicians in the effort to improve BP control and related clinical outcomes. With current treatment algorithms, control rates among treated patients are unlikely to exceed 70%. Thus, newer approaches to selecting therapy are attractive *(73,74)*. While the validity of new approaches are being verified, it is critical for providers to employ established best practice approaches to the control of hypertension in older Americans *(75)*.

The provider has a major impact on compliance with medication and lifestyle advice *(76–79)*. Changes in provider behavior as a result of

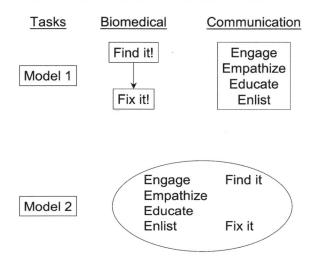

Fig. 1. A new model for patient–physician communication. The traditional approach to medicine utilizes lineal and strategic questions to "find it" (i.e., diagnose the problem) to "fix it." In other words, the focus of communication is finding and fixing problems. The traditional approach appears to work well for approximately half the patients *(32)*. An alternative approach focuses on communication that engages and empathizes with the patient to find it and then educates and enlists the patient to fix it. The alternative model may work better for the other half of patients who are not adhering well with the traditional approach. (From ref. *94*.)

medical education and feedback on performance have significant potential for enhancing patient adherence and improving outcomes *(79)*.

ASSESSING ADHERENCE

Clinicians have difficulty assessing patient adherence in the usual clinical setting, which has led to a variety of studies and tools to detect nonadherence. If a patient admits to anything less than complete adherence, the vast majority of the time (>85%) they are in fact taking less than 75% of the prescribed medication *(70)*. However, approximately 40% of patients reporting perfect, that is, 100%, adherence were also taking less than 75% of their medication. There are some specific clinical clues to nonadherence and factors the provider can use to assess adherence (Table 3) *(80,81)*.

ASSESSING READINESS TO CHANGE

The transtheoretical model recognizes that patients are at varying degrees of readiness to change (Table 4) *(82)*. The patient who has not

Table 3
Clues to Nonadherence and Assessment of Adherence in Clinical Practice

Clues to nonadherence	Assessing adherence
• Young, very elderly • Lack social support, low socio- economic status • Multiple health problems • Depression, anxiety • Complex regimen, side effects • Finance, drug, alcohol problems • Lack regular primary care • Missed appointments • Blood pressure uncontrolled	• Treatment result • Patient self-report • Family report • Provider opinion • Prescription refill history • Pill counts

Table 4
Application of the Transtheoretical Model of Readiness
to Change in Clinical Practice

Stage of change	Stage-appropriate action
• Precontemplative (have not thought about it) benefits of change	• Encouraging statements about
• Contemplative	• Assist in resolving barriers
• Planning	• Assist in refining plan, including restarting action after relapse
• Action	• Encourage, reinforce, clarify
• Maintenance	• Document and discuss impact of change; encourage
• Relapse	• Review plan to restart after relapse; reassure; discuss positives and negatives of change

considered beginning an exercise program requires a different approach than one who is just getting started or another person who stopped exercising 3 months earlier. With some simple questions, the physician can rapidly assess the readiness of the patient to change and tailor the education and advice to help move the patient toward effective maintenance of the desired behavior (83).

If goal BP remains elusive, providers may need to take several steps to assess adherence to therapy (Table 3) as well as the adequacy of treatment and possible secondary causes of hypertension, including renovascular disease. Providers can reinforce the goals of therapy by using the prescription as an educational tool. For example, "Take one tablet every morning to get BP to less than 140/90 mmHg" can be written on the bottle. Patients need to be instructed early in their treatment that, although the initial drug will probably lower their BP, it may not control BP to goal. Selected combination agents may also enhance adherence and control *(84)*. The Seventh Report of the Joint National Committee on the Prevention, Detection, Evaluation, and Treatment of High Blood Pressure recommends beginning with a two-medication regimen for hypertensive patients with BP 20/10 mmHg or greater from goal *(85)*.

ASSESSING OUT-OF-OFFICE BLOOD PRESSURE

Several studies found that BP measurements outside the office increase adherence with treatment and BP control, especially among uncontrolled hypertensive patients who have difficulty remembering to take their medication *(86,87)*. The use of a home monitoring service with twice weekly automated feedback to providers was associated with better BP control than when providers did not receive similar feedback on home BP monitoring *(88)*. Programs with pharmacists monitoring out-of-office BP appear highly effective and may be logistically more convenient for some patients *(86)*.

ASSESSING LIFESTYLE, COMPLICATING FACTORS, AND ALTERNATIVE THERAPIES

The patient–provider interaction is critical in several ways. A focused history is often essential to BP control. Habits of patients that lessen response to antihypertensive therapy include a diet high in sodium; alcohol; possibly caffeine; smoking cigarettes within 15 minutes of the BP measurement; nonsteroidal anti-inflammatory drugs, including the selective cyclooxygenase-2 inhibitors *(89,90)*; and use of alternative therapies *(91)*. Patients who use home remedies are less likely to adhere to traditional therapeutic regimens.

IMPROVING ADHERENCE

Efforts to improve compliance long term is formidable, complex, and of limited efficacy *(92,93)*. McDonald et al. concluded that, "The full benefits of medications cannot be realized at currently achievable levels of adherence; therefore, more studies of innovative approaches to assist patients to adhere with prescriptions medications are needed" *(92)*.

PROVIDER EDUCATION CAN IMPROVE PATIENT ADHERENCE

A relatively brief 1- to 2-hour tutorial for primary care providers on patient compliance raised adherence of their patients in taking more than 75% of medication from 32% to 61% and improved BP control from

36% to 60%—changes that were not observed in the control group *(79)*. Compared to providers in the control group who did not receive the tutorial, the "trained" physicians spent more time in patient education and less time in the traditional history and physical examination.

The reallocation of time is consistent with a different model of provider–patient communication than is traditionally taught in medical school (i.e., diagnose and treat or "find it, fix it"). The alternative model is centered on communication in which the provider strives to engage and empathize the patient to facilitate diagnosis and educate and enlist the individual to enhance treatment (Fig. 1) *(94)*. Although clinicians generally endorse the notion that better patient communication and education improve outcomes, they also indicate that current reimbursement patterns make it impractical to spend less time on the history and physical evidence and more time on patient communication and education. Changes in health care reimbursement and incentives are required to translate this important research information into clinical practice.

INTERVIEW STYLES AND COMMUNICATION PATTERNS

Traditional education programs train physicians to diagnose and treat medical conditions but typically do not emphasize the structure of questions and principles of communication. In general, physicians utilize lineal and strategic questions. The literature on patient counseling suggests that circular and reflexive questions such as "How have your activities changed?", and "How would (or does) a low salt diet affect you?" tend to generate better patient rapport and to enlist patients more actively in their own care *(95)*. Moreover, the capacity to diagnose a medical problem can be improved when clinicians engage and empathize with patients, and the effectiveness of the therapeutic plan can be enhanced when providers educate and enlist their participation in the treatment program *(94)*.

PROVIDER STRATEGIES FOR ENHANCING PATIENT SATISFACTION AND ADHERENCE

A list of things providers can do to enhance patient adherence is provided in Table 5. Physicians who provide more information derive greater patient satisfaction and adherence *(96)*. Of interest, physicians who were determined to be highly competent by their peers also achieved greater patient satisfaction and better outcomes. Older patients and Caucasians tend to ask more questions and receive more information *(96)*. Therefore, the physician may be more successful in fostering patient adherence by greater efforts to engage, empathize, educate, and enlist the patient's cooperation, especially when the patient is less interactive.

Table 5
Provider Approaches to Enhancing Patient Adherence

- Educate patient and family
  - Enlist patient (and family) participation
  - Self-monitoring of blood pressure, diabetes, weight as appropriate
- Visual and written instructions, contracts, incentives, engage family
- Simplify regimens; use combination tablets when possible; address cost when it is an issue
- Monitor adherence; have patient bring prescription bottles and check refills remaining against date of prescription
- Ask about side effects; discuss alternatives, likely outcomes

The list of provider suggestions for enhancing adherence is self-evident. However, time pressures on clinicians continue to escalate and can erode the capacity to include simple yet very practical and important patient counseling. Establishing educational procedures, using pre-printed patient education materials, and delegating some components of patient education to staff can help address these system barriers to better BP control in the practice setting.

The Treatment Factor Amplified: A Ceiling to Better Blood Pressure Control

The limitation of treatment efficacy represents a major impediment to the Healthy People 2010 goals for BP control. Only about 43% of treated hypertensive patients 60 years and older have a BP less than 140/90 mmHg. The uncontrolled portion includes many who are adherent with an effective regimen. The hypertension control rates achieved in clinical trials, in which providers and patients are motivated and all visits, diagnostic testing, and medications are paid by the research grant, are in the range of about 62 to 70% *(13,14,34)*. Thus, given the existing relatively high proportions of unaware and/or untreated patients, novel and more effective therapeutic tools and/or strategies are required to raise control rates in patients under treatment to reach the goal of controlling BP in 50% of all hypertensive patients.

CONCLUSIONS

Hypertension is controlled to less than 140/90 mmHg in about one in four hypertensive patients 60 years and older *(5)*. The absolute benefits of treating hypertension are greatest in those at highest risk, including those with isolated systolic hypertension, diabetes, dyslipidemias, and

Table 6
Some Steps to Attaining the Healthy People 2010 Blood Pressure Control
Goal

- Increasing awareness will require public health efforts to educate patients about systolic hypertension and providers to inform patients with readings above 140 mmHg that these are high
- Increasing treatment requires provider commitment to diagnose, manage, and control stage 1 systolic hypertension
- New therapeutic tools and strategies are needed to raise control rates above the current ceiling of 70% of treated patients
- Changes in health care reimbursement are vital to ensure continuity of care, incentives for effective patient education, and access to essential medications

target organ damage, who are disproportionately older patients. The importance of hypertension control becomes even more important in the years ahead given the rapid growth in the numbers of older Americans. This reality provides compelling rationale for a concerted effort to achieve the Healthy People 2010 goal of controlling BP in 50% of all hypertensive patients. Attaining that goal will be a tremendous challenge (Table 6).

Increasing Hypertension Awareness Is Vital

Because 30% of hypertensive patients are unaware of the diagnosis *(4,5)*, it will be nearly impossible for health care providers alone to achieve the Healthy People 2010 goal for hypertension control by treating more aggressively. Awareness must be increased and can be most readily attained in older patients because they are seen more frequently in the health care system. Reinforcement of the risks of systolic hypertension and the benefits of treatment, including healthy lifestyle patterns, from the public health sector is essential to reaching the Healthy People 2010 goal.

Providers Play a Pivotal Role in Achieving
the 2010 Blood Pressure Control Goal

Clinicians are largely responsible for diagnosing hypertension, recommending lifestyle changes, prescribing an effective antihypertensive regimen, and taking steps to optimize patient adherence. Many older patients with untreated and/or uncontrolled hypertension have SBPs in the range 140–159 mmHg. Greater clinician commitment to diagnosing, treating, and controlling stage 1 systolic hypertension is critical in improving BP control rates.

Newer Therapeutic Tools or Strategies Are Needed

Given current approaches to managing hypertension, control rates in excess of 70% in the usual clinical setting are unlikely *(12,13,34)*. Currently, only fewer than 50% of older hypertensive patients on treatment have a BP less than 140/90 mm Hg. However, another 20% to 25% have BPs of less than 150/95 mmHg *(7,97)*. A reduction of less than 10/5 mmHg in patients who are close to goal would raise control rates to approximately 70%. Detecting and documenting the substantial subset of patients with office hypertension will be important in achieving these control rates. Newer therapeutic strategies also hold significant promise for significantly increasing control rates among treated hypertensive patients *(73,74)*, as do novel opportunities for extending the academic mission of excellence in patient care, education, and research to the community through a growing network of nationally certified clinical hypertension specialists *(97)*. Until newer strategies and approaches are established, it is vital that clinicians commit to applying evidence-based, best-practice approaches to the management of hypertension in older patients, with attention to special considerations in minorities *(75,98)*.

Changes in Health Care Reimbursement

Providers can play a vital role in educating patients and improving both adherence and outcomes *(76–79)*. However, current patterns of health care reimbursement represent a disincentive to effective patient education. Changes in reimbursement based in part on patient outcomes rather than principally on written documentation would provide greater incentive for effective patient education. Reimbursement paradigms that enhance continuity of primary care and access to essential medications are likewise vital in efforts to optimize hypertension control.

A More Consumer- and Wellness-Oriented Health Care System

The health care system is not working well for 45% to 61% of hypertensive patients *(32)*. Providers, payers, and policymakers should be more attuned to the impact of health literacy, discount rates, and alternative therapeutic approaches in addressing national goals for improving health and reducing health disparities.

Putting It All Together

Achieving the Healthy People 2010 goal of controlling BP to less than 140/90 mmHg in 50% of all hypertensive patients will be incredibly challenging but particularly important in older individuals. The population of elderly patients is growing rapidly, and this group has the highest rates of costly target organ complications. As outlined in this chapter, nothing short of an aggressive, integrated, multilateral effort will be required to attain the Healthy People 2010 BP objective.

ACKNOWLEDGMENTS

This work was supported in part by grants P01HS1087 (EXCEED) from the Agency for Healthcare Research and Quality; HL58794, HL04290, and P60-MD00267 (EXPORT) from the National Heart, Lung, and Blood Institute; and the Duke Foundation.

REFERENCES

1. Kannel WB, Dawber TR, McGee DL. Perspectives on systolic hypertension. *Circulation* 1980;61:1179–1182.
2. Psaty BM, Furberg CD, Kuller LH, et al. Association between blood pressure level and the risk of myocardial infarction, stroke, and total mortality. *Arch Intern Med* 2001;161:1181–1192.
3. Perry HM, Miller JP, Fornoff JR, et al. Early predictors of 15-year end-stage renal disease in hypertensive patients. *Hypertension* 1995;25(pt 1):587–594.
4. Burt VL, Whelton P, Roccella EJ, et al. Prevalence of hypertension in the US adult population: results from the Third National Health and Nutrition Examination Survey, 1988–1991. *Hypertension* 1995;25:305–313.
5. Hajjar I, Kotchen TA. Trends in prevalence, awareness, treatment, and control of hypertension in the United States, 1988–2000. *JAMA* 2003;290:199–206.
6. Franklin SS, Larson MG, Khan SA, et al. Does the relation of blood pressure to coronary heart disease risk change with aging? The Framingham Study. *Circulation* 2001;103:1188–1190.
7. Hyman DJ, Pavlik VN. Characteristics of patients with uncontrolled hypertension in the United States. *N Engl J Med* 2001;345:479–486.
8. Healthy People 2010. US Government Printing Office No. 017-001-00547–9. Available at: www.healthypeople.gov/publications/. Accessed July 2003.
9. Ford ES, Giles WH, Dietz WH. Prevalence of the metabolic syndrome among US adults: findings from the third National Health and Nutrition Examination Survey. *JAMA* 2002;287:356–359.
10. Lakka H-M, Laaksonen DE, Lakka TA, et al. The metabolic syndrome and total and cardiovascular disease mortality in middle-aged men. *JAMA* 2002;288:2790–2716.
11. O'Connell JB, Bristow MR. Economic impact of heart failure in the United States: time for a different approach. *J Heart Lung Transplant* 1994;13:S107–S112.
12. Kostis JB, Davis BR, Cutler J, et al. Prevention of heart failure by antihypertensive drug treatment in older persons with isolated systolic hypertension. *JAMA* 1997;278:212–216.
13. Cushman WC, Ford CE, Cutler JA, et al. Success and predictors of blood pressure control in diverse North American settings: the Antihypertensive and Lipid-Lowering Treatment to Prevent Heart Attack Trial (ALLHAT). *J Clin Hypertens* 2002;4:393–405.
14. Black HR, Elliott WJ, Neaton JD, et al. Baseline characteristics and early blood pressure control in the CONVINCE Trial. *Hypertension* 2001;37:12–18.

15. Egan BM, Lackland DT, Cutler NE. Awareness, knowledge and attitudes of older Americans about high blood pressure: Implications for healthcare policy, education and research. *Arch Intern Med* 2003;163:681–687.

16. Vasan RS, Beiser A, Seshadri S, et al. Residual lifetime risk for developing hypertension in middle-aged women and men: the Framingham Heart Study. *JAMA* 2002;287:1003–1010.

17. Egan BM, Basile JN. Controlling blood pressure in 50% of all hypertensive patients: an achievable goal in the Healthy People 2010 Report? *J Invest Med* 2003;51:373–385.

18. Hyman DJ, Pavlik VN. Self-reported hypertension treatment practices among primary care physicians: blood pressure thresholds, drug choices, and the role of guidelines and evidence-based medicine. *Arch Intern Med* 2000;160:2281–2286.

19. Berlowitz DR, Ash AS, Hickey EC, et al. Inadequate management of blood pressure in a hypertension population. *N Engl J Med* 1998;339:1957–1963.

20. Oliveria SA, Lapuerta P, McCarthy BD, L'Italien GJ, Berlowitz DR, Asch SM. Physician-related barriers to the effective management of uncontrolled hypertension. *Arch Intern Med* 2002;162:413–420.

21. SHEP Cooperative Research Group. Prevention of stroke by antihypertensive drug treatment in older persons with isolated systolic hypertension. *JAMA* 1991;265:3255–3264.

22. Benetos A, Thomas F, Bean K, Gautier S, Smulyan H, Guize L. Prognostic value of systolic and diastolic blood pressure in treated hypertensive men. *Arch Intern Med* 2002;162:577–581.

23. The Antihypertensive Lipid-Lowering Treatment to Prevent Heart Attack Trial (ALLHAT). Major outcomes in high-risk hypertensive patients randomized to angiotensin-converting enzyme inhibitor or calcium channel blocker vs diuretic. *JAMA* 2002;288:2981–2997.

24. Pickering TG, James GD, Boddie C, Harshfield GA, Blank S, Laragh JH. How common is white coat hypertension? *JAMA* 1988;259:225–228.

25. Mejia A, Egan B, Schork N, Zweifler A. Importance of blood pressure measurement artifacts and lack of target organ involvement in the assessment of patients with treatment resistant hypertension. *Ann Intern Med* 1990;112:270–277.

26. Brown MA, Buddle ML, Martin A. Is resistant hypertension really resistant? *Am J Hypertens* 2001;14:1263–1269.

27. Khattar RS, Senior R, Lahiri A. Cardiovascular outcome in white-coat vs sustained mild hypertension: a 10-year follow-up study. *Circulation* 1998;98:1892–1897.

28. Staessen JA, Thijs L, Fagard R, et al. Predicting cardiovascular risk using conventional vs ambulatory blood pressure in older patients with systolic hypertension. *JAMA* 1999;282:539–546.

29. Clement DL, DeBuyzere ML, DeBacquer DA, et al. Prognostic value of ambulatory blood-pressure recordings in patients with treated hypertension. *N Engl J Med* 2003;348:2407–2415.

30. Yegian JM, Pockell DG, Smith MD, Murray EK. The nonpoor uninsured in California, 1998. *Health Aff (Millwood)* 2000;19:171–177.

31. Solberg LI, Brekke ML, Kottke TE. Are physicians less likely to recommend preventive services to low-SES patients? *Prev Med* 1997;26:350–357.

32. Weir MR, Maibach EW, Bakris GL, et al. Implications of a health lifestyle and medication analysis for improving hypertension control. *Arch Intern Med* 2000;160:481–490.

33. Townsend RR, Shulkin DJ, Bernard D. Improved outpatient hypertension control with disease management guidelines. *Am J Hypertens* 1999;12(4 pt 2):88A.

34. Julius S, Kjeldsen SE, Brunner H, et al. VALUE Trial: long-term blood pressure trends in 13,449 patients with hypertension and high cardiovascular risk. *Am J Hypertens* 2003;16:544–548.
35. Weinick RM, Zuvekas SH, Cohen JW. Racial and ethnic differences in access to and use of health care services. *Med Care Res Rev* 2000;57(suppl 1):36–54.
36. Cabana MD, Rand CS, Powe NR, et al. Why don't physicians follow clinical practice guidelines? A framework for improvement. *JAMA* 1999;282:1458–1465.
37. Lackland D, Egan B, Cheek D, Dunbar J. Racial differences in the use of office-based medical services for blood pressure assessment. *Am J Hypertens* 1993;6:88A.
38. Wheeler FC, Lackland DT, Mace ML, Reddick A, Hogelin G, Remington PL. Evaluating South Carolina's community cardiovascular disease prevention project. *Public Health Rep* 1991;106:536–543.
39. Rigaud AS, Seux ML, Staessen JA, Birkenhager WH, Forette F. Cerebral complications of hypertension. *J Hum Hypertens* 2000;14:605–616.
40. LaCroix AZ, Ott SM, Ichikawa L, Scholes D, Barlow WE. Low-dose hydrochlorothiazide and preservation of bone mineral density in older adults: a randomized, double-blind, placebo-controlled trial. *Ann Intern Med* 2000;133:516–526.
41. Applegate WB, Pressel S, Wittes J, et al. Impact of the treatment of isolated systolic hypertension on behavioral variables. *Arch Intern Med* 1994;154:2154–2160.
42. Wiklund I, Halling K, Ryden-Bergsten T, Fletcher A. Does lowering blood pressure improve the mood? Quality-of-life results from the Hypertension Optimal Treatment (HOT) study. *Blood Press* 1997;6:357–364.
43. Houston MC. The role of vascular biology, nutrition, and nutraceuticals in the prevention and treatment of hypertension. *J Am Nutraceut Assoc* 2002;April(suppl 1):5–71.
44. Andrus MR, Roth MT. Health literacy: a review. *Pharmacotherapy* 2002;22:282–302.
45. Weiss BD. Health literacy: an important issue for communicating health information to our patients. *Chinese Med J* 2001;64:603–608.
46. Parikh NS, Parker RM, Nurss JR, Baker DW, Williams MV. Shame and health literacy: the unspoken connection. *Patient Educ Couns* 1996;27:33–39.
47. Trento M, Passera P, Tomalino M, et al. Group visits improve metabolic control in type 2 diabetes: a 2-year follow-up. *Diabetes Care* 2001;24:995–1000.
48. van der Pol M, Cairns J. Estimating time preferences for health using discrete choice experiments. *Soc Sci Med* 2001;52:1459–1470.
49. Enemark U, Lyttkens CH, Troeng T, Weibull H, Ranstam J. Implicit discount rates of vascular surgeons in the management of abdominal aortic aneurysms. *Med Decis Making* 1998;18:168–177.
50. Ganiats TG, Carson RT, Hamm RM, et al. Population-based time preferences for future health outcomes. *Med Decis Making* 2000;20:263–270.
51. Meland E, Maeland JG, Laerum E. The importance of self-efficacy in cardiovascular risk factor change. *Scand J Public Health* 1999;27:11–17.
52. Skelly AH, Marshall JR, Haughey BP, Davis PJ, Dunford RG. Self-efficacy and confidence in outcomes as determinants of self-care practices in inner-city, African-American women with non-insulin-dependent diabetes. *Diabetes Educ* 1995:21:38–46.
53. Jackson AL. Operation Sunday School—educating caring hearts to be healthy hearts. *Public Health Rep* 1990;105:85–88.
54. Ahluwalia JS, McNagny SE, Rask KJ. Correlates of controlled hypertension in indigent, inner-city hypertensive patients. *J Gen Intern Med* 1997;23:7–14.
55. Shea S, Misra D, Ehrlich MH, Field L, Francis CK. Correlates of nonadherence to hypertension treatment in an inner-city minority population. *Am J Public Health* 1992;82:1607–1612.

56. David SK, Winkleby MA, Farquhar JW. Increasing disparity in knowledge of cardiovascular disease risk factors and risk-reduction strategies by socioeconomic status: Implications for policymakers. *Am J Prev Med* 1995;11:318–323.
57. Gates G, McDonald M. Comparison of dietary risk factors for cardiovascular disease in African-American and white women. *J Am Diet Assoc* 1997;97:1394–1400.
58. Kayrooz K, Moy TF, Yanek JL, Becker DM. Dietary fat patterns in urban African-American women. *J Community Health* 1998;23:453–469.
59. Karanja NM, McCullough ML, Kumanyika SK, et al. Pre-enrollment diets of dietary approaches to stop hypertension trial participants. *J Am Diet Assoc* 1998;99(8 suppl):S28–S34.
60. Keli SO, Hertog MGL, Feskens EJM, Kromhout D. Dietary flavonoids, antioxidant vitamins and incidence of stroke. *Arch Intern Med* 1996;154:637–642.
61. Joshipura KJ, Ascherio A, Manson JE, et al. Fruit and vegetable intake in relation to risk of ischemic stroke. *JAMA* 1999;282:1233–1239.
62. Appel JL, Moore TJ, Obarzanek E, et al. A clinical trial of the effects of dietary patterns on blood pressure. *N Engl J Med* 1997;336:1117–1124.
63. Svetkey LP, Moore TJ, Simons-Morton DG, et al. Angiotensinogen genotype and blood pressure response in the Dietary Approaches to Stop Hypertension (DASH) study. *J Hypertens* 2001;19:1949–1956.
64. DiMatteo MR, Lepper HS, Croghan TW. Depression is a risk factor for noncompliance with medical treatment. *Arch Intern Med* 2000;160:2101–2107.
65. Lang T, Degoulet P, Aime F, Devries C, Jacquinet-Salord MC, Fouriaud C. Relationship between alcohol consumption and hypertension prevalence and control in a French population. *J Chron Dis* 1987;40:713–720.
66. Langfield S. Hypertension. Deficient care in the medically served. *Ann Intern Med* 1973;78:19–23.
67. Haynes RB, Taylor W, Sackett DL, et al. Can simple clinical measurements detect patient noncompliance? *Hypertension* 1980;2:656–664.
68. Inui TS, Carter WB, Pecoraro RE. Screening for noncompliance among patients with hypertension: is self-report the best available measure? *Med Care* 1981;19:1061–1064.
69. Alexander M, Tekawa I, Hunkeler E, et al. Evaluating hypertension control in a managed care setting. *Arch Intern Med* 1999;159:2673–2677.
70. Meissner I, Whisnant JP, Sheps SG, et al. Detection and control of high blood pressure in the community: do we need a wake-up call? *Hypertension* 1999;34:466–471.
71. Ferguson RP, Wetle T, Dubitzky D, Winsemius D. Relative importance to elderly patients of effectiveness, adverse effects, convenience and cost of antihypertensive medications. A pilot study. *Drugs Aging* 1994;4:56–62.
72. Larme AC, Pugh JA. Attitudes of primary care providers toward diabetes: barriers to guideline implementation. *Diabetes Care* 1998;21:1391–1396.
73. Blumenfeld JD, Laragh JH. Renin system analysis: a rational method for the diagnosis and treatment of the individual patient with hypertension. *Am J Hypertens* 1998;11:894–896.
74. Taler S J, Textor SC, Augustine JE. Resistant hypertension: comparing hemodynamic management to specialist care. *Hypertension* 2002;39:982–988.
75. Prisant LM, Moser M. Hypertension in the elderly: can we improve the results of therapy? *Arch Intern Med* 2000;160:283–289.
76. Sanson-Fisher RW, Campbell EM, Redman S, Hennrikus DJ. Patient-provider interactions and patient outcomes. *Diabetes Educ* 1989;15:134–138.
77. Shank JC, Powell T, Llewelyn J. A 5-year demonstration project associated with improvement in physician health maintenance behavior. *Fam Med* 1989;21:273–278.

78. Sciamanna CN, Tate DF, Lang W, Wing RR. Who reports receiving advice to lose weight? Results from a multistate survey. *Arch Intern Med* 2000;160:2334–2339.
79. Inui TS, Yourtee EL, William JW. Improved outcomes in hypertension after physician tutorials: a controlled trial. *Ann Intern Med* 1976;84:646–651.
80. Schoenberger JA. *Topics in Hypertension: Patient Compliance in Antihypertensive Therapy.* New York: American Society of Hypertension; 1997:2–7.
81. Dunbar JM, Stunkard AJ. Adherence to diet and drug regimen. In: Levy R, Rifkin B, Dennis B, Ernst N, eds. *Nutrition, Lipids and Coronary Heart Disease.* New York: Raven Press; 1979:391–423.
82. Beesesen DH. Applying stages of change theory to office-based counseling. In: Beesesen DH, Kushner R, eds. *Evaluation and Management of Obesity.* Philadelphia: Hanley and Belfus; 2002:33–39.
83. Diehl NS, Evenson KR. Exercise: Getting your patient going in 3 minutes or less. In: Egan BM, Basile JN, Lackland DT, eds. *Hot Topics in Hypertension: A TRIP With the Experts.* Philadelphia: Hanley and Belfus; 2003:215–222.
84. Ruzicka M, Leenen FHH. Monotherapy vs combination therapy as first line treatment of uncomplicated arterial hypertension. *Drugs* 2001;61:944–954.
85. Chobanian AV, Bakris GL, Black HR, et al. Seventh report of the Joint National Committee on Prevention, Detection, Evaluation, and Treatment of High Blood Pressure. *Hypertension* 2003;42:12067–1252.
86. Johnson AL, Taylor W, Sackett DL, Dunnett CW, Shimizu AG. Self-recording of blood pressure in the management of hypertension. *Can Med Assoc J* 1978;119: 1034–1039.
87. Rogers MA, Small D, Buchan DA, et al. Home monitoring service improves mean arterial pressure in patients with essential hypertension. A randomized, controlled trial. *Ann Intern Med* 2001;134:1024–1032.
88. Mehos BM, Saseen JJ, MacLaughlin EF. Effect of pharmacist intervention and initiation of home blood pressure monitoring in patients with uncontrolled hypertension. *Pharmacotherapy* 2000;20:1384–1389.
89. Frishman WH. Effects of nonsteroidal anti-inflammatory drug therapy on blood pressure and peripheral edema. *Am J Cardiol* 2002;89:18D–25D.
90. Blackshear JL, Schwartz GL. Step care therapy for hypertension in diabetic patients. *Mayo Clin Proc* 2001;76:1266–1274.
91. Brown CM, Segal R. The effects of health and treatment perceptions on the use of prescribed medication and home remedies among African-American hypertensives. *Soc Sci Med* 1996;43:903–917.
92. McDonald HP, Garg AX, Haynes RB. Interventions to enhance patient adherence to medication prescriptions: Scientific Review. *JAMA* 2002;288:2868–2879.
93. Haynes RB, McDonald HP, Garg AX. Helping patients follow prescribed treatment. *JAMA* 2002;288:2880–2883.
94. Keller VF, Carroll JG. A new model for physician–patient communication. *Patient Educ Couns* 1994;23:131–140.
95. Ryan D, Carr A. A study of the differential effects of Tomm's questioning styles on therapeutic alliance. *Fam Process* 2001;40:67–77.
96. Hall JA, Roter DL, Katz NR. Meta-analysis of correlates of provider behavior in medical encounters. *Med Care* 1988;26:657–675.
97. Egan BM, Lackland DT, Basile JN. American Society of Hypertension Regional Chapters: leveraging the impact of the clinical hypertension specialist in the local community. *Am J Hypertens* 2002;15:372–379.
98. Douglas JG, Bakris GL, Epstein M, et al. Management of high blood pressure in African Americans: consensus statement of the hypertension in African Americans Working Group of the International Society of Hypertension in Blacks. *Arch Intern Med* 2003;163:525–541.

INDEX